AF478319

AIRWAY SECRETION

LUNG BIOLOGY IN HEALTH AND DISEASE

Executive Editor

Claude Lenfant
Director, National Heart, Lung and Blood Institute
National Institutes of Health
Bethesda, Maryland

AIRWAY SECRETION

PHYSIOLOGICAL BASES FOR THE CONTROL OF MUCOUS HYPERSECRETION

Edited by

Tamotsu Takishima

Sanae Shimura

Tohoku University School of Medicine
Sendai, Japan

Marcel Dekker, Inc.   **New York•Basel•Hong Kong**

Library of Congress Cataloging-in-Publication Data

Airway secretion: physiological bases for the control of mucous hypersecretion / edited by Tamotsu Takishima, Sanae Shimura.
        p.   cm. -- (Lung biology in health and disease; v. 72)
     Includes bibliographical references and indexes.
     ISBN: 0-8247-8843-5 (alk. paper)
     1. Airway (Medicine)--Secretions. 2. Mucus. 3. Airway (Medicine)--
Pathophysiology. I. Takishima, Tamotsu. II. Shimura, Sanae. III. Series.
     [DNLM: 1. Exocrine Glands--physiology. 2. Mucus--physiology. 3. Res-
piratory System--physiology.   W1 LU62 v. 72 1994 / WF 101 A298 1994]
QP123.A36 1994
612.2--dc20
DNLM/DLC
for Library of Congress   93-38784
                                                                        CIP

The publisher offers discounts on this book when ordered in bulk quantities. For more information, write to Special Sales/Professional Marketing at the address below.

This book is printed on acid-free paper.

MARCEL DEKKER, INC.
270 Madison Avenue, New York, New York 10016

Current printing (last digit):
10 9 8 7 6 5 4 3 2 1

PRINTED IN THE UNITED STATES OF AMERICA

INTRODUCTION

For generations, the topic of airway secretion has inspired most interesting observations and intense discussions, if not controversies. It is noteworthy that the Yellow Emperor (2000 BC) and Maimonides (1135–1204) described expectoration in terms unrecognizable today. Shakespeare referred to it as "spit." However, its medical significance was not understood. In fact, in ancient times, respiration's perceived purpose was only to cool the blood, and nasal mucus was thought to be a discharge from the brain.

In the fiftieth monograph of the series "Lung Biology in Health and Disease," entitled *Respiratory Defense Mechanisms*, D. F. Proctor reports a fascinating page of history. He points out that it was Schneider, in 1755, who demonstrated that fluids cannot travel from the brain to the nose. However, he did it in such an expansive fashion that, in 1898, J. Wright remarked that "never was the kernel of an important fact so wrapped up in the husks of verbosity."

It appears that credit for pointing out the medical significance of bronchial secretions and the biological value of the exocrine function of the lungs belongs to Laennec. In *Diseases of the Chest*, he described the condition "dry catarrh" as "inflammations of the bronchi which are attended with little or no expectorations." Then he went on to describe the "chronic idiopathic pituitous catarrh" known today as bronchorrhea, which is characterized by paroxysms of expectoration.

The importance of all this is that airway secretions, and their alternations, became one of the cardinal signs of many respiratory diseases. From this followed a flurry of observations and research activities to uncover the origin, the nature, and the role of mucous secretions in health and in disease. Contributions from important disciplines such as electron microscopy, biochemistry, molecular biology, and genetics have led to an explosion of knowledge. Still, we must recognize that the field of airway secretion retains much of its secrecy.

This volume, edited by Drs. Tamotsu Takishima and Sanae Shimura from the prestigious Tohoku University in Japan, brings the reader up to date, but it also points to directions that need to be explored. It assembles a multinational roster of talented and pioneering investigators. All of them, editors and authors, have made a major contribution to this volume and to the series of monographs as a whole. As the editor of the series, I am grateful for their participation in this landmark work.

Claude Lenfant, M.D.
Bethesda, Maryland

PREFACE

The lung is characterized as an exocrine organ because airway and alveolar epithelial cells that cover all surfaces of the lungs possess some exocrine functions; however, airway secretion seems to be much more complex in origin than secretion from other exocrine glands. The lung's function of respiration or ventilation, necessary for the maintenance of life, also subjects it to negative events such as inhalation of pathogens and other harmful substances.

Airway secretion plays a primary role in mucociliary clearance and, as such, acts as a defense mechanism against these inhaled particles. Disturbance of this defense mechanism leads to intraluminal mucus accumulation in the airways associated with mucous hypersecretion, and creates a clinical problem in almost all pulmonary and some nonpulmonary diseases. Airway mucous hypersecretion is an important determinant in the prognosis and clinical features of various pulmonary diseases such as chronic bronchitis, pulmonary emphysema, and bronchial asthma, in addition to cystic fibrosis, which is a disease of exocrine glands.

Medical doctors in intensive care units experience difficulty in treating excessive bronchial mucus, which can lead to suffocation, respiratory failure, and bacterial infection. Some asthmatic patients die in spite of treatment with powerful bronchodilators and anti-inflammatory medicines, including glucocorticoids. At autopsy, lungs from such patients show the presence of excessive bronchial mucus and mucus plugging. However, to date, there have been few useful medications or therapies to treat this condition. One reason for lack of useful therapies seems to be a lack of knowledge of the physiological aspects of airway secretion, which is complex in origin.

Exocrine glands, including their morphology, functions, and molecular aspects, have been extensively studied in salivary glands, lacrimal glands, and the pancreas. Their dynamic cellular and intracellular mechanisms have attracted a number of investigators to exocrine gland studies, and the knowledge gained from these studies can now be applied to other cells and tissues. The examination of receptors and intracellular second messengers, using exocrine cells and tissues, has resulted in the recent discovery of the cystic fibrosis transmembrane conductance regulator gene. And, at the same time, this knowledge is also useful for the study of airway secretion. Hence we asked two outstanding exocrine gland researchers to describe molecular and cellular concepts that are fundamentally similar to those of airway secretion.

Basic, molecular, and physiological aspects of airway secretion will be described (Chaps. 1–5), including morphology, biochemistry, rheology, and gene expression of mucus (Chaps. 6–8). Because of its complexity of origin, it is important to know the various kinds of cells or tissues and how they contribute to airway secretion. The importance of the rheological or flow properties of airway mucus has been recognized in relation to mucociliary and cough clearance, and these properties are defined by their chemical structures. Furthermore, airway secretion is known to contain some antibacterial and anti-inflammatory substances, which play some role in the defense mechanism. These rheological and biochemical aspects are described in Chapters 6 and 7. Secretory responses are described in chapters devoted to submucosal gland secretion (Chap. 9); ion (or fluid) transport across the epithelium (Chap. 10); and surface goblet cell secretion (Chap. 11).

The physiological aspects of diseased lungs are abnormal, and Chapters 12–16 on airway secretion in pathological conditions address this issue. Hypertrophy and/or hyperplasia of airway secretory cells (bronchial glands and epithelial goblet cells) are characteristic of chronic airway diseases, including chronic bronchitis, that are associated with chronic airway inflammation. Sputum, or pathological mucus, is airway secretion contaminated by secretions other than bronchial secretion (cell debris, tissue exudate, saliva, etc.). Airway inflammation induces hypersecretion through various mechanisms, including the release of chemical mediators from surrounding tissues and cells. In addition to the secretion, mucosal exudation, which comes from the paracellular route in the epithelium, is important for understanding airway secretion in diseased lungs. These findings are described in Chapters 12 and 13; sputum is treated in Chapter 16. We have selected three representative diseases—cystic fibrosis (Chap. 14), chronic bronchitis (Chap. 16), and bronchial asthma (Chap. 15)—in which airway hypersecretion is the most dominant and determinant clinical feature. These pathological conditions must be compared with normal physiological features. Finally, Chapter 17 is concerned with the possibility of treating airway hypersecretion.

The purpose of this book is to provide an update on current knowledge and understanding of airway secretion and to identify some of the blanks on the map where further exploration is needed. The final goal is to control airway hypersecretion. There have been few monographs or textbooks concerning airway secretion. Thus, airway secretion seems to be an immature and undiscovered field of research that is important and universally relevant to almost all pulmonary diseases. We hope this book will help to attract investigators to this field.

Tamotsu Takishima
Sanae Shimura

CONTRIBUTORS

Matthew P. Anderson, Ph.D.   Department of Internal Medicine and Physiology and Biophysics, Howard Hughes Medical Institute, University of Iowa College of Medicine, Iowa City, Iowa

Carol Basbaum, Ph.D.   Associate Professor, Anatomy and Cardiovascular Research Institute, University of California, San Francisco, California

Herbert A. Berger, M.D.   Pulmonary Associate, Department of Internal Medicine, Howard Hughes Medical Institute, University of Iowa College of Medicine, Iowa City, Iowa

Thomas F. Boat, M.D.   Professor and Chairman, Department of Pediatrics, University of Cincinnati School of Medicine, Cincinnati, Ohio

Pi-Wan Cheng, Ph.D.   Associate Professor, Department of Pediatrics, University of North Carolina School of Medicine, Chapel Hill, North Carolina

Sanford Chodosh, M.D.   Chief of Staff and Pulmonary, Veterans Administration Outpatient Clinic and Associate Professor of Medicine, Boston University School of Medicine, Boston, Massachusetts

Gerene M. Denning, Ph.D.   Research Scientist, Department of Medicine, Howard Hughes Medical Institute, University of Iowa College of Medicine, Iowa City, Iowa

David Vincent Gallacher, B.Sc., B.D.S.   Senior Lecturer, Department of Physiology, University of Liverpool, Liverpool, England

Berthold H. Jany, M.D.   Privat Dozent, Medizinische Poliklinik Universität, Würzburg, Germany

Peter K. Jeffery, M.Sc., Ph.D.   Reader, Department of Lung Pathology, Royal Brompton Hospital, National Heart and Lung Institute, London, England

Kwang Chul Kim, Ph.D.   Associate Professor, Department of Pharmacology and Toxicology, University of Maryland School of Pharmacy, Baltimore, Maryland

Malcolm King, Ph.D.   Professor, Department of Medicine, University of Alberta, Edmonton, Alberta, Canada

Pierre Larivée, M.D.   Assistant Professor, Department of Medicine, Pulmonology Division, Centre Hospitalier Universitaire de Sherbrooke, Sherbrooke, Quebec, Canada

Margaret Warren Leigh, M.D.   Associate Professor, Department of Pediatrics, University of North Carolina School of Medicine, Chapel Hill, North Carolina

Stewart J. Levine, M.D.   Medical Staff Fellow, Department of Critical Care Medicine, National Institutes of Health, Bethesda, Maryland

Lynda S. Ostedgaard, Ph.D.   Howard Hughes Medical Institute, University of Iowa College of Medicine, Iowa City, Iowa

Carl G. A. Persson   Professor, Department of Clinical Pharmacology, University Hospital of Lund, Lund, Sweden

Charles G. Plopper, Ph.D.   Professor, Veterinary Anatomy and Cell Biology, University of California, Davis, California

Devra P. Rich, Ph.D.   Postdoctoral Associate, Department of Internal Medicine, Howard Hughes Medical Institute, University of Iowa College of Medicine, Iowa City, Iowa

Rafel Dwaine Rieves, M.D.   Assistant Professor, Division of Pulmonary Medicine, University of Mississippi School of Medicine, Jackson, Mississippi

Bruce K. Rubin, M.D.   Associate Professor, St. Louis University School of Medicine, St. Louis, Missouri

Tsukasa Sasaki, M.D., Ph.D.   Assistant Professor, First Department of Internal Medicine, Tohoku University School of Medicine, Sendai, Japan

James H. Shelhamer, M.D.   Deputy Chief, Department of Critical Care Medicine, Clinical Center, National Institutes of Health, Bethesda, Maryland

David N. Sheppard, Ph.D.   Postdoctoral Associate, Department of Internal Medicine, Howard Hughes Medical Institute, University of Iowa College of Medicine, Iowa City, Iowa

Sanae Shimura, M.D., Ph.D.   Associate Professor, First Department of Internal Medicine, Tohoku University School of Medicine, Sendai, Japan

Peter M. Smith, B.Sc., Ph.D.   Department of Clinical Dental Sciences, University of Liverpool, Liverpool, England

Judith A. St. George, Ph.D.   Senior Scientist, Genzyme Corporation, Framingham, Massachusetts

Lawrence A. Tabak, D.D.S., Ph.D.   Professor, Department of Dental Research and Biochemistry, University of Rochester, Rochester, New York

Kazuhiko Takeuchi, M.D.   Assistant Professor, Department of Otorhinolaryngology, Mie University School of Medicine, Tsu, Mie, Japan

Jean-Marie Tournier, Ph.D.   INSERM Unite 314, C.H.R., Reims, France

Tamotsu Takishima, M.D., Ph.D.   Professor and Chairman, First Department of Internal Medicine, Tohoku University School of Medicine, Sendai, Japan

Tohru Tsuda, M.D., Ph.D.   Assistant Professor, Division of Respiratory Disease, University of Occupational and Environmental Health, Kitakyushu City, Japan

Pedro Verdugo, M.D.   Professor, Department of Bioengineering, University of Washington, Seattle, Washington

Shiping Wang, M. Phil.   Lecturer, Department of Animal Science and Veterinary Medicine, Huazhong Agricultural University, Wuhan, People's Republic of China

Adam Wanner, M.D.   Professor of Medicine, Chief, Pulmonary Division, Department of Medicine, University of Miami, Miami, Florida

Michael J. Welsh, M.D.   Investigator, Howard Hughes Medical Institute and Professor of Medicine and Physiology and Biophysics, Department of Internal Medicine, University of Iowa College of Medicine, Iowa City, Iowa

Jonathan H. Widdicombe, D.Phil.   Senior Member, Cardiovascular Research Institute, University of California–San Francisco, San Francisco, California

CONTENTS

1

Electrolyte and Fluid Secretion in Exocrine Acinar Cells

PETER M. SMITH
and DAVID VINCENT GALLACHER

University of Liverpool
Liverpool, England

TSUKASA SASAKI

Tohoku University School of Medicine
Sendai, Japan

I. Introduction

A. Fluid and Electrolyte Secretion in Exocrine Acinar Cells

The aim of this short review is to outline the current understanding of the mechanisms by which the major exocrine (such as salivary, lacrimal, and pancreatic) acinar cells achieve the unidirectional secretion of the isotonic, plasmalike fluid that constitutes the primary secretion. The minute-to-minute regulation of exocrine secretion is under the control of the secretomotor, autonomic innervation of the glands and also, most significantly for the exocrine pancreas, by circulating hormones. A potent stimulus for exocrine secretion is the release of acetylcholine (ACh) from the postganglionic parasympathetic nerve endings. Acetylcholine acts on muscarinic cholinergic receptors (blocked by the pharmacological antagonist atropine) to initiate the secretory mechanisms that result in the translocation of electrolytes and fluid from the interstial space across the acinar epithelium and into the luminal space. This primary fluid is plasmalike (high in sodium and chloride), isotonic, and essentially of constant composition at all flow rates. Thus, the role of nervous or hormonal stimulation is to alter the rate of production of the primary acinar secretion, rather than its composition. The nature of the primary fluid is, however, considerably altered—in particular, sodium is reabsorbed and potassium is secreted—in its passage along the system of ductules and ducts that ultimately lead the fluid to drain into or onto their respective target tissues. This secondary modification of the primary fluid by the ductal system is a rate-dependent process and the secondary transport mechanisms of the ducts also vary in nature and capacity among different glands and, particularly, among different species. In this way the final exocrine secretion is modified to subserve the individual dietry and specialist (e.g., evaporation of saliva for temperature regulation) requirements of all the different species. The unifying concept is that, in the major exocrine glands of all species, the acinar cells that constitute the blind endings of the ductal tree secrete, in immediate response to nervous or hormonal stimulation, a primary plasmalike fluid (Thaysen et al., 1954). It is in this knowledge that we seek a mechanism, common to all major exocrine acinar cells, that will achieve the transepithelial transport of an isotonic fluid. This review will not consider the mechanism of secretion of macromolecules, which will be covered in a separate chapter in this volume. It should also be stated that the review will not cover the active and secondary active transports that are components of fluid secretion. These will be presented only as in a model outlining the overall transports associated with fluid and electrolyte secretion.

It is now recognized that fluid and electrolyte secretion is initiated by a family of receptors that regulate a common transduction mechanism in exocrine acinar cells. In general, these receptors share a common structure with seven domains passing through the membrane from external to internal surfaces. They are not directly coupled to their effector enzyme, but operate by regulatory G proteins. These G proteins, activated by binding to a cytoplasmic domain on the receptor, in turn, stimulate the activity of the enzyme phosphoinositidase C to promote the hydrolysis of a phospholipid in the membrane to yield two second-messenger products (detailed later), the effect of which is to give rise to an elevation in intracellular calcium. This rise in cytosolic calcium is the trigger for the activation of electrolyte and fluid transport. The role of calcium is to activate ion channels (calcium-activated ion channels) in the acinar membranes, which leads to the movement of ions that represent the earliest event in electrolyte secretion. In this chapter we will provide an overview of the electrophysiological characterization of the ion channels identified in the cell membranes of the acinar cells of the major exocrine glands and describe their respective roles in the secretory process. We will also describe the nature of the calcium signals arising in exocrine acinar cells and discuss the mechanisms whereby neurotransmitter activation leads to mobilization of intracellular calcium. The final scheme for the secretion of fluid and electrolytes that is to be presented is applicable to all the major exocrine acinar cells [including human salivary (Morris et al., 1987a) and human pancreatic (Petersen et al., 1985) acinar cells] yet investigated; with only one notable exception. The rodent pancreatic acinar cells do not conform to the secretory model we will present. The rat and mouse pancreatic acinar cells differ from all other acini, and from the pancreatic acinar cells of other species (e.g., human) so far investigated, in that they alone have no demonstrable K^+-selective conductance pathway. This, as will be detailed, is an essential component of the secretory model formulated for all other acinar cells, and the rodent pancreata must secrete by a different mechanism. They are then the exception to the general scheme to be presented.

B. Signal Transduction

A variety of neurotransmitters and hormones are known to promote electrolyte and fluid transport in exocrine acinar cells by mobilizing calcium and, thereby, activating calcium-dependent ionic conductances. In salivary acinar cells, the cholinergic muscarinic, the α-adrenergic and peptidergic (substance P) receptors are the most extensively investigated. In the other major exocrine glands, these and other agonists acting in a similar manner have been identified; for instance, the gastrointestinal hormone cholecystokinin acts on the exocrine pancreatic acinar cells to elevate intracellular calcium to promote electrolyte and fluid secretion. All these agonists that couple stimulus to secretion by means of Ca^{2+} mobilization employ a common signal transduction pathway to generate the Ca^{2+} signal. Different agonists may modify the resultant Ca^{2+} signal in various ways (Yule et al., 1991), but the initial transduction mechanism is universal, whether activated by neurotransmitters, such as ACh or norepinephrine, or local hormones, such as cholecystokinin. The initial step in signal transduction after binding of agonist to receptor is activation of a G protein (GTP-binding protein). The binding of the agonist to the receptor increases the affinity of the receptor for the G protein complex. The G protein in the resting state binds GDP, but upon activation, the GDP dissociates and GTP is bound. It is in this state that the G protein, in turn, activates the effector enzyme. The calcium-mobilizing agonists result in the activation of the enzyme phosphoinositidase C. This enzyme promotes hydrolysis of a membrane-bound phospholipid, phosphatidylinositol 4,5-biphosphate producing two highly reactive breakdown products, diacylglycerol (DAG) and inositol 1,4,5-triphosphate [Ins(1,4,5)P$_3$] (see Berridge, 1993). Diacylglycerol remains membrane-bound and activates protein kinase C. The DAG is thought to have a modulatory role in Ca^{2+} mobilization (Yule et al., 1991), but so far as fluid secretion is concerned, its role is secondary to Ins(1,4,5)P$_3$ and its metabolites. It is now established that Ins(1,4,5)P$_3$ binds to a specific receptor on intracellular organelles that constitute a store of sequestered calcium and open a calcium channel in their membrane allowing the efflux of Ca^{2+} into the cytosol. This release of calcium from intracellular stores can support only a transient secretory response, and the calcium signal and secretion is sustained only by an influx of

Ca^{+2} across the cell surface membrane from the extracellular to intracellular fluid. The mechanism of second-messenger-mediated Ca^{+2} influx, as opposed to release, is still not well understood, but is undoubtedly related to the $Ins(1,4,5)P_3$-induced release of calcium from intracellular stores and may involve both $Ins(1,4,5)P_3$ and the more highly charged inositol polyphosphate, $Ins(1,3,4,5)P_4$, which is produced by phosphorylation of $Ins(1,4,5)P_3$.

II. Electrophysiology of Exocrine Glands

A. Introduction to Patch–Clamp Electrophysiology

The patch–clamp technique has two modes of operation, both of which offer unique opportunities in the study of the ionic permeabilities of the plasma membrane (Hamill et al., 1981). In one type of experiment, the movement of charge is measured across a small patch of membrane that is electrically isolated from the rest of the cell. Protocols of this type offer the opportunity to measure current flow through individual ion channels in the membrane. Thus, the precise *conductivity* (the greater the conductance the larger the current passing for a given electrochemical gradient) and *selectivity* (preference of the channel for one ionic species compared with another) of each ion channel present in the membrane may be determined. An alternative patch–clamp technique, whole-cell current recording, measures a composite current that is the sum of the individual ionic currents activated over the whole-cell surface membrane. The discrete single-channel current events are no longer resolved, but the overall conductance changes associated with secretion are recorded, accurately reflecting their relative magnitude and time course of activation.

B. Single-Channel Experiments

Introduction

The patch–clamp technique is perhaps best known for measurement of single-channel events in a small patch of membrane. The membrane patch is electrically isolated from the rest of the cell by placing a patch–clamp pipette with a tip diameter of 1–5 μm on to the cell surface and applying gentle suction. An Ω-shaped patch of membrane is sucked into the pipette (Fig. 1a) and the border of this patch seals to the surface of the glass pipette. This is termed the cell-attached configuration because the membrane patch is still attached to the body of the cell. The electrical resistance across the seal between glass and cell membrane may be in excess of 30 gigaohms (30×10^9 ohms); therefore, the only effective route for current flow is across the membrane patch. Because the patch is so small, it contains only a very few ion channels and the opening of a single ion channel causes a significant and measurable increase in the conductance of the membrane patch. These currents are recorded as steplike deflections in the traces corresponding directly to the opening and closing of individual channels.

Potassium (K⁺) Conductance

Voltage Activation

Figure 1b shows a record made across a patch of membrane from a submandibular acinar cell in the cell-attached configuration. The rectangular deflections of the trace represent openings of a high-conductance (maxi-) K^+ channel; the size of the current deflection is a direct measurement of the conductance of this channel. If two channels are open simultaneously, then the current is twice that expected from the unit conductance of the channel. Figure 1b shows that there were at least three channels in this particular patch because there are three current levels. Any one patch may contain none or several channels, depending on the density of channels [which varies with the type of channel under study, the cell type and, probably, the part of the cell membrane, (apical or basolateral) from which the patch was formed] and also on the diameter of the patch pipette. Ion channels may be distinguished from one another on the basis of this characteristic unit conductance, on the duration of each opening (open time), and on the probability of the channel being open (open probability) under a given set of conditions. The successive traces in Figure 1b were obtained by injecting current into the pipette using the patch–clamp amplifier altering the potential difference across the patch of membrane. These data show that the activity (open probability) of this channel is increased at depolarizing voltages (i.e., the channel opens more frequently at depolarizing voltages). Figure 1c shows the current voltage relationship (a plot of the current amplitude, I, as a function of the transmembrane potential difference, V) for the maxi-K^+ channel measured when the patch pipette contained a high-concentration K^+ saline intended to mimic the high-concentration K^+ conditions within the cell, and the cell was depolarized by a high-concentration K^+ bathing solution. (In this high-K^+ concentration solution, the cell has no resting membrane potential, and the potential difference across the patch of isolated membrane is entirely dictated by the voltage set in the recording pipette.) Under these conditions the I/V plot is a straight line with zero current flow at zero voltage—at this point there is no electrical potential difference or chemical concentration gradient to promote net movement of ions in any direction. The slope of the line gives the unit conductance of the individual ion channel (by application of Ohm's law). The unit conductance of the maxi-K^+ channel is 120–260 pS, depending on the species and cell type; this is a very high conductance value, which gives the channel its name.

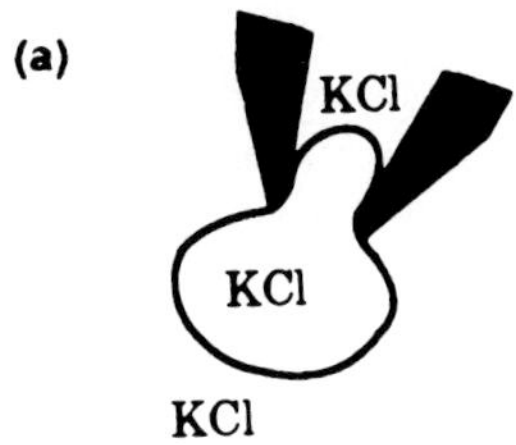

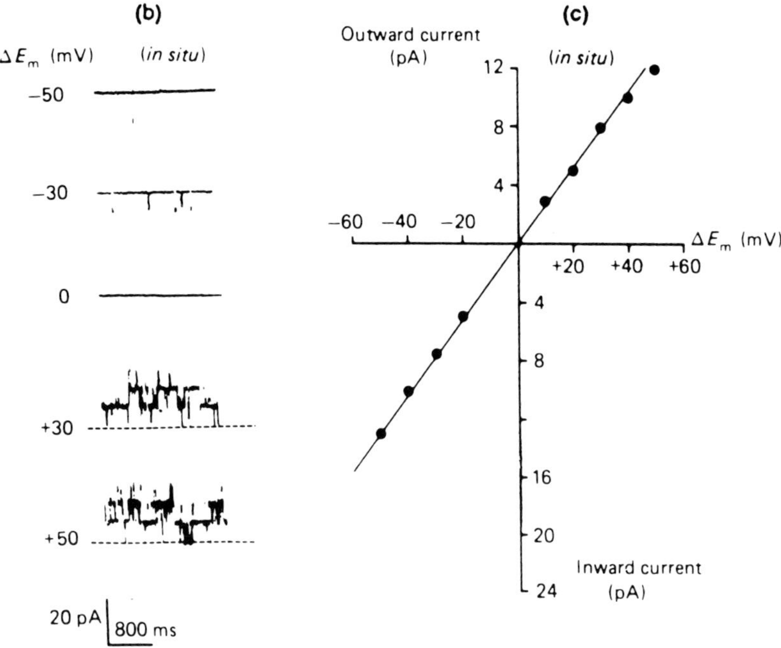

Figure 1 (a) Cartoon showing the cell-attached configuration. The Ω-shaped membrane patch that is sucked into the patch pipette seals to the glass around the circumference of the patch (seal resistance $> 10^{10}$ ohm) and, therefore, is electrically isolated from the rest of the cell. The inside of the patch is bathed by the high K^+ concentration of the cytosol and the outside by the solution contained in the patch pipette. (b) Single-channel currents and current–voltage plot for cell attached (i.e., in situ patches of basolateral membrane from mouse submandibular cells). The patch pipettes were filled with a high-concentration K^+ (145 mM KCl) solution with 1 mM EGTA, but no added Ca^{2+}. What is shown is the effect of changing the potential across the patch (ΔE_m) on the amplitude and frequency of single-channel currents. The patch is cell-attached and at 0-mV change in the pipette potential

Selectivity Over Sodium (Na+)

Figure 2 shows the same experiment carried out with a high-concentration Na^+ saline solution in the pipette; when the voltage gradient across the patch is drawing K^+ from the cell, the I/V relationship is linear, and the conductance approaches that shown in the experiment in Figure 1c; however, when the voltage gradient is reversed, such that it will now tend to promote the influx of Na^+ from the pipette to the cell, there is no current flow (i.e., the channel will not allow Na^+ to pass). Between these two extremes, we observe a gradual reduction in the slope conductance. This sort of I/V profile is characteristic of an ion channel that is highly selective for K^+, as compared with Na^+. Consequently, when activated, it will allow K^+ ions to pass, but not Na^+ ions; this is important because, at normal intracellular membrane potentials, in most acinar cells the electrochemical gradients are such that both K^+ and Na^+ would move (out and into the cell, respectively) if a nondiscriminating aqueous pore (ion channel) were to open. The opening of this highly selective channel, therefore, is a mechanism to allow potassium efflux in the absence of a concomitant Na^+ influx. This will also result in a hyperpolarization of the membrane, rather than depolarization and, as we shall discuss later, the transmembrane potential must be maintained, as it is an essential motive force in the translocation of electrolytes to achieve secretion.

Direct Activation by Calcium

We have described the recording of single-channel currents in cell-attached patches. If, however, after making a "gigaseal" the patch–clamp pipette is rapidly withdrawn from the surface of the cell, the patch of membrane in the pipette is torn away from the cell surface, away from the cell, but remains inside the pipette with the gigaseal intact. What has been formed is an isolated inside-out patch (Fig. 3a), so-called because what was facing the inside of the cell (the cytosolic membrane face) is now exposed to the external bathing solution. This technique allows direct access to the cytoplasmic aspect of the plasma membrane, and thus the role of second messengers in the regulation of ion channels can now be investigated directly by applying the appropriate second messengers to the intracellular membrane surface. The trace in Figure 3b was derived from a patch isolated into a solution in which the free Ca^{2+} was initially buffered to less than 10^{-9} M. In this

---

$(\Delta E_m = 0)$ the transmembrane potential across the patch corresponds to the membrane potential of the cells. These cells are K^+-depolarized so that the membrane potential of the cell was 0 mV The patches are then either hyperpolarized $(\Delta E_m < 0)$ or depolarized $(\Delta E_m > 0)$. (c) Current voltage relationship for the single-channel currents measured in (b). Outward current is positive charge leaving the cell and inward current the reverse. The plot is linear, and the unit conductance of the channel, as measured from the slope of the line, is 257 pS. (b and c modified from Gallacher and Morris, 1986.)

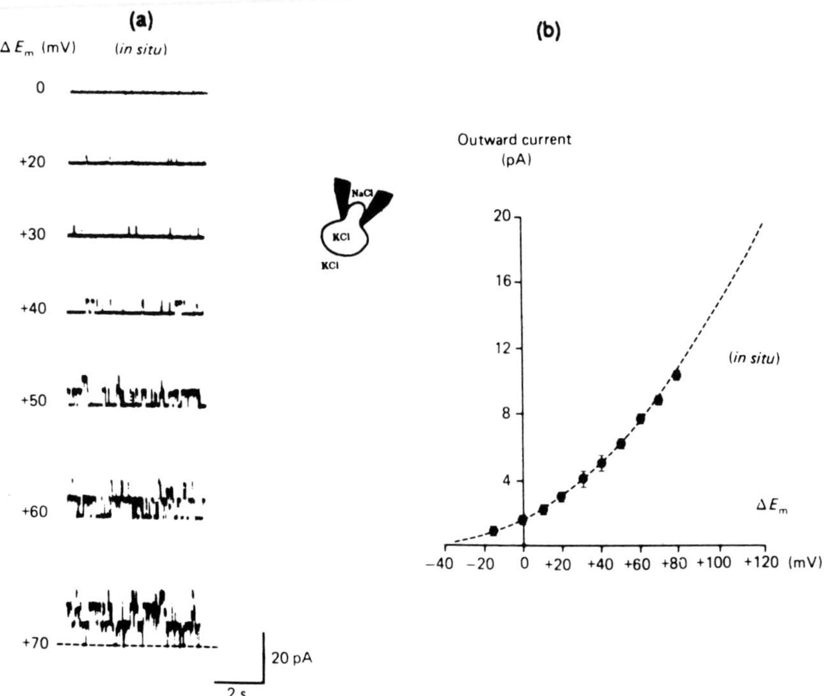

Figure 2   (a) Amplitude and frequency of single-channel currents for cell-attached in situ patch in mouse submandibular acinar cells as a function of changing transmembrane patch potential. The recording situation (inset) was as in Figure 1, with the exception that the pipette was filled with a high-concentration Na^+ solution (NaCl 145 mM) containing 1 mM EGTA and no added Ca^{2+}. Only outward currents were observed in this situation. (b) Current voltage relationship for the single-channel currents measured in (a). The plot deviates from linearity and shows a marked rectification. The dotted line is the current voltage relationship predicted by the constant field equation. (Modified from Gallacher and Morris, 1986.)

experiment, the successive traces were obtained by increasing the free Ca^{2+} in the bathing solution. A significant degree of activation was seen at a free Ca^{2+} concentration of 60 nM, and the channel was maximally activated by a Ca^{2+} concentration of 100 nM–1 μM.

Response to Stimulation by Physiological Agonist

Figure 4 shows how the activity of the maxi-K^+ channel in submandibular cells was increased by application of the muscarinic agonist ACh to the solution bathing

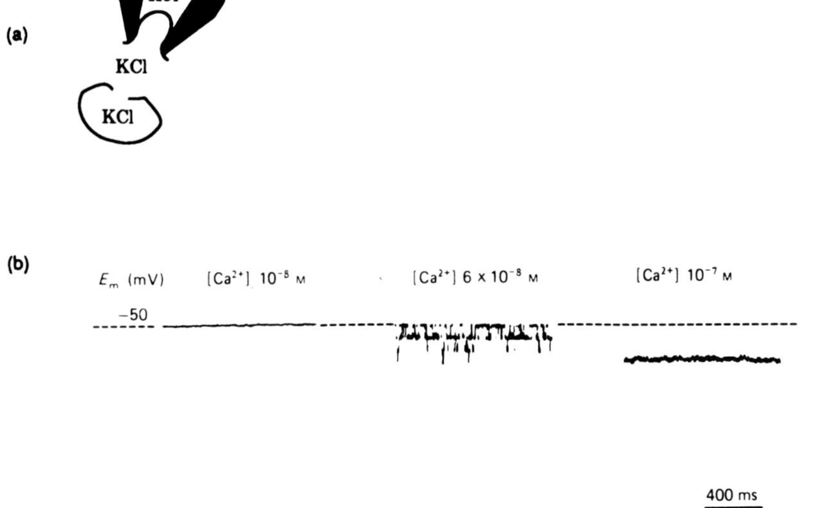

Figure 3 (a) Cartoon showing the inside-out excised patch configuration. The pipette and the patch of membrane sealed to it have been withdrawn from the cell. The cytoplasmic face of the patch is bathed by the external bathing solution and the extracellular face by the solution contained in the patch pipette. (b) Sections of a recording from a single excised inside-out patch of basolateral membrane from a mouse submandibular acinar cell. The pipette contained a 145 mM K⁺ solution, with 1 mM EGTA and no added Ca^{2+}. The external bathing solution was identical, except that sufficient Ca^{2+} had been added to raise the free [Ca^{2+}] to between 10^{-8} and 10^{-7} M. When the patch was clamped to −50 mV (close to the spontaneous resting potential of the intact cell) ion channel activity was stimulated by [Ca^{2+}] between 60 and 100 nM. (Modified from Gallacher and Morris, 1986.)

the cell. The patch pipette prevents the agonist from directly reaching the patch of membrane from which the channel currents are being recorded: it is only the cell surface membrane outside the patch pipette that is stimulated. One can see that the ion channels in the patch are, after a delay, activated. These experiments show that the agonist-stimulated channel openings in exocrine cells must be mediated by some diffusable intracellular second messenger(s), since there was no possibility of any direct interaction of the agonist with the channels in the isolated patch membrane.

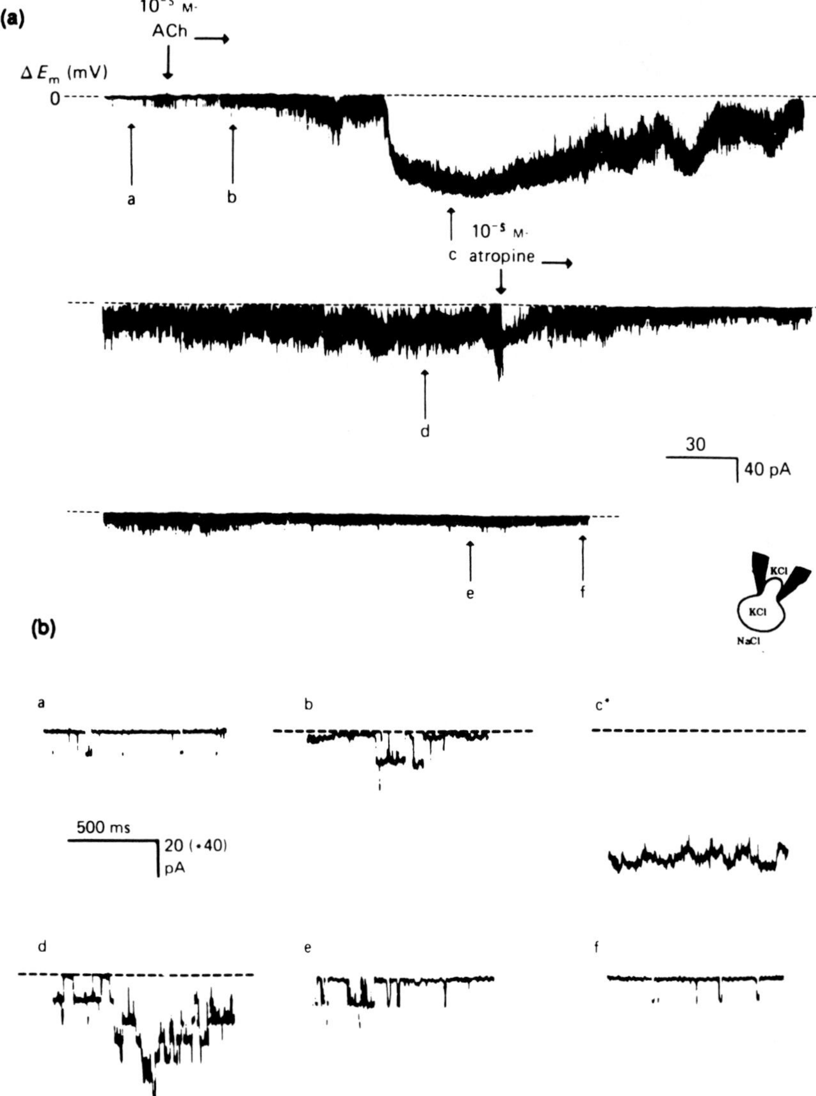

Figure 4 Continuous recording from a cell-attached membrane patch derived from mouse submandibular cells. The patch pipette contained high-concentration K solution (145 mM KCl) with 1 mM EGTA, but no Ca^{2+} added. The patch was clamped at the spontaneous resting potential of the acinar cells (ΔE_m=0). The cells were bathed in a high (145 mM) concentration Na^+ solution containing 1.2 mM Ca^{2+}. At the point indicated, ACh was added to the external bathing medium to give a final concentration of 10 μM. The ACh was then present for the duration of the experiment. The muscarinic receptor antagonist atropine was added after 7 min. The Ach has no direct access to the patch of membrane inside

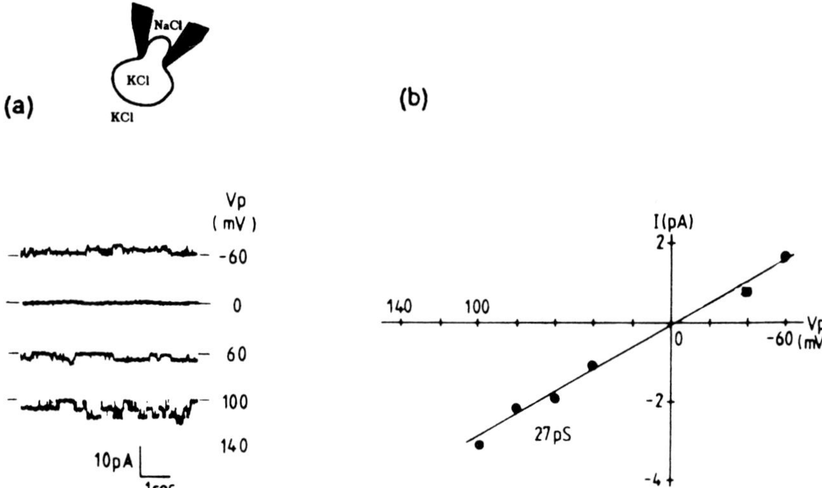

Figure 5   (a) Single-channel currents recorded from cell-attached patches derived from mouse lacrimal cells. The recording situation (inset) was identical with that in Figure 3, and the cells were potassium-depolarized. (b) Current–voltage relationship for the single-channel currents measured in (a). Both outward and inward currents were observed, the plot is linear through zero, and the unit conductance of the channel, as measured from the slope of the line, is 27 pS. This channel cannot discriminate between Na^+ and K^+; in this experiment the inward current was carried by Na^+ and the outward current by K^+. (Modified from Sasaki and Gallacher, 1990.)

Nonselective Cation Conductance

Figure 5 shows another experiment in a membrane patch derived from a mouse lacrimal acinar cell. Lacrimal cells also have the maxi-K^+ channel, but this patch was chosen because it did not contain that channel; hence, activation of a smaller conductance channel could be more easily observed (this channel is also readily observed in salivary acinar cells). The I/V relationship for this channel is measured with protocols similar to those already described for the K^+-selective channel. A

---

the recording pipette and any change in ion channel activity must be mediated via the cell cytosol, i.e., second messenger-mediated. The ACh caused a pronounced increase in the number, frequency, and duration of the single-channel currents and this effect was reversed by atropine. (b) Oscilloscope photographs taken at the points indicated in the continuous recording of (a) (i.e., a,b,c,d,e, and f). At the faster time base the single-channel currents are resolved before, at various times during, and after stimulation by ACh. (Modified from Gallacher and Morris, 1986.)

high-concentration Na^+ solution is contained in the pipette (Fig. 5b). The I/V is a straight line (contrast this with Fig. 2b), with a slope conductance of 27 pS which reverses through zero, even with asymmetric solutions bathing either side of the membrane. This channel clearly passes current, regardless of whether the gradient favors the movement of K^+ or Na^+. The channel conducts K^+ and Na^+ with equal ease and is referred to as a nondiscriminating cation channel. This channel has also been observed in both cell-attached and cell-isolated patches derived from salivary gland cells and is also found in pancreatic acinar cells (Petersen and Gallacher, 1988). It, similar to the maxi-K^+ channel, is Ca^{2+}-activated, but much higher concentrations of Ca^{2+} (in the micromolar to millimolar range) are required. It also differs from the maxi-K^+ channel in that it displays no voltage sensitivity.

Anion Channel

Epithelial cells derived from the intestine or the trachea have a cAMP- or Ca^{2+}-activated Cl^- conductance, which may be resolved using single-channel techniques (Frizell et al., 1986; Hayslet et al., 1987), and a smaller cAMP-activated Cl^- channel has been demonstrated in pancreatic ducts (Gray et al., 1989, 1990). However, no single-channel currents have been recorded in enzymatically isolated salivary acinar cells. Noise analysis of Cl^- channel activity in lacrimal acinar cells estimates the size of this channel to be 1–2 pS (Marty et al., 1984), which is at the limit of resolution for patch–clamp techniques, and it is possible that these channels have been missed in patch recordings. An alternative explanation is that the Cl^- channels are localized specifically to the luminal membrane of the acinar cells. The luminal membrane represents only a very small component of the entire surface membrane, and by far the majority of excised patches would be of basolateral, as opposed to luminal, origin. This is not an unreasonable proposal, since patch–clamp studies in other secretory epithelia have identified Cl^- channels specifically in the luminal membranes (Frizzel et al., 1986). There is very little information, at the level of single-channel current recording, on the anionic permeabilities of the exocrine acinar cells. However, there is no doubt that agonist activation results in a marked increased in the anionic conductance (Cl^- permeability) of exocrine acinar cell membranes. This is made clear in the application of the patch–clamp technique to record whole-cell, as opposed to single-channel, currents.

C. Patch–Clamp Whole-Cell Technique

Introduction

The patch–clamp whole-cell configuration, as its name suggests, measures the integral of all channel openings over the whole-cell membrane. The first step in achieving this configuration is again obtaining a gigaseal between the pipette and the cell membrane. However, the patch of membrane under the pipette, which is the focus of attention in the single-channel experiments, is destroyed to make the interior of the pipette continuous with the interior of the cell. This allows measurements of the currents across the entire plasma membrane to be made (Fig. 6a). A great advantage of the whole-cell current-recording technique is that, on disruption of the patch of membrane underneath the recording pipette, the solution in the pipette will enter into and equilibrate with the cell interior. The rate of equilibration or dialysis of the cell will naturally vary with the size of both the molecule under consideration and the size of the hole made which, in turn, is dependent on the pipette diameter. It is clear that small ions equilibrate within seconds, rather than minutes. In the whole-cell recording mode, the ionic composition of both the external (bathing) and internal (pipette) solutions may then be determined. In this manner, the electrochemical equilibrium, the driving force for ion movement, is not only known very precisely, but it can be manipulated during the course of an experiment. This is of fundamental importance in whole-cell recording because the currents measured are generally a mixture of currents arising from the simultaneous activation of more than one conductance pathway. It is with the knowledge of, and the ability to, manipulate the electrochemical equilibrium potentials that it is possible to develop experimental protocols in which the different current elements can be identified and investigated. Another advantage of the whole-cell technique again relates to the property of dialysis of the cell interior by the solution filling the recording pipette. This approach can be employed to introduce putative second messengers into cells, to investigate their effect on currents in situ, and to directly compare these responses with those evoked in the same cells by the natural neurotransmitter agonists.

Pulse Protocol Measurements

Figure 6 illustrates the methods by which the control over ionic conditions offered by the patch–clamp technique may be exploited in salivary and lacrimal acinar cells to measure changes in two different conductance pathways almost simultaneously. The first step is to separate, as far as possible, the current flowing across the membrane into its individual components. The easiest way to achieve this is to create ionic conditions at which K^+ and Cl^- have different reversal potentials. By using a high-concentration KCl solution inside the pipette and a high-concentration NaCl solution outside the cell, the Nernst equation gives an equilibrium potential for Cl^- or 0 mV (the Cl^- concentration is the same inside and outside the cell; hence, at 0 mV, there is neither a chemical nor electrical gradient to support net Cl^- movement; i.e., no Cl^- current at 0 mV). Neither can the nondiscriminating cation channels contribute to the current at 0 mV because, as for Cl^-, in this ionic situation their equilibrium potential is 0 mV. Thus, at 0 mV we are exclusively monitoring the outward K^+ currents. The same considera-

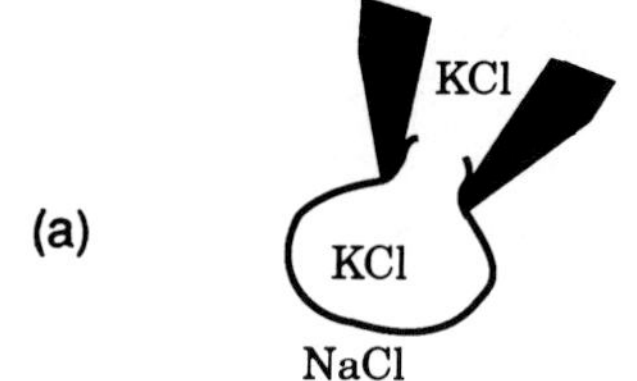

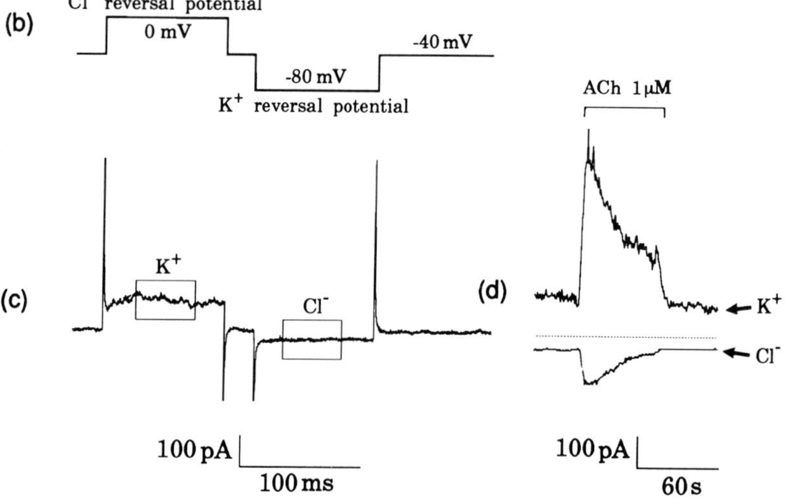

Figure 6 (a) Cartoon showing the whole-cell configuration. The patch of membrane sealed to the pipette has been ruptured (by a sharp application of suction pressure). The interior of the patch pipette is now continuous with the cell interior, and ion exchange can occur. Typically, the cell interior was dialyzed with a high-concentration K^+ solution, containing 0.5 mM EGTA and no added Ca^{2+}. The cell exterior was bathed by a high-concentration Na^+ solution containing 1.2 mM Ca^{2+}. (b) Voltage–pulse protocol used for discriminating between changes in K^+ and Cl^- conductance using the intra- and extracellular solutions described in (a). This voltage protocol was repeated twice each second. (c) Current trace measured at high-sampling frequency (5 kHz) in response to the voltage protocol described in (b). (d) Transient and sustained outward K^+ current (top line) and inward Cl^- currents measured in response to ACh stimulation using the pulse protocol shown in (a) in mouse submandibular cells. The dotted line represents the zero current level. Both currents were rapidly activated, and the K^+ current showed a biphasic response, similar to the response seen using microfluorimetric methods to measure changes in $[Ca^{2+}]_i$. The activation of the Cl^- current was transient, however, and typically, the Cl^- conductance returned to prestimulus values within 2–3 min. As the voltage protocol was repeated twice per second, the time resolution of these traces is 500 ms.

tions can be applied to selectively eliminate K^+ currents from the recordings. The reversal potential for K^+ is about -80 mV. Consequently, if a cell is voltage-clamped to have a membrane potential of -80 mV, there is no driving force for K^+ movement, and so there can be no contribution of K^+ to the net current, regardless of the number of open K^+ channels. The net inward current recorded at -80 could still be due to either Cl^- or nondiscriminating cation channel activation. However, the nonselective cation channel in patches excised from salivary glands requires $[Ca^{2+}]_i$ to be increased into the millimolar range before it is activated. There has been no demonstration in salivary or lacrimal acinar cells that this nondiscriminat-ing channel can be activated in situ by the Ca^{2+} rise induced by neurotransmitters. It appears that the increase in $[Ca^{2+}]_i$ in response to ACh stimulation does not reach levels sufficient to activate the nonselective cation channels. At -80 mV it can be demonstrated that the inward current is entirely due to an increase in Cl^- conductance, because the current is totally abolished by replacing Cl^- in the pipette and the external bathing solution with an impermeant anion. If the Ach-evoked inward current were, even in part, due to Na^+ influx by the nonselective channel, it would persist in the absence of Cl^-. Both the K^+ and Cl^- currents can then be measured nearly simultaneously by pulsing from the K^+ reversal potential (measure Cl^- current) to the Cl^- reversal potential (measure K^+ current). This is illustrated in Figure 6c, which shows the current response obtained to a voltage protocol that stepped from the K^+ reversal potential to the Cl^- reversal potential before returning to a holding potential (-40 mV), close to the resting membrane potential of these cells under these conditions. As explained in the chapter introduction, the rodent pancreatic acinar cells differ from those of all other major exocrine cells, including pancreatic acinar cells of other species, in that they do not possess any K^+-selective conductance pathways. In these cells the non-discriminating cation channel is activated during the response to physiological agonists. Here, the rodent pancreatic acinar cells are once again exceptional and do not conform to the overall scheme presented. A different mechanism must be invoked to explain rodent pancreatic fluid secretion. Attempts have been made to formulate models (Kasai and Augustine, 1990) for these tissues, but they are as yet unproved.

The Electrophysiological Response to Acetylcholine Stimulation

Figure 6d shows that K^+ and Cl^- currents in submandibular cells, measured with a voltage pulse protocol in the patch–clamp whole-cell technique, were both rapidly increased following stimulation by ACh. The increase in K^+ current is biphasic, following an initial rapid rise in current to a maximum, it declines to a lower, but still elevated, level that was maintained for the duration of ACh stimulation. It is possible to confirm that the action of ACh in these cells is mediated by Ca^{2+} by increasing the concentration of the Ca^{2+} buffer, EGTA, within the patch–clamp pipette to 2.5 mM, so that any ACh-evoked Ca^{2+} release from internal stores or

Ca^{2+} influx across the plasma membrane will be rapidly chelated before it could give rise to any effective increase in $[Ca^{2+}]_i$. Experimental evidence has supported this prediction, and ACh did not evoke any increase in K^+ or Cl^- current (Morris et al., 1987b; Smith and Gallacher, 1992).

The patch–clamp technique in its single-channel and whole-cell recording modes has proved to be invaluable in the characterization of the ion channels that exist in salivary, lacrimal, and pancreatic exocrine acinar cell membranes and in revealing the conductances activated by agonists. The agonists regulating ion channel activity do so by means of the second messenger-mediated Ca^{2+} signals that they give rise to. The patch–clamp recording of Ca^{2+}-activated conductances is thus also a powerful tool to indirectly measure and monitor the agonist-induced changes in Ca^{2+}. Recently, however, it has become possible to directly measure the Ca^{2+} signals induced by neurotransmitters, even in single, isolated acinar cells. This is the technique of microfluorimetry.

D. Microfluorimetric Measurements of Intracellular Calcium Ions

Fura-2 is one of the latest in a series of fluorescent Ca^{2+}-sensitive dyes that have been designed to indicate Ca^{2+} in the physiological range (50–1000 nM; Grynkiewicz et al., 1985). The dye is readily loaded into isolated cells in a membrane-permeable acetoxymethyl ester (AM) form. Cytosolic enzymes cleave the AM groups from the fura-2, which is then lipid-insoluble and trapped inside the cell. The dye fluorescence is a function of the free Ca^{2+} concentration. Importantly, however, the spectral sensitivity of the dye shifts on binding Ca^{2+}. At low Ca^{2+} levels the maximum fluorescence is obtained at an excitation wavelength of near 380 nm. As Ca^{2+} is bound toward saturation, this emission maximum shifts to an excitation wavelength of 340 nm. The significance of this is that by alternately monitoring the emission intensity at these two wavelengths, a ratio value for emission can be calculated that can be converted to $[Ca^{2+}]_i$. This ratio value, being independent of the concentration, leakage or photobleaching of the dye, overcomes what were serious problems with earlier single-wavelength excitation dyes. Exocrine acinar cells have been extensively investigated using the single-cell microfluorometric technique (Yule and Gallacher, 1988; Gray, 1988; Osipchuk et al., 1990; Yule et al., 1991; Toescu et al., 1992). Figure 7 shows a Ca^{2+} signal evoked in a pancreatic acinar cell that is typical of the elevations in Ca^{2+} induced by phosphoinositidase-coupled agonists. The initial rapid rise in Ca^{2+} is due to release of Ca^{2+} from internal stores, and this persists, even in the absence of Ca^{2+} from the external medium. However, the sustained, or plateau, phase is dependent on extracellular Ca^{2+}, and if Ca^{2+} is absent or removed from the extracellular fluid, then the $[Ca^{2+}]_i$ very rapidly returns to prestimulus levels. The initial Ca^{2+} release is thus followed by Ca^{2+} influx across the cell surface membrane.

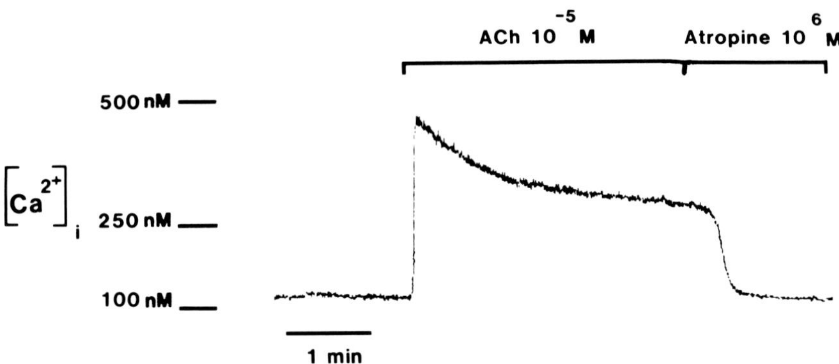

Figure 7   Changes in $[Ca^{2+}]_i$ in a pancreatic acinar cell on stimulation by ACh at 10 μM. The response is biphasic. There was an initial rapid rise in $[Ca^{2+}]_i$ to a maximum, after which it declined to a lower, but still elevated level that was sustained for the period of ACh application or until the muscarinic antagonist atropine was applied. (Modified from Yule and Gallacher, 1988.)

E.   The Role of Calcium-Activated Ion Conductances in a Model for Secretion

Figure 8 shows a model for secretion in which the secretory process depends on activation of the Cl^- and K^+ conductances. The ubiquitous Na^+/K^+-ATPase on the basolateral membrane maintains a high intracellular $[K^+]$ and creates an inwardly directed Na^+ gradient. The Na^+ gradient energizes Cl^- uptake by a basolaterally situated $Na^+/K^+/2Cl^-$ cotransporter, so that Cl^- is also maintained in the cell above its electrochemical potential. Therefore, if a Cl^- channel opens on the luminal membrane, Cl^- will leave the cell and enter the acinar lumen down its electrochemical gradient.

Sodium crosses the epithelium, probably by a paracellular route (tight junctions are much more cation- than anion-permeable) to maintain electrical neutrality, and this creates an osmotic gradient for fluid movement across the cell. This system, however, would rapidly run down as electrochemical gradients are dissipated. The function of the K^+ conductance is to maintain the electrochemical gradient for Cl^- efflux. A increasing Cl^- conductance depolarizes the cells and reduces the driving force for Cl^- efflux: an increasing K^+ conductance hyperpolarizes the cell membrane potential and restores the driving force for Cl^- efflux. The efflux of K^+ across the basolateral membrane into the interstitial space is probably also important in further driving the activity of the inwardly directed $Na^+/K^+/2Cl^-$ cotransporter (see Petersen and Maruyama, 1984; Petersen and Gallacher, 1988). Thus, simultaneous activation of both channels can generate and sustain the luminal Cl^- efflux, which underlies acinar cell secretion and the

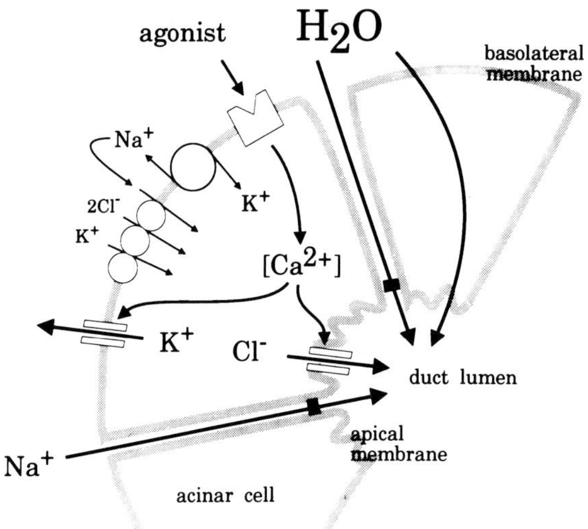

Figure 8   A model for fluid and electrolyte secretion: K$^+$ and Cl$^-$ are maintained above electrochemical equilibrium by the combined action of Na$^+$/K$^+$-ATPase and the Na$^+$–K$^+$-2Cl$^-$ cotransport system. Increased [Ca^{2+}]$_i$ following agonist stimulation (and increased inositolphosphate metabolism) activates an apical membrane anion conductance and a basolateral K$^+$ conductance. The Cl$^-$ exits across the apical membrane, and Na$^+$ follows, probably by a paracellular route. This generates an osmotic gradient and, thereby, fluid secretion. Increased efflux of K$^+$ across the basolateral membrane serves to maintain the cell membrane potential (and, thereby, the driving force for Cl$^-$ efflux) in the face of increased Cl$^-$ conductance.

formation of the primary fluid. This model is applicable to salivary (including human; Morris et al., 1987a) and lacrimal acinar cells of all species yet tested. It is also applicable to pancreatic acinar cells, such as in the human (Petersen et al., 1985), but not to the acinar cells of the rodent pancreas.

III.   Calcium Concentration Homeostasis and the Control of Fluid Secretion

A.   A Critical Assessment of the Secretory Model

Although there is a superficial agreement between the agonist-evoked Ca^{2+} signals, the increases in K$^+$ and Cl$^-$ conductance (see Fig. 6d), and the requirements of the model for secretion, there are two outstanding problems. The first relates to the time course of Cl^- current activation. The data shown for Cl^- current activation fall short of the requirements of the model in one important respect. The agonist-evoked increase in Cl^- conductance is only transient. If, as these data suggest, the Cl^- conductance returns close to control levels within 3–5 min of exposure to agonist, there cannot be sustained electrolyte and fluid secretion by this mechanism. The observation that agonist-stimulated increases in ionic conductivity decline rapidly toward control values is not unique to this preparation, nor to patch–clamp experiments (Putney, 1977; Iwatsuki et al., 1985; Gray, 1988). Previously, it has been ascribed to a loss of some vital factor in the in vitro preparation; for example, the patch–clamp whole-cell technique is particularly vulnerable to loss of soluble cytoplasmic constituents through the patch–clamp pipette. There may well be an alternative explanation, and this is outlined below. The second problem with the model is really one of omission. One of the ion channel species is missing; the model does not incorporate the nondiscriminating cation channels. Indeed, the model need not include this channel, since in situ it has never been shown to be activated by agonists on salivary or lacrimal acinar cells. The rodent pancreas, which lacks the K^+-selective ion channels, in fact, is the only tissue for which activation of the nondiscriminating ion channels has been reported during the physiological response to agonist stimulation. The question arises of whether there is, then, any role for these nondiscriminating cation channels in the secretion of fluid and electrolytes in tissues that have the K^+-selective ion channels: are they not functionally redundant? We will report recent investigations that highlight an important new role for these channels in salivary and lacrimal acinar cells.

B. Transient Increases in Intracellular Calcium Concentration

The Disappearing Chloride Conductance: Are Transients the Solution?

Figure 9 shows the change in $[Ca^{2+}]_i$ of pancreatic acinar cells to low ACh concentrations. Instead of a sustained increase in $[Ca^{2+}]_i$ seen in response to the micromolar concentrations of ACh normally employed, 100 nM ACh caused a series of increases in $[Ca^{2+}]_i$ (i.e., an oscillating $[Ca^{2+}]_i$ signal). These are manifest as rapid narrow spikes in Ca^{2+}, often superimposed on an increase in the steady-state $[Ca^{2+}]_i$ level. Combined measurement of $[Ca^{2+}]_i$ and Ca^{2+}-activated currents show a precise correspondence between large-amplitude oscillations in $[Ca^{2+}]$ and activation of the Cl^- current in pancreatic acinar cells (Osipchuk et al., 1990). That study also revealed that the electrophysiological technique is more sensitive to very small or very local changes in $[Ca^{2+}]$ than the fura-2 measurements. Doses of agonist that produce a threshold response in electrophysiological measurements could not be detected using microfluorimetry (Osipchuk et al., 1990; Marty, 1991). This arises because the microfluorimetric technique of photon

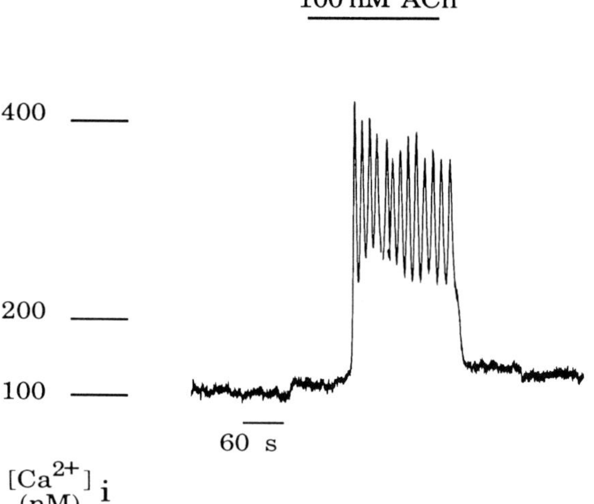

Figure 9   Changes in [Ca^{2+}]$_i$ in a single pancreatic acinar cell on stimulation by ACh at 100 nM. The response to ACh consists of a series of transient increases in [Ca^{2+}]$_i$ on top of a raised baseline [Ca^{2+}]$_i$ that persisted for the duration of ACh application. (Modified from Yule et al., 1991.)

counting provides a measure of the average Ca^{2+} over the entire cell volume. The local discrete Ca^{2+} spikes that appear to be activated at the lowest concentrations of agonists, although giving rise to Ca^{2+}-dependent current activation, do not give rise to any measurable change in the mean [Ca^{2+}]$_i$ throughout the cell. This problem of microfluorimetry can be offset to some extent by the technique of digital videoimaging, which provides both spatial and temporal resolution of Ca^{2+} within the cells. This technique has recently been applied to pancreatic and lacrimal acinar cells (Kasai and Augustine, 1990; Toescu et al., 1992) to reveal that the initial rise in Ca^{2+} in response to maximal concentrations of phosphoinositidase-coupled agonists arises at the luminal pole of the cells, then spreads out to elevate Ca^{2+} throughout the cell.

Until recently, studies of electrolyte and fluid secretion in exocrine glands had, as for the Ca^{2+} measurements, employed micromolar concentrations of agonist, to which the cells responded with only a transient activation of the Cl$^-$ current, despite the sustained elevation in intracellular Ca^{2+}. However, the data in Figure 10 show that when the ACh concentration was reduced to 50 nM, the submandibular acinar cells responded, not with a single transient activation of the Cl$^-$ current, but rather, with a series of transient activations corresponding to the pattern of repetitive transient increases in [Ca^{2+}]$_i$ measured using microfluorimetry. Furthermore, as these repetitive transients and, in particular, the Cl$^-$ current

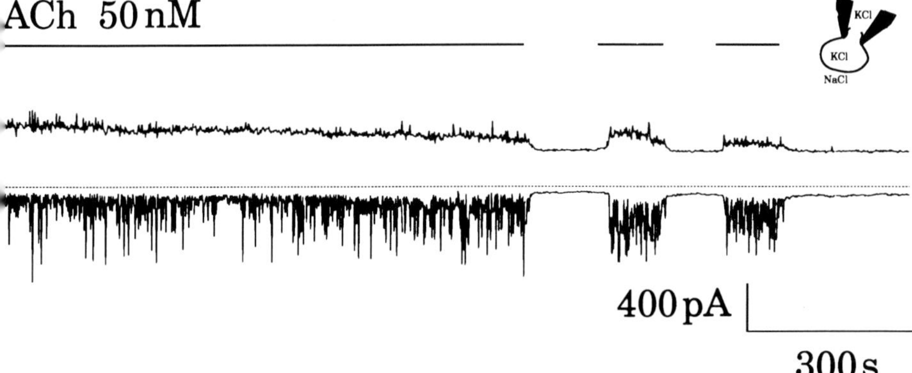

Figure 10 Repetitive transient activation of the outward K$^+$ current (top line) and inward Cl$^-$ currents measured in response to ACh (50 nM) stimulation using pulse protocol in mouse submandibular cells. The dotted line represents the zero current level and the recording configuration is shown in the inset. The response to low agonist concentration was not a single transient activation of the K$^+$ and the Cl$^-$ currents, but a series of rapid transient activations that repeat with a frequency of 1–2 s. Both K$^+$ and Cl$^-$ current transients persist for the duration of agonist application, shown here for 15–20 min. Therefore, the mean Cl$^-$ conductivity can remain elevated for extended periods.

component, could be maintained for the duration of the exposure to agonist. This pattern of activation provides, in the long term, for a Cl$^-$ current activation that now meets the requirements of the model of secretion. It may well be that this response evoked by low concentrations (most probably more physiological concentrations) reflects the pattern of conductance changes that sustain secretion.

The Mechanism Underlying the Calcium Transients

It is now clear that in exocrine acinar cells the phosphoinositidase-coupled agonists can give rise to oscillating Ca^{2+} signals that are reflected in oscillating conductance changes. The simplest explanation of these oscillating second–messenger-mediated Ca^{2+} signals would be that the concentration of the second messenger, Ins(1,4,5)P$_3$, is oscillating. This has indeed been suggested, and the scheme proposed is that Ins(1,4,5)P$_3$ promotes Ca^{2+} release, whereas diacylglycerol stimulates protein kinase C to inhibit Ins(1,4,5)P$_3$ and diacylglycerol formation, thereby giving rise to oscillating Ca^{2+} signals. There is evidence of an inhibitory effect of protein kinase C stimulation on Ca^{2+} mobilization (Woods et al., 1986; Llano and Marty, 1987; Yule et al., 1991); however, other lines of evidence indicate that this is not the mechanism underlying Ca^{2+} oscillations. Repetitive transient or oscillatory increases in [Ca^{2+}]$_i$-dependent ion currents may be achieved in response to infusion of $Ins(1,4,5)P_3$ by the patch–clamp pipette in pancreatic (Wakui et al., 1989) and submandibular cells (Smith, P. M., and Gallacher, D. V., unpublished data). Whereas the $Ins(1,4,5)P_3$ concentration induced in response to agonist activation might have oscillated, that induced by infusion will not. These data suggest that oscillations are intrinsic to the process involved in Ca^{2+} homoeostasis and not a response to oscillating levels of $Ins(1,4,5)P_3$.

Several hypotheses have been advanced to account for the patterns of Ca^{2+} signaling that have been observed in lacrimal (Horn and Marty, 1989; Smith, 1992b), salivary (Gray, 1988; Smith and Gallacher, 1992), and other exocrine (Petersen et al., 1991) and nonexocrine cell types (Woods et al., 1986; Jacob et al., 1988). There are still too many unknowns to be able to propose a definitive model for these processes (but see Goldbeter et al., 1990). Although the $Ins(1,4,5)P_3$ receptor–Ca^{2+} channel complex has been identified from liver and brain cells (Spat et al., 1986; Theibert et al., 1990; Challis et al., 1991) and there is consensus that this receptor regulates Ca^{2+} release from an $Ins(1,4,5)P_3$-sensitive fraction of stored intracellular Ca^{2+}, the morphological site of the $Ins(1,4,5)P_3$-sensitive Ca^{2+} pool is still undetermined. Parts of the endoplasmic reticulum (Streb et al., 1984), more diffuse and less organized structures termed calciosomes (Volpe et al., 1988), and even the secretory granules found at the luminal pole of the cells, have been proposed (Marty, 1991). The situation is unresolved, but it is clear that the intracellular stores for Ca^{2+} most probably comprise a heterogeneous group (Meldolesi et al., 1990). The $[Ca^{2+}]_i$, K^+, and Cl^- current transients have a very abrupt rising phase that is characteristic of a regenerative Ca^{2+} signal (Marty, 1991). One explanation for this is that part of the Ca^{2+}-mobilizing mechanism is a Ca^{2+}-induced Ca^{2+}-release (CICR) process that amplifies the Ca^{2+} signal in response to $Ins(1,4,5)P_3$ (Marty and Tan, 1989; Wakui et al., 1990; Osipchuk et al., 1990; Smith and Gallacher, 1992; Toescu et al., 1992). The idea is that $Ins(1,4,5)P_3$ accumulates to promote release of Ca^{2+} from an $Ins(1,4,5)P_3$-sensitive store, this Ca^{2+}, in turn, results in the rapid and regenerative release of Ca^{2+} from another store by means of CICR. The signal is terminated when the CICR pool is depleted, and it cannot be retriggered until these stores have refilled; hence, the delay until the next Ca^{2+} spike can be generated, and so on. This concept of CICR is not novel. In skeletal muscle Ca^{2+} is released from the sarcoplasmic reticulum, primarily by a process of CICR, and the CICR Ca^{2+} channel has been identified. The CICR response can also be induced pharmacologically with caffeine (Weber and Herz, 1968). Caffeine is thought to stimulate CICR by lowering the threshold for activation of the Ca^{2+}-sensitive Ca^{2+} channel by Ca^{2+} (Goldbeter et al., 1990). The data in Figure 11 show that caffeine is able to stimulate repetitive transient activation of both the K^+ and the Cl^- currents in submandibular acinar cells in the absence of any $Ins(1,4,5)P_3$-linked agonist, which is consistent with a role for caffeine in stimulating CICR. In pancreatic acinar cells, injection of Ca^{2+} into the

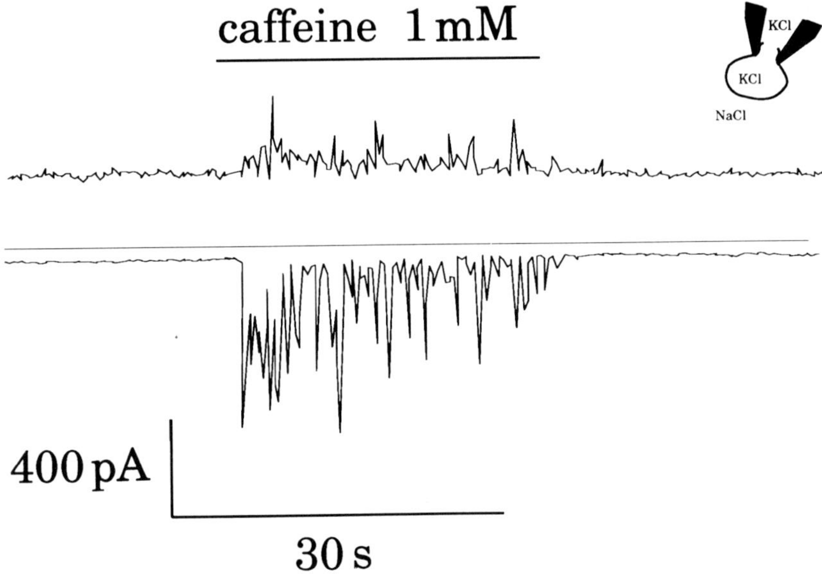

Figure 11 Repetitive transient activation of the outward K^+ current (top line) and inward Cl^- currents, measured in a submandibular acinar cell in response to caffeine (1 mM) stimulation using pulse protocol. The dotted line represents the zero current level, and the recording configuration is shown inset. Caffeine, at low dose, evokes repetitive transient increases in both K^+ and Cl^- current, identical with those induced by low concentrations of ACh. This stimulation is consistent with enhancement of Ca^{2+}-induced Ca^{2+} release by caffeine.

cells, through a whole-cell patch–clamp recording pipette, can induce Ca^{2+} and current transients (Osipchuk et al., 1990; Wakui et al., 1990). Both of these findings, therefore, support the hypothesis that CICR both amplifies $Ins(1,4,5)P_3$-evoked Ca^{2+} signal and may be the key to the mechanism of transient generation.

C. Calcium Influx

So far we have considered only the process of Ca^{2+} release from internal stores, it is clear, however, that even the transient or oscillating Ca^{2+} signals are ultimately dependent on extracellular Ca^{2+} (i.e., Ca^{2+} influx from the extracellular to intracellular fluid). There are two sources of Ca^{2+} normally available to the cell, a finite Ca^{2+} store, held within intracellular Ca^{2+} pools, and Ca^{2+} in the extracellular compartment. Over the short term, repetitive transient activation of the K^+ and Cl^- currents in submandibular cells is generated by mobilization and resequestration of intracellular Ca^{2+} and is independent of extracellular Ca^{2+}. This is illustrated in Figure 12, which shows repetitive transient activation of these currents for over 10 min in the absence of extracellular Ca^{2+}. Recent work in pancreatic acinar cells suggests that Ca^{2+} extrusion from the cell is a part of the mechanism by which $[Ca^{2+}]_1$ is returned to resting levels (Tepikin et al., 1992a,b); therefore, the cycle of release and reuptake is not completely closed, and there is almost certainly some Ca^{2+} loss from the cell with each transient increase in $[Ca^{2+}]_i$. By the end of a 10-min incubation period in Ca^{2+}-free solution (see Fig. 12), there is some evidence that there is a cumulative shortfall in Ca^{2+} resequestration, which manifests as a reduction in the size of the K^+ and Cl^- current transients. Presumably, under more normal conditions when Ca^{2+} is present in the extracellular bathing solution, this shortfall would be supplemented by Ca^{2+} influx across the plasma membrane. The data in Figure 12 also support the hypothesis that the response to agonist becomes more dependent on extracellular Ca^{2+} over time as readmission of Ca^{2+} to the extracellular bathing solution restored the magnitude of both Ca^{2+}-dependent currents.

There are several hypotheses to account for the control of Ca^{2+} influx (Irvine, 1990; Putney, 1990), but a common feature in these models is that Ca^{2+} influx is in some way secondary to, and controlled by, emptying of the intracellular Ca^{2+} pools. This fits with the gradual dependence of the repetitive transients on extracellular Ca^{2+} and also predicts that an easier way to study Ca^{2+} influx would be to increase agonist dose to empty the intracellular pools more rapidly.

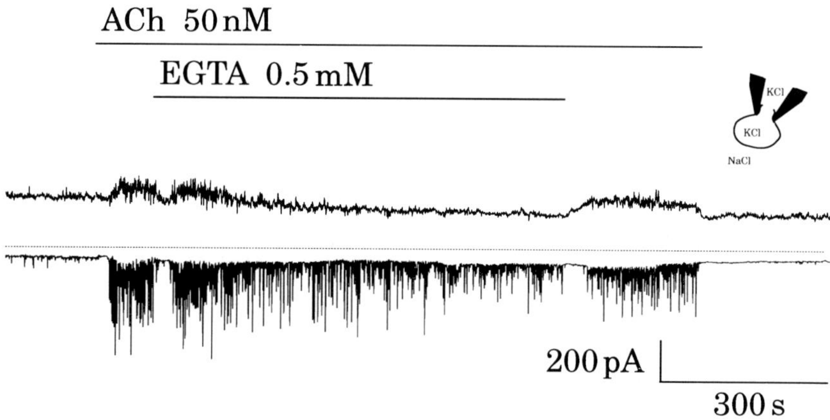

Figure 12 Repetitive transient activation of the outward K^+ current (top line) and inward Cl^- currents measured in response to ACh (50 nM) stimulation using pulse protocol in mouse submandibular cells. The dotted line represents the zero current level, and the recording configuration is shown inset. The repetitive transient activation of the K^+ and Cl^- currents are not critically dependent on extracellular Ca^{2+} as they persist for many minutes when Ca^{2+} in the bathing solution is replaced by 0.5 mM EGTA.

Indeed, the Ca^{2+} signal during the sustained response to high concentrations of agonists is critically dependent on extracellular Ca^{2+}. The intracellular stores can also be depleted by high concentrations of $Ins(1,4,5)P_3$ in the recording pipette. The question that arises is whether $Ins(1,4,5)P_3$-induced depletion of intracellular Ca^{2+} stores is, in itself, the complete stimulus for Ca^{2+} entry. The data available in exocrine cells is controversial. One study in rat lacrimal acinar cells reported that $Ins(1,4,5)P_3$ could promote both Ca^{2+} release and influx, although the effects were transient (Llano et al., 1987). Another report, in mouse lacrimal acinar cells, showed that in addition to $Ins(1,4,5)P_3$ there was also a requirement for the $Ins(1,4,5)P_3$ metabolite $Ins(1,3,4,5)P_4$ to effect Ca^{2+} influx (Morris et al., 1987b; Changya et al., 1989). $Ins(1,3,4,5)P_4$ is produced during agonist activation by the action of a specific $Ins(1,4,5)P_3$-3-kinase phosphorylating $Ins(1,4,5)P_3$ to generate $Ins(1,3,4,5)P_4$. A more recent study of mouse lacrimal acinar cells (Bird et al., 1991) employed extremely high concentrations of $Ins(1,4,5)P_3$ (500 μM, much higher than can be considered to be in the physiological range), and these authors reported that $Ins(1,4,5)P_3$ was itself adequate to fully promote Ca^{2+} influx and achieve sustained activation of K^+ currents, thereby precluding any requirement for $Ins(1,3,4,5)P_4$ in the Ca^{2+} influx process.

Figure 13a shows the result of a very recent series of experiments using the same mouse lacrimal cells to reinvestigate this problem, employing the very high concentrations of $Ins(1,4,5)P_3$, but this time looking at both K^+ and Cl^- currents. After an initial large transient increase in both currents, which may be the product of release of intracellular Ca^{2+} and independent of extracellular Ca^{2+} (Smith, 1992b), the remaining sustained Ca^{2+}-dependent K^+ current was briefly dependent on extracellular Ca^{2+} [i.e., $Ins(1,4,5)P_3$ had promoted Ca^{2+} influx]. Note, however, that the Cl^- current is, as it is for high concentrations of agonists, very transient. Figure 13b shows that the additional presence of only 50 μM $Ins(1,3,4,5)P_4$ with the 500 μM $Ins(1,4,5)P_3$ was sufficient to stimulate a sustained Cl^- current component that was also critically dependent on extracellular Ca^{2+}. It is clear that, even at these very high concentrations of $Ins(1,4,5)P_3$, there is an additional and important role for $Ins(1,3,4,5)P_4$, although its precise mode of action is unclear. There can be no doubt that $Ins(1,3,4,5)P_4$ is a biologically active compound involved in Ca^{2+} mobilization. $Ins(1,3,4,5)P_4$ has been shown to cause Ca^{2+} release independently of $Ins(1,4,5)P_3$ in some cell types (Ely et al., 1990; Ivorra et al., 1991; Ferguson, 1991) and enhance $Ins(1,4,5)P_3$-induced Ca^{2+} mobilization (Morris et al., 1987b; Changya et al., 1989; Cullen et al., 1990; Smith, 1992b). Furthermore, most recently, $Ins(1,3,4,5)P_4$, in the presence of $[Ca^{2+}]_i$ has been shown to directly activate a Ca^{2+} influx pathway in the surface membrane of endothelial cells (Luckhoff and Clapham, 1992). If one bears in mind that depletion of intracellular stores is what probably stimulates Ca^{2+} influx, it is difficult to determine the precise mechanism by which $Ins(1,3,4,5)P_4$ stimulates Ca^{2+} entry in these cells, whether it is a direct action at a

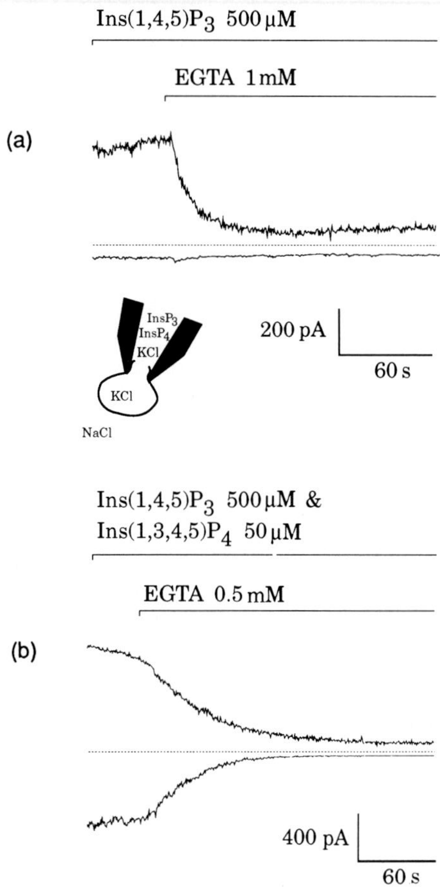

Figure 13 (a) Sustained phase of the biphasic response of mouse lacrimal cells to 500 µM Ins(1,4,5)P$_3$ and (b) 500 µM Ins(1,4,5)P$_3$ and 50 µM Ins(1,3,4,5)P$_4$ together. The dotted line represents the zero current level, and the recording configuration is shown inset. Ins(1,4,5)P$_3$ evokes a sustained increase in the K$^+$ current (upper line) that is abolished by removing extracellular Ca^{2+} and replacing it with the Ca^{2+} chelator EGTA (a). Ins(1,4,5)P$_3$ and Ins(1,3,4,5)P$_4$ together cause a sustained increase in both the K$^+$ and the Cl$^-$ current, both of which are critically dependent on extracellular Ca^{2+}.

plasma membrane Ins(1,3,4,5)P$_4$ receptor or is secondary to an enhancement of release of intracellular Ca^{2+}. Figure 14 combines a model for repetitive transient increases in [Ca^{2+}]$_i$ with one relating the depletion of intracellular Ca^{2+} pools to Ca^{2+} influx. A role for the Ins(1,4,5)P$_3$ derivative Ins(1,3,4,5)P$_4$ is included on the model.

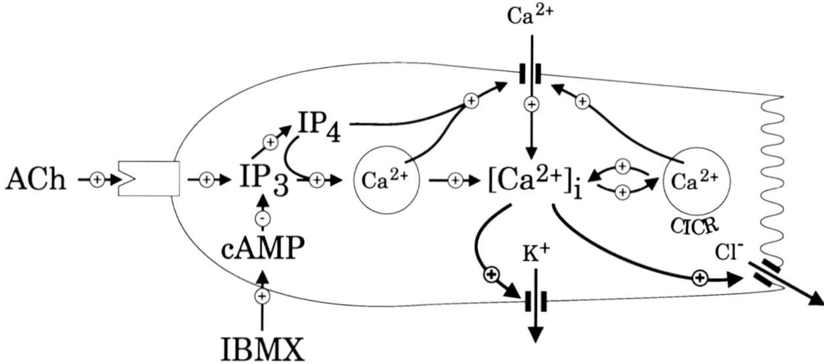

Figure 14   A model for Ca^{2+} mobilization to give repetitive transient increases in $[Ca^{2+}]_i$. Muscarinic receptor activation stimulates inositolphosphate metabolism and production of Ins(1,4,5)P$_3$. Ins(1,4,5)P$_3$ causes Ca^{2+} release from Ins(1,4,5)P$_3$-sensitive intracellular stores. This Ca^{2+} signal is amplified by further release of Ca^{2+} by Ca^{2+}-induced Ca^{2+} release (CICR). Resequestration and rerelease of Ca^{2+} by the Ins(1,4,5)P$_3$-sensitive pool and the CICR pool form the basis for the mechanism of oscillations in $[Ca^{2+}]_i$. Gradual depletion of both the Ins(1,4,5)P$_3$-sensitive and the CICR Ca^{2+} pool activates the influx process. Agents that increase cytosolic cAMP are able to inhibit ACh-induced repetitive transient increases in $[Ca^{2+}]_i$ by inhibiting Ins(1,4,5)P$_3$ production.

D.   A Role for Nondiscriminating Cation Channels

Receptor-Operated, Phosphoinositidase-Independent, Calcium Influx

In 1982, Gallacher reported that ATP, acting as an extracellular agonist, could evoke electrophysiological responses in salivary acinar cells. In the microelectrode recordings of that time, the potential changes induced by ATP resembled those evoked by either ACh or α-adrenergic agonists. The roles of phosphoinositides and Ins(1,4,5)P$_3$ were then not yet known, but the general conclusion was that all of these agonist probably activated essentially the same receptor transduction mechanism. We now know that this is incorrect. In 1988, ATP-induced current responses were reported in rat parotid acinar cells, and an elevation in Ca^{2+} was directly demonstrated (McMillan et al., 1988). Surprisingly, those authors reported that this activation and Ca^{2+} rise was not associated with the generation of Ins(1,4,5)P$_3$. Sasaki and Gallacher (1990) investigated the ATP-induced effects in mouse lacrimal acinar cells and demonstrated that ATP activated a novel transduction mechanism that promoted Ca^{2+} influx in the absence of phosphoinositide metabolism.

In lacrimal and submandibular cells, the nonselective cation channel is not activated in response to Ca^{2+}-mobilizing agents, such as ACh or Ins(1,4,5)P$_3$.

However, it is activated directly by ATP (Sasaki and Gallacher, 1990). Figure 15 shows the effect of ATP on whole-cell currents, note that ATP evoked both inward and outward currents in a pattern superficially like those induced by ACh. However, a close examination of the ATP-evoked currents reveals that the inward current is not a Cl^- current, as it may be obtained in Cl^- free solutions (see Fig. 15b), but rather, is a Na^+ current through the nonselective cation channel. The nonselective cation channel can also conduct Ca^{2+} (Sasaki and Gallacher, 1990), so that Ca^{2+} as well as Na^+ enters the cell in response to ATP stimulation, and this rise in Ca^{2+} triggers the K^+ current by a mechanism entirely separate from phosphoinositide metabolism. The outward current is then a tetraethylammonium (TEA)-sensitive K^+ current through the Ca^{2+}-dependent maxi-K^+ channel. The data in Figure 15c show that, unlike the ACh response for which the initial transient K^+ current was independent of extracellular Ca^{2+}, both the transient and sustained phases of the ATP-activated K^+ current were abolished when Ca^{2+} was omitted from the bathing solution. The inward current persists because it is carried predominantly by Na^+. Analysis of the initial seconds of the response to both ACh and ATP in these cells is consistent with this hypothesis, as it may be observed that in the response to ACh the more Ca^{2+}-sensitive K^+ current rises in advance of the Cl^- current, but when stimulated by ATP, the inward current (of which some component represents Ca^{2+} entry) precedes the activation of the K^+ current (Sasaki and Gallacher, 1990). The ATP effect in directly activating receptor-operated channels to promote Ca^{2+} influx could at least provide a role for nondiscriminating cation channels in salivary and lacrimal acinar cells.

E. Interaction Between Cyclic-AMP and Electrolyte and Fluid Secretion Pathways

No mention has yet been made of those agonists that stimulate adenylate cyclase to generate the second-messenger cyclic adenosine monophosphate (cAMP). The cAMP pathway is not associated with marked effects, if any, on electrolyte and fluid secretion. It is classically considered to promote protein secretion by stimulation of exocytosis. (This secretion of macromolecules is considered elsewhere in this volume.) However, there is recent evidence of interactions between the cAMP pathway and the phosphoinositide and receptor-operated mechanisms, described in the foregoing for fluid secretion.

Figure 16 shows the effect of pharmacological agents known to increase intracellular cAMP on repetitive transient activation of Ca^{2+}-dependent K^+ and Cl^- currents in mouse submandibular cells. Membrane-permeable chlorophenyl-thio (CPT)-cAMP and isobutylmethylxanthine (IBMX, an inhibitor of cAMP phosphodiesterase) reversibly inhibit the current transients induced by ACh. It has been proposed that this is accomplished by an inhibition of $Ins(1,4,5)P_3$ production by cAMP (Bianca et al., 1986; Neylon and Summers, 1988; Rasmussen et al.,

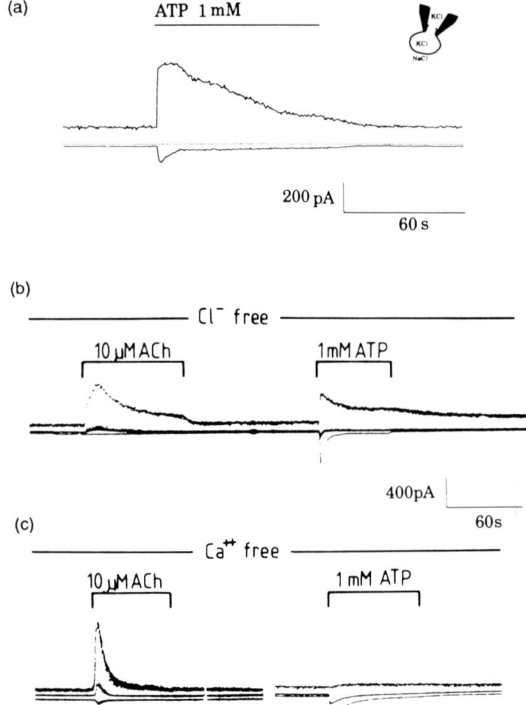

Figure 15 (a) Outward (upper line) and inward currents in a single mouse lacrimal cell response to stimulation by 1 mM ATP. The biphasic response is superficially similar to that evoked by micromolar concentrations of ACh (cf. Fig. 6d). (b) Comparison of outward (upper line) and inward currents induced by ATP and ACh in the absence of extracellular and intracellular Cl^-. The inward Cl^- current induced by ACh is abolished, whereas the inward current induced by ATP is not. Therefore, the inward current induced by ATP is not a Cl^-, but rather, an inward Na^+ current through the nonselective cation channels. (c) Comparison of outward (upper line) and inward currents induced by ATP and ACh in the absence of extracellular Ca^{2+}. The transient, but not the sustained, phase of the ACh response could be elicited in the absence of extracellular Ca^{2+}, which is consistent with the hypothesis that this component of the response to ACh follows release of intracellular Ca^{2+}. Both the transient and the sustained phase of the outward current response to ATP were abolished in the absence of extracellular Ca^{2+}. This is consistent with activation of the K^+ current following influx of Ca^{2+} by the nonselective cation channels. (b and c modified from Sasaki and Gallacher, 1990.)

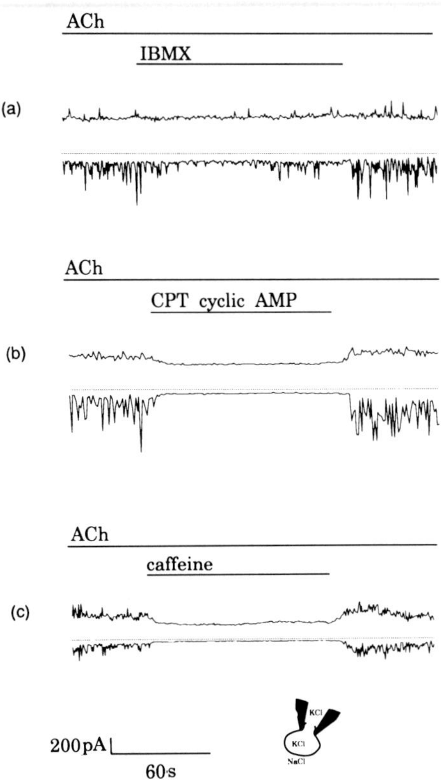

Figure 16 Repetitive transient activation of the outward K^+ current (top line) and inward Cl^- currents measured in response to ACh (50 nM) stimulation using pulse protocol. The dotted line represents the zero current level, and the recording configuration is shown inset. (a) Inhibition by 100 μM isobutylmethylxanthine; (b) inhibition by 10 μM chlorophenylthio cAMP; (c) inhibition by 10 mM caffeine. All three of these agents increase cAMP levels within the cell, either following direct application of a membrane-permeable form as in (c) or by inhibition of cAMP phosphodiesterase. These data are all consistent with inhibition by cAMP or a cAMP-mediated process of ACh-induced $Ins(1,4,5)P_3$ production. (Modified from Smith and Gallacher, 1992)

1990; Smith and Gallacher, 1992), and this has been supported by data from pancreatic acinar cells in which IBMX is able to inhibit the transients in response to ACh, but not in response to $Ins(1,4,5)P_3$ (Smith and Gallacher, unpublished data). We have demonstrated earlier that caffeine could induce current transients in the absence of any agonist. This effect of caffeine is achieved at low, 1 mM, concentrations. At higher concentrations, caffeine will inhibit the agonist-induced responses in a manner similar to cAMP or IBMX. Caffeine is unique in that it is able to stimulate transients at low concentration by CICR and inhibit at higher doses by phosphodiesterase inhibition (caffeine like IBMX is a phosphodiesterase inhibitor at higher concentrations) and increased cAMP levels. However, interpretation of data involving caffeine is further complicated because caffeine is also able to inhibit both the transient and the sustained responses to direct infusion by $Ins(1,4,5)P_3$ and, in this respect, it does not mimic cAMP or IBMX (Osipchuk et al., 1990; Smith and Gallacher, unpublished data). A possible mechanism by which caffeine could inhibit Ca^{2+} mobilization in response to $Ins(1,4,5)P_3$ is a direct block of CICR through an inhibitory effect at the same channel it activates at lower concentrations.

There is also an interaction between cAMP and the Ca^{2+} influx induced by ATP activation of the nondiscriminating cation channels. Isoproterenol, which stimulates cAMP production by β-adrenergic receptors, has no effect on the resting currents in lacrimal acinar cells. Isoproterenol does, however, dramatically potentiate both the outward and inward current responses to ATP (Sasaki and Gallacher, 1992). The mechanism whereby this is achieved is thought to be phosphorylation of the channel or some associated regulatory protein, such that the sensitivity of the channel to cytosolic Ca^{2+} is increased. The effect is that when ATP opens the channels and promotes Ca^{2+} influx in the presence of cAMP the elevation in $[Ca^{2+}]_i$ will itself promote further Ca^{2+} influx. However, the Ca^{2+} influx is always under the control of ATP, because cAMP phosphorylation cannot itself open the channels. At the extracellular receptor, ATP is an absolute requirement. When the ATP is removed the Ca^{2+} influx will cease, even in the presence of cAMP-generating agonists.

IV. Conclusions

The objective of this chapter was to review the mechanisms regulating fluid and electrolyte transport across the acinar epithelium of the major exocrine glands. The most potent stimulus for electrolyte transport is provided by a group of neurotransmitters and hormones that activate a common transduction mechanism. The receptors for these agonists are coupled to the effector enzyme, phosphoinositidase C, through G proteins. When stimulated by the agonist–receptor-activated–G protein complex, this enzyme promotes the hydrolysis of the membrane phospholipid, phosphatidylinositol 4,5-bisphosphate to generate two second messengers, $Ins(1,4,5)P_3$ and diacylglycerol. The $Ins(1,4,5)P_3$ releases Ca^{2+} from intracellular stores and ultimately, in doing so, or in association with other inositol polyphosphates arising from $Ins(1,4,5)P_3$, promotes the influx of Ca^{2+} across the cell surface membrane that is essential to maintain the secretory response. The Ca^{2+}, in turn, activates K^+ (on the basolateral) and Cl^- (at the luminal) channels in the membrane to trigger the movement of electrolytes that initiate the secretory process. The polarization of the different channels to these morphologically and functionally distinct membrane components is fundamental to the unidirectional transport of the electrolytes and fluid that constitutes formation of the primary secretion. We have also reported the complex nature of the Ca^{2+} signals that can be generated and the conductance changes that parallel them. The possible significance of oscillating Ca^{2+} and membrane conductance in terms of exocrine secretion has been discussed, as have the intracellular mechanisms that underlie such oscillating signals. There is strong evidence that the role of the $Ins(1,4,5)P_3$-induced Ca^{2+} release is to promote, by means of Ca^{2+}-induced Ca^{2+} release, a rapidly developing Ca^{2+} signal that will then be propagated throughout the cell. Digital videoimaging of the Ca^{2+} signals has already revealed that the earliest rise in Ca^{2+} in response to maximal concentrations of agonists is located at one—the luminal—pole of the cell. We have also reported a very recently observed transduction pathway in salivary and lacrimal acinar cells that stimulates Ca^{2+} influx in the absence of the production of the inositol polyphosphate second messengers. As an extracellular agonist, ATP directly activates the nondiscriminating cation channels (already known to exist, but with no role being ascribed for them in terms of exocrine secretion in response to phosphoinositidase-coupled agonists) to promote Ca^{2+} influx and the activation of Ca^{2+}-dependent currents. The physiological role of ATP has yet to be fully evaluated. These are very active areas of research, with the major exocrine glands being used as model systems in the investigation of problems that are of wide and very general physiological interest. We can look forward to many exciting new developments further increasing our understanding of the mechanisms that underlie acinar secretion.

References

Berridge, M. J. (1993). Inositol trisphosphate and diacylglycerol: Calcium signaling. *Nature* 361: 315–325.

Bianca, V. D., de Togni, P., Grzeskowiak, M., Vincenti, L. M., and di Virgilio, F. (1986). Cyclic AMP inhibition of phosphoinositide turnover in human neutrophils. *Biochim. Biophys. Acta* 886: 441–447.

Bird G. St. J., Rossier, M. F., Hughes, A. R., Shears, S. B., Armstrong, D. L., and Putney, J. W., Jr. (1991). Activation of Ca^{2+} entry into acinar cells by a non-phosphorylatable inositol trisphosphate. *Nature* 352: 162–165.

Challis, R. A. J., Wicocks, A. L., Mulloy, B., Potter, B. V. L., and Nahorski, S. R. (1991). Characterization of inositol 1,4,5-trisphosphate and inositol 1,3,4,5-tetrakis-phosphate binding sites in rat cerebellum. *Biochem. J.* 274: 861–867.

Changya, L., Gallacher, D. V., Irvine, R. F., Potter, B. V. L., and Petersen, O. H. (1989). Inositol 1,3,4,5-tetrakisphosphate and inositol 1,4,5-trisphosphate act by different mechanisms when controlling Ca^{2+} in mouse lacrimal cells. *J. Membr. Biol.* 109: 85–93.

Cullen P. J., Irvine, R. F., and Dawson, A. P. (1990). Synergistic control of Ca^{2+} mobilization in permeabilized mouse L1210 lymphoma cells by inositol 2,4,5-trisphosphate and inositol 1,3,4,5-tetrakisphosphate. *Biochem. J.* 271: 549–553.

Ely, J. A., Hunyady, L., Baukal, A. J., and Catt, K. J. (1990). Inositol 1,3,4,5-tetrakisphosphate stimulated calcium release from bovine adrenal microsomes by a mechanism independent of the inositol 1,4,5-trisphosphate receptor. *Biochem. J.* 268: 333–338.

Ferguson, J. E., Han, J. K., Kao, J. P. Y., and Nuccitelli, R. (1991). The effects of inositol trisphosphates and inositol tetrakisphosphates on Ca^{2+} release and Cl$^-$ current pattern in the *Xenopus laevis* oocyte. *Exp. Cell. Res.* 192: 352–356.

Frizzell, R. A., Rechkemmer, G., and Shoemaker, R. L. (1986). Altered regulation of airway epithelial cell chloride channels in cystic fibrosis. *Science* 233: 558–560.

Gallacher, D. V. (1982). Are there purinergic receptors on parotid acinar cells? *Nature* 296: 83–86.

Gallacher, D. V., and Morris, A. P. (1986). A patch clamp study of potassium currents in resting and acetylcholine-stimulated mouse submandibular acinar cells. *J. Physiol. (Lond.)* 373: 379–395.

Goldbeter, A., Dupont, G., and Berridge, M. J. (1990). Minimal models for signal-induced Ca^{2+} oscillations and their frequency encoding through protein phosphorylation. *Proc. Natl. Acad. Sci. USA* 87: 1461–1465.

Gray, P.T. (1988). Oscillations of free cytosolic calcium evoked by cholinergic and catecholaminergic agonists in rat parotid acinar cells. *J. Physiol. (Lond.)* 406: 35–53.

Gray, M. A., Harris, A., Coleman, L., Greenwell, J. R., and Argent, B. E. (1989). Two types of chloride channel on duct cells cultured from human fetal pancreas. *Am. J. Physiol.* 257: C240–C251.

Gray, M. A., Pollard, C. E., Harris, A., Coleman, L., Greenwell, J. R., and Argent, B. E. (1990). Anion selectivity and block of the small conductance chloride channel on pancreatic duct cells. *Am J. Physiol.* 259: C752–C761.

Grynkiewicz, G., Poenie, M., and Tsien, R. Y. (1985). A new generation of Ca^{2+} indicators with greatly improved fluorescence properties. *J. Biol. Chem.* 260: 3440–3450.

Hamil, O. P., Marty, A., Neher, E., Sackman, B., and Sigworth, J. (1981). Improved patch clamp techniques for high resolution current recordings from cells and cell free membrane patches. *Eur. J. Physiol.* 381: 85–100.

Hayslet, J. P., Gogelein, H., Kunzelman, K., and Greger, R. (1987). Characteristics of apical chloride channels in human colonic cells (HT$_{29}$). *Eur. J. Physiol.* 410: 487–494.

Horn, R., and Marty, A. (1989). Muscarinic activation of ionic currents measured by a new whole cell recording method. *J. Gen. Physiol.* 92: 145–149.

Irvine, R. F. (1990). Quantal release and the control of Ca^{2+} entry by inositol phosphates—a possible mechanism. *FEBS Lett.* 263: 5–9.

Ivorra, I., Gigg, R., Irvine, R. F., and Parker, I. (1991). Inositol 1,3,4,6-tetrakisphosphate mobilizes calcium in xenopus oocytes with high potency. *Biochem. J.* 273: 317–321.

Iwatsuki, N., Maruyama, Y., Matsumoto, O., and Nishiyama, A. (1985). Activation of calcium dependent Cl^- and K^+ conductances in rat and mouse parotid acinar cells. *Jpn. J. Physiol.* 35: 933–944.

Jacob, R., Merrit, J. E., Hallam, T. J., and Rink, T. J. (1988). Repetitive spikes in cytoplasmic calcium evoked by histamine in human endothelial cells. *Nature* 335: 40–45.

Kasai, H., and Augustine, G. J. (1990). Cytosolic Ca^{2+} gradients triggering unidirectional fluid secretion from exocrine pancreas. *Nature* 348: 735–738.

Llano, I., and Marty, A. (1987). Protein kinase-C activators inhibit the inositol trisphosphate-mediated muscarinic current response in rat lacrimal cells. *J. Physiol. (Lond.)* 394: 239–248.

Llano, I., Marty, A., and Tanguy, J. (1987). Dependence of intracellular effects of GTPγS and inositol trisphosphate on cell membrane potential and on extracellular Ca^{2+} ions. *Pflugers Arch.* 409: 499–506.

Luckoff, A., and Clapham, D. E. (1992). Inositol 1,3,4,5-tetrakisphosphate activates an endothelial Ca^{2+}-permeable channel. *Nature* 355: 356–358.

Marty, A. (1991). Calcium release and internal calcium regulation in acinar cells of exocrine glands. *J. Membr. Biol.* 124: 189–197.

Marty, A., and Tan, Y. P. (1989). The initiation of calcium release following muscarinic stimulation in rat lacrimal glands. *J. Physiol. (Lond.)* 419: 665–688.

Marty, A., Tan, Y. P., and Trautmann, A. (1984). Three types of calcium dependent channel in rat lacrimal glands. *J. Physiol. (Lond.)* 357: 293–325.

McMillan, M. K., Soltoff, S. P., Lechleiter, J. D., Cantley, L. C., and Talamo, B. R. (1988). Extracellular ATP increases free cytosolic calcium in rat parotid acinar cells. *Biochem. J.* 255: 291–300.

Meldolesi, J., Madeddu, L., and Pozzan, T. (1990). Intracellular calcium storage organelles in non-muscle cells: Heterogeneity and functional assignment. *Biochim. Biophys. Acta* 1055: 130–140.

Morris, A. P., Gallacher, D. V., Fuller, C. M., and Scott, J. (1987a). Cholinergic receptor-regulation of K^+ channels and K^+ transport in human submandibular acinar cells. *J. Dent. Res.* 66: 541–546.

Morris, A. P., Gallacher, R. F., Irvine, R. F., and Petersen, O. H. (1987b). Synergism of inositol trisphosphate and tetrakisphosphate in activating Ca^{2+}-dependent K^+ channels. *Nature* 330: 653–655.

Neylon, C. B., and Summers, R. J. (1988). Inhibition by cAMP of the phosphoinositide response to α_1 adrenoreceptor stimulation in rat kidney. *Eur. J. Pharmacol.* 148: 441–444.

Osipchuk, Y. V., Wakui, M., Yule, D. I., Gallacher, D. V., and Petersen, O. H. (1990). Cytoplasmic Ca^{2+} oscillations invoked by receptor stimulation, G-protein activation, internal activation of inositol trisphosphate or Ca^{2+}: Simultaneous microfluorimetry and Ca^{2+}-dependent chloride channel recording in a single pancreatic acinar cell. *EMBO J.* 9: 697–704.

Peterson, O. H., and Maruyama, Y. (1984). Calcium-activated potassium channels and their role in secretion. *Nature* 307: 693–696.

Petersen, O. H., Findlay, I., Iwatsuki, N., Singh, J., Gallacher, D. V., Fuller, C. M.,

Pearson, G. T., Dunne, M. J., and Morris, A. P. (1985). Human pancreatic acinar cells: Studies of stimulus–secretion coupling. *Gastroenterology* 89: 109–117.

Petersen, O. H., and Gallacher, D. V. (1988). Electrophysiology of pancreatic and salivary acinar cells. *Annu. Rev. Physiol.* 5: 65–80.

Petersen, O. H., Gallacher, D. V., Wakui, M., Yule, D. I., Petersen, C. C. H., and Toescu, E. C. (1991). Receptor-activated cytoplasmic Ca^{2+} oscillations in pancreatic acinar cells: Generation and spreading of Ca^{2+} signals. *Cell Calcium* 12: 135–144.

Putney, J. W. (1977). Role of calcium in the fate of potassium release response in the rat parotid gland. *J. Physiol. (Lond.)* 281: 383–394.

Putney, J. W., Jr. (1986). Identification of cellular activation mechanisms associated with salivary secretion. *Annu. Rev. Physiol.* 48: 75–88.

Putney, J. W., Jr. (1990). Capacitive calcium entry revisited. *Cell Calcium* 11: 611–624.

Rasmussen, H., Kelley, G., and Douglas, J. S. (1990). Interaction between Ca^{2+} and cAMP messenger systems in regulation of airway smooth muscle contraction. *Am. J. Physiol.* 258: L279–L288.

Sasaki, T., and Gallacher, D. V. (1990). Extracellular ATP activates receptor-operated cation channels in mouse lacrimal acinar cells to promote calcium influx in the absence of phosphoinositide metabolism. *FEBS Lett.* 264: 130–134.

Smith, P. M. (1992). Patch–clamp whole-cell pulse protocol measurements using a microcomputer. *J. Physiol. (Lond.)* 446: 72P.

Smith, P. M. (1992). Ins(1,4,5)P$_3$ promotes sustained activation of the Ins(1,4,5)P$_3$-dependent Cl^- current in isolated mouse lacrimal cells. *Biochem. J.* 283: 27–30.

Smith, P. M., and Gallacher, D. V. (1992). Acetylcholine and caffeine evoked repetitive transient Ca^{2+}-activated K^+ and Cl^- currents in mouse submandibular cells. *J. Physiol. (Lond.)* 449: 109–120.

Spat, A., Bradford, P. G., McKinney, J. S., Rubin, R. P., and Putney, J. W., Jr. (1986). A saturable receptor for ^{32}P-1,4,5-trisphosphate in hepatocytes and neutrophils. *Nature* 319: 514–516.

Streb, H., Beyerdorffer, E., Haase, W., Irvine, R. F., and Schulz, I. (1984). Effect of inositol-1,4,5-trisphosphate on isolated subcellular fractions of rat pancreas. *J. Membr. Biol.* 81: 241–253.

Tepikin, A. V., Voronina, S. G., Gallacher, D. V., and Petersen, O. H. (1992). Acetylcholine-evoked increase in the cytosolic Ca^{2+} concentration and Ca^{2+} extrusion measured simultaneously in single mouse pancreatic acinar cells. *J. Biol. Chem.* 267: 3569–3572.

Tepikin, A. V., Veronina, S. G., Gallacher, D. V., and Petersen, O. H. (1992). Pulsatile Ca^{2+} extrusion from single pancreatic acinar cells during receptor-activated cytosolic Ca^{2+} spiking. *J. Biol. Chem.* 269: 3569–3572.

Thaysen, J. H., Thorn, N. A., and Schwartz, I. L. (1954). Excretion of sodium, potassium chloride and carbon dioxide in human parotid saliva. *Am. J. Physiol.* 178: 155–159.

Theibert, A. B., Supattapone, S., Ferris, C. D., Danoff, S. K., Evans, R. K., and Snyder, S. H. (1990). Solubilization and separation of inositol 1,3,4,5-tetrakisphosphate- and inositol 1,4,5-trisphosphate-binding proteins and metabolizing enzymes in rat brain. *Biochem. J.* 268: 441–445.

Toescu, E. C., Lawrie, A. M., Petersen, O. H., and Gallacher, D. V. (1992). Spatial and temporal distribution of agonist evoked cytoplasmic Ca^{2+} signals in exocrine acinar cells analyzed by digital image microscopy. *EMBO J.* 11: 1623–1629.

Volpe, P., Krause, K. H., Hashimoto, S., Zorato, F., Pozzan, T., Meldolesi, J., and Lew, D. P. (1988). Calcoisome, a cytoplasmic organelle: The inositol 1,4,5 trisphosphate-sensitive calcium store of non-muscle cells? *Proc. Natl. Acad. Sci. USA* 85: 1091–1095.

Wakui, M., Potter, B. V. L., and Petersen, O. H. (1989). Pulsatile intracellular calcium release does not depend on fluctuations in inositol trisphosphate concentration. *Nature* 339: 317–320.

Wakui, M., Osipchuk, Y. V., and Petersen, O. H. (1990). Receptor-activated cytoplasmic Ca^{2+} spiking mediated by inositol trisphosphate is due to Ca^{2+}-induced Ca^{2+} release. *Cell* 63: 1025–1032.

Weber, A., and Herz, R. (1968). The relationship between caffeine contracture of intact muscle and the effect of caffeine on the reticulum. *J. Gen. Physiol.* 52: 750–759.

Woods, N. M., Cuthbertson, K. S. R., and Cobold, P. H. (1986). Repetitive transient rises in cytoplasmic free calcium in hormone stimulated hepatocytes. *Nature* 319: 600–602.

Yule, D. I., and Gallacher, D. V. (1988). Oscillations of cytotolic calcium in single pancreatic acinar cells stimulated by acetylcholine. *FEBS. Lett.* 239: 358–362.

Yule, D. I., Lawrie, A. M., and Gallacher, D. V. (1991). Acetylcholine and cholecystokinin induce different patterns of oscillating calcium signals in pancreatic acinar cells. *Cell Calcium* 12: 145–151.

2

Molecular Biology of Protein Secretion in Exocrine Cells

LAWRENCE A. TABAK

University of Rochester
Rochester, New York

I. Introduction

The function of exocrine tissue is to synthesize and secrete large quantities of proteins and glycoproteins. Palade (1975) proposed a subcellular model of protein secretion that consisted of six successive processes (Table 1). This model, which emerged as a result of technological advances in electron microscopy and improvement in cell fractionation procedures, emphasized the vectorial flow of secretory products.

At that time Palade remarked that the (then) current research trend was to move from a subcellular analysis of exocytosis toward a more molecular view. This view proved prophetic with the explosion of new experimental strategies and information made available by recombinant DNA approaches.

Great advances have been made in our understanding of what controls the expression of genes and, thus, a much clearer understanding of the events that regulate the biosynthesis of secretory proteins is now available. Current evidence indicates that the biosynthesis of secretory proteins is coupled (by signal transduction pathways) to cellular machinery responsible for secretion.

The mechanisms that control secretory protein segregation and trafficking within a cell have been examined through the detailed study of baker's yeast,

Table 1 The Stages of Secretion

1. Synthesis of secreted proteins
2. Segregation of secreted proteins
3. Intracellular transport
4. Concentration
5. Intracellular storage
6. Discharge

Saccharomyces cerevisiae. This organism is a lower eukaryote in which genetic manipulation has proved to be relatively facile (Sherman et al., 1974). Investigators have exploited this model system through the use of combined genetic and biochemical approaches. The central strategy was to isolate temperature-sensitive growth mutants of *S. cerevisiae* that failed to secrete marker proteins (invertase and acid phosphatase) at nonpermissive temperature (37°C), but could function normally at the permissive temperature (Schekman, 1982). In this way, potentially lethal mutant pathways could be studied. Many of these organisms carrying the secretory (*sec*) mutation have been isolated, and the nature of their mutational defect determined. This has provided insight into the structure and function of several key factors in the secretory process. Through the use of "double" mutants, the vectorial events along the secretory pathway was established (Schekman, 1982). It has also provided a valuable tool whereby analogues of these factors can be identified in other systems, such as mammalian cells.

Molecular cloning has enabled investigators to gain insight into the structure and function of diverse proteins that were intractable to conventional approaches of purification and characterization. In particular, great advances have been made in our understanding of receptors and the proteins responsible for transducing signals into the cell. Once complementary DNAs (cDNAs) encoding the relevant protein have been identified, they are amenable to various forms of analysis. Conceptual translation of these cDNAs allows analysis of homology among related proteins (e.g., Argos et al., 1991), predictions to be made about protein structure, and, from homologies and structure predictions, guesses about protein function. Much has been written about the limitations in predicting protein structure from primary amino acid sequence. It is estimated that, at best, predictions are only 65% accurate when standard methods of secondary structure analysis are used (Garnier, 1990). However, advantage can be made by considering the structure of homologous proteins of known structure. This permits assignment of amino acids that occupy equivalent (and conserved) spatial positions, which enables a more accurate modeling of the unknown protein. Most recently, an attempt has been made to match sequences with protein topology of defining sequences that are most compatible with environments found in the tertiary structure of known proteins (Bowie et al., 1991).

There is also the opportunity to test proposed structure–function relationships of a protein by mutating the protein and then testing the recombinant protein for altered function. Several caveats must be considered, however, in this type of analysis (Schimmel, 1990). For example, one must consider the potential for novel interactions between a mutated protein and an unknown partner, which could confound activity measurements. Similarly, a mutated transcript may be unstable, and this could be misinterpreted as loss of activity owing to alteration of critical amino acids. There is also the possibility of an artifact arising from recombination of a plasmid-based sequence with a chromosomal locus. Despite these potential pitfalls, these approaches have been exploited to provide an enormous insight into the mechanisms that underlie the process of protein secretion.

Another type of experiment that molecular biological approaches have made possible is the targeted "knockout" experiment. Whereas the testing of temperature-sensitive yeast mutants involves a random mutagenesis and screening procedure to uncover phenotypes of a desired type, in this approach the expression of a specific gene product is inhibited. Two approaches are commonly used. In the first, a null allele for the gene of interest is created and expressed by recombination, and the resultant phenotype is characterized. Many experiments of this type have been performed in *S. cerevisiae* owing to the ease of genetic manipulation in that organism, although recent advances in transgenic technology have made it feasible to perform similar studies in mammals (Capecchi, 1989). The second method that has been used in cell lines is the injection or expression of complementary RNA or DNA sequences (so-called antisense) that prevent either the processing, transcription, or translation of the relevant transcript (van der Krol et al., 1988).

The intent of this review is to provide a brief "update" of the Palade model, with emphasis on molecular mechanisms that underlie the six stages of secretion originally proposed. Thus, in preparing this review, we have highlighted studies that have used molecular biological approaches, and we refer the reader to pertinent reviews of work in which a more pharmacological or physiological approach has been applied. Although this distinction is, at best, arbitrary, it is hoped that some appreciation for the power of the molecular biological approaches to the problem of protein secretion will be gained from this exercise.

II. Stage 1: Regulation of Secretory Protein Biosynthesis

Many of the proteins and glycoproteins that are destined for secretion are expressed in a tissue- or cellular-restricted manner. Multiple levels of control have been identified that potentially contribute to this tissue- or cellular-specific expression (Table 2). The labyrinth of control points and circuits undoubtedly contributes to a fine-tuning of the system. Additionally, there is likely to be some

Table 2 Control of Secretory
Protein Expression

1.	Transcriptional initiation
2.	Posttranscriptional processing
3.	Translation
4.	Posttranslational modifications

redundancy to this system, leading to backup systems in the event of primary system failure.

A gene sequence is written in a 5′ to 3′ direction. By convention, reading a sequence right-to-left is *upstream*, whereas a sequence read from the left-to-right direction is *downstream*. The transcriptional start site (designated +1) represents the first nucleotide that is transcribed. The protein-coding regions of most eukaryotic genes, termed *exons*, are discontinuous (i.e., they are interrupted by noncoding sequences, termed *introns*). These regions must be removed before formation of the final transcript.

In general, the concentration of a protein is directly related to the steady-state level of the transcript that encodes it. Transcript concentration reflects the net balance between the rate of transcription and the stability of the resultant mRNA. In theory, therefore, the level of a gene product can be regulated at either the initiation stage of transcription, or posttranscriptionally.

A. Transcriptional Initiation

Compelling evidence points to the importance of transcriptional initiation in regulating the expression of tissue-specific gene products (reviewed in Maniatis et al., 1987; Mitchell and Tjian, 1989). The enzymatic engine that drives the transcription of messenger RNA (mRNA) from the DNA template is RNA polymerase II. The function of this enzyme is dependent on a group of proteins, termed transcription factors, that help align the enzyme–template complex. Short sequences (typically 8–12 base pairs [bp]) of the DNA template, termed *cis*-elements, act as specific target sites for the transcription factors, which may enhance or inhibit gene transcription. Thus, eukaryotic transcription factors are characterized by a DNA-binding domain that accounts for their sequence-specific interaction with DNA (Freemont et al., 1991) and an effector domain that interacts with other transcription factors (TF) or RNA polymerase II to effect a stimulatory or inhibitory influence on transcription (Latchman, 1990). The *cis*-elements that function upstream and within several hundred base pairs of the transcriptional start site are referred to as *promoters*. *Enhancers* are *cis*-elements that function at a distance from the transcriptional start site and in an orientation-independent fashion.

Several *cis*-elements and their corresponding transcription factors are common among many eukaryotic cell types and constitute the basal transcriptional apparatus (Mitchell and Tjian, 1989; Roeder, 1991). A key basal element consists of an alternating sequence of thymidines (T) and adenines (A), the so-called TATA box, placed about 30 nucleotides upstream from the transcriptional start site. Other sequences conserved among many eukaryotic cells include (C(cytosine)-AAT and G(guanine)C(cytosine). The preinitiation complex assembles about these core elements through an ordered set of protein–protein and protein–DNA interactions (Roeder, 1991). At least six discrete factors have now been identified that participate in the formation of this supramolecular complex. Thus, factor TFIID recognizes and binds to the TATA box, whereas other factors bind to the RNA polymerase II, each other, or help stabilize the interaction of the TFIID to the core promoter sequence (Roeder, 1991). The process that leads to the assembly of this preinitiation complex is thus a complex regulatory point for the expression of eukaryotic genes.

In contrast to "shared" basal *cis*-elements and transcriptional factors, other *cis*-elements and transcription factors are expressed in a restricted manner (i.e., they are tissue- or cellular-specific). The restricted expression of these elements and factors is thought to play a central role in the acquisition of unique tissue-specific phenotypes (Falvey and Schibler, 1991).

Although satisfying in concept, it seems unlikely that all tissue-specific gene products merely share identical *cis*-elements that are activated by a master transcription factor. Rather, tissue-specific expression appears to reflect the interplay of multiple factors at one or more DNA sites. Some *cis*-elements are indeed shared among specific gene products; for example, related enhancer sequences have been identified within genes expressed in the exocrine pancreas (Boulet et al., 1986), and this sequence has been termed the *core enhancer*. However, several discrete nuclear proteins bind to similar regions of this core enhancer (e.g., Cockell et al., 1989; Howard et al., 1989; Roux et al., 1989; Meisler et al., 1989; Weinrich et al., 1991; Sommer et al., 1991), suggesting that discrete transcription factors converge on common or related *cis*-elements. Furthermore, many transcription factors are common to genes expressed in multiple tissues; the potential hierarchical import of these different factors in specific cell or tissue types remains to be defined.

B. Posttranscriptional Events

Once formed, the primary transcript (pre-mRNA) in eukaryotes undergoes posttranscriptional processing within a macromolecular complex termed the spliceosome (Maniatis and Reed, 1987). Intronic regions, which are designated by specific nucleotide sequences at their 5′ (donor splice site) and 3′ (acceptor splice site) boundaries (Mount, 1982), are selectively removed by *splicing* reactions, leaving the mature message. In alternative-splicing reactions, specific exons are removed from the final mRNA, whereas others are retained, yielding a mosaic of different exons that are patched together to yield the final transcript. The mixing and matching of exons that results from differential splicing markedly enhances the diversity of resultant protein products (Andreadis et al., 1987). Many secretory protein families are generated in this manner.

In contrast with tissue-specific genes, which are regulated at the level of transcriptional initiation, several housekeeping genes are regulated at the level of mRNA maturation or stability (e.g., Carneiro and Schibler, 1984). Transcript half-life ranges from a few minutes for products that require a quick turnoff (e.g., cytokines, oncogenes) to 4 days when transcription rate and translation efficiency are uncoupled (Hentze, 1991; Hargrove and Schmidt, 1989). In general, transcripts for secreted proteins tend to be stable relative to the time frame required for their release (Hargrove and Schmidt, 1989).

Posttranscriptional control may be engaged in instances for which the speed of response is critical, since such control points could be called into play more rapidly than those employed at the transcriptional level.

C. Translation

A currently held view of translational initiation is represented by the "scanning model" (Kozak, 1991). A 40S ribosomal subunit, charged with a set of initiation factors and carrying a Met-tRNA^{met}, binds to the 5' of a capped mRNA. The subunit migrates in a 3' direction until it encounters an AUG sequence. At this point, a 60S ribosomal subunit joins the assembly, and this results in the synthesis of the initial peptide bond in the nascent protein. There are several structural features of eukaryotic transcripts that modulate translational initiation (Kozak, 1991); these include the following: a 5' 7-methylguanosine triphosphate cap (m^7 cap) at the 5' end of the transcript; the position of, and the flanking sequence about, the AUG initiation codon; secondary structure of the transcript; and the length of the sequence between the cap and the first available AUG codon. It has also been argued that the 3' sequence of polyadenylic acid [poly(A) tail], added posttranscriptionally to messages, also plays a role by enhancing translational initiation, presumably by facilitating the binding of an initiation factor at the mRNA 5' end (Munroe and Jacobson, 1990).

Several protein factors that participate in the regulation of protein synthesis have been identified and the roles established. Available evidence indicates that the phosphorylation state of these factors regulates the initiation of protein synthesis (Hershey, 1989). For example, methionyl-tRNA binding to the 40S ribosomal subunit represents the first stage of protein synthesis initiation. This step requires the participation of a complex consisting of eukaryotic initiation factor—2(eIF-2)·GTP·Met-tRNA. Following an initiation event, eIF-2 is released from the 40S ribosomal subunit as an eIF-2·GDP complex. To regenerate the eIF-2·GTP·Met-tRNA complex, GDP must be replaced in eIF-2·GDP by a reaction mediated by eIF-2B. However, when eIF-2 is phosphorylated at Ser-51, it is unable to undergo the GDP–GTP exchange reaction, with the overall effect being an inhibition of protein synthesis (Rowlands et al., 1988).

The factor that recognizes the m^7 cap at the 5' terminus of transcripts is eIF-4F. Dephosphorylation of the α-subunit of the eIF-4F correlates with an inhibition of protein synthesis. Similarly, the phosphorylated form of eIF-4B, an mRNA-binding protein that is involved in melting transcript secondary structure, is correlated with protein synthesis activation.

III. Segregation and Posttranslational Modification of Secretory Proteins

Proteins destined for export from a cell begin their extracellular journey by translocation across the endoplasmic reticulum membrane. The framework for these events was elegantly outlined by Blobel and Dobberstein (1975a,b) in their *signal hypothesis*. The key elements of this process include (1) recognition of the subset of proteins that contain a *signal sequence* (i.e., a contiguous stretch of amino acids that sorts the protein to the secretory path); (2) targeting of the secretory protein to the endoplasmic reticulum membrane; (3) transport of the secretory protein through the membrane of the endoplasmic reticulum; and (4) cleavage of the signal peptide from the preprotein. During this time frame, posttranslational modifications of secretory proteins begins, principally in the form of *N*-glycosylation.

Many secreted proteins are modified by the addition of carbohydrate side chains, termed oligosaccharides. Eukaryotic oligosaccharides may contain galactose (Gal), fucose (Fuc), mannose (Man), xylose (Xyl), *N*-acetylgalactosamine (GalNAc), *N*-acetylglucosamine (GlcNac), and sialic acids. Protein-bound oligosaccharides are classified according to the nature of the amino acid–carbohydrate linkage. *N*-linked glycoproteins are those in which GlcNAc is attached to the amide nitrogen of asparagine. This process begins within the endoplasmic reticulum. *N*-Glycans are subdivided into three categories: high mannose, hybrid, and complex (Kornfeld and Kornfeld, 1985).

A. Signal Sequences

Most secretory proteins are synthesized in precursor form (i.e., a preprotein) that contains an NH_2-terminal sequence of between 15 and 30 amino acids, termed the signal sequence (Gierasch, 1989). Exhaustive comparison of known signal sequences reveals no specific consensus sequence of amino acids. Rather, what emerges are similarities in patterns. Three discrete regions have been identified in eukaryotic cells; the n (NH$_2$-most terminal) region is variable in length, but carries a net positive charge; the h (hydrophobic core) region is about ten residues long and is rich in hydrophobic amino acids; and the c (COOH-terminal) region, which contains the cleavage site, is about five to seven amino acids (Von Heijne, 1985).

B. Targeting the Secretory Protein to the Endoplasmic Reticulum

As the signal peptide of the nascent protein emerges from the ribosome, it is recognized by the 54-kd protein subunit of the signal recognition particle (Gilmore et al., 1982a,b; Kurzchalia et al., 1986; Kreig et al., 1986). The signal recognition particle consists of six polypeptide subunits (72, 68, 54, 19, 14, and 9 kd), which are organized about a 7S RNA scaffold (Siegel and Walter, 1988). As a result of the signal recognition particle–signal peptide interaction, the affinity of the signal recognition particle for the ribosome is increased by three to four orders of magnitude (Walter et al., 1981), and the translation is arrested (Walter and Blobel, 1981). This is thought to prevent premature folding of the nascent polypeptide, thereby giving it more time to interact with the endoplasmic reticulum membrane and the necessary components of the translocation engine (Bernstein et al., 1989). The initial step of translocation involves attachment of the signal recognition particle–ribosome complex to the signal recognition particle receptor, a heterodimeric endoplasmic reticulum protein (the *docking protein*, Meyer et al., 1982). For translocation to proceed, a GTP-binding–dependent release of the signal sequence from the signal recognition particle occurs, followed by GTP hydrolysis, which releases the signal recognition particle from the docking protein (Connolly et al., 1991). The ribosome then appears to bind to integral membrane proteins of the endoplasmic reticulum membrane (Savitz and Meyer, 1990; Tazawa et al., 1991) and, thus, the signal recognition peptide and its receptor are not part of the ultimate ribosome–endoplasmic reticulum complex (Bernstein et al., 1989).

C. Translocation of the Secretory Protein Across the Endoplasmic Reticulum

The events surrounding the actual passage of secretory protein through the endoplasmic reticulum membrane are unclear. Recently, evidence for a protein-conducting channel in the endoplasmic reticulum membrane was detected electrophysiologically (Simon and Blobel, 1991). Puromycin-induced chain termination results in channel closure. This may mimic physiological gating of the channel following a round of translation in vivo. The signal to open this putative channel may be the attachment of the signal sequence after its GTP-dependent displacement from the signal recognition peptide. Several candidate proteins of the endoplasmic reticulum could be responsible for this and related surrogate activities, including the signal recognition peptide receptor itself.

Translocation-defective mutants of *S. cerevisiae* were developed by targeting the enzyme that converts histidinol to the histidine enzyme on the lumen of the endoplasmic reticulum. This intentional "missorting" proves fatal to wild-type cells when grown on histidinol, since the enzyme is sequestered from the substrate. Temperature-sensitive mutants that fail to sort the enzyme are selected from the survivors of growth on minimal medium supplemented with histidinol. In this manner, the gene mutations *SEC61*, *SEC62*, and *SEC63* were identified (Deshaies and Schekman, 1987, 1989a; Stirling et al., 1992); each gene encodes a membrane protein resident within the endoplasmic reticulum. Cross-linkage studies have suggested that the nascent protein contacts with the SEC61 protein in an ATP, SEC62, SEC63, and BiB protein-dependent manner (Sanders et al., 1992; Müsch et al., 1992). BiP is then required at some point distal in this process to advance the secretory protein from its interaction with the SEC61 protein to its translocation across the endoplasmic reticulum membrane (Sanders et al., 1992).

Although the exact role played by these proteins has yet to be defined, clearly, at least some of them bind, preventing misfolding of the newly formed proteins and, thus, are part of the general class of proteins referred to as chaperones (Bernstein et al., 1989). In contrast, the signal recognition particle functions as a translocator. It seems likely that the two classes of proteins function synergistically (i.e., the chaperones prevent preproteins from entering a conformation that would preclude their interaction with the signal recognition particle). It is clear that these proteins are essential; unless newly synthesized secretory proteins attain their correct tertiary and quarternary structure, they fail to traffic properly within the cell and are ultimately degraded (Bienkowski, 1983; Gething and Sambrook, 1992). BiP (Grp 78), a member of the superfamily of stress-70 proteins (Gething and Sambrook, 1992), binds to unfolded secretory proteins in the endoplasmic reticulum and prevents them from misfolding or aggregating. Secretory proteins in native conformation remain unrecognized. Members of the stress-70 family of proteins have weak intrinsic ATPase activity; it has been suggested that ATP hydrolysis provides a timed release of the stress-70 protein from its substrate, thereby allowing the substrate to continue the following process (Rothman, 1989). The peptide-binding site of BiP accommodates a stretch of seven amino acids, with a bias toward aliphatic residues (i.e., this mimics the interior of a globular protein). This property enables BiP to coat newly translocated polypeptides and prevents them from premature folding (Flynn et al., 1991).

Several enzymes also play a role in proper folding of nascent polypeptides within the endoplasmic reticulum (Freedman, 1989). Protein disulfide isomerase catalyzes thiol–disulfide exchange and, thereby, facilitates the formation of the correct set of disulfide bonds by promoting rapid reshuffling of incorrect disulfide bridges. This enzyme is particularly abundant in cells that engage in a high level of secretory activity (Freedman, 1984), and cross-linking studies demonstrate that protein disulfide isomerase binds to peptides within the endoplasmic reticulum lumen (Noiva and Lennarz, 1992). Moreover, when endoplasmic reticulum microsomes are stripped of their luminal contents with alkali or detergent, proteins synthesized in vitro do not form disulfide linkages correctly. However, when purified protein disulfide isomerase is added back to such microsomes, proper folding of in vitro translated proteins occurs (Bulleid and Freedman, 1988). Protein disulfide isomerase appears to have dual function; it is identical with the β-subunit of prolyl-4-hydroxylase, the endoplasmic reticulum enzyme involved in the cotranslational hydroxylation of proline in collagens (Freedman, 1989).

The second enzyme implicated in proper folding of proteins is peptidyl-prolyl *cis–trans* isomerase. This enzyme catalyzes the interconversion of *cis–trans* conformers of the peptide backbone about the imide bond in the sequence X-Pro (Freedman, 1989). Treatment of chick embryonic fibroblasts with a peptidyl-prolyl *cis-trans* isomerase inhibitor (cyclosporine) delays the formation of the type I collagen triple-helix (Bachinger and Compton, 1991) and, thus, it is likely that this enzyme helps to catalyze the initial steps of folding. Evidence for the interdependence of peptidyl-prolyl *cis–trans* isomerase and protein disulfide isomerase was recently obtained; the efficiency of protein disulfide isomerase is enhanced when peptidyl-prolyl *cis–trans* isomerase is present (Schönbrunner and Schmid, 1992).

D. Proteolytic Processing of Preproteins in the Endoplasmic Reticulum Lumen

Almost all secretory proteins are synthesized as part of a larger precursor molecule that includes the signal sequence required for transport across the rough endoplasmic reticulum. Following entry into the endoplasmic reticulum, the signal sequence is cleaved by a specific signal peptidase, an integral membrane protein of the endoplasmic reticulum. No consensus sequence has been identified for the signal peptidase. However, an analysis of amino acids that flank the signal peptidase cleavage sites of 78 eukaryotic signal sequences led to the formulation of the −3, −1 "rule"; that is, the signal sequence must have Ala, Ser, Gly, Cys, Thr, or Gln in position −1, and must not have an aromatic, charged, or polar amino acid at position −3, as well as no proline in the region spanning −3 to +1 (Von Heijne, 1983; Perlman and Halvorson, 1983). Refinements have been made, and a method that predicts cleavage sites with an accuracy of about 75% has been described (von Heijne, 1986).

The signal peptidase in *S. cerevisiae* has been demonstrated to be the product of the *SEC11* gene, a locus that has been shown to be essential for growth

(Böhni et al., 1988). Signal peptidases have been characterized from both canine pancreas and hen oviduct. In contrast with the peptidases found in prokaryotes, the signal peptidases of these eukaryotic sources are multisubunit in structure (Baker and Lively, 1987; Evans et al., 1986; Shelness et al., 1988). Nevertheless, the substrate specificity of prokaryotic and eukaryotic signal peptidases are quite similar (Deshaies et al., 1989b).

Secretory proteins with mutated cleavage sites accumulate as core-*N*-glycosylated precursors in the lumen of the endoplasmic reticulum. Translocation is unaffected; however, transport from the endoplasmic reticulum is severely compromised (Deshaies et al., 1989b). Moreover, removal of the signal sequence is necessary for the correct conformational development of pancreatic secretory proteins (Scheele and Jacoby, 1982) and the expression of their biological activities (Scheele and Jacoby, 1983).

E. *N*-Glycosylation of the Translocated Protein

The synthesis of *N*-glycans occurs cotranslationally within the endoplasmic reticulum. The initial steps are identical in yeast and higher eukaryotic cells; differences between mammalian and yeast pathways occur in the final stages of processing. A core oligosaccharide ($Glc_3Man_9GlcNAc_2$) is built stepwise on a long-chained polyisoprenoid lipid (dolichyl phosphate) carrier molecule (Abeijon and Hirschberg, 1992). The initial step of this process is the formation of *N*-acetylglucosaminylpyrophosphoryl dolichol (GlcNAc-P-P-dolichol), which is under control of UDP-GlcNAc:dolichol phosphate GlcNAc-1-phosphate transferase (GPT). This represents the committed step in the synthesis of asparagine-linked oligosaccharides (Lehrman, 1991) and is thus a key enzyme in the regulation of *N*-glycosylation. The GPT enzyme is membrane-bound in the endoplasmic reticulum. It is strongly inhibited by the *Streptomyces lysosuperficus* antibiotic tunicamycin, which is structurally homologous to UDP-GlcNAc (Elbein, 1987). Thus, this antibiotic has found widespread use as a specific inhibitor of *N*-linked glycosylation, although homologues of tunicamycin inhibit protein synthesis (Duksin and Mahoney, 1982), and at high concentrations (e.g., 150–200 μg/ml) the synthesis of gangliosides may be affected (Yusuf et al., 1984). Tunicamycin has also been the key reagent in cloning GPT (Lehrman, 1991); because the expression of GPT is so ubiquitous, the usual strategy of expression cloning in a cell lacking GPT was discarded in favor of isolating cDNAs that conferred resistance to tunicamycin (Lehrman et al., 1988; Zhu and Lehrman, 1990). The first such clone was identified in *S. cerevisiae* and mapped to the *ALG7* gene of this yeast (Rine et al., 1983); this gene was demonstrated to be essential for growth, since a null mutation resulted in cell lethality (Kukuruzinska and Robbins, 1987). The level of *ALG7* transcript in yeast may be controlled by the production of two transcripts that differ only in their 3′ end (Kukuruzinska and Robbins, 1987).

Homologues to the *ALG7* gene have been identified in Chinese hamster ovary (CHO) cells (Zhu and Lehrman, 1990; Scocca and Krag, 1990), and several lines of evidence have been presented indicating that these clones do indeed encode the GPT enzyme (Zhu et al., 1992).

The core oligosaccharide is completed by the addition of another GlcNAc (donated from UDP-GlcNAc), five residues of mannose from GDP-Man, four residues of mannose from Man-P-dolichol and three residues of glucose from glucose-P-dolichol (Lehrman, 1991). Considerable progress has been made in the molecular characterization of the enzymes involved in these steps. Yeasts with an *SEC53* mutation lack a phosphomannomutase, the enzyme that is responsible for the formation of Man-1-P, a precursor of GDP-Man (Kepes and Schekman, 1988). The yeast gene *ALG1* encodes the mannosyltransferase that catalyzes the formation of ManGlcNAc$_2$P-P-dolichol from GlcNAc$_2$-P-P-dolichol and GDP-Man (Albright and Robbins, 1990). The *ALG1* gene is transcribed into two classes of mRNA that differ at their 5′ ends. The long form of the transcript is preponderant in stationary cells, whereas the short form is abundant in cells that are actively growing, suggesting that transcript initiation or stability is important in the regulatory control of this enzyme. In contrast, dolichol phosphate-Man-synthase, which has been cloned from yeast (*DPM1* gene), appears to be regulated by phosphorylation (Banerjee et al., 1987; Orlean et al., 1988). Phosphorylation of microsomal membranes, in vitro, by a cAMP-dependent protein kinase led to a twofold increased GPT V_{max}. Alkaline phosphatase treatment of these membrane preparations led to substantial reduction of dolichol phosphate-Man-synthase activity (Banerjee et al., 1987). The product of dolichol phosphate-Man-synthase, Man-P-dolichol, activates GPT, thereby ensuring that GlcNAc-P-P-dolichol is formed when sufficient Man-P-dolichol is available (Lehrman, 1991). Conversely, high levels of the completed core oligosaccharide inhibit GPT activity. In this way, the finite pool of dolichol phosphate is made available for other biosynthetic pathways (Rosenwald et al., 1990).

The pre-formed oligosaccharide is then transferred, en bloc, from the lipid carrier to an Asn-X-Ser/Thr sequence (where X can be any amino acid but proline) on the nascent polypeptide (Kornfeld and Kornfeld, 1985). This sequon has been shown to be a necessary, but insufficient, signal for *N*-linked oligosaccharide attachment. The enzyme that catalyzes this transfer is dolicholdiphosphoryloligosaccharide:protein oligosaccharyltransferase (oligosaccharyltransferase). This enzyme appears to correspond to the previously characterized ribophorin I, a relatively abundant integral membrane glycoprotein that is expressed exclusively in the rough endoplasmic reticulum (Kelleher et al., 1992). The gene encoding yeast oligosaccharyltransferase (or an essential component of the enzyme) has been identified as *WBP* (te Heesen et al., 1992); the protein product of this gene is essential for yeast viability (te Heesen et al., 1991).

The core oligosaccharide is then subjected to a series of modifications whereby glucose residues are removed stepwise by the sequential actions of α-glucosidases I and II which are localized to the rough endoplasmic reticulum (Kornfeld and Kornfeld, 1985). Remodeling continues with the removal of all four of the α1,2,-linked mannosyl residues to yield a core $Man_5GlcNAc_2$ structure. This core structure can be further processed within the Golgi system to yield high-mannose, hybrid, or complex *N*-glycans.

IV. Intracellular Transport of Secretory Proteins

A. Transport of Secretory Proteins from the Endoplasmic Reticulum to the Golgi System

Secretory proteins are exported from the endoplasmic reticulum at different rates (Lodish et al., 1983; Fries et al., 1984; Scheele and Tartakoff, 1985; Yeo et al., 1985). These differences may reflect variation in protein folding and assembly, core *N*-glycosylation, or selective interaction with specific transport receptors within the endoplasmic reticulum (Lodish and Kong, 1990). Thus, two models have been proposed to define protein export from the endoplasmic reticulum. One view is that transport from the endoplasmic reticulum occurs by a default (i.e., no signal) pathway (Rothman, 1987). The alternative model invokes a signal-dependent exit from the endoplasmic reticulum; rapid movement would require interaction with some transport receptor (Lodish, 1988).

The bulk flow rate of a model glycopeptide from the endoplasmic reticulum to the cell surface has been determined to be approximately 10 min (Wieland et al., 1987). Because it is unlikely that such a simple glycopeptide has any intrinsic signal, this result supports the argument that no signal is needed for the vectorial flow of secretory proteins. The default model further predicts that proteins destined for retention in intracellular compartments contain retention signals. Such a signal has been identified for three proteins that remain resident in the endoplasmic reticulum lumen of COS cells, BiP, GRP94, and protein disulfide isomerase; common to each is a COOH-terminal Lys-Asp-Glu-Leu (KDEL) sequence, which experimentally, has been necessary and sufficient for their retention within the endoplasmic reticulum (Munro and Pelham, 1987). A similar system has been found in *S. cerevisiae* in which the COOH-terminal sequence of His-Asp-Glu-Leu (HDEL) is the signal (Pelham et al., 1988). Luminal endoplasmic reticulum proteins appear to be sorted from secreted proteins in a postendoplasmic reticulum compartment. For example, when cathepsin D, a lysosomal enzyme, is modified by attachment of the KDEL sequence, it accumulates within the lumen of the endoplasmic reticulum, but in a mannose 6-phosphorylated form (Pelham, 1988). The enzyme responsible for this phosphorylation is in a postendoplasmic reticulum site. This indicates that KDEL-tagged proteins are retrieved from a postendoplasmic reticulum compartment. Similarly, an invertase fusion protein that contains the HDEL sequence is localized to yeast endoplasmic reticulum, but in a partially mannosylated form (Pelham et al., 1988). The mannosyl transferase responsible for this modification has been localized to the *trans*-Golgi compartment. Collectively, these two observations support the view that targeting to the endoplasmic reticulum is achieved by continuous retrieval of proteins from the Golgi system.

Smooth vesicles have been identified morphologically (e.g., Jamieson and Palade, 1967; Nowack et al., 1987; Morré et al., 1989) that are thought to shuttle newly synthesized proteins from the endoplasmic reticulum to the Golgi system (Palade, 1975). From enzyme marker activity and protein profiles, subcellular fractions have been characterized that differ from both the endoplasmic reticulum and the Golgi system (Paulik et al., 1988; Lodish et al., 1987; Schweizer et al., 1990; 1991). It remains to be determined if any of these represent the morphological site of the biochemical events underlying transport from the endoplasmic reticulum to the Golgi system.

Numerous gene products have been identified that are thought to play some role in the trafficking of secretory proteins from the endoplasmic reticulum to the first elements of the Golgi system (Newman et al., 1990). In yeast, temperature-sensitive mutants in nine (*sec12*, *sec13*, *sec16*, *sec17*, *sec18*, *sec20*, *sec21*, *sec22*, and *sec23*; Novick et al., 1980) *Sec* (secretory) and two (*bet 1* and *bet 2*; Newman et al., 1990) *bet* (blocked early in transport) genes have now been detected in which secretory proteins remain in the endoplasmic reticulum at nonpermissive temperatures. These cells also accumulate an extensive network of endoplasmic reticulum membrane, which suggested that the products of these genes were involved in the processes of vesicle bud formation and fusion. The numerous separate gene products implicated in these events suggest that macromolecular assemblies may be required to effect vesicular transport. Additionally, factors may require posttranslational modifications to be converted from inactive to active form (Newman et al., 1990). The striking homology among yeast and mammalian components involved in protein secretion reflects the highly conserved nature of the secretory apparatus in evolution (Ossig et al., 1991).

Analysis of stains carrying the *sec* mutation indicates that vesicle budding and fusion are discrete events (Newman et al., 1990). The products of *sec12*, *13*, *16*, and *23* are implicated in the former process; whereas *sec17*, *18*, *22*, and *bos1* products are thought to be involved in vesicle fusion events. The sec23 (Ruohola et al., 1988; Hicke and Schekman, 1989), and sec13 (d'Enfert et al., 1991) proteins are hydrophilic and are found in both cytoplasmic and membrane-bound forms. Functional sec23 protein purifies as a complex of about 400 kd (Hicke and Shekman, 1989), although the gene encodes a product that is 85 kd in size. The sec12 protein is an integral membrane protein found in both the endoplasmic reticulum and Golgi system (Nakano et al., 1988), which is thought to facilitate formation of a membrane-associated macromolecular complex of some of the hydrophilic sec proteins. This view is supported by genetic interactions observed among *sec12*, *sec13*, *sec16*, *sec23*, and *Sar1* gene products (Kaiser and Schekman, 1990; d'Enfert et al., 1991), and by the restricted localization of the mammalian homologue of the sec23 protein to the endoplasmic reticulum transitional cytoplasm (Orci et al., 1991a).

Mutation in *sec17*, *sec8*, *sec23* (Novick et al., 1980), or *Bos1* (Shim et al., 1991) genes results in the accumulation of 50-nm vesicles, suggesting a defect in the ability of these structures to fuse with the *cis-* compartment of the Golgi system. *bos1* encodes a 27-kd protein that is required for endoplasmic reticulum to Golgi transport and apparently suppresses the function of the *bet1* and *sec22* gene products (Newman et al., 1990). However, the function of these proteins is not yet known. The activity of the protein encoded by *sec18* is abolished by exposure to the disulfide bond alkylating agent, *N*-ethylmaleimide (Beckers et al., 1989), and is homologous (Wilson et al., 1989) to a mammalian protein of identical function, termed *N*-ethylmaleimide-*sensitive factor* (NSF). It has been proposed that NSF functions as a general component of the intracellular transport machinery, which is required for membrane fusion; thus, this protein has also been implicated in interorganelle transport among the various Golgi system compartments (Block et al., 1988; Weidman et al., 1989; Graham and Emr, 1991). The *sec17* gene product, a peripheral membrane protein, has also been implicated in vesicle fusion by its homology to mammalian *soluble NSF attachment protein* (SNAP), a factor that is required to bind NSF to Golgi membranes (Weidman et al., 1989). In yeast extracts, sec17 protein binds to sec18 protein with a 1:1 stoichiometry (Griff et al., 1992). Morphological localization suggests that sec17 and sec18 are needed for vesicle consumption in vivo (Kaiser and Schekman, 1990). Each protein appears to act at a point distal to a step in the vesicle pathway that is inhibited by an inhibitor of GTP hydrolysis (at the same point of NSF-mediated blockade).

Hydrolysis of GTP is required for the transport of protein between the endoplasmic reticulum and the Golgi system in both mammalian (Melancon et al., 1987; Beckers and Balch, 1989) and yeast (Baker et al., 1988) cells. By analogy to elongation factor Tu, it has been suggested that GTP hydrolysis functions to ensure unidirectionality of the secretory process (Bourne et al., 1990). In the presence of GTPγS, a nonhydrolyzable GTP analogue, or the AlF$_4$-complex, transport is blocked irreversibly, and precursor proteins accumulate in a pre-Golgi compartment [defined by incubation of CHO cells at reduced (15°C) temperature; Beckers and Balch, 1989]. Several GTP-binding proteins have been implicated, including members of the *rab*, *sar*, and *arf* gene families. The *rab* family is a member of the *ras* superfamily and consists of at least 20 related members (Goud and McCaffrey, 1991). Transport between the endoplasmic reticulum and the *cis*-Golgi compartment requires the rab1 protein in mammalian cells (Plutner et al., 1990, 1991).

Thus, the transport of vesicular stomatitis virus G protein is inhibited in CHO cells in the presence of a synthetic peptide that is homologous to the rab 1 protein effector domain (Schwaninger et al., 1991). Similarly, when *YPT1*, the yeast homologue of mammalian *rab 1*, is mutated in yeast, invertase fails to traffic from the endoplasmic reticulum to the Golgi system, apparently owing to a defect in vesicle fusion (Segev et al., 1988; Schmitt et al., 1988; Segev, 1991). The product of the *sar1* gene, which is required for vesicle budding, represents a second group of GTP-binding proteins (Nakano and Muramatsu, 1989; Nishikawa and Nakano, 1991). This interacts with the *sec12* gene product, as described in the preceding section. The third group of GTP-binding proteins implicated in vesicular trafficking are members of the ARF (*ADP-ribosylation factor*) family (Kahn, 1991). Addition of peptides encoding the NH_2-terminal domain of ARF, inhibit protein transport between the endoplasmic reticulum and the *cis*-Golgi compartment at a step that is late in vesicle fusion (Balch et al., 1992). Temporally, this corresponds to a discrete Ca^{2+}-dependent step just distal to the GTPγS-sensitive point in the pathway (Beckers and Balch, 1989), which also is inhibited by a rab effector domain peptide (Schwaninger et al., 1991).

Some insight into the mechanisms that regulate the expression of the GTP-binding proteins is beginning to emerge. *bet2* encodes a protein that is required for the membrane attachment of the Ypt1 protein (Rossi et al., 1991). Sequence analysis of the bet2 protein reveals that it is related to the *Dpr1* gene product, an essential component of a protein phenyltransferase that modifies RAS, enabling it to attach to membranes. On the basis of this homology, it has been suggested that bet2 protein performs a similar function for the Ypt1 protein (Rossi et al., 1991). Defects in the GTP-binding protein Ypt1 can be overcome by expression of yeast *SLY* gene products (Ossig et al., 1991). None of these suppressors encodes a GTP-binding protein that merely substitutes for the *ypt1* product and, thus, their mode of action is yet to be delineated.

The endoplasmic reticulum is a major site of intracellular calcium storage. Release of calcium from this reservoir by inositol triphosphates represents a central event in signal transduction pathways. It has been suggested that perturbation of the luminal calcium levels within the endoplasmic reticulum compromises the ability of some secretory proteins to fold properly, and that such malformed proteins are retained within this compartment (Lodish and Kong, 1990; Lodish et al., 1992).

B. Transport and Modification of Secretory Proteins Within the Golgi Complex

It has been useful to consider the Golgi complex as consisting of at least three discrete compartments, termed the *cis*-Golgi network, medial-Golgi or the Golgi stack, and the *trans*-Golgi (Mellman and Simons, 1992; Rothman and Orci, 1992), although increasing evidence argues that there are distinctive *trans*-Golgi and *trans*-Golgi network compartments (Chege and Pfeffer, 1990; Reaves and Banting, 1992; Reaves et al., 1992). Experimental evidence in support of this model is largely based upon localization of glycosyltransferases by either immunohistochemical or cell fractionation procedures. In some cells, these enzymes are found in discrete subfractions of the Golgi complex (Roth, 1987) and appear to be "ordered" in a manner that is consistent with oligosaccharide processing. Temperature "blocks" at 20° and 15–16°C lead to buildup of precursors within the *trans*-Golgi network and *cis*-Golgi network, respectively, supporting the discrete functional nature of these compartments (Saraste et al., 1986; Rothman and Orci, 1992).

The *cis*-Golgi network receives newly formed protein from the endoplasmic reticulum. *O*-Glycosylation is initiated within this compartment, and the processing of *N*-linked glycans continues. In addition, proteins destined for permanent residence in the endoplasmic reticulum may find their way here temporarily before they are recycled back by a KDEL-recognition mechanism. Thus, some workers have come to view this compartment as a salvage compartment.

Posttranslational Modifications in the cis-*Golgi Network*

Biosynthesis of *N*-Linked Glycoproteins

Following transfer of the preformed core oligosaccharide, newly formed *N*-linked glycoprotein enters the *cis*-Golgi. The enzyme that regulates subsequent modifications is GlcNAc transferase I, which can add a single GlcNAc residue yielding a GlcNAcMan$_5$GlcNAc$_2$ structure. This GlcNAcMan$_5$GlcNAc$_2$ is a substrate for α-mannosidase II, which is localized within the *cis*-compartment of the Golgi complex. Two mannosyl residues are removed, resulting in the formation of an oligosaccharide that can then be further modified into more complex or hybrid structures. In the absence of GlcNAc transferase I activity, oligosaccharide processing becomes limited to the high-mannose path of structures. Thus, GlcNAc transferase I plays a key role in *N*-glycan biosynthesis (Schachter, 1991).

Biosynthesis of *O*-Linked Glycoproteins

O-Linked glycoproteins are those in which GalNAc, GlcNAc, or Xyl are attached to the hydroxyl group of serine or threonine. Mucin glycoproteins, which are the principal organic constituent of mucus, are characterized by large numbers of *O*-linked carbohydrate side chains (Tabak et al., 1982).

In most systems studied, *O*-glycosylation is a posttranslational event which initiates in the *cis*-compartment of the Golgi apparatus (Moreira et al., 1989; Deschuyteneer et al., 1988; Hanover et al., 1980; Johnson and Spear, 1983) and requires no lipid intermediate (Babczinski, 1980; Hanover et al., 1980). Thus, sugars are added stepwise to the growing oligosaccharide chain, under the control of glycosyltransferases. The most common initiator of *O*-glycosylation is UDP-GalNAc: polypeptide α-GalNAc transferase (polypeptide GalNAc transferase), which catalyzes the addition of a single GalNAc residue to either serine or threonine in an α-anomeric linkage.

In contrast with *N*-linked glycosylation, no consensus *O*-glycosylation sequon has yet been identified (Aubert et al., 1976; Wilson et al., 1991; O'Connell et al., 1991). Nevertheless, some patterns have emerged by testing sets of synthetic peptides based on a known glycosylation site in human von Willebrand's factor for their ability to act as substrates for the polypeptide GalNAc transferase (O'Connell et al., 1991). Positions -1, -2, -3, and $+3$ relative to the glycosylation site were sensitive to changes in amino acids. For example, substitution of a charged residue at positions -1, -2, or -3 abolished the ability of the peptide to act as a substrate. The presence of proline at position $+3$ within this sequence context appeared necessary for glycosylation to occur. Addition of a second proline at positions $+2$ or $+4$ enhanced incorporation of GalNAc (O'Connell et al., 1991, 1992). Particularly intriguing is the observation that serinyl-containing peptides act as poor substrates (e.g., Hughes et al., 1988; O'Connell et al., 1991, 1992; Wang et al., 1992). This suggests that there is a separate serinyl polypeptide GalNAc transferase. Indeed, by analogy to protein kinases, it is plausible that there are multiple threonyl and serinyl polypeptide GalNAc transferases, each with its own unique specificities. Alternatively, there may be inhibitors of serinyl *O*-glycosylation. Either possibility would help explain why no clear consensus sequon has emerged, for all work to date has looked at mixtures of enzymic activity.

Transfer of Secretory Proteins Within the Golgi Complex

Transport from one Golgi compartment to the next is mediated by vesicles (75 nm) that are observed to form from Golgi in the presence of ATP and cytosolic factors. Much of our current understanding of vesicular transport in the Golgi is based on the analysis of protein traffic, as monitored by transport-coupled glycosylation (Balch et al., 1984a,b). Golgi fractions from cells that lack GlcNAc transferase activity (donor compartment) are mixed with Golgi fractions from wild-type cells that have this activity (acceptor compartment). Transport is measured by the incorporation of GlcNAc into a marker protein, such as vesicular stomatitis virus G protein. The acquisition of new sugars or linkages has been exploited in a similar manner to mark transport throughout the Golgi system.

Coat proteins α-(corresponding to yeast sec16 protein), β-, γ-(sec23 protein), and δ-(sec21 protein) "COPs"; p36 (sec13 protein); p20 (sec12 protein); together with ADP-ribosylation factor (ARF) assemble on the cisternae of the *cis*-Golgi network or the Golgi stack to yield a coated vesicle by an ATP-, GTP-, and palmitoyl–CoA-dependent process (Waters et al., 1991; Rothman and Orci, 1992).

In contrast with vesicles found in the *trans*-Golgi network that are coated with clathrin and protein complexes referred to as *adaptors*, COP-coated vesicles do not contain clathrin (Orci et al., 1986a), although β-COP is homologous to β-adaptin found in clathrin-coated vesicles (Serafini et al., 1991). The lack of clathrin seems reasonable on functional grounds. Clathrin-coated vesicles are selective in nature (Pearse and Bretscher, 1981; Pearse, 1987) and, therefore, are used at the *trans*-Golgi network where multiple and significant sorting events occur (Griffiths and Simons, 1986; Orci et al., 1987). The COP-coated vesicles do not select their passengers, since proteins destined for localization in a Golgi subcompartment must be excluded from these carriers through the recognition of an appropriate retention signal (Mellman and Simons, 1992).

Formation of COP-coated vesicles is essential for the vectorial transport of proteins to and through the Golgi system. The elements that regulate the formation of these vesicles form a potentially significant control point of secretory regulation. Much insight into this potential control process has been gained through the use of a fungal antibiotic, brefeldin A. Exposure of cells to brefeldin A results in complete disruption of Golgi architecture and a redistribution of Golgi enzymes to the endoplasmic reticulum owing to retrograde (i.e., Golgi to endoplasmic reticulum) transport (Fujiwara et al., 1988). The earliest detectable brefeldin A-induced alteration is the displacement from the Golgi stacks of β-COP (Donaldson et al., 1990). Subsequently, an extensive tubular network forms by an ATP and NSF-dependent reaction that connects both the endoplasmic reticulum and the Golgi subcompartments (Lippincott-Schwartz et al., 1989, 1990; Orci et al., 1991b). It has been proposed that by blocking incorporation of coat subunits and, thereby, the formation of anterograde coated vesicles, brefeldin A treatment leads to the exclusive use of transport components for the formation of retrograde tubules (Orci et al., 1991b). It remains controversial whether this represents an exaggerated form of the normal physiological system used for retrograde transport from the Golgi to the endoplasmic reticulum (Lippincott-Schwartz et al., 1989, 1990) or a brefeldin A-induced aberration (Pelham, 1991). Some insight into the physiological relevance of the brefeldin A effect has been obtained. Down regulation of the yeast receptor for the HDEL endoplasmic reticulum retention sequence, *ERD-2* (Semenza et al., 1990), in yeast results in accumulation of Golgi-derived intracellular membrane. On this basis, it was proposed that the HDEL receptor functions not only to retrieve wayward endoplasmic reticulum proteins, but also to maintain the Golgi architecture (Semenza et al., 1990). Overexpression of human homologue of *ERD-2*, *ELP-1* (Hsu et al., 1992) results in a brefeldin A-like phenotype (i.e., redistribution of Golgi coat proteins, loss of Golgi architecture, and retrograde transport of resident Golgi proteins to the endoplasmic reticulum). Collectively, the data are consistent with the view that the endoplasmic reticulum retention receptors are responsible for the regulation of retrograde traffic between the Golgi and the endoplasmic reticulum (Hsu et al., 1992).

Vesicle content is transferred to the adjacent Golgi cisternae by sequential GTP-dependent uncoating (Melancon et al., 1987) and NSF-dependent fusion (Block et al., 1988). NSF and two auxiliary proteins, α-SNAP and γ-SNAP, bind to the Golgi membrane through a SNAP receptor to yield a 20S particle that serves as the "core" for fusion events (Rothman and Orci, 1992). The *sec7* gene encodes a high-molecular-mass yeast protein that is thought to be a structural scaffold and appears to be required for all stages of intraorganelle transport (Achstetter et al., 1988; Franzusoff and Schekman, 1989). The *myo2* gene of yeast encodes an essential myosin protein that is required for the vectorial transport of vesicles along actin cables (Johnston et al., 1991).

Numerous GTP-binding proteins, belonging to the subfamily of *Ras*-like genes termed *rab*, have been implicated in vesicular transport. It is envisioned that a vesicle surface-bound GTP-binding protein directs delivery of the vesicle to an appropriate target site. Once docking occurs, the GTP-binding protein undergoes a conformational change, GTP is hydrolyzed and the GTP-binding protein is released (Bourne et al., 1990). Several candidate proteins have emerged that display the necessary pro. These include the proteins encoded by the yeast gene *sec4* (Walworth et al., 1992), and its mammalian homologues, members of the *Rab* family of genes (Chavrier et al., 1990). Significant homology between the sec4 and ypt1 protein has been found; this latter protein has been implicated in transport between the endoplasmic reticulum and the *cis*-Golgi network. Thus, several of the gene products implicated in intra-Golgi transfer of material are common to the events underlying transport of newly synthesized proteins from the endoplasmic reticulum to the *cis*-Golgi network.

Posttranslational Modifications in the Medial, trans-*Golgi and* trans-*Golgi Network*

Elongation and Completion of Oliogosaccharides

Subsequent processing or elongation of the oligosaccharide side chains appears to be dictated by availability of enzymes, their substrate specificity (i.e., the product of the first glycosyltransferase reaction becomes the substrate for the second (Roseman, 1970; Beyer et al., 1979; Williams and Schachter, 1980; Williams et al., 1980), and the protein context of the given glycosylation site (Dahms and Hart, 1986; Hubbard, 1988; Bielinkska et al., 1989; Yet and Wold, 1990). It has been proposed that interactions between carbohydrate and peptide backbone influences oligosaccharide conformation which, in turn, may help dictate which of several competing enzymes will process the *N*- or *O*-glycan next (Carver and Cumming, 1987; Brockhausen et al., 1990; Schachter, 1991; Shakin-Eshleman, 1992; Nemansky et al., 1992).

Brefeldin A treatment preferentially disrupts addition of sialic acid to *N*-linked glycans; sialylation of *O*-glycans appears unaffected (Shite et al., 1990).

This implies that the sialyl transferases involved in asparagine-linked biosynthesis are localized in the *trans*-Golgi, whereas those responsible for mucin-type linkages are within the brefeldin A-insensitive compartment of the *trans*-Golgi network (Chege and Pfeffer, 1990).

Sulfation

Studies with brefeldin A suggest that sulfation occurs in the brefeldin A-insensitive compartment of the *trans*-Golgi network (Rosa et al., 1992). The presence of sulfate has been reported for both *N*- and *O*-linked oligosaccharides of several secretory proteins including Gal-3-SO$_4$ and GlcNAc-6-SO$_4$ on thyroglobulin (Spiro and Bhoyroo, 1988); GlcNAc-6-SO$_4$ on rat (Green and Embery, 1987) salivary mucin glycoprotein; GlcNAc-4-SO$_4$ on monkey (Tabak and Levine, 1981) or canine (Lombart and Winzler, 1974) salivary mucin glycoproteins; and the pituitary hormones lutropin and thyrotropin (Green and Baenziger, 1988).

The mechanism underlying the biosynthesis of lutropin-sulfated oligosaccharides has been examined in some detail, since the half-life of the hormone is regulated by the presence of the SO$_4$-4GalNAc β1,4GlcNAcβ1,2Manα sequence, which is recognized by a receptor found in Kupffer cells (Baenziger et al., 1992; Fiete et al., 1991). Transfer of sulfate occurs within the Golgi system. 3′Phosphoadenosine 5′-phosphosulfate (PAPS) enters the Golgi by a specific transporter (Schwarz et al., 1984; Capasso and Hirschberg, 1984) and serves as the sulfate donor. A sulfotransferase responsible for the 4-*O*-sulfation of terminal β-GalNAc in lutropin and thyrotropin has been identified (Skelton et al., 1991). The key control point appears to be the addition of the GalNAcβ1,4. The GalNAc transferase responsible for this recognizes the tripeptide sequence Pro-Leu-Arg (Smith and Baenziger, 1992); once this is added, it serves as the substrate for the sulfyltransferase. A similar scheme has recently been unraveled for the synthesis of another pituitary glycoprotein, proopiomelanocortin, which contains asparagine-linked glycans that terminate with SO$_4$-GalNAcβ1,4GlcNAcβ1,2Man. A tripeptide recognition sequence Pro-Val-Lys is required for the action of the hormone-specific GalNAc transferase (Skelton et al., 1992).

V. Concentration of Secretory Proteins

A. Secretory Protein Sorting in the *trans*-Golgi Network

Following their arrival in the *trans*-Golgi network, protein destined for transport to the lysosomes (Farquhar, 1985) and the plasma membrane (Orci et al., 1987) are diverted from the secretory pathway.

Two distinct types of secretory pathways have been identified: constitutive and regulated (Kelly, 1985). In the constitutive pathway, secretory product is released as it is synthesized by bulk flow. In regulated secretion, proteins are concentrated (some ninefold in exocrine cells and as much as 200-fold in endocrine cells) within the Golgi-condensing vacuoles and are ultimately stored in secretory granules until an appropriate signal is received for release.

Because many cells can use both modes of transport, some segregation of proteins destined for one path or the other must occur. Although most models envision the process of selection occurring within the *trans*-Golgi network (Pfeffer and Rothman, 1987; Burgess and Kelly, 1987; Orci et al., 1987; Tooze and Huttner, 1990), several mechanisms have been proposed to account for sorting including selective aggregation (Tooze and Huttner, 1990; Gerdes et al., 1989; Chanat and Huttner, 1991), recognition of specific carriers (Chung et al., 1989) or storage in specific membrane carriers (von Zastrow and Castle, 1987; Hashimoto et al., 1987; Castle et al., 1992).

No sequon has yet been identified that represents a universal sorting signal to secretory granules. Thus, whereas the secretory granule targeting information of trypsinogen is not present at the NH_2-terminus of the protein (Burgess et al., 1987), a 13-amino acid NH_2-terminal domain of a basic salivary proline-rich protein was demonstrated to be necessary for storage in secretory granules (Castle et al., 1992). This domain is encoded by a region (the transition region) that is well conserved among the superfamily of proline-rich proteins (Carlson et al., 1991; Cooper et al., 1991).

B. Properties of Secretory Granules

Secretory granules must store and concentrate proteins destined for export. In response to some external signal, these granules must fuse with the plasma membrane, typically at the apical face of the cell. Following release, membrane components are recycled to the Golgi complex for subsequent reuse (Farquhar and Palade, 1981). Comparative analysis of secretion granules, derived from parotid, lacrimal, submandibular glands, and pancreas, revealed that there is a common set of membrane proteins (Cameron et al., 1986). Indeed, three membrane proteins (apparent M_r, 31, 33, and 35 ka) termed *secretory carrier membrane proteins* (SCAMPS), have been identified as being common to both exocrine and endocrine granule membranes, as well as synaptic vesicle membranes (Brand et al., 1991). Similarly, monoclonal antibodies have been used to detect a family of integral membrane glycoproteins that are localized on the luminal side of secretory granules of both exocrine and endocrine cells (Yamashita and Yasuda, 1992).

Few studies have been conducted on the molecular organization of secretory granules. Electron micrographs reveal a spectacular diversity of patterns, at least some of which have been attributed to fixation and processing artifact (e.g., Simson, 1977; Cutler and Chaudhry, 1974). Secretory granules usually contain a mixture of all the protein secreted by that cell type (Bendayan, 1982; Kraehenbuhl et al., 1977), although they may be in different proportions in individual granules (Mroz and Lechene, 1986). Furthermore, there are some data to suggest that supramolecular organization exists within the granule. For example, in secretory granules prepared from rat islets of Langerhans, insulin is contained largely in an electron-dense central core in a crystalline state, whereas the C peptide is dissolved in the outer fluid of the granule that bathes the central core region (Michael et al., 1987). Electron microscopic immunolocalization of rat submandibular gland mucin and glutamine–glutamic acid-rich proteins (GRP) revealed that, although both proteins colocalize to the same secretory granule, mucin is detected mainly over the electron-lucent matrix of the granules, whereas GRP localized primarily over the electron-dense regions of the granules (Moreira et al., 1989). It has been speculated that the GRP (Mirels et al., 1987) are the functional equivalents of endocrine cell chromagranins, which have been implicated in granule packaging by acting as charge shields and modulators of peptide processing (Huttner et al., 1991).

C. Posttranslational Processing in Secretory Vesicles

Many secretory proteins often require additional proteolytic processing before the active form of the protein is obtained (Schwartz, 1986). Most commonly, such proteins belong to the general class of regulatory peptides (e.g., hormones, growth factors, neuropeptides) and, thus, are typical products of neural or endocrine cells. However, increasing evidence suggests that these processes also occur within exocrine cells (von Zastrow et al., 1986). The precursor protein is cleaved by an endoproteinase, the resultant COOH-terminal basic amino acid is removed by the action of a carboxypeptidase, and the new COOH-terminal residue is often amidated (Fisher and Scheller, 1988). In general, these processing steps occur within secretory vesicles, although, in yeast, some of these events occur in the *trans*-Golgi network (Redding et al., 1991). Superimposed over the specific regulatory elements dictated by the enzymes responsible for processing events is the general control of pH. A relationship between processing and a low pH environment has been demonstrated for several systems. For example, conversion of proinsulin to insulin occurs coordinately with the acidification of maturing secretory vesicles (Orci et al., 1986b); thus, ionophores that disrupt intracellular H^+ gradients inhibit conversion of the proinsulin.

Typically, endoproteinase cleavage signals are dibasic amino acids; in a survey of 35 different peptide hormone and neuropeptide precursors, Lys-Arg (70%) was most commonly used, followed by Arg-Arg (15%), Lys-Lys (10%), and Arg-Lys (5%) (Stoller and Shields, 1989). Tri- and tetrabasic sites have also been identified (Fisher and Scheller, 1988). None of these signals are absolute, however; not all dibasic sites are processed, and many examples of monobasic cleavage sites of attack are known (Schwartz, 1986). For example, many Pro-Arg or Arg-Pro participate in proline-directed arginyl cleavage reactions. The observation that identical precursor protein can be processed in a unique tissue-specific manner argues for a distinct regulatory role for the tissue-specific expression of the processing enzymes.

Purification of the proteinases involved in the posttranslational modification of secretory proteins has proved challenging. The best-characterized enzymes are those in *S. cerevisiae* (Jones, 1991). Kex2 proteinase is an endoproteinase that cleaves on the COOH-terminal side of Lys-Arg or Arg-Arg. It is an integral membrane glycoprotein that is localized to the *trans*-regions of the Golgi system (Redding et al., 1991). This proteinase is involved in the processing of killer toxin (*k*iller *ex*pression) and the α-mating factor. Interestingly, in yeast mutants defective in clathrin, Kex2 proteinase missorts to the plasma membrane, suggesting that clathrin is required for the retention of Kex2 proteinase in the Golgi compartment (Payne and Schekman, 1989). Kex1 carboxypeptidase removes COOH-terminal lysine or arginine residues. It, too, is an integral membrane protein found in the late Golgi system. Dipeptidyl aminopeptidase catalyzes the scission of Glu-Ala or Asp-Ala bonds in the α-mating factor precursor. From sequence homologies, it is thought that this enzyme is localized within the Golgi system. Several endopeptidases have been identified within secretory granules. For example, an endopeptidase, which is implicated in the processing of proocytocin–neurophysin peptide, was detected in highly purified bovine pituitary neurosecretory granules (Clamgirand et al., 1986). Similarly, an endoproteinase from rat small intestinal mucosal secretory granules has been partially purified that generates somatostatin from prosomatostatin by cleavage of an Arg-Ser site (Beinfeld et al., 1989). Such purifications represent the initial step toward understanding the mechanisms that regulate the expression of these enzymatic activities.

VI. Discharge of Secretory Proteins

A. Regulation of Constitutive Release

Available evidence indicates that constitutive release does not require the active synthesis of new proteins (Wieland et al., 1987). Rather, the recycling of vesicle components is sufficient to ensure release through this pathway (Brion et al., 1992). This is in contrast with the regulated secretion of glycosaminoglycans (Brion et al., 1992), for which inhibition of protein synthesis severely impairs release of the product.

B. Regulated Secretion

In the regulated secretory pathway, the release of stored product is under the control of signal transduction pathways. These pathways allow external stimuli received at the cell plasma membrane to be transduced intracellularly, resulting in the physical release of the secretory store. Although the pathways are remarkably diverse in terms of specific participants, each involves the same general elements: namely, receptors, signal transducers, second messengers, and effectors.

Receptors

Extracellular stimuli are detected at the level of the plasma membrane by a cell surface receptor. Classically, receptor types have been defined pharmacologically (i.e., on the basis of their affinity for standard agonist and antagonists; Ahlquist, 1948). The recent cloning, sequencing, and functional expression of many receptors has allowed these classification schemes to be refined to reflect the structure of the receptors themselves (Hollenberg, 1991) and the nature of the signal transducer molecules to which they are coupled (Strosberg, 1991; Savarese and Fraser, 1992).

Adrenergic and Cholinergic Receptors

Receptors that bind epinephrine and related catecholamines are termed adrenergic receptors (O'Dowd et al., 1989; Dohlman et al., 1991). Acetylcholine signals through two distinct types of receptors, the nicotinic and muscarinic cholinergic receptors. The adrenergic and muscarinic cholinergic receptors belong to the superfamily of GTP-binding regulatory protein-coupled receptors. Once occupied with agonist, these receptors undergo a conformational change that evokes the transmembrane signal. Thus, the receptors themselves contain the key structural element that transduces the signal intracellularly (Hollenberg, 1991). In contrast, the nicotinic cholinergic receptor belongs to the superfamily of receptor-gated channels. Acetylcholine binds to the subunit of the receptor that opens a cation channel; thus, the transported cation represents the signal (Hosey, 1992).

There are at least ten unique adrenergic receptors, belonging to either α- ($\alpha_{1a,b,c}$ and $\alpha_{2a,b,c,d}$) or β- (β_1,β_2, and β_3) subgroups. Agonist occupancy of β-receptors activates G_s (GTP-binding stimulatory protein), which causes stimulation of adenylate cyclase, thereby leading to an increase in the level of intracellular cAMP. α_2-Adrenergic receptors inhibit adenylate cyclase through activation of G_i (GTP-binding inhibitory protein) and may also stimulate an Na^+/H^+ antiporter. Activation of α_1-adrenergic receptors stimulates the enzyme phospholipase C through activation of G_o which, in turn, generates second messengers, such as diacylglycerol. Diacylglycerol activates both protein kinase C and inositol triphosphate, which leads to mobilization of intracellular Ca^{2+} (Lefkowitz and Caron, 1988; Strosberg, 1991; Savarese and Fraser, 1992).

There are at least five discrete muscarinic cholinergic receptors, designated m_1, m_2, m_3 m_4, and m_5. Subtypes m_1, m_3, and m_5 stimulate formation of phosphatidylinositol by activation of G_o, whereas m_2 and m_4 inhibit adenylate cyclase through G_i (Strosberg, 1991; Savarese and Fraser, 1992; Hosey, 1992).

From biochemical analysis of purified receptors and conceptual translation of cDNA sequences encoding each subtype, it has been shown that members of the superfamily of GTP-binding regulatory protein-coupled receptors share considerable structural homology with each other and with the light-sensitive pigment rhodopsin (Dohlman et al., 1991). They consist of a single polypeptide chain that contains seven transmembrane domain segments (20–28 amino acids), with the intervening regions forming domains that are exposed either intra- or extra-cellularly. The NH_2-terminal portion of the receptors is exposed extracellularly and contains potential sites for *N*-linked glycans. The COOH-terminal domain of the receptors is located intracellularly. Several discrete functional domains have been identified, including the ligand-binding domain, the activation domain, and the coupling domain. Most is known about the adrenergic receptors, although emerging work suggests that the general principles may be applicable to the other members of this receptor superfamily (Savarese and Fraser, 1992).

Ligand-Binding Domains. Available evidence indicates that the ligand-binding domain of adrenergic receptors is encoded by the seven transmembrane domains. Several key aspartate and serine residues within these transmembrane domains have been identified by site-directed mutagenesis experiments as being necessary for ligand interaction. Additionally, cysteine residues from the second and third extracellular domains appear to form a critical disulfide bond. From this type of study, several general conclusions have been reached. First, binding sites for antagonists and agonists do not appear to be coincident, but rather, they seem to overlap. Second, although α- and β-adrenergic receptors share common structural domains, agonist interactions within this region are not identical. Third, the disulfide bond that forms between the second and third extracellular domain may be necessary for correct sorting of the receptor. Fourth, the sequence of transmembrane domain IV appears to encode the determinants of agonist specificity (Savarese and Fraser, 1992).

The Activation Domain. By analogy to bacteriorhodopsin, it has been argued that conserved aspartate residues in the second transmembrane domain of G-coupled receptors play a significant role in the conformational change that the receptor undergoes with agonist occupancy (Venter et al., 1989). For example, there are data implicating Asp-79 in the Na^+-mediated allsoteric alterations of these receptors (Horstman et al., 1990).

Domains Interacting With G Proteins. Deletion analysis has revealed that intracellular loop III (residues 240–270 of the well-studied β_2-receptor), which forms between the V and VI transmembrane domains, is essential for coupling the receptor to G proteins. In general, deletion or substitution of residues from the COOH-terminal region of this segment greatly diminished agonist-induced adenylate cyclase activity in β_2-receptors. These residues are predicted to form amphiphilic α-helices. However, no specific sequon has been detected for G protein-specificity (Strosberg, 1991).

Peptidergic Receptors

Many peptide receptors have been identified that are involved in the regulation of protein secretion and belong to the general class of G protein-coupled receptors (Strosberg, 1991). Among these are hormones (e.g., luteinizing hormone, chorio-gonadotropin), neuropeptides, such as the tachykinins (e.g., substance P, substance K), and vasoactive intestinal peptide. The substance P receptor has been cloned, and it shares the structural features outlined in the foregoing for adrenergic and cholinergic muscarinic receptors (Hershey and Krause, 1990). Stimulation of substance P receptor results in the activation of phospholipase C through G_p, which in turn generates phosphatidylinositol.

Desensitization of Receptors

Many of the G protein-coupled receptors share in their ability to become desensitized (i.e., they become refractory to further stimulation after an initial response; Dohlman et al., 1991). Temporally, there are two discrete phases of desensitization: short-term or long-term.

Short-term exposure (within seconds) results in either homologous or heterologous desensitization of the receptor, such that coupling with its G protein becomes compromised. In heterologous desensitization, receptors become unresponsive to any stimuli following exposure to low levels (nM) of agonist. This involves phosphorylation of the β-adrenergic receptor by the cAMP-dependent protein kinase. Available evidence suggests that the phosphorylation of the consensus sequence [Lys/Arg-Arg-X-(Xaa)-Ser] at position 259–262 on the third cytoplasmic loop is sufficient for phosphokinase A-mediated desensitization (Hausdorff et al., 1990). This phosphorylation may serve to decrease the ability of the receptor to couple with its appropriate G protein (Lefkowitz and Caron, 1988).

In homologous desensitization, which occurs following exposure of high levels (μM) of agonist, only the desensitizing agent loses stimulatory activity. In this instance, the β-adrenergic receptor is phosphorylated by both the cAMP-dependent protein kinase A and a cAMP-independent protein kinase, termed βARK (Benovic et al., 1987). The target site for this kinase occurs in the COOH-terminal of the β-adrenergic receptor between amino acids 355 and 364. The phosphorylated receptor then binds to the protein β-arrestin, which is thought to interfere with the coupling between the receptor and its G protein. This results in the inhibition of receptor function (Hausdorff et al., 1990, 1991; Lohse et al., 1992).

G Proteins: Signal Transducers of Protein Secretion

There are two families of signal-transducing GTP-binding proteins, the "small" G proteins, which consist of single polypeptide chains (M_r 20 kd) and function in vesicular formation and transport, and the heterotrimeric G proteins consisting of α-, β-, and γ-subunits, that function as "relay" switches in signal transduction pathways (Freissmuth et al., 1989; Bourne et al., 1990).

The G proteins cycle between active (GTP) and inactive (GDP) forms. Interaction of a G protein with an activated receptor induces exchange of α-subunit-bound GDP for GTP, with the subsequent dissociation of the α–GTP complex from the remaining βγ-heterodimer. Both the α–GTP complex and the βγ-heterodimer can modulate the activity of various effectors, described in the next section. Because one receptor can activate multiple G proteins, the signal of one ligand binding to its receptor can be amplified manyfold. The intrinsic GTPase activity of the α-subunit catalyzes conversion of the bound GTP to GDP, at which point the subunit is inactivated (Simon et al., 1991).

Classically, G proteins were classified according to their susceptibility to ADP-ribosylation; that is, cholera toxin substrates were thought to stimulate adenylate cyclase (G_s), whereas pertussis toxin substrates inhibited adenylate cyclase (G_i). Subsequently, substrates susceptible to both toxins or insusceptible to either toxin were identified (Neer and Clapham, 1988).

α-Subunit

The α-subunit is the functional arm of the G proteins; it expresses a GTPase activity and contains high-affinity-binding sites for guanine nucleotides and Mg^{2+}. A daunting number of G protein α-subunits have been uncovered by molecular cloning (Bourne et al., 1990, 1991; Simon et al., 1991; Olate and Allende, 1991). Indeed, it has been observed that the number of G proteins exceeds the number of known G protein functions, indicating that cells contain different G proteins of similar function that can couple to distinct receptors (Ashkenazi et al., 1989). Most variants have been cloned from neural (e.g., brain) or sensory (olfactory epithelium, retina) tissues (Olate and Allende, 1991), and several distinct subclasses have emerged on the basis of amino acid homologies (G_s, G_i, G_2, and G_{12}; Simon et al., 1991), and each subclass contains multiple isoforms. However, few studies of this type have been performed in secretory tissues, per se. Rather, identification of the G proteins implicated in protein secretion has been made indirectly through the use of toxins (e.g., Fleming et al., 1989), photoaffinity-labeling procedures (e.g., Schnefel et al., 1990), western blot analysis using antisera directed against specific isoforms (e.g., Miyamoto et al., 1992), or reconstitution studies using purified G proteins (e.g., MacDonald and Boyd, 1989).

Members of the G_s ($G_{\alpha s}$) and G_i ($G_{\alpha i1}$, $G_{\alpha i2}$, $G_{\alpha i3}$, $G_{\alpha o}$, $G_{\alpha x}$) classes of G proteins (Simon et al., 1991) are found in many cell types and are among the best-characterized G proteins. $G_{\alpha s}$ activates adenylate cyclase to increase intracellular levels of cAMP, whereas members of the G_i class can inhibit adenylate cyclase (to decrease intracellular levels of cAMP), activate phospholipase C (to increase levels of inositol triphosphate and diacyglycerol), activate phospholipase A_2 (to increase release of arachidonate), activate K^+ channels, or inhibit Ca^{2+} channels (Bourne et al., 1990). Although it is convenient to think of G protein-coupling in terms of "one G protein–one effector system," there is sufficient data to suggest that G proteins are promiscuous (i.e., they are able to couple with more than one effector system; Yatani et al., 1988).

Models of G_α subunit structure have been proposed on the basis of homology with the p21*ras* G protein for which a crystal structure has been solved (Bourne et al., 1991). The NH_2-terminal region of the G_α subunit has been implicated in binding to the $\beta\gamma$-subunits and is the site for myristoylation, which is a post-translational modification that adds a 14-carbon myristic acid to an NH_2-terminal glycine following cleavage of the NH_2-terminal methionine. This modification enhances the formation of the heterotrimeric complex (Spiegel et al., 1991). The COOH-terminal region of the G_α subunit is thought to be the site of G protein–receptor interaction (Masters et al., 1988). The stretch of amino acids between 100 and 230 dictates GTPase activity; several mutations have been localized to this region that can alter this enzymatic activity by as much as two orders of magnitude (Simon et al., 1991).

βγ-Heterodimer

There now are at least four distinct β- and six unique γ-subunits known in mammalian G proteins (Simon et al., 1991). Recent evidence suggests that different combinations of these subunits are involved in controlling signaling events. For example, β-γ-heterodimers appear to regulate the activity of adenylate cyclase (Tang and Gilman, 1991; Federman et al., 1992) and phospholipase A_2 (Kim et al., 1989). Thus, it seems unlikely that the βγ-heterodimers are passive bystanders in signal transduction and are able to play an active role in the process.

Effectors of Protein Secretion

Adenylate Cyclase

Protein $G_{\alpha s}$ interacts with the catalytic subunit of adenylate cyclase, leading to a marked enhancement of its activity. This results in an increased conversion of ATP to cAMP. The increase in intracellular cAMP concentration promotes protein kinase A-mediated phosphorylation of several intracellular proteins involved in protein secretion.

Molecular cloning has uncovered five distinct forms of mammalian adenylate cyclase thus far, which appear to be expressed in tissue-restricted patterns. Types I and II are highly expressed in brain (Krupinski et al., 1989; Feinstein et al., 1991; Bakalyar and Reed, 1990). Type III is highly expressed in olfactory tissues and is thought to mediate odorant detection (Bakalyar and Reed, 1990). Type IV adenylate cyclase is expressed in a wide range of tissues (Gao and Gilman, 1991), and type V transcripts are abundant in heart and brain, but are not expressed in testis, skeletal muscle, kidney, or lung (Ishikawa et al., 1992). Sequence homology argues that these enzymes are members of a superfamily of genes that includes the products of both the cystic fibrosis gene (*CFTR*; Riordan et al., 1989) and the multidrug-resistance gene (P glycoprotein; Gros et al., 1986). Common to all these gene products is a motif that consists of two alternating sets of hydrophobic and hydrophilic domains. The hydrophobic regions are composed of six transmembrane domains, whereas the hydrophilic region forms a large intracellular loop and is characterized by a sequence that is homologous to guanylate cyclases and thus likely nucleotide-binding sites. The structure terminates with a second hydrophilic domain in the form of a large intracellular tail (Krupinski et al., 1989). There is some homology with the *S. cerevisiae* adenylate cyclase in the region that contains the catalytic domain; however, the yeast enzyme lacks transmembrane domains, which indicates that the two proteins have diverged considerably (Krupinski et al., 1989).

Phospholipases

Phospholipase A_2.   The hydrolysis of phosphatidylcholine by phospholipase A_2 releases arachidonic acid from cell membranes (Dennis et al., 1991). Sequence comparison of all known phospholipase A_2 enzymes reveals that they consist of a single polypeptide chain of about 120 amino acids. The enzyme requires Ca^{2+} for activity, and there is conservation of a calcium-binding loop, as well as cysteine residues in all forms studied.

There is some data to suggest that G proteins control phospholipase A_2 activity (Exton, 1990), and a novel G protein G_E has been proposed as a potential candidate (Cockcroft and Stutchfield, 1988), although this form has not yet been isolated.

Phospholipase C.   Phospholipase C (PLC) catalyzes the conversion of phosphatidylinositol into 1,2-diacylglycerol and inositol phosphates (Majerus et al., 1990). 1,2-Diacylglycerol activates protein kinase C, which includes threonine–serine kinases that phosphorylate several target substrates implicated in protein secretion (Nishizuka, 1986). Inositol triphosphates promote the release of intracellular Ca^{2+} stores (Berridge and Irvine, 1989).

It has been proposed that a family of G proteins, termed G_p, which is a substrate for pertussis toxin in some cells (neutrophils, platelets), but not others (pancreas), couples phospholipase C to its receptor (Cockcroft and Stutchfield, 1988). However, confirmation of this awaits purification or cloning of this form.

Four distinct types of phospholipase C, termed PLC-α, PLC-β, PLC-γ and PLC-δ, have been detected on the basis of conceptual translations or immunological relatedness (Majerus et al., 1990; Dennis et al., 1991). All isoforms of the enzyme share similar substrate specificity; that is, they hydrolyze phosphatidylinositol, phosphatidylinositol 4-phosphate, and phosphatidylinositol 4,5-diphosphate, although there is some variation in the Ca^{2+} requirement of these reactions (Dennis et al., 1991). Moreover, there is little amino acid sequence homology among this group; two domains, designated X and Y (150 and 240 amino acids, respectively) that are essential for catalysis (Emori et al., 1989), are 60 and 40% identical among PLC-β, PLC-γ, and PLC-δ. Sequences related to src homology regions 2 and 3 (SH$_2$ and SH$_3$) are inserted between the X and Y domains in PLC-γ. Deletion of the SH domains diminishes, but does not abolish, PLC activity (Emori et al., 1989). Phospholipase C-α is dissimilar to these other three forms; interestingly, it displays homology with protein disulfide isomerase (Crooke and Bennett, 1989).

Phosphatidylcholine can be metabolized by unique forms of phospholipase C into diacylglycerol (Dennis et al., 1991). Available evidence indicates that the breakdown of phosphatidylcholine is agonist-induced, and it has been suggested that this is under the control of either protein kinase C or intracellular Ca^{2+} (Exton, 1990). Because the levels of phosphatidylcholine are so high in cells, this pathway can yield significant levels of diacylglycerol for an extended period. By contrast, hydrolysis of phosphatidylinositol 4,5-biphosphate produces a relatively small amount of diacylglycerol for a short time frame. Consequently, it has been speculated that phosphatidylcholine metabolism is involved in regulatory processes that require a sustained activation of protein kinase C, such as transcription (Exton, 1990).

Phospholipase D. Phosphatidylcholine can also be metabolized by unique forms of phospholipase D into phosphatidic acid (Dennis et al., 1991). This pathway appears to occur more rapidly than the phospholipase C-mediated formation of diacylglycerol. Tumor-promoting phorbol esters activate phospholipase D, suggesting that the system is under control of protein kinase C pathway (Exton, 1990). Phosphatidic acid could play several potential regulatory roles within a cell. For example, phosphatidic acid appears to mobilize intracellular Ca^{2+} stores (Murayama and Ui, 1985; Moolenaar et al., 1986). It may also inhibit adenylate cyclase by interaction with G$_i$ (Murayama and Ui, 1985), perhaps explaining the inhibitory effects of Ca^{2+}-mobilizing agonists on intracellular levels of cAMP (Exton, 1990).

Ion Channels

Ion channels form pores that permit ion flow across membranes. Several forms of ion channels have been identified, including, gap junctions, which are involved in intracellular communication; ligand-gated channels, which allow passage of ions into a cell ' en the channel is occupied by a specific agonist; and voltage-gated ion channels, which mediate ion flux in response to membrane depolarization (Jan and Jan, 1989; Catterall, 1991).

Indirect regulatory influence of G protein-mediated signal transduction pathways on ion channels is well established. For example, phosphorylation of Ca^{2+} channels by cAMP-dependent protein kinase A reaction results in a stimulation of Ca^{2+} currents in cardiac tissue, hippocampal neurons, and GH$_3$ cells (Rosenthal et al., 1988). However, it is now apparent that there is a direct control of both K$^+$ and Ca^{2+} ion channels by G protein-coupled receptors (Rosenthal et al.,

1988; Brown and Birnbaumer, 1988; Kleuss et al., 1991). For example, in rat pituitary cells, intracellular Ca^{2+} levels are regulated by a voltage-sensitive Ca^{2+} channel. Inhibition of this channel is mediated by G_{o1} and G_{o2}, through muscarinic and somatostatin receptors, respectively (Kleuss et al., 1991). Thus, secretion by this cell is regulated, in part, by this G protein-gated channel. Similarly, galanin, a 29-amino acid neuropeptide that inhibits insulin secretion in the perfused pancreas, activates a G protein-gated K^+ channel (Dunne et al., 1989).

Second Messengers and Regulatory Molecules of Protein Secretion

Second messengers, such as cAMP or diacylglycerol, act as allosteric effectors to directly activate a wide range of protein kinases (Harper, 1988). Kinase-mediated phosphorylation of target proteins represents a final common pathway for many biological regulatory schemes, including secretion of proteins (Greengard, 1978; Nishizuka, 1984; Shenolikar, 1988). Numerous candidate protein and peptide substrates have been proposed as being important in secretory events (e.g., Baum et al., 1981; Freedman and Jamieson, 1982a,b; Quissell et al., 1983, 1985; Marino et al., 1990; Söling et al., 1989; Sobel, 1991). Although it is clear that these candidate molecules are modified in a temporally correct manner, none have yet been proved to be necessary for secretion to occur. Indeed, there are some data that argue against a causal relationship between protein secretion and phosphorylation (e.g., Takuma, 1990). Moreover, little is known about the potential role played by protein phosphatases (Shenolikar, 1988) in modulating secretory events.

Other second messengers, such as the inositol phosphates, modulate intracellular levels of Ca^{2+} (Berridge and Irvine, 1984; Harper, 1988). These intracellular concentrations have been shown to oscillate (i.e., vary in time and space within the cell; Berridge and Irvine, 1989). Although several calcium-dependent pathways have been identified in formation of the primary secretory fluid (Petersen, 1992), the precise role of Ca^{2+} in regulating protein secretion is still unclear (Quissell and Tabak, 1989). Potential roles include activation of calmodulin-dependent pathways, activation of protein kinase C, and interaction with calcium-binding proteins implicated in secretory granule–plasma membrane fusion (Harper, 1988).

Protein Kinases

The protein kinases represent a large superfamily of molecules with more than 200 members identified (Hanks et al., 1988). Two broad classes of substrate specificity have been defined: serine–threonine-specific and tyrosine-specific. All protein kinases consist of two domains, the regulatory domain, which responds to the second messenger, and the catalytic domain. The primary sequence of the catalytically active domains of these enzymes has been compared in some detail.

Eleven major subdomains within the catalytic domain have been identified as being highly conserved, and invariant amino acids within each subdomain are predicted to play important roles in catalysis (Hanks et al., 1988). Within subdomain I is found the consensus sequence Gly-X-Gly-X-X-Gly, which is characteristic of many nucleotide-binding proteins. It is envisioned that this sequence forms an elbow around the nucleotide, with the first glycine contacting ribose and the second lying near the terminal pyrophosphate. In subdomain II is a catalytically essential lysine residue, which appears to be directly involved in proton transfer. The area including subdomains VI–IX, which corresponds to the central core of the catalytic domain, is the most highly conserved region of the enzyme. Subdomain VII contains the invariant Ala-Pro-Glu sequence, which lies close to the active site of the enzyme.

The information for the recognition of the hydroxyamino acid substrate is located in subdomains VI and VIII. Within subdomain VI, the consensus Asp-Leu-Lys-Pro-Glu-Asn is characteristic of a serine–theonine enzyme whereas, the sequence Asp-Leu-Arg-Ala-Ala-Asn or Asp-Leu-Ala-Ala-Arg-Asn is found in the tyrosine enzyme (Hanks et al., 1988). In subdomain VIII, the protein–tyrosine kinase consensus sequence is Pro-Ile-/Val-Lys/Arg-Trp-Thr/Met-Ala-Pro-Glu and the corresponding sequence for the serine–theonine kinase is Gly-Thr/Ser-X-X-Try/Phe-X-Ala-Pro-Glu.

Because of the many similarities observed in sequence among the many family members, the structure of one protein kinase will enable reasonable predictions to be made about all the others. The crystal structure of the catalytic subunit of a cAMP-dependent protein kinase has been solved (Knighton et al., 1991), which should pave the way for substantial progress in modeling attempts of the other kinase family members.

Cyclic AMP-Dependent Protein Kinase.   Unlike other protein kinases, the functional domains of cAMP-dependent protein kinase A are found on two discrete subunit structures, the regulatory subunit (R) which binds cAMP and the catalytic subunit (C) (Taylor et al., 1988). In the absence of cAMP, the enzyme is found in an inactive tetrameric state, R_2C_2. Upon binding of cAMP, an R_2 $(cAMP)_4$ dimer dissociates from the holoenzyme, leaving two free catalytically active subunits (Bramson et al., 1983).

The crystal structure of the catalytic subunit of cAMP-dependent protein kinase consists of two lobes of unequal size, with a deep cleft between them (Knighton et al., 1991). The smaller lobe binds ATP, and it takes the form of an antiparallel β-sheet. The larger lobe is the site of substrate binding and has a largely helical architecture, with a single β-sheet at the domain interface. Transfer of phosphate actually occurs within the intralobular cleft.

Two distinct types of regulatory subunits can bind to the catalytic subunit of cAMP-dependent protein kinase A, yielding either type I or type II holoenzyme (Taylor et al., 1988). Both regulatory subunits form dimers. The COOH-terminal region of the protein is the site of cAMP binding and is highly conserved. The NA_2-terminal region of the regulatory subunit is more variable and is the site of subunit dimer formation. In the type II holoenzyme, it is also the site (Arg-Arg-Val-Ser(P)-Val-Cys) of autophosphorylation (Taylor, 1989). A model of the cAMP-binding site has been built, drawing upon the known structure of the cAMP-binding region of the *Escherichia coli* catabolite gene activator protein (CAP). It is envisioned as a β-barrel structure in which Arg-82 interacts with the negative charge on the cyclic phosphate ring and Glu-72 hydrogen bonds to the 2′OH of ribose. These two residues are invariant in all known regulatory subunits (Taylor, 1989).

Diacylglycerol Protein Kinase C.   Protein kinase C is a calcium- and phospholipid-dependent theonine–serine kinase that can be activated by diacylglycerol. Thus, diacylglycerol acts as a second messenger linking muscarinic cholinergic-mediated phosphatidylinositol turnover with protein kinase C (El-Fakahany et al., 1988). Experimentally, it has been shown that the tumor-promoting phorbol esters can also activate protein kinase C (Blumberg et al., 1984). This has intensified interest in this class of protein kinases, with the view that inappropriate phosphorylation yields some of the tumor characteristics induced by the phorbol esters (Nishizuka, 1988).

Nine distinct isoforms of protein kinase C have now been identified by molecular cloning (Bell and Burns, 1991). Structure–function studies of these variants argue that each has discrete function and, thus, the differential expression of these enzymes has significant functional import (Nishizuka, 1988; Parker et al., 1989).

In structure, protein kinase C is a single polypeptide, containing an NH_2-terminal regulatory domain and a COOH-terminal catalytic domain, connected by a flexible hinge region. Sequence comparisons show that there are four highly conserved and five variable regions spread across these two functional domains. The regulatory domain comprises the first and second variable (V_1, V_2) and conserved (C_1, C_2) regions. The phorbol-, diacylglycerol-, and calcium-binding sites, as well as a pseudosubstrate site are contained within this domain. C_1 is characterized by a tandem repeat of a cystine-rich sequence, $Cys\text{-}X_2\text{-}Cys\text{-}X_{13\text{-}14}\text{-}Cys\text{-}X_2\text{-}Cys\text{-}X_7\text{-}Cys\text{-}X_7\text{-}Cys$, which is similar to the zinc finger motif found in DNA-binding proteins (Bell and Burns, 1991). The catalytic domain contains an ATP-binding site (Gly-X-Gly-X-X-Gly . . . Lys) in C_3, and the protein substrate-binding sites in C_4 and V_5.

Inactive protein kinase C has substrate bound to the pseudosubstrate site. After binding, diacylglycerol protein kinase C undergoes a conformational change that dislocates the substrate from the pseudosubstrate site in the regulatory domain and makes it available to bind to the substrate site in the catalytic domain (Bell and Burns, 1991). Activation by diacylglycerol is stereospecific, requiring the *sn*1,2-diacylglycerol form. Phosphatidylinositol 4,5-biphosphate can also activate protein kinase C in a calcium- and phosphatidylserine-dependent manner and, thus, is similar to the action of diacylglycerol (Bell and Burns, 1991). The usual requirement of calcium and phospholipid can be bypassed under acidic conditions; between pH 4 and 6 protein kinase C undergoes autophosphorylation (McFadden et al., 1989).

Inositol Phosphate and the Regulation of Calcium Signaling

Inositol 1,4,5-triphosphate is a second messenger that regulates levels of intracellular Ca^{2+} by mobilizing it from internal stores and stimulating entry of extracellular ion (Berridge and Irvine, 1984, 1989; Putney et al., 1989). The inositol 1,4,5-triphosphate-mediated release of intracellular Ca^{2+} involves an extramitochondrial store, which is thought to be localized within the endoplasmic reticulum or within a calciosome (Volpe et al., 1988).

The intracellular receptor that mediates inositol 1,4,5-triphosphate-stimulated Ca^{2+} mobilization has been purified and sequenced by conceptual translation of cDNAs that encode it (Taylor and Richardson, 1991). These receptors are tetrameric, with subunits characterized by an M_r between 220 and 330 ka. Immunohistological localization reveals that the receptor is found mainly in the nuclear envelope and endoplasmic reticulum (Ross et al., 1989). Inositol 1,4,5-triphosphate binds to the NH_2-terminal (cytoplasmically localized) domain of a receptor subunit. This results in a conformational change that is transduced by a long, linking domain to the COOH-terminal membrane-spanning domain, which functions as part of the Ca^{2+} channel. The linking domain contains several potential target sites for cAMP-dependent protein kinase-mediated phosphorylation, as well as a cyclic nucleotide-binding site (Mignery and Südhof, 1990), providing one means of crosstalk between the protein kinase A- and Ca^{2+}-activated signal transduction pathways (Houslay, 1991). These findings are consistent with the observation that inositol 1,4,5-triphosphate-mediated release of Ca^{2+} is potentiated by the action of cAMP-dependent protein kinase A (Burgess et al., 1991).

The metabolism of inositol phosphates has proved more complex than originally thought (Berridge and Irvine, 1989), and this has generated considerable interest in the potential roles played by other inositol phosphates in Ca^{2+} mobilization (e.g., Berridge and Irvine, 1989; Putney et al., 1989); however, there is as yet no clear proof linking these other forms to specific roles.

VII. Coupling of Secretory Protein Biosynthesis with Secretion

Physiologically, secretory tissues must continually replenish their stores of exportable product. For efficiency, the machinery responsible for secretion must be coupled to the cellular apparatus that controls the biosynthesis of the secretate (Cooper et al., 1991). Available evidence suggests that coupling is effected by elements of the signal transduction pathway and that it occurs at the level of gene transcription and posttranslational modifications, such as glycosylation.

A. Gene Transcription

*The Protein Kinase A and C Signal Transduction Pathways Converge
on Similar cis-Elements to Provide a Direct Mechanism to Couple
Transcription with Secretion*

The transcription of many genes has been shown to be influenced by second
messengers, such as cAMP (reviewed in Roesler et al., 1988), Ca^{2+} (Stratowa and
Rutter, 1986; Bandyopadhyay and Bancroft, 1989; Rodland et al., 1990; Preston
et al., 1990), or diacylglycerol (Auwerx et al., 1989), which serve to activate
protein kinase A or protein kinase C. Thus, inhibition (Grove et al., 1987; Mellon
et al., 1989; Grove et al., 1989) or overexpression (Mellon et al., 1989; Maurer,
1989) of protein kinase A results in inhibition or potentiation of cAMP-dependent
gene transcription. However, increasing evidence argues that the signal transduction pathways merge, thereby allowing crosstalk at the level of gene transcription
(Karin, 1989; Ziff, 1990; Habener, 1990; Miner and Yamamoto, 1991; Karin,
1992).

Two discrete classes of genes that are modulated by cAMP have been
identified (Roesler et al., 1988). Group I genes respond within minutes by a
cyclohexamide-insensitive process. This implies that, mechanistically, regulation
depends on the modification of preexisting protein, rather than on the synthesis
of new transcription factors. Group II genes respond after several hours of
exposure to cAMP by a cyclohexamide-sensitive mechanism.

Two discrete classes of *cis*-elements have been found in the family of group I
genes. The first to be defined functionally was the 8-bp palindromic sequence
TGACGTCA, termed the *c*AMP *r*egulatory *e*lement (CRE). This has been shown
to be necessary for cAMP induction for several genes, but requires surrounding
sequences for activity (Montminy et al., 1986; Delegeane et al., 1987; Deutsch
et al., 1988a). Transcription factors termed *c*AMP *r*esponsive *e*lement-*b*inding
proteins (CREB; Montminy and Bilezikjian, 1987; Gonzalez et al., 1991) and
*a*ctivation *t*ranscription *f*actor (ATF-1; Rehfuss et al., 1991) bind to this element
and activate transcription. The regulatory site of CREB is phosphorylated
(Ser-133) by both Ca^{2+} (Sheng et al., 1991) and cAMP-dependent kinases
(Gonzalez et al., 1991); thus, CREB can mediate a transcriptional response to
either Ca^{2+} or cAMP. Additional crosstalk is achieved through the similarity
between CRE and *cis*-element that has been shown to be responsive to protein
kinase C activators, such as phorbol esters, TGAC/GTCA (Deutsch et al., 1988b;
Fink et al., 1991). Further control of CRE is achieved through the differential
expression of the *c*AMP-*r*esponsive *e*lement *m*odulator (CREM) gene, which can
act as negative regulator (Foulkes et al., 1991). The second *cis*-element that has
been identified in class I cAMP regulatory genes is the element *a*ctivator *p*rotein
(AP-2), CCCCAGGC, which was first described as a basal transcription enhancer

in the SV40 and human metallothionein II_A promoters (Roesler et al., 1988). This element differs from the CRE in that it is responsive to both cAMP and activators of protein kinase C, such as phorbol esters (e.g., Hyman et al., 1989).

Even though there are many examples of group I genes (Roesler et al., 1988), only two examples of group II genes have been identified; thus, this group remains poorly characterized. The β-subunit of human chorionic gonadotropin is the most thoroughly studied to date (Milsted et al., 1987; Fuh et al., 1989; Ferstermaker et al., 1989). No consensus sequence for response to cAMP has yet been defined, although it seems likely that it will differ from the CRE motif (Ferstermaker et al., 1989).

Activation of salivary gland β_1-adrenergic receptors leads to a pronounced glandular hyperplasia and hypertrophy, coupled with profound alterations in the expression of a large family of proteins, termed proline-rich proteins (PRP) (Carlson et al., 1991). Given the time frame required for isoproterenol (a β-adrenergic agonist)-mediated regulation of PRPs (Carlson et al., 1991; Cooper et al., 1991) and the sensitivity of PRP induction to cyclohexamide (Wright et al., 1990), we argue that this superfamily of salivary proteins is likely to be group II cAMP response genes (Cooper et al., 1991). Because of the diversity of PRPs (Carlson et al., 1991) and the differential effects of isoproterenol on their expression (Cooper et al., 1991), examination of PRP gene regulation may provide considerable insight into the mechanisms that underlie group II gene expression.

Functional analysis of a macaque PRP gene revealed that salivary-specific and cAMP-regulatory elements localize to a region between nucleotides (nt) -107 and $+5$ of the promoter. A sequence, AGGTGTCA, homologous to the CRE element (5/8 nt match) was found at nt -51 to -44, although it is not yet known if this sequence is functional. The CRE-related sequences have been found in several PRP, but their function has yet to be determined (Carlson et al., 1991). A 28-nt sequence that is common to several members of the PRP superfamily of genes has been identified; it is conserved across species (rat, mouse, hamster, and human PRP genes) and is found in constitutively expressed (rat GRP-Ca, human PRPs), isoproterenol-inducible (mouse and hamster PRPs), and androgen-inducible (rat SMR 2) genes (Cooper et al., 1991; Roberts et al., 1991). Mobility shift assay have indicated that isoproterenol-induced, mouse parotid nuclear proteins interact with an NF-κB/rel-like site that is embedded in this conserved sequence (Roberts et al., 1991). NF-κB is structurally related to both the *rel* oncoprotein and the *dorsal* homeotic protein (Gilmore, 1990), and thus plays a central role in cytokine regulation of cell growth and proliferation (Lenardo and Baltimore, 1989). When complexed to IκB in the cytoplasm, NF-κB is rendered inactive. Upon induction (perhaps owing to phosphorylation of a putative protein kinase C site on IκB; Ghosh and Baltimore, 1990), IκB dissociates from NK-κB to target the nucleus, where it binds DNA (Lenardo and Baltimore, 1989). Thus, NF-κB may play a role in both the isoproterenol-mediated hypertrophy of rodent salivary glands and the cAMP modulation of PRP gene expression.

The Modulation of Receptor Expression Provides an Indirect Means
to Couple the Biosynthesis of Secretory Proteins with Secretion

Regulation of Genes That Encode the GTP-Binding Coupled Receptors

No introns are found in the genes that code for the three β-adrenergic, the two α-adrenergic, and the five muscarinic cholinergic receptors (Strosberg, 1991). Several consensus sequences of *cis*-elements have been identified in the flanking regions of adrenergic receptor genes. The cAMP response elements (CRE) have been identified in the 5′ flanking regions of several genes (Collins et al., 1991). Thus, the genes encoding these receptors are subject to autoregulation. Therefore, short-term exposure to epinephrine modulates the rate of transcription of the β_2-adrenergic gene resulting in a three- to fourfold increase in the steady-state level of transcript (Collins et al., 1989). Four potential CRE sequences were found in the gene that encodes the β_3-adrenergic receptor, suggesting that this gene may also be upregulated by the end product (cAMP) of its pathway (Thomas et al., 1992). Cyclic AMP enhances the transcription of the α_2-adrenergic receptor gene, resulting in an increased number of these receptors (Sakaue and Hoffman, 1991). The increased number of α_2-adrenergic receptors leads to an inhibition of intracellular levels of cAMP.

There is a single glucocorticoid response element in the β_1- and β_3-adrenergic receptor genes, whereas there are multiple elements of this type in the β_2-adrenergic receptor gene (Strosberg, 1991). This is thought to account for the increased rate of transcription of β_2-adrenergic receptor message in response to glucocorticoid exposure (Collins et al., 1988).

The substance P receptor gene contains four introns; it has been suggested that this arrangement helps accommodate the larger ligands of the tachykinin class (Hershey et al., 1991). The 5′ flanking region of this gene contains sequences that are homologous to Ca^{2+}-inducible elements, as well as a consensus CRE sequence (Hershey et al., 1991). However, it is not yet known if any of these sequences are functional.

Down Regulation

After prolonged exposure (hours) of the agonist, there is a progressive loss of β_1- or β_2-adrenergic receptors by a process referred to as down regulation (Collins et al., 1992). As much as 70% of these receptors can be lost (Hausdorff et al., 1990). In part, this decrease is mediated by a decreased transcription of the mRNA that encodes the receptors. In contrast, similar treatment leads to an up regulation of β_3-adrenergic receptors (Thomas et al., 1992) to a level 165% of the basal value.

B. Posttranslational Processing of Secretory Proteins Is Coupled to Their Release by Elements of the Signal Transduction Pathway

Glycosylation Is Regulated Indirectly

In contrast to proteins and nucleic acids, which are synthesized by highly accurate template mechanisms, much of the genetic control required for the synthesis of glycoproteins is transferred by indirect pathways (Schachter, 1986). Thus, although the expression of the unglycosylated precursor protein (the apoprotein) represents the initial level of control in glycoprotein biosynthesis, one must also consider the regulation of the many genes that are required for the co- and posttranslation modifications to occur. For example, sugars must first be converted to a sugar nucleotide form for use in biosynthesis of glycoproteins. Sugar nucleotides are produced within the cytoplasm of a cell, except for CMP-sialic acid, which forms in the nucleus (Hirschberg and Snider, 1987). Translocation of nucleotide sugars across intramembranous boundaries of the rough endoplasmic reticulum and Golgi system occurs by a facilitated transport process (Barthelson and Roth, 1985) that is thought to involve antiport proteins that span membrane domains. Thus, availability of the appropriate sugar nucleotide pool represents a second potential control point in glycosylation. The expression and activity of the glycosyltransferases, which are responsible for the transfer of the sugars from the nucleotide donors to the growing oligosaccharide, must also be considered. Studies with highly purified enzymes have supported a one-linkage–one-enzyme concept (Beyer et al., 1979; Williams and Schachter, 1980; Williams et al., 1980).

"Leakiness" in the integration among these multiple pathways may well account for the variation (termed microheterogeneity) observed in the oligosaccharide structures of a glycoprotein (Tabak, 1991). How contrived microheterogeneity is has been debated for many years (Gottschalk, 1969; Gallagher and Cornfield, 1978; Tabak et al., 1982); nevertheless, until a specific function can be attributed to each specific carbohydrate variant, the arguments remain speculative at best (Tabak, 1991).

Structural Modulation: Regulation of Glycosylation by Elements of the Signal Transduction Pathway

The posttranslational modification of glycoproteins is subject to a wide range of extrinsic controls. These controls form the basis of a mechanism that enables a cell to modify the structure of a glycoconjugate in response to a new functional demand. We refer to these control mechanisms as *structural modulation* (Tabak et al., 1982; Tabak, 1991). Thus, the biosynthesis of secretory proteins is coupled to secretion at two levels, transcription and posttranslational modifications.

Secretagogues Influence the Glycosylation of Secretory Glycoproteins

Extended exposure to the β-adrenergic agonist isoproterenol leads to an increased sialic acid content of submandibular glands (Curbelo et al., 1968), whereas adrenalectomy has the opposite effect (Curbelo, 1973). Variation in the content of fucose and sialic acid in the submandibular gland mucins of dogs was dependent on the intensity of pilocarpine (a cholinergic agonist) stimulus used to elicit secretion (Dische et al., 1969; Lombart and Winzler, 1974). It was suggested that these two residues compete with each other to terminate the growing oligosaccharide (Dische et al., 1969), or maintain charge by substitution of sulfate residues for sialic acid (Lombart and Winzler, 1974). Incorporation of carbohydrate (as measured by N-acetyl[^{14}C]mannosamine) was enhanced two- to threefold by extended exposure to isoproterenol and three- to fourfold by treatment with pilocarpine (Amerongen et al., 1984). Increases in intracellular cAMP levels result in an enhancement of N-linked glycosylation mediated, in part, by an increase in mannosyl phosphodolichol synthase activity (Banerjee et al., 1987). Other hormones, such as estrogen (Chilton et al., 1988; Carson and Tang, 1989; Carson et al., 1990), prolactin (Bradshaw et al., 1985), and thyrotropin (Di Jeso et al., 1992), enhance glycosylation or influence glycosylation processing. Activation of protein kinase C by exposure to phorbol esters alters the glycosylation of fibronectin cell surface receptors (Symington et al., 1989).

Expression of Protooncogenes Induces Modifications of N- and O-Linked Glycosylation

Cell surface carbohydrates undergo a wide range of structural alterations in malignant cells (Hakomori, 1985). Transformation of cells by oncogenes produces similar alterations, which have been traced, in general, to an increased activity of specific glycosyltransferases of the N-linked pathway. For example, sarcoma virus, or H-*ras* transformation of fibroblasts, results in an increased branching of asparagine-linked glycans induced by increased activity of UDP-GlcNAc:αMan β1,6N-acetylglucosaminyl transferase (GlcNAc transferase V) (Hubbard, 1987; Dennis et al., 1989; Easton et al., 1991). The tetra-antennary asparagine-linked glycans, found on NIH 3T3 cells, that normally terminate in Galα1,3Gal linkages, acquire sialic acid, linked α2,3 to galactose in H-*ras*-transformed cells (Santer et al., 1989), presumably from enhanced activity of an α2,3-sialyltransferase. Similarly, H-*ras* transformation, (but not v-*src*, polyoma middle T, or BPV1) of rat fibroblasts led to a marked increase in the expression (i.e., transcript) and activity of β-galactoside α2,6-sialyltransferase (Le Marer et al., 1992).

The mechanisms that underlie these observations are unclear. However, the protein products encoded by many oncogenes can participate in the signal transduction pathways of the cell (Cantley et al., 1991). For example, the *ras* genes belong to the superfamily of genes that encode GTP-binding proteins and, accordingly, are related to the heterotrimeric G proteins (Lowy et al., 1991).

Therefore, it seems plausible that *ras* acts in a manner similar to that observed for secretagogues, thereby further strengthening the argument that the biosynthesis of secretory proteins is coupled to their secretion by the signal transduction pathways.

Acknowledgments

I wish to thank Ms. Patricia Noonan for her help in preparing this chapter. Original work from my laboratory was supported, in part, by grants from the National Institute of Dental Research (DE-08511 and DE-08108).

References

Abeijon, C., and Hirschberg, C. B. (1992). Topography of glycosylation reactions in the endoplasmic reticulum. *Trends Biochem. Sci.* 17: 32–36.

Achstetter, T., Franzusoff, A., Field, C., and Schekman, R. (1988). *SEC7* encodes an unusual, high molecular weight protein required for membrane traffic from the yeast Golgi apparatus. *J. Biol. Chem.* 263: 11711–11717.

Ahlquist, R. P. (1948). A study of the adrenotropic receptors. *Am. J. Physiol.* 153: 586–600.

Albright, C. F., and Robbins, P. W. (1990). The sequence and transcript heterogeneity of the yeast gene *ALG1*, an essential mannosyltransferase involved in *N*-glycosylation. *J. Biol. Chem.* 265: 7042–7049.

Amerongen, A. V. N., Aarsman, M. E. G., Bos-Vreugdenhil, A. P., and Roukema, P. A. (1984). Influence of autonomic agonists on the in vitro incorporation of [³H]leucine and *N*-acetyl[¹⁴C]mannosamine into submandibular mucin of the mouse. *Biochim. Biophys. Acta* 798: 103–110.

Andreadis, A., Gallego, M. E., and Nadal-Ginard, B. (1987). Generation of protein isoform diversity by alternative splicing: mechanistic and biological implications. *Annu. Rev. Cell Biol.* 3: 207–242.

Argos, P., Vingron, M., and Vogt, G. (1991). Protein sequence comparison: Methods and significance. *Protein Eng.* 4: 375–383.

Ashkenazi, A., Peralta, E. G., Winslow, J. W., Ramachandran, J., and Capon, D. J. (1989). Functionally distinct G proteins selectively couple different receptors to P1 hydrolysis in the same cycle. *Cell* 56: 487–493.

Aubert, J. P., Biserte, G., and Loucheux-Lefebvre, M. H. (1976). Carbohydrate–peptide linkage in glycoproteins. *Arch. Biochem. Biophys.* 175: 410–418.

Auwerx, J. H., Chait, A., Wolfbauer, G., and Deeb, S. S. (1989). Involvement of second messengers in regulation of the low-density lipoprotein receptor gene. *Mol. Cell. Biol.* 9: 2298–2302.

Babczinski, P. (1980). Evidence against the participation of lipid intermediates in the in vitro biosynthesis of serine-(threonine)-*N*-acetyl-D-galactosamine linkages in submaxillary mucin. *FEBS Lett.* 117: 207–211.

Bachinger, H. P., and Compton, L. A. (1991). Characterization of *E. coli* peptiyl-prolyl *cis*–

trans isomerases (ppiase) and the influence of cyclosporin A on the in vivo folding of the collagen triple helix. *J. Cell. Biochem. [Suppl.]* 15G(Abstr. R203): 188.

Baenziger, J. U., Kumar, S., Brodbeck, R. M., Smith, P. L., and Beranek, M. C. (1992). Circulating half-life but not interaction with the lutropin/chorionic gonadotropin receptor is modulated by sulfation of bovine lutropin oligosaccharides. *Proc. Natl. Acad. Sci. USA* 89: 334–338.

Bakalyar, H. A., and Reed, R. R. (1990). Identification of a specialized adenylyl cyclase that may mediate odorant detection. *Science* 250: 1403–1406.

Baker, K., Hicke, L., Rexach, M., Schleyer, M., and Schekman, R. (1988). Reconstitution of SEC gene product-dependent intercompartmental protein transport. *Cell* 54: 335–344.

Baker, R. K., and Lively, M. O. (1987). Purification and characterization of hen oviduct microsomal signal peptidase. *J. Biochem.* 26: 8561–8567.

Balch, W. E., Dunphy, W. G., Braell, W. A., and Rothman, J. E. (1984a). Reconstitution of the transport of protein between successive compartments of the Golgi measured by the coupled incorporation of *N*-acetylglucosamine. *Cell* 39: 405–416.

Balch, W. E., Glick, B. S., and Rothman, J. E. (1984b). Sequential intermediates in the pathway of intercompartmental transport in a cell-free system. *Cell* 39: 525–536.

Balch, W. E., Kahn, R. A., and Schwaninger, R. (1992). ADP-ribosylation factor is required for vesicular trafficking between the endoplasmic reticulum and the *cis*-Golgi compartment. *J. Biol. Chem.* 267: 13053–13061.

Bandyopadhyay, S. K., and Bancroft, C. (1989). Calcium induction of the mRNAs for prolactin and c-*fos* is independent of protein kinase C activity. *J. Biol. Chem.* 264: 14216–14219.

Banerjee, D. K., Kousvelari, E. E., and Baum, B. J. (1987). cAMP-mediated protein phosphorylation of microsomal membranes increases mannosylphosphodolichol synthase activity. *Proc. Natl. Acad. Sci. USA* 84: 6389–6393.

Barthelson, R., and Roth, S. (1985). Topology of UDP-galactose cleavage in relation of *N*-acetyl-lactosamine formation in Golgi vesicles. *Biochem. J.* 225: 67–75.

Baum, B. J., Freiberg, J. M., Ito, H., Roth, G. S., and Filburn, C. R. (1981). β-Adrenergic regulation of protein phosphorylation and its relationship to exocrine secretion in dispersed rat parotid gland acinar cells. *J. Biol. Chem.* 256: 9731–9736.

Beckers, C. J. M., and Balch, W. E. (1989). Calcium and GTP: Essential components in vesicular trafficking between the endoplasmic reticulum and Golgi apparatus. *J. Cell. Biol.* 108: 1245–1256.

Beckers, C. J. M., Block, M. R., Glick, B. S., Rothman, J. E., and Balch, W. E. (1989). Vesicular transport between the endoplasmic reticulum and the Golgi stack requires the NEM-sensitive fusion protein. *Nature* 339: 397–398.

Beinfeld, M. C., Bourdais, J., Kuks, P., Morel, A., and Cohen, P. (1989). Characterization of an endoprotease from rat small intestinal mucosal secretory granules which generates somatostatin-28 from prosomatostatin by cleavage after a single arginine residue. *J. Biol. Chem.* 264: 4460–4465.

Bell, R. M., and Burns, D. J. (1991). Lipid activation of protein kinase C. *J. Biol. Chem.* 266: 4661–4664.

Bendayan, M. (1982). Double immunocytochemical labeling applying the protein A–gold technique. *J. Histochem. Cytochem.* 30: 81–85.

Benovic, J. L.,Kuhn, H., Weyand, I., Codina, J., Cron, M. G., and Lefkowitz, R. J. (1987). Functional desensitization of the isolated β-adrenergic receptor by the β-adrenergic receptor kinase: Potential role of an analog for the retinal protein arrestin (48-kDa protein). *Proc. Natl. Acad. Sci. USA* 84: 8879–8882.

Bernstein, H. D., Rapoport, T. A., and Walter, P. (1989). Cytosolic protein translocation factors: Is SRP still unique? *Cell* 58: 1017–1019.

Berridge, M. J., and Irvine, R. F. (1984). Inositol trisphosphate, a novel second messenger in cellular signal transduction. *Nature* 312: 315–321.

Berridge, M. J., and Irvine, R. F. (1989). Inositol phosphates and cell signalling. *Nature* 341: 197–205.

Beyer, T. A., Rearick, J. I., Paulson, J. C., Priels, J.-P., Sadler, J. E., and Hill, R. L. (1979). Biosynthesis of mammalian glycoproteins. *J. Biol. Chem.* 254: 12531–12541.

Bielinska, M., Matzuk, M. M., and Boime, I. (1989). Site-specific processing of the N-linked oligosaccharides of the human chorionic gonadotropin α subunit. *J. Biol. Chem.* 264: 17113–17118.

Bienkowski, R. S. (1983). Intracellular degradation of newly synthesized secretory proteins. *Biochem. J.* 214: 1–10.

Blobel, G., and Dobberstein, B. (1975a). Transfer of proteins across membranes. I. Presence of proteolytically processed and unprocessed nascent immunoglobulin light chains on membrane-bound ribosomes of murine myeloma. *J. Cell Biol.* 67: 835–851.

Blobel, G., and Dobberstein, B. (1975b). Transfer of proteins across membranes. II. Reconstitution of functional rough microsomes from heterologous components. *J. Cell Biol.* 67: 852–862.

Block, M. R., Glick, B. S., Wilcox, C. A., Wieland, F. T., and Rothman, J. E. (1988). Purification of an N-ethylmaleimide-sensitive protein catalyzing vesicular transport. *Proc. Natl. Acad. Sci. USA* 85: 7852–7856.

Blumberg, P. M., Jaken, S., Konig, B., Sharkey, N. A., Leach, K. L., Jeng, A. Y., Yeh, E. (1984). Mechanism of action of the phorbol ester tumor promoters: Specific receptors for lipophilic ligands. *Biochem. Pharmacol.* 33: 933–940.

Böhni, P. C., Deshaies, R. J., and Shekman, R. (1988). SEC11 is required for signal peptide processing and yeast cell growth. *J. Cell Biol.* 106: 1035–1042.

Boulet, A. M., Erwin, C. R., and Rutter, W. J. (1986). Cell-specific enhancers in the rat exocrine pancreas. *Proc. Natl. Acad. Sci. USA* 83: 3599–3603.

Bourne, H. R., Sanders, D. A., and McCormick, F. (1991). The GTPase superfamily: Conserved structure and molecular mechanism. *Nature* 349: 117–127.

Bourne, H. R., Sanders, D. A., and McCormick, F. (1990). The GTPase superfamily: a conserved switch for diverse cell functions. *Nature* 348: 125–132.

Bowie, J. U., Lüthy, R., and Eisenberg, D. (1991). A method to identify protein sequences that fold into a known three-dimensional structure. *Science* 253: 164–170.

Bradshaw, J. P., Hatton, J., and White, D. A. (1985). The hormonal control of protein N-glycosylation in the developing rabbit mammary gland and its effect upon transferrin synthesis and secretion. *Biochim. Biophys. Acta* 847: 344–351.

Bramson, H. N., Kaiser, E. T., and Mildvan, A. S. (1983). Mechanistic studies of cAMP-dependent protein kinase actions. *CRC Crit. Rev. Biochem.* 15: 93–124.

Brand, S., Laurie, S. M., Mixon, M. B., and Castle, J. D. (1991). Secretory carrier membrane proteins 31–35 define a common protein composition among secretory carrier membranes. *J. Biol. Chem.* 266: 18949–18957.

Brion, C., Miller, S. G., and Moore, H.-P. H. (1992). Regulated and constitutive secretion: Differential effects of protein synthesis arrest on transport of glycosaminoglycan chains to the two secretory pathways. *J. Biol. Chem.* 267: 1477–1483.

Brockhausen, I., Möller, G., Merz, G., Adermann, K., and Paulsen, H. (1990). Control of mucin synthesis: The peptide portion of synthetic *O*-glycopeptide substrates influences the activity of *O*-glycan core 1 UDP galactose:*N*-acetyl-α-galactosaminyl-*R* β3-galactosyltransferase. *Biochemistry* 29: 10206–10212.

Brown, A. M., and Birnbaumer, L. (1988). Direct G protein gating of ion channels. *Am. J. Physiol.* 254: H401–H410.

Bulleid, N. J., and Freedman, R. B. (1988). Defective co-translational formation of disulfide bonds in protein disulfide–isomerase-deficient microsomes. *Nature* 335: 649–651.

Burgess, G. M., Bird, G. S. J., Obie, J. F., and Putney, J. W., Jr. (1991). The mechanism for synergism between phospholipase C- and adenylylcyclase-linked hormones in liver: Cyclic AMP-dependent kinase augments inositol trisphosphate-mediated Ca^{2+} mobilization without increasing the cellular levels of inositol polyphosphates. *J. Biol. Chem.* 266: 4772–4781.

Burgess, T. L., and Kelly, R. B. (1987). Constitutive and regulated secretion of proteins. *Annu. Rev. Cell Biol.* 3: 243–293.

Burgess, T. L., Craik, C. S., Matsuuchi, L., and Kelly, R. G. (1987). In vitro mutagenesis of trypsinogen: Role of amino terminus in intracellular protein targeting to secretory granules. *J. Cell Biol.* 105: 659–668.

Cameron, R. S., Cameron, P. L., and Castle, J. D. (1986). A common spectrum of polypeptides occurs in secretion granule membranes of different exocrine glands. *J. Cell Biol.* 103: 1299–1313.

Cantley, L. C., Auger, K. R., Carpenter, C., Duckworth, B., Graziani, A., Kapeller, R., and Soltoff, S. (1991). Oncogenes and signal transduction. *Cell* 64: 281–302.

Capasso, J. M., and Hirschberg, C. B. (1984). Effect of atractylosides, palmitoyl coenzyme A, and anion transport inhibitors on translocation of nucleotide sugars and nucleotide sulfate into Golgi vesicles. *J. Biol. Chem.* 259: 4263–4266.

Capecchi, M. R. (1989). The new mouse genetics: Altering the genome by gene targeting. *Trends Genet.* 5: 70–76.

Carlson, D. M., Zhou, J., and Wright, P. S. (1991). Molecular structure and transcriptional regulation of the salivary gland proline-rich protein multigene families. *Prog. Nucleic Acids Res. Mol. Biol.* 41: 1–22.

Carneiro, M., and Schibler, U. (1984). Accumulation of rare and moderately abundant mRNAs in mouse L-cells is mainly post-transcriptionally regulated. *J. Mol. Biol.* 178: 869–880.

Carson, D. D., and Tang, J.-P. (1989). Estrogen induces *N*-linked glycoprotein expression by immature mouse uterine epithelial cells. *Biochemistry* 28: 8116–8123.

Carson, D. D., Farrar, J. D., Laidlaw, J., and Wright, D. A. (1990). Selective activation of the *N*-glycosylation apparatus in uteri by estrogen. *J. Biol. Chem.* 265: 2947–2955.

Carver, J. P., and Cumming, D. A. (1987). Site-directed processing of N-linked oligosaccharides: the role of three-dimensional structure. *Pure Appl. Chem.* 59: 1465–1476.

Castle, A. M., Stahl, L. E., and Castle, J. D. (1992). A 13-amino acid N-terminal domain of a basic proline-rich protein is necessary for storage in secretory granules and facilitates exit from the endoplasmic reticulum. *J. Biol. Chem.* 267: 13093–13100.

Catterall, W. A. (1991). Functional subunit structure of voltage-gated calcium channels. *Science* 253: 1499–1500.

Chanat, E., and Huttner, W. B. (1991). Milieu-induced, selective aggregation of regulated secretory proteins in the *trans*-Golgi network. *J. Cell Biol.* 115: 1505–1519.

Chavrier, P., Vingron, M., Sander, C., Simons, K., and Zerial, M. (1990). Molecular cloning of *YPT1/SEC4*-related cDNAs from an epithelial cell line. *Mol. Cell. Biol.* 10: 6578–6585.

Chege, N. W., and Pfeffer, S. R. (1990). Compartmentation of the Golgi complex: Brefeldin-A distinguishes *trans*-Golgi cisternae from the *trans*-Golgi network. *J. Cell Biol.* 111: 893–899.

Chilton, B. S., Kaplan, H. A., and Lennarz, W. J. (1988). Estrogen regulation of the central enzymes involved in *O*- and *N*-linked glycoprotein assembly in the developing and the adult rabbit endocervix. *Endocrinology* 123: 1237–1244.

Chung, K.-N., Walter, P., Aponte, G. W., and Moore, H.-P. H. (1989). Molecular sorting in the secretory pathway. *Science* 243: 192–197.

Clamgirand, C., Camier, M., Boussetta, H., Fahy, C., Morel, A., Nicolas, P., and Cohen, P. (1986). An endopeptidase associated with bovine neurohypophysis secretory granules cleaves pro-ocytocin/neurophysin peptide at paired basic residues. *Biochem. Biophys. Res. Commun.* 134: 1190–1196.

Cockcroft, S., and Stutchfield, J. (1988). G-proteins, the inositol lipid signalling pathway, and secretion. *Philos. Trans. R. Soc. Lond.* B320: 247–265.

Cockell, M., Stevenson, B. J., Strubin, M., Hagenbüchle, O., and Wellauer, P. K. (1989). Identification of a cell-specific DNA-binding activity that interacts with a transcriptional activator of genes expressed in the acinar pancreas. *Molec. Cell. Biol.* 9: 2464–2476.

Collins, S., Bouvier, M., Bolanowski, M. A., Caron, M. G., and Lefkowitz, R. J. (1989). cAMP stimulates transcription of the β_2-adrenergic receptor gene in response to short-term agonist exposure. *Proc. Natl. Acad. Sci. USA* 86: 4853–4857.

Collins, S., Caron, M. G., and Lefkowitz, R. J. (1988). β_2-Adrenergic receptors in hamster smooth muscle cells are transcriptionally regulated by glucocorticoids. *J. Biol. Chem.* 263: 9067–9070.

Collins, S., Caron, M. G., and Lefkowitz, R. J. (1991). Regulation of adrenergic receptor responsiveness through modulation of receptor gene expression. *Annu. Rev. Physiol.* 53: 497–508.

Collins, S., Caron, M. G., and Lefkowitz, R. J. (1992). From ligand binding to gene expression: New insights into the regulation of G-protein-coupled receptors. *Trends Biochem. Sci.* 17: 37–39.

Connolly, T., Rapiejko, P. J., and Gilmore, R. (1991). Requirement of GTP hydrolysis for dissociation of the signal recognition particle from its receptors. *Science* 252: 1171–1172.

Cooper, L. F., Elia, D. M., and Tabak, L. A. (1991). Secretagogue-coupled changes in the expression of glutamine/glutamic acid-rich proteins (GRPs): Isoproterenol induces changes in GRP transcript expression and changes in isoforms secreted. *J. Biol. Chem.* 266: 3532–3539.

Crooke, S. T., and Bennett, C. F. (1989). Mammalian phosphoinositide-specific phospholipase C isoenzymes. *Cell Calcium* 10: 309–323.

Curbelo, H. M., Devalle, J. J., Houssay, A. B., Gamper, C. H., and Tocci, A. A. (1968). Effects of isoproterenol upon the sialic acid content of salivary glands in the rat. *J. Oral Ther. Pharmacol.* 4: 431–438.

Curbelo, H. M., Houssay, A. B., Gamper, C. H., and Sancho, O. (1973). Influence of the adrenal glands on the sialic acid content of submaxillary and retrolingual glands in the rat. *J. Dent. Res.* 52: 1265–1267.

Cutler, S., and Chaudhry, A. P. (1974). Cytodifferentiation of the acinar cells of the rat submandibular gland. *Dev. Biol.* 41: 31–41.

Dahms, N. M., and Hart, G. W. (1986). Influence of quaternary structure on glycosylation: Differential subunit association affects the site-specific glycosylation of the common β-chain from Mac-1 and LFA-1. *J. Biol. Chem.* 261: 13186–13196.

Delegeane, A. M., Ferland, L. H., and Mellon, P. L. (1987). Tissue-specific enhancer of the human glycoprotein hormone α-subunit gene: Dependence on cyclic AMP-inducible elements. *Mol. Cell. Biol.* 7: 3994–4002.

d'Enfert, C., Barlowe, C., Nishikawa, S.-I., Nakano, A., and Schekman, R. (1991). Structural and functional dissection of a membrane glycoprotein required for vesicle budding from the endoplasmic reticulum. *Mol. Cell. Biol.* 11: 5727–5734.

Dennis, E. A., Rhee, S. G., Billah, M. M., and Hannun, Y. A. (1991). Role of phospholipases in generating lipid second messengers in signal transduction. *FASEB J.* 5: 2068–2077.

Dennis, J. W., Kosh, K., Bryce, D.-M., and Breitman, M. L. (1989). Oncogenes conferring metastatic potential induce increase branching of Asn-linked oligosaccharides in rat2 fibroblasts. *Oncogene* 4: 853–860.

Deschuyteneer, M., Eckhardt, A. E., Roth, J., and Hill, R. L. (1988). The subcellular localization of apomucin and non-reducing terminal *N*-acetylgalactosamine in porcine submaxillary glands. *J. Biol. Chem.* 263: 2452–2459.

Deshaies, R. J., and Schekman, R. (1987). A yeast mutant defective at an early stage in import of secretory protein into the endoplasmic reticulum. *J. Cell Biol.* 105: 633–645.

Deshaies, R. J., and Schekman, R. (1989a). *sec62* encodes a membrane protein required for protein translocation into the yeast endoplasmic reticulum. *J. Cell Biol.* 109: 2653–2664.

Deshaies, R. J., Kepes, F., and Böhni, P. C. (1989b). Genetic dissection of the early stages of protein secretion in yeast. *Trends Glycobiol.* 5: 87–93.

Deutsch, P. J., Hoeffler, J. P., Jameson, J. L., and Habener, J. F. (1988b). Cyclic AMP and phorbol ester-stimulated transcription mediated by similar DNA elements that bind distinct proteins. *Proc. Natl. Acad. Sci. USA* 85: 7922–7926.

Deutsch, P. J., Hoeffler, J. P., Jameson, J. L., Lin, J. C., and Habener, J. F. (1988a). Structural determinants for transcriptional activation by cAMP-responsive DNA elements. *J. Biol. Chem.* 263: 18466–18472.

Di Jeso, B., Liguoro, D., Ferranti, P., Marinaccio, M., Acquaviva, R., Formisano, S., and Consiglio, E. (1992). Modulation of the carbohydrate moiety of thyroglobulin by thyrotropin and calcium in Fisher rat thyroid line-5 cells. *J. Biol. Chem.* 267: 1938–1944.

Dische, Z., Burgher, C. M., Danilchenko, A., and Rothschild, C. (1969). Variations in the composition of glycoproteins of the submaxillary and parotid saliva of the dog in relation to intensity of secretory stimulus. *Arch. Biochem. Biophys* 135: 1–9.

Dohlman, H. G., Caron, M. G., and Lefkowtiz, R. J. (1991). Model systems for the study of seven-transmembrane-segment receptor. *Annu. Rev. Biochem.* 60: 653–688.

Donaldson, J. G., Lippincott-Schwartz, J., Bloom, G. S., Kreis, T. E., and Klausner, R. D. (1990). Dissociation of a 110 kD peripheral membrane protein from the Golgi apparatus is an early event in brefeldin A action. *J. Cell Biol.* 111: 2295–2306.

Duksin, D., and Mahoney, W. C., (1982). Relationship of the structure and biological activity of the natural homologues of tunicamycin. *J. Biol. Chem.* 257: 3105–3109.

Dunne, M. J., Bullet, M. J., Li, G., Wollheim, C. B., and Petersen, O. H. (1989). Galanin activates nucleotide-dependent K^+ channels in insulin-secreting cells via a pertussis toxin-sensitive G-protein. *EMBO J.* 8: 413–420.

Easton, E. W., Bolscher, J. G. M., and van den Eijnden, D. H. (1991). Enzymatic amplification involving glycosyltransferases forms the basis for the increased size of asparagine-linked glycans at the surface of NIH 3T3 cells expressing the N-*ras* proto-oncogene. *J. Biol. Chem.* 266: 21674–21680.

El-Fakahany, E. E., Alger, B. E., Lai, W. S., Pitler, T. A., Worley, P. F., and Baraban, J. M. (1988). Neuronal muscarinic responses: Role of protein kinase C. *FASEB J.* 2: 2575–2583.

Elbein, A. D. (1987). Inhibitors of the biosynthesis and processing of *N*-linked oligosaccharide chains. *Annu. Rev. Biochem.* 56: 497–534.

Emori, Y., Homma, Y., Sarimachi, H., Kawasaki, H., Nakanishi, O., Suzuki, K., and Takenawa, T. (1989). A second type of rat phosphoinositide-specific phospholipase C containing a *src* related sequence not essential for phosphoinositide-hydrolyzing activity. *J. Biol. Chem.* 264: 21885–21890.

Evans, E. A., Gilmore, R., and Blobel, G. (1986). Purification of microsomal signal peptidase as a complex. *Proc. Natl. Acad. Sci. USA* 83: 581–585.

Exton, J. H. (1990). Signaling through phosphatidylcholine breakdown. *J. Biol. Chem.* 265: 1–4.

Falvey, E., and Schibler, U. (1991). How are regulators regulated? *FASEB J.* 5: 309–314.

Farquhar, M. G., and Palade, G. E. (1981). The Golgi apparatus (complex)—(1954–1981)—from artifact to center stage. *J. Cell Biol.* 97: 77s–103s.

Farquhar, M. G. (1985). Progress in unraveling pathways of Golgi traffic. *Annu. Rev. Cell Biol.* 1: 447–488.

Federman, A. D., Conklin, B. R., Schrader, K. A., Reed, R. R., and Bourne, H. R. (1992). Hormonal stimulation of adenylyl cyclase through Gi-protein βγ subunits. *Nature* 356: 159–161.

Feinstein, P. G., Schrader, K. A., Bakalyar, H. A., Tang, W.-J., Krupinski, J., Gilman, A. G., and Reed, R. R. (1991). Molecular cloning and characterization of a Ca^{2+}/calmodulin insensitive adenylyl cyclase from rat brain. *Proc. Natl. Acad. Sci. USA* 88: 10173–10177.

Fenstermaker, R. A., Milsted, A., Virgin, J. B., Miller, W. L., and Nilson, J. H. (1989). The transcriptional response of the human chorionic gonadotropin β-subunit to cAMP is cycloheximide sensitive and is mediated by cis-acting sequences different from that found in the α-subunit gene. *Molec. Endocrin.* 3: 1070–1076.

Fiete, D., Srivastava, V., Hindsgaul, O., and Baenziger, J. U. (1991). A hepatic reticuloendothelial cell receptor specific for SO_4-4GalNAcβ1,4GlcNAcβ1,2Manα that mediates rapid clearance of lutropin. *Cell* 67: 1103–1110.

Fink, J. S., Verhave, M., Walton, K., Mandel, G., and Goodman, R. H. (1991). Cyclic AMP- and phorbol ester-induced transcriptional activations are mediated by the same enhancer element in the human vasoactive intestinal peptide gene. *J. Biol. Chem.* 266: 3882–3887.

Fisher, J. M., and Scheller, R. H. (1988). Prohormone processing and the secretory pathway. *J. Biol. Chem.* 263: 16515–16518.

Fleming, N., Sliwinski-Lis, E., and Burke, D. N. (1989). G regulatory proteins and muscarinic receptor signal transduction in mucous acini of rat submandibular gland. *Life Sci.* 44: 1027–1035.

Flynn, G. C., Pohl, J., Flocco, M. T., and Rothman, J. E. (1991). Peptide-binding specificity of the molecular chaperone BiP. *Nature* 353: 726–730.

Foulkes, N. S., Borrelli, E., and Sassone-Corsi, P. (1991). *CREM* gene: Use of alternative DNA-binding domains generates multiple antagonists of cAMP-induced transcription. *Cell* 64: 739–749.

Franzusoff, A., and Schekman, R. (1989). Functional compartments of the yeast Golgi apparatus are defined by the *sec7* mutation. *EMBO J.* 8: 2695–2702.

Freedman, R. B. (1984). Native disulfide bond formation in protein biosynthesis: Evidence for the role of protein disulfide isomerase. *Trends Biochem. Sci.* 9: 438–441.

Freedman, R. B. (1989). Protein disulfide isomerase: Multiple roles in the modification of nascent secretory proteins. *Cell* 57: 1069–1072.

Freedman, S. D., and Jamieson, J. D. (1982a). Hormone-induced protein phosphorylation. I. Relationship between secretagogue action and endogenous protein phosphorylation in intact cells from the exocrine pancreas and parotid. *J. Cell Biol.* 95: 903–908.

Freedman, S. D., and Jamieson, J. D. (1982b). Hormone-induced protein phosphorylation. II. Localization to the ribosomal fraction from rat exocrine pancreas and parotid of a 29,000-dalton protein phosphorylated in situ in response to secretagogues. *J. Cell Biol.* 95: 909–917.

Freemont, P. S., Lane, A. N., and Sanderson, M. R. (1991). Structural aspects of protein–DNA recognition. *Biochem. J.* 278: 1–23.

Freissmuth, M., Casey, P. J., and Gilman, A. G. (1989). G proteins control diverse pathways of transmembrane signaling. *FASEB J.* 3: 2125–2131.

Fries, E., Gustaffson, L., and Peterson, P. A. (1984). Four secretory proteins synthesized by hepatocytes are transported from endoplasmic reticulum to Golgi complex at different rates. *EMBO J.* 3: 147–152.

Fuh, V. L., Burrin, J. M., and Jameson, J. L. (1989). Cyclic AMP (cAMP) effects on chorionic gonadotropin gene transcription and mRNA stability: Labile proteins mediate basal expression whereas stable proteins mediate cAMP stimulation. *Mol. Endocrinol.* 3: 1148–1155.

Fujiwara, T., Oda, K., Yokota, S., Takatsuki, A., and Ikehara, Y. (1988). Brefeldin A causes disassembly of the Golgi complex and accumulation of secretory proteins in the endoplasmic reticulum. *J. Biol. Chem.* 263: 18545–18552.

Gallagher, J. T., and Cornfield, A. P. (1978). Mucin-type glycoproteins: new perspectives on their structure and synthesis. *Trends Biochem. Sci.* 3: 38–41.

Gao, P., and Gilman, A. G. (1991). Cloning and expression of a widely distributed (type IV) adenylyl cyclase. *Proc. Natl. Acad. Sci. USA* 88: 10178–10182.

Garnier, J. (1990). Protein structure prediction. *Biochimie* 72: 513–524.

Gerdes, H.-H., Rosa, P., Phillips, E., Baeuerle, P. A., Frank, R., Argos, P., and Huttner, W. B. (1989). The primary structure of human secretogranin II; a widespread tyrosine-sulfated secretory protein that exhibits low pH and a calcium-induced aggregation. *J. Biol. Chem.* 264: 12009–12015.

Gething, M. J., and Sambrook, J. (1992). Protein folding in the cell. *Nature* 355: 33–44.

Ghosh, S., and Baltimore, D. (1990). Activation in vitro of NF-κB by phosphorylation of its inhibitor I-κB. *Nature* 344: 678–682.

Gierasch, L. M. (1989). Signal sequences. *Biochemistry* 28: 923–930.

Gilmore, R., Blobel, G., and Walter, P. (1982a). Protein translocation across the endoplasmic reticulum. I. Detection in the microsomal membrane of a receptor for the signal recognition particle. *J. Cell Biol.* 95: 463–469.

Gilmore, R., Walter, P., and Blobel, G. (1982b). Protein translocation across the endoplasmic reticulum. II. Isolation and characterization of the signal recognition particle receptor. *J. Cell Biol.* 95: 470–477.

Gilmore, T. D. (1990). Nf-κB, KBF1, *dorsal* and *rel*ated matters. *Cell* 62: 841–843.

Gonzalez, G. A., Menzel, P., Leonard, J., Fischer, W. H., and Montminy, M. R. (1991). Characterization of motifs which are critical for activity of the cyclic AMP-responsive transcription factor CREB. *Mol. Cell. Biol.* 11: 1306–1312.

Gottschalk, A. (1969). Biosynthesis of glycoproteins and its relationship to heterogeneity. *Nature* 222: 452–454.

Goud, B., and McCaffrey, M. (1991). Small GTP-binding proteins and their role in transport. *Curr. Opin. Cell Biol.* 3: 626–633.

Graham, T. R., and Emr, S. D. (1991). Compartmental organization of Golgi-specific protein modification and vacuolar protein sorting events defined in a yeast sec 18 (NSF) mutant. *J. Cell Biol.* 114: 207–218.

Green, D. R. J., and Embery, G. (1987). Isolation chemical and biological characterization of sulphated glycoproteins synthesized by rat buccal and palatine minor salivary glands in vivo and in vitro. *Arch. Oral Biol.* 32: 391–399.

Green, E. D., and Baenziger J. U. (1988). Asparagine-linked oligosaccharides on lutropin, follitropin, and thyrotropin. I. Structural elucidation of the sulfated and sialylated oligosaccharides on bovine, ovine, and human pituitary glycoprotein hormones. *J. Biol. Chem.* 263: 25–35.

Greengard, P. (1978). Phosphorylated proteins as physiological effectors. *Science* 199: 146–151.

Griff, I. C., Schekman, R., Rothman, J. E., and Kaiser, C. A. (1992). The yeast *SEC17* gene product is functionally equivalent to mammalian α-SNAP protein. *J. Biol. Chem.* 267: 12106–12115.

Griffiths, G., and Simons, K. (1986). The *trans* Golgi network: Sorting at the exit site of the Golgi complex. *Science* 234: 438–442.

Gros, P., Croop, J., and Housman, D. (1986). Mammalian multidrug resistance gene: Complete cDNA sequence indicates strong homology to bacterial transport proteins. *Cell* 47: 371–380.

Grove, J. R., Deutsch, P. J., Price, D. J., Habener, J. F., and Avruch, J. (1989). Plasmids encoding PKI(1–31), a specific inhibitor of cAMP-stimulated gene expression, inhibit the basal transcriptional activity of some but not all cAMP-regulated DNA response elements in JEG-3 cells. *J. Biol. Chem.* 264: 19506–19513.

Grove, J. R., Price, D. J., Goodman, H. M., and Avruch, J. (1987). Recombinant fragment of protein kinase inhibitor blocks cyclic AMP-dependent gene transcription. *Science* 238: 530–533.

Habener, J. F. (1990). Cyclic AMP response element binding proteins: A cornucopia of transcription factors. *Mol. Endocrinol.* 4: 1087–1094.

Hakomori, S. I. (1985). Aberrant glycosylation in cancer cell membranes as focused on glycolipids: Overview and perspectives. *Cancer Res.* 45: 2405–2414.

Hanks, S. K., Quinn, A. M., and Hunter, T. (1988). The protein kinase family: Conserved features and deduced phylogeny of the catalytic domains. *Science* 241: 42–52.

Hanover, J. A., Lennarz, W. J., and Young, J. (1980). Synthesis of *N*- and *O*-linked glycopeptides in oviduct membrane preparations. *J. Biol. Chem.* 255: 6713–6716.

Hargrove, J. L., and Schmidt, F. H. (1989). The role of mRNA and protein stability in gene expression. *FASEB J.* 3: 2360–2370.

Harper, J. F. (1988). Stimulus-secretion coupling: Second messenger-regulated exocytosis. *Adv. Second Mess. Phosph. Res.* 22: 193–318.

Hashimoto, S., Fumagalli, G., Zanini, A., and Meldolesi, J. (1987). Sorting of three secretory proteins to distinct secretory granules in acidophilic cells of cow anterior pituitary. *J. Cell Biol.* 105: 1579–1586.

Hausdorff, W. P., Campbell, P. T., Ostrowski, J., Yu, S. S., Caron, M. G., and Lefkowitz, R. J. (1991). A small region of the β-adrenergic receptor is selectively involved in its rapid regulation. *Proc. Natl. Acad. Sci. USA* 88: 2979–2983.

Hausdorff, W. P., Caron, M. G., and Lefkowitz, R. J. (1990). Turning off the signal: Desensitization of β-adrenergic receptor function. *FASEB J.* 4: 2881–3049.

Hentze, M. W. (1991). Determinants and regulation of cytoplasmic mRNA stability in eukaryotic cells. *Biochim. Biophys. Acta* 1090: 281–292.

Hershey, J. W. B. (1989). Protein phosphorylation controls translation rates. *J. Biol. Chem.* 264: 20823–20826.

Hershey, A. D., and Krause, J. E. (1990). Molecular characterization of a functional cDNA encoding the rat substance P receptor. *Science* 247: 958–962.

Hershey, A. D., Dykema, P. E., and Krause, J. E. (1991). Organization, structure, and expression of the gene encoding the rat substance P receptor. *J. Biol. Chem.* 266: 4366–4374.

Hicke, L., and Schekman, R. (1989). Yeast Sec23p acts in the cytoplasm to promote protein transport from the endoplasmic reticulum to the Golgi complex in vivo and in vitro. *EMBO J.* 8: 1677–1684.

Hirschberg, C. B., and Snider, M. D. (1987). Topography of glycosylation in the rough endoplasmic reticulum and Golgi apparatus. *Annu. Rev. Biochem.* 56: 63–87.

Hollenberg, M. D. (1991). Structure–activity relationships for transmembrane signaling: The receptor's turn. *FASEB J.* 5: 178–186.

Horstman, D. A., Brandon, S., Wilson, A. L., Guyer, C. A., Cragoe, E. J., Jr., and Limbird, L. E. (1990). An aspartate conserved among G-protein receptors confers allosteric regulation of α_2-adrenergic receptors by sodium. *J. Biol. Chem.* 265: 21590–21595.

Hosey, M. M. (1992). Diversity of structure, signaling and regulation within the family of muscarinic cholinergic receptors. *FASEB J.* 6: 845–852.

Houslay, M. D. (1991). "Crosstalk": A pivotal role for protein kinase C in modulating relationships between signal transduction pathways. *Eur. J. Biochem.* 195: 9–27.

Howard, G., Keller, P. R., Johnson, T. M., and Meisler, M. H. (1989). Binding of a pancreatic nuclear protein is correlated with amylase enhancer activity. *Nuc. Acids Res.* 17: 8185–8195.

Hsu, V. W., Shah, N., and Klausner, R. D. (1992). A brefeldin A-like phenotype is induced by the overexpression of a human ERD-2-like protein, ELP-1. *Cell* 69: 625–635.

Hubbard, S. C. (1987). Differential effects of oncogenic transformation of *N*-linked oligosaccharide processing at individual glycosylation sites of viral glycoproteins. *J. Biol. Chem.* 262: 16403–16411.

Hubbard, S. C. (1988) Regulation of glycosylation: The influence of protein structure on *N*-linked oligosaccharide processing. *J. Biol. Chem.* 263: 19303–19317.

Hughes, R. C., Bradbury, A. F., and Smyth, D. G. (1988). Substrate recognition by UDP-*N*-acetylgalactosaminyltransferase: Effects of chain length and disulfide bonding of synthetic peptide substrates. *Carbohydr. Res.* 178: 259–269.

Huttner, W. B., Gerdes, H.-H., and Rosa, P. (1991). The grain (chromogranin/secretogranin) family. *Trends Biochem. Sci.* 16: 27–30.

Hyman, S. E., Comb, M., Pearlberg, J., and Goodman, H. M. (1989). An AP-2 element acts synergistically with the cyclic AMP- and phorbol ester-inducible enhancer of the human proenkephalin gene. *Mol. Cell. Biol.* 9: 321–324.

Ishikawa, Y., Katsushika, S., Chen, L., Halnon, N. J., Kawabe, J. I., and Homcy, C. J. (1992). Isolation and characterization of a novel cardiac adenylylcyclase cDNA. *J. Biol. Chem.* 267: 13553–13557.

Jamieson, J. D., and Palade, G. E. (1967). Intracellular transport of secretory proteins in the pancreatic exocrine cell. I. Role of peripheral elements of the Golgi complex. *J. Cell Biol.* 34: 577–596.

Jan, L. Y., and Jan, Y. N. (1989). Voltage-sensitive ion channels. *Cell* 56: 13–25.

Johnson, D. C., and Spear, P. G. (1983). O-linked oligosaccharides are acquired by herpes simplex virus glycoproteins in the Golgi apparatus. *Cell* 32: 987–997.

Johnston, G. C., Prendergast, J. A., and Singer, R. A. (1991). The *Saccharomyces cerevisiae MYO2* gene encodes an essential myosin for vectorial transport of vesicles. *J. Cell Biol.* 113: 539–551.

Jones, E. W. (1991). Three proteolytic systems in the yeast *Saccharomyces cerevisiae*. *J. Biol. Chem.* 266: 7963–7966.

Kahn, R. A. (1991). Fluoride is not an activator of the smaller (20–25 kDa) GTP-binding proteins. *J. Biol. Chem.* 266: 15595–15597.

Kaiser, C., and Schekman, R. (1990). Distinct sets of *SEC* genes govern transport vesicle formation and fusion early in the secretory pathway. *Cell* 61: 723–733.

Karin, M. (1989). Complexities of gene regulation by cAMP. *Trends Genet.* 5: 65–67.

Karin, M. (1992). Signal transduction from cell surface to nucleus in development and disease. *FASEB J.* 6: 2581–2590.

Kelleher, D. J., Kreibich, G., and Gilmore, R. (1992). Oligosaccharyltransferase activity is associated with a protein complex composed of ribophorins I and II and a 48 kd protein. *Cell* 69: 55–65.

Kelly, R. B. (1985). Pathways of protein secretion in eukaryotes. *Science* 230: 25–32.

Kepes, F., and Schekman, R. (1988). The yeast *SEC53* gene encodes phosphomannomutase. *J. Biol. Chem.* 263: 9155–9161.

Kim, D., Lewis, D. L., Graziadei, L., Neer, E. J., Bar-Sagi, D., and Clapham, D. E. (1989). G-protein $\beta\gamma$-subunits activate the cardiac muscarinic K^+ channel via phospholipase A_2. *Nature* 337: 557–560.

Kleuss, C., Hescheler, J., Ewel, C., Rosenthal, W., Schultz, G., and Wittig, B. (1991). Assignment of G-protein subtypes to specific receptors inducing inhibition of calcium currents. *Nature* 353: 43–48.

Knighton, D. R., Zheng, J., Ten Eyck, L. F., Ashford, V. A., Xuong, N.-H., Taylor, S. S., and Sowadski, J. M. (1991). Crystal structure of the catalytic subunit of cyclic adenosine monophosphate-dependent protein kinase. *Science* 253: 407–414.

Kornfeld, R., and Kornfeld, S. (1985). Assembly of asparagine-linked oligosaccharides. *Annu. Rev. Biochem.* 54: 631–664.

Kozak, M. (1991). Structural features in eukaryotic mRNAs that modulate the initiation of translation. *J. Biol. Chem.* 266: 19867–19870.

Kraehenbuhl, J. P., Racine, L., and Jamieson, J. D. (1977). Immunocytochemical localization of secretory proteins in bovine pancreatic exocrine cells. *J. Cell Biol.* 72: 406–423.

Kreig, U. C., Walter, P., and Johnson, A. E. (1986). Photocrosslinking of the signal sequence of nascent preprolactin to the 54 kD polypeptide of the signal recognition particle. *Proc. Natl. Acad. Sci. USA* 83: 8604–8608.

Krupinski, J., Coussen, F., Bakalyar, H. A., Tang, W.-J., Feinstein, P. G., Orth, K., Slaughter, C., Reed, R. R., and Gilman, A. G. (1989). Adenylyl cyclase amino acid sequence: Possible channel- or transporter-like structure. *Science* 244: 1558–1564.

Kukuruzinska, M. A., and Robbins, P. W. (1987). Protein glycosylation in yeast: Transcript heterogeneity of the *ALG7* gene. *Proc. Natl. Acad. Sci. USA* 84: 2145–2149.

Kurzchalia, T. V., Wiedmann, M., Girshovich, A. S., Bochkareva, E. S., Bielka, H., and Rapoport, T. A. (1986). The signal sequence of nascent preprolactin interacts with the 54 kD polypeptide of the signal recognition particle. *Nature* 320: 634–636.

Latchman, D. S. (1990). Eukaryotic transcription factors. *Biochem. J.* 270: 281–289.

Le Marer, N., Laudet, V., Svensson, E. C., Cazlaris, H., Van Hille, B., Lagrou, C., Stehelin, D., Montreuil, J., Verbert, A., and Delannoy, P. (1992). The *c-Ha-ras* oncogene induces increased expression of β-galactoside α-2,6-sialyltransferase in rat fibroblast (FR3T3) cells. *Glycobiology* 2: 49–56.

Lefkowitz, R. J., and Caron, M. G. (1988). Adrenergic receptors: Models for the study of receptors coupled to guanine nucleotide regulatory proteins. *J. Biol. Chem.* 263: 4993–4996.

Lehrman, M., Zhu, X., and Khounlo, S. (1988). Amplification and molecular cloning of the hamster tunicamycin-sensitive *N*-acetylglucosamine-1-phosphate transferase gene. *J. Biol. Chem.* 263: 19796–19803.

Lehrman, M. A. (1991). Biosynthesis of *N*-acetylglucosamine-P-P-dolichol, the committed step of asparagine-linked oligosaccharide assembly. *Glycobiology* 1: 553–562.

Lenardo, M. J., and Baltimore, D. (1989). NF-κB: A pleiotropic mediator of inducible and tissue-specific gene control. *Cell* 58: 227–229.

Lippincott-Schwartz, J., Donaldson, J. G., Schweizer, A., Berger, E. G., Hauri, H.-P., Yuan, L. C., and Klausner, R. D. (1990). Microtubule-dependent retrograde transport of proteins into the ER in the presence of brefeldin A suggest an ER recycling pathway. *Cell* 60: 821–836.

Lippincott-Schwartz, J., Yuan, L. C., Bonifacino, J. S., and Klausner, R. D. (1989). Rapid redistribution of Golgi proteins into the ER in cells treated with brefeldin A: Evidence for membrane cycling from Golgi to ER. *Cell* 56: 801–813.

Lodish, H. F., Kong, N., Snider, M., and Strous, G. J. A. M. (1983). A vesicular intermediate in the transport of hepatoma secretory proteins from the rough endoplasmic reticulum to the Golgi complex. *Nature* 304: 80–83.

Lodish, H. F. (1988). Transport of secretory and membrane glycoproteins from the rough endoplasmic reticulum to the Golgi. *J. Biol. Chem.* 263: 2107–2110.

Lodish, H. F., and Kong, N. (1990). Perturbation of cellular calcium blocks exit of secretory proteins from the rough endoplasmic reticulum. *J. Biol. Chem.* 265: 10893–10899.

Lodish, H. F., Kong, N., and Wikström, L. (1992). Calcium is required for folding of newly made subunits of the asialoglycoprotein receptor within the endoplasmic reticulum. *J. Biol. Chem.* 267: 12753–12760.

Lodish, H. F., Kong, N., Hirani, S., and Rasmussen, J. (1987). A vesicular intermediate in the transport of hepatoma secretory proteins from the rough endoplasmic reticulum to the Golgi complex. *J. Cell Biol.* 104: 221–230.

Lohse, M. J., Andexinger, S., Pitcher, J., Trukawinski, S., Codina, J., Faure, J.-P., Caron, M. G., and Lefkowitz, R. J. (1992). Receptor-specific desensitization with purified proteins: Kinase dependence and receptor specificity of β-arrestin and arrestin in the $β_2$-adrenergic receptor and rhodopsin systems. *J. Biol. Chem.* 267: 8558–8564.

Lombart, C. G., and Winzler, R. J. (1974). Isolation and characterization of oligosaccharides from canine submaxillary mucin. *Eur. J. Biochem.* 45: 77–86.

Lowy, D. R., Zhang, K., Declue, J. E., and Willumsen, B. M. (1991). Regulation of p21^{ras} activity. *Trends Genet.* 7: 346–351.

MacDonald, A. S., and Boyd, N. D. (1989). Regulation of substance P receptor affinity by guanine nucleotide-binding proteins. *J. Neurochem.* 53: 264–271.

Majerus, P. W., Ross, T. S., Cunningham, T. W., Caldwell, K. K., Jefferson, A. B., and Bansal, V. S. (1990). Recent insights in phosphatidylinositol signaling. *Cell* 63: 459–465.

Maniatis, T., and Reed, R. (1987). The role of small nuclear ribonucleoprotein particles in pre-mRNA splicing. *Nature* 325: 673–678.

Maniatis, T., Goodbourn, S., and Fischer, J. A. (1987). Regulation of inducible and tissue-specific gene expression. *Science* 236: 1237–1245.

Marino, C. M., Castle, J. D., and Gorelick, F. S. (1990). Regulated phosphorylation of secretory granule membrane proteins of the rat parotid gland. *Am. J. Physiol.* 259: G70–G77.

Masters, S. B., Sullivan, K. A., Miller, R. T., Beiderman, B., Lopez, N. G., Ramachandran, J., and Bourne, H. R. (1988). Carboxyl terminal domain of GS_α specifies coupling of receptors to stimulation of adenylyl cyclase. *Science* 241: 448–451.

Maurer, R. A. (1989). Both isoforms of the cAMP-dependent protein kinase catalytic subunit can activate transcription of the prolactin gene. *J. Biol. Chem.* 264: 6870–6873.

McFadden, P. N., Mandpe, A., and Koshland, D. E., Jr. (1989). Calcium- and lipid-independent protein kinase C autophosphorylation: Activation by low pH. *J. Biol. Chem.* 264: 12765–12771.

Meister, A., Weinrich, S. L., Nelson, C., and Rutter, W. J. (1989). The chymotrypsin enhancer core: specific factor binding and biological activity. *J. Biol. Chem.* 264: 20744–20751.

Melancon, P., Glick, B. S., Malhotra, V., Weidman, P. J., Serafini, T., Gleason, M. L., Orci, L., and Rothman, J. E. (1987). Involvement of GTP-binding "G" proteins in transport through the Golgi stack. *Cell* 51: 1053–1062.

Mellman, I., and Simons, K. (1992). The Golgi complex: In vitro veritas? *Cell* 68: 829–840.

Mellon, P. L., Clegg, C. H., Correll, L. A., and McKnight, G. S. (1989). Regulation of transcription by cyclic AMP-dependent protein kinase. *Proc. Natl. Acad. Sci. USA* 86: 4887–4891.

Meyer, D. I., Krause, E., and Dobberstein, B. (1982). Secretory protein translocation across membranes—the role of the "docking protein." *Nature* 297: 647–650.

Michael, J., Carroll, R., Swift, H. H., and Steiner, D. F. (1987). Studies on the molecular organization of rat insulin secretory granules. *J. Biol. Chem.* 262: 16531–16535.

Mignery, G. A., and Südhof, T. C. (1990). The ligand binding site and transduction mechanism in the inositol-1,4,5-triphosphate receptor. *EMBO J.* 9: 3893–3898.

Milsted, A., Cox, R. P., and Nilson, J. H. (1987). Cyclic AMP regulates transcription of the genes encoding human chorionic gonadotropin with different kinetics. *DNA* 6: 213–219.

Miner, J. N., and Yamamoto, K. R. (1991). Regulatory crosstalk at composite response elements. *Trends Biochem. Sci.* 16: 423–426.

Mirels, L., Bedi, G. S., Dickinson, D. P., Gross, K. W., and Tabak, L. A. (1987). Molecular characterization of glutamine/glutamic acid-rich secretory proteins from rat submandibular glands. *J. Biol. Chem.* 262: 7289–7297.

Mitchell, P. J., and Tjian, R. (1989). Transcriptional regulation in mammalian cells by sequence-specific DNA binding proteins. *Science* 245: 371–378.

Miyamoto, A., Villalobos-Molina, R., Kowatch, M. A., and Roth, G. S. (1992). Altered coupling of α_1-adrenergic receptor-G protein in rat parotid during aging. *Am. J. Physiol.* 262: C1181–C1188.

Montminy, M. R., and Bilezikjian, L. M. (1987). Binding of a nuclear protein to the cyclic-AMP response element of the somatostatin gene. *Nature* 328: 175–178.

Montminy, M. R., Sevarino, K. A., Wagner, J. A., Mandel, G., and Goodman, R. H. (1986). Identification of a cyclic-AMP-responsive element within the rat somatostatin gene. *Proc. Natl. Acad. Sci. USA* 83: 6682–6686.

Moolenaar, W. H., Kruijer, W., Tilly, B. C., Verlaan, I., Bierman, A. J., and de Laat, S. W. (1986). Growth factor-like action of phosphatidic acid. *Nature* 323: 171–173.

Moreira, J. E., Tabak, L. A., Bedi, G. S., Culp, D. J., and Hand, A. R. (1989). Light and electron microscopic immunolocalization and rat submandibular gland mucin-glycoprotein and glutamine/glutamic acid-rich proteins. *J. Histochem. Cytochem.* 37: 515–528.

Morré, D. J., Minnifield, N., and Paulik, M. (1989). Identification of the 16°C compartment of the ER in rat liver and cultured hamster kidney cells. *Biol. Cell* 67: 51–60.

Mount, S. M. (1982). A catalogue of splice junction sequences. *Nucleic Acids Res.* 10: 459–472.

Mroz, E. A., and Lechene, C. (1986). Pancreatic zymogen granules differ markedly in protein composition. *Science* 232: 871–873.

Munro, S., and Pelham, H. R. B. (1987). A C-terminal signal prevents secretion of terminal ER proteins. *Cell* 48: 899–907.

Munroe, D., and Jacobson, A. (1990). mRNA poly(A) tail, a 3′ enhancer of translational initiation. *Mol. Cell. Biol.* 10: 3441–3455.

Murayama, T., and Ui, M. (1985). Receptor-mediated inhibition of adenylate cyclase and stimulation of arachidonic acid release in 3T3 fibroblasts. Selective susceptibility to islet-activating protein, pertussis toxin. *J. Biol. Chem.* 260: 7226–7233.

Müsch, A., Wiedmann, M., and Rapoport, T. A. (1992). Yeast Sec proteins interact with polypeptides traversing the endoplasmic reticulum membrane. *Cell* 69: 343–352.

Nakano, A., and Muramatsu, M. (1989). A novel GTP-binding protein, Sar1p, is involved in transport from the endoplasmic reticulum to the Golgi apparatus. *J. Cell Biol.* 109: 2677–2691.

Nakano, A., Brada, D., and Schekman, R. (1988). A membrane glycoprotein, Sec12p, required for protein transport from the endoplasmic reticulum to the Golgi apparatus in yeast. *J. Cell Biol.* 109: 2677–2691.

Neer, E. J., and Clapham, D. E. (1988). Roles of G protein subunits in transmembrane signalling. *Nature* 333: 129–134.

Nemansky, M., Edzes, H. T., Wijnands, R. A., and Van den Eijnden, D. H. (1992). The polypeptide part of human chorionic gonadotrophin affects the kinetics of α6-sialylation of its *N*-linked glycans but does not alter the branch of specificity of CMP-NeuAc:Galβ1-4GlcNAc-*R* α2-6-sialyltransferase. *Glycobiology* 2: 109–117.

Newman, A. P., Shim, J., and Ferro-Novick, S. (1990). *BET1*, *BOS1*, and *SEC22* are members of a group of interacting yeast genes required for transport from the endoplasmic reticulum to the Golgi complex. *Mol. Cell. Biol.* 10: 3405–3414.

Nishikawa, J., and Nakano, A. (1991). The GTP-binding Sar1 protein is localized to the early compartment of the yeast secretory pathway. *Biochim. Biophys. Acta* 1093: 135–143.

Nishizuka, Y. (1984). Turnover of inositol phospholipids and signal transduction. *Science* 225: 1365–1370.

Nishizuka, Y. (1986). Studies and perspectives of protein kinase C. *Science* 233: 305–312.

Nishizuka, Y. (1988). The molecular heterogeneity of protein kinase C and its implications for cellular regulation. *Nature* 334: 661–665.

Noiva, R., and Lennarz, W. J. (1992). Protein disulfide isomerase: A multifunctional protein resident in the lumen of the endoplasmic reticulum. *J. Biol. Chem.* 267: 3553–3556.

Novick, P., and Schekman, R. (1980). Identification of 23 complementary groups required for post-translational events in the yeast secretory pathway. *Cell* 21: 205–215.

Nowack, D. D., Morré, D. M., Paulik, M., Keenen, T. W., and Morré, D. J. (1987). Intracellular membrane flow: Reconstitution of transitional vesicle formation and function in a cell-free system. *Proc. Natl. Acad. Sci. USA* 84: 6098–6102.

O'Connell, B. C., Hagen, F. K., and Tabak, L. A. (1992). The influence of flanking sequence on the *O*-glycosylation of threonine in vitro *J. Biol. Chem.* 267:25010–25018.

O'Connell, B., Tabak, L. A., and Ramasubbu, N. (1991). The influence of flanking sequences in *O*-glycosylation. *Biochem. Biophys. Res. Commun.* 180: 1024–1030.

O'Dowd, B. F., Lefkowitz, R. J., and Caron, M. G. (1989). Structure of the adrenergic and related receptors *Annu. Rev. Neurosci.* 12: 67–83.

Olate, J., and Allende, J. E. (1991). Structure and function of G proteins. *Pharmacol. Ther.* 51: 403–419.

Orci, L., Glick, B. S., and Rothman, J. E. (1986a). A new type of coated vesicular carrier that appears not to contain clathrin: Its possible role in protein transport within the Golgi stack. *Cell* 46: 171–184.

Orci, L., Ravazzola, M., Amherdt, M., Madsen, O., Perrelet, A., Vassalli, J.-D., and Anderson, R. G. W. (1986b). Conversion of proinsulin to insulin occurs coordinately with acidification of maturing secretory vesicles. *J. Cell Biol.* 103: 2273–2281.

Orci, L., Ravazzola, M., Amherdt, M., Perrelet, A., Powell, S. K., Quinn, D. L., and Moore, H.-P. H. (1987). The *trans*-most cisternae of the Golgi complex: A compartment for sorting of secretory and plasma membrane proteins. *Cell* 51: 1039–1051.

Orci, L., Ravazzola, M., Meda, P., Holcomb, C., Moore, H.-P., Hicke, L., and Schekman, R. (1991a). Mammalian Sec23p homologue is restricted to the endoplasmic reticulum transitional cytoplasm. *Proc. Natl. Acad. Sci. USA* 88: 8611–8615.

Orci, L., Tagaya, M., Amherdt, M., Perrelet, A., Donaldson, J. G., Lippincott-Schwartz, J., Klausner, R. D., and Rothman, J. E. (1991b). Brefeldin A, a drug that blocks secretion, prevents the assembly of non-clathrin-coated buds on Golgi cisternae. *Cell* 64: 1183–1195.

Orlean, P., Albright, C., and Robbins, P. W. (1988). Cloning and sequencing of the yeast gene for dolichol phosphate mannose synthase, an essential protein. *J. Biol. Chem.* 263: 17499–17507.

Ossig, R., Dascher, C., Trepte, H.-H., Schmitt, H. D., and Gallwitz, D. (1991). The yeast *SLY* gene products, suppressors of defects in the essential GTP-binding Ypt1 protein, may act in endoplasmic reticulum-to-Golgi transport. *Mol. Cell. Biol.* 11: 2980–2993.

Palade, G. (1975). Intracellular aspects of the process of protein synthesis. *Science* 189: 347–358.

Parker, P. J., Kour, G., Marais, R. M., Mitchell, F., Pears, C., Schaap, D., Stabel, S., and Webster, C. (1989). Protein kinase C—a family affair. *Mol. Cell. Endocrinol.* 65: 1–11.

Paulik, M., Nowack, D. D., and Morré, D. J. (1988). Isolation of a vesicular intermediate in the cell-free transfer of membrane from transitional elements of the endoplasmic reticulum to Golgi apparatus cisternae of rat liver. *J. Biol. Chem.* 263: 17738–17748.

Payne, G. S., and Schekman, R. (1989). Clathrin: A role in the intracellular retention of a Golgi membrane protein. *Science* 245: 1358–1365.

Pearse, B. M. F. (1987). Clathrin and coated vesicles. *EMBO J.* 6: 2507–2512.

Pearse, B. M. F., and Bretscher, M. S. (1981). Membrane recycling by coated vesicles. *Annu. Rev. Biochem.* 50: 85–101.

Pelham, H. R. B. (1988). Evidence that luminal ER proteins are sorted from secreted proteins in a post-ER compartment. *EMBO J.* 7: 913–918.

Pelham, H. R. B. (1991). Multiple targets for brefeldin A. *Cell* 67: 449–451.

Pelham, H. R. B., Hardwick, K. G., and Lewis, M. J. (1988). Sorting of soluble ER proteins in yeast. *EMBO J.* 7: 1757–1762.

Perlman, D., and Halvorson, H. O. (1983). A putative signal peptidase recognition site and sequence in eukaryotic and prokaryotic signal peptides. *J. Mol. Biol.* 167: 391–409.

Petersen, O. H. (1992). Stimulus-secretion coupling: Cytoplasmic calcium signals and the control of ion channels in exocrine acinar cells. *J. Physiol.* 448: 1–51.

Pfeffer, S. R., and Rothman, J. E. (1987). Biosynthetic protein transport and sorting by the endoplasmic reticulum and the Golgi. *Annu. Rev. Biochem.* 56: 829–852.

Plutner, H., Cox, A. D., Pind, S., Khosravi-Far, R., Bourne, J. R., Schwaninger, R., Der, C. J., and Balch, W. E. (1991). Rab1b regulates vesicular transport between the endoplasmic reticulum and successive Golgi compartments. *J. Cell Biol.* 115: 31–43.

Plutner, H., Schwaninger, R., Pind, S., and Balch, W. E. (1990). Synthetic peptides of the Rab effector domain inhibit vesicular transport through the secretory pathway. *EMBO J.* 9: 2375–2383.

Preston, G. M., Billis, W. M., and White, B. A. (1990). Transcriptional and posttranscriptional regulation of the rat prolactin gene by calcium. *Mol. Cell. Biol.* 10: 442–448.

Putney, J. W., Jr., Takemura, H., Hughes, A. R., Horstman, D. A., and Thastrup, O. (1989). How do inositol phosphates regulate calcium signaling? *FASEB J.* 3: 1899–1905.

Quissell, D. O., and Tabak, L. A. (1989). Salivary mucin secretion. In: Handbook of Physiology. Salivary, Pancreatic, Gastric, and Hepatobiliary Secretions. Edited by J. G. Forte. Bethesda, American Physiological Society, pp. 79–91.

Quissell, D. O., Deisher, L. M., and Barzen, K. A. (1983). Role of protein phosphorylation in regulating rat submandibular mucin secretion. *Am. J. Physiol.* 245: G44–G53.

Quissell, D. O., Deisher, L. M., and Barzen, K. A. (1985). The rate determining step in cyclic AMP-mediated exocytosis in the rat parotid and submandibular glands appears to involve analogous 26-kDa integral membrane phosphoproteins. *Proc. Natl. Acad. Sci. USA* 82: 3237–3241.

Reaves, B., and Banting, G. (1992). Perturbation of the morphology of the trans-Golgi network following brefeldin A treatment: redistribution of a TGN-specific integral membrane protein, TGN38. *J. Cell. Biol.* 116: 85–94.

Reaves, B., Wilde, A., and Banting, G. (1992). Identification, molecular characterization and immunolocalization of an isoform of the *trans*-Golgi-network (TGN)-specific integral membrane protein TGN38. *Biochem. J.* 283: 313–316.

Redding, K., Holcomb, C., and Fuller, R. S. (1991). Immunolocalization of Kex2 protease identifies a putative late Golgi compartment in the yeast *Saccharomyces cerevisiae*. *J. Cell Biol.* 113: 527–538.

Rehfuss, R. P., Walton, K. M., Loriaux, M. M., and Goodman, R. H. (1991). The cAMP-regulated enhancer-binding protein ATF-1 activates cAMP-dependent protein kinase A. *J. Biol. Chem.* 266: 18431–18434.

Rine, J., Hansen, W., Hardeman, E., and Davis, R. W. (1983). Targeted selection of recombinant clones through gene dosage effects. *Proc. Natl. Acad. Sci. USA* 80: 6750–6754.

Riordan, J. R., Rommens, J. M., Kerem, B.-S., Alon, N., Rozmahel, R., Grzelczak, Z., Zielenski, J., Lok, S., Plavsic, N., Chou, J.-L., Drumm, M. L., Iannuzzi, M. C., Collins, F. S., and Tsui, L.-C. (1989). Identification of the cystic fibrosis gene: Cloning and characterization of complementary DNA. *Science* 245: 1066–1073.

Roberts, S. G. E., Layfield, R., and McDonald, C. J. (1991). The mouse proline-rich protein MP6 promoter binds isoprenaline-inducible parotid nuclear proteins via a highly conserved NFκB/rel-like site. *Nucleic Acids Res.* 19: 5205–5211.

Rodland, K. C., Muldoon, L. L., Lenormand, P., and Magun, B. E. (1990). Modulation of RNA expression by intracellular calcium: Existence of a threshold calcium concentration for induction of VL30 RNA by epidermal growth factor, endothelin, and protein kinase C. *J. Biol. Chem.* 265: 11000–11007.

Roeder, R. G. (1991). The complexities of eukaryotic transcription initiation: Regulation of preinitiation complex assembly. *Trends Biochem. Sci.* 16: 402–407.

Roesler, W. J., Vandenbark, G. R., and Hanson, R. W. (1988). Cyclic AMP and the induction of eukaryotic gene transcription. *J. Biol. Chem.* 263: 9063–9066.

Rosa, P., Mantovani, S., Rosboch, R., and Huttner, W. B. (1992). Monensin and brefeldin A differentially affect the phosphorylation and sulfation of secretory proteins. *J. Biol. Chem.* 267: 12227–12232.

Roseman, S. (1970). The synthesis of complex carbohydrates by multiglycosyltransferase systems and their potential function in intercellular adhesion. *Chem. Phys. Lipids* 5: 270–297.

Rosenthal, W., Hescheler, J., Trautwein, W., and Schultz, G. (1988). Control of voltage-dependent Ca^{2+} channels by G protein-coupled receptors. *FASEB J.* 2: 2784–2790.

Rosenwald, A. G., Stoll, J., and Krag, S. S. (1990). Regulation of glycosylation. *J. Biol. Chem.* 265: 14544–14553.

Ross, C. A., Meldolesi, J., Milner, T. A., Satoh, T., Supattapone, S., and Snyder, S. H. (1989). Inositol 1,4,5-trisphosphate receptor localized to endoplasmic reticulum in cerebellar Purkinje neurons. *Nature* 339: 468–470.

Rossi, G., Jiang, Y., Newman, A. P., and Ferro-Novick, S. (1991). Dependence of Ypt1 and Sec4 membrane attachment on Bet2. *Nature* 351: 158–161.

Roth, J. (1987). Subcellular organization of glycosylation in mammalian cells. *Biochim. Biophys. Acta* 906: 405–436.

Rothman, J. E. (1987). Protein sorting by selective retention in the endoplasmic reticulum and Golgi stack. *Cell* 50: 521–522.

Rothman, J. E. (1989). Polypeptide chain binding proteins: Catalysts of protein folding and related processes in cells. *Cell* 59: 591–601.

Rothman, J. E., and Orci, L. (1992). Molecular dissection of the secretory pathway. *Nature* 355: 409–415.

Roux, E., Strubin, M., Hagenbüchle, O., and Wellauer, P. K. (1989). The cell-specific transcription factor PTF1 contains two different subunits that interact with the DNA. *Gene Dev.* 3: 1613–1624.

Rowlands, A. G., Panniers, R., and Henshaw, E. C. (1988). The catalytic mechanism of guanine nucleotide exchange factor action and competitive inhibition by phosphory-lated eukaryotic initiation factor. *J. Biol. Chem.* 263: 5526–5533.

Ruohola, H., Kabcenell, A. K., and Ferro-Novick, S. (1988). Reconstitution of protein transport from the endoplasmic reticulum to the Golgi complex in yeast: The acceptor Golgi compartment is defective in the sec23 mutant. *J. Cell Biol.* 107: 1465–1476.

Sakaue, M., and Hoffman, B. B. (1991). cAMP regulates transcription of the α_{2A} adrenergic receptor gene in HT-29 cells. *J. Biol. Chem.* 266: 5743–5749.

Sanders, S. L., Whitfield, K. M., Vogel, J. P., Rose, M. D., and Schekman, R. W. (1992). Sec61p and BiP directly facilitate polypeptide translocation into the ER. *Cell* 69: 353–365.

Santer, U. V., DeSantis, R., Hard, K. J., van Kuik, J. A., Vliegenthart, J. F. G., Won, B., and Glick, M. C. (1989). *N*-linked oligosaccharide changes with oncogenic transforma-tion require sialylation of multiantennae. *Eur. J. Biochem.* 181: 249–260.

Saraste, J., Palade, G. E., and Farquhar, M. G. (1986). Temperature-sensitive steps in the transport of secretory proteins through the Golgi complex in exocrine pancreatic cells. *Proc. Natl. Acad. Sci. USA* 83: 6425–6429.

Savarese, T. M., and Fraser, C. M. (1992). In vitro mutagenesis and the search for structure–function relationships among G protein-coupled receptors. *Biochem. J.* 283: 1–19.

Savitz, A. J., and Meyer, D. I. (1990). Identification of a ribosome receptor in the rough endoplasmic reticulum. *Nature* 346: 540–544.

Schachter, H. (1986). Biosynthetic controls that determine the branching and micro-heterogeneity of protein-bound oligosaccharides. *Biochem. Cell Biol.* 64: 163–181.

Schachter, H. (1991). The "yellow brick road" to branched complex *N*-glycans. *Glycobiol-ogy* 1: 453–461.

Scheele, G., and Jacoby, R. (1982). Conformational changes associated with proteolytic processing of presecretory proteins allow glutathione-catalyzed formation of native disulfide bonds. *J. Biol. Chem.* 257: 12277–12282.

Scheele, G., and Jacoby, R. (1983). Proteolytic processing of presecretory proteins is required for development of biological activities in pancreatic exocrine proteins. *J. Biol. Chem.* 258: 2005–2009.

Scheele, G., and Tartakoff, A. (1985). Exit of non-glycosylated secretory proteins from the rough endoplasmic reticulum is asynchronous in the exocrine pancreas. *J. Biol. Chem.* 260: 926–931.

Schekman, R. (1982). The secretory pathway in yeast. *Trends Biochem. Sci.* 7: 243–246.

Schimmel, P. (1990). Hazards and their exploitation in the applications of molecular biology to structure–function relationships. *Biochemistry* 29: 9495–9502.

Schmitt, H. D., Puzicha, M., and Gallwitz, D. (1988). Study of a temperature-sensitive mutant of the *ras*-related *YPT1* gene product in yeast suggests a role in the regula-tion of intracellular calcium. *Cell* 53: 635–647.

Schnefel, S., Pröfrock, A., Hinsch, K. D., and Schultz, I. (1990). Cholecystokinin activates Gi_1, Gi_2, and Gi_3 and several G_s proteins in rat pancreatic acinar cells. *Biochem. J.* 269: 483–488.

Schönbrunner, E. R., and Schmid, F. X. (1992). Peptidyl-prolyl *cis–trans* isomerase improves the efficiency of protein disulfide isomerase as a catalyst of protein folding. *Proc. Natl. Acad. Sci. USA* 89: 4510–4513.

Schwaninger, R., Beckers, C. J. M., and Balch, W. E. (1991). Sequential transport of protein between the endoplasmic reticulum and successive Golgi compartments in semi-intact cells. *J. Biol. Chem.* 266: 13055–13063.

Schwartz, T. W. (1986). The processing of peptide precursors: "Proline-directed arginyl cleavage" and other monobasic processing mechanisms. *FEBS Lett.* 200: 1–10.

Schwarz, J. K., Capasso, J. M., and Hirschberg, C. B. (1984). Translocation of adenosine 3'-phosphate 5'-phosphosulfate into rat liver Golgi vesicles. *J. Biol. Chem.* 259: 3554–3559.

Schweizer, A., Fransen, J., Matter, K., Kreis, T. E., Ginsel, L., and Hauri, H. P. (1990). Identification of an intermediate compartment involved in protein transport from ER to Golgi apparatus. *Eur. J. Cell Biol.* 53: 185–196.

Schweizer, A., Matter, K., Ketcham, C. M., and Hauri, H.-P. (1991). The isolated ER–Golgi intermediate compartment exhibits properties that are different from ER and *cis*-Golgi. *J. Cell Biol.* 113: 45–54.

Scocca, J. R., and Krag, S. S. (1990). Sequence of a cDNA that specifies the uridine diphosphate N-acetyl-D-glucosamine:dolichol phosphate N-acetylglucosamine-1-phosphate transferase from Chinese hamster ovary cells. *J. Biol. Chem.* 265: 20621–20626.

Segev, N. (1991). Mediation of the attachment or fusion step in vesicular transport by the GTP-binding Ypt1 protein. *Science* 252: 1553–1556.

Segev, N., Mulholland, J., and Botstein, D. (1988). The yeast GTP-binding YPT1 protein and a mammalian counterpart are associated with the secretion machinery. *Cell* 52: 915–924.

Semenza, J. C., Hardwick, K. G., Dean, N., and Pelham, H. R. B. (1990). *ERD2* a yeast gene required for the receptor-mediated retrieval of luminal ER proteins from the secretory pathway. *Cell* 61: 1349–1357.

Serafini, T., Stenbeck, G., Brecht, A., Lottspeich, F., Orci, L., Rothman, J. E., and Wieland, F. T. (1991). A coat subunit of Golgi-derived nonclathrin-coated vesicles with homology to the clathrin-coated vesicle coat protein β-adaptin. *Nature* 349: 215–220.

Shakin-Eshleman, S. H., Remaley, A. T., Eshleman, J. R., Wunner, W. H., and Spitalnik, S. L. (1992). N-Linked glycosylation of rabies virus glycoprotein. *J. Biol. Chem.* 267: 10690–10698.

Shelness, G., Kanwar, Y. S., and Blobel, G. (1988). cDNA-derived primary structure of the glycoprotein component of canine microsomal signal peptidase complex. *J. Biol. Chem.* 263: 17063–17070.

Sheng, M., Thompson, M. A., and Greenberg, M. E. (1991). CREB: a Ca^{2+}-regulated transcription factor phosphorylated by calmodulin-dependent kinases. *Science* 252: 1427–1430.

Shenolikar, S. (1988). Protein phosphorylation: Hormones, drugs, and bioregulation. *FASEB J.* 2: 2753–2764.

Sherman, F., Fink, G., and Lawrence, C. (1974). *Methods in Yeast Genetics.* Cold Spring Harbor, N.Y., Cold Spring Harbor Laboratory Press.

Shim, J., Newman, A. P., and Ferro-Novick, S. (1991). The *BOS1* gene encodes an essential

27-kD putative membrane protein that is required for vesicular transport from the ER to the Golgi complex in yeast. *J. Cell Biol.* 113: 55–64.

Shite, S., Seguchi, T., Mizoguchi, H., Ono, M., and Kuwano, M. (1990). Differential effects of brefeldin A on sialylation of *N*- and *O*-linked oligosaccharides in low density lipoprotein receptor and epidermal growth factor receptor. *J. Biol. Chem.* 265: 17385–17388.

Siegel, V., and Walter, P. (1988). Each of the activities of signal recognition particle (SRP) is contained within a distinct domain: Analysis of biochemical mutants of SRP. *Cell* 52: 39–49.

Simon, M. I., Strathmann, M. P., and Gautam, N. (1991). Diversity of G proteins in signal transduction. *Science* 252: 802–808.

Simon, S., and Blobel, G. (1991). A protein-conducting channel in the endoplasmic reticulum. *Cell* 65: 371–380.

Simson, J. A. (1977). The influence of fixation on the carbohydrate cytochemistry of rat salivary gland secretory granules. *Histochem. J.* 9: 645–657.

Skelton, T. P., Hooper, L. V., Srivastava, V., Hindsgaul, O., and Baenziger, J. U. (1991). Characterization of a sulfotransferase responsible for the 4-*O*-sulfation of terminal β-*N*-acetyl-D-galactosamine on asparagine-linked oligosaccharides of glycoprotein hormones. *J. Biol. Chem.* 266: 17142–17150.

Skelton, T. P., Kumar, S., Smith, P. L., Beranek, M. C., and Baenziger, J. U. (1992). Proopiomelanocortin synthesized by corticotrophs bears asparagine-linked oligosaccharides terminating with SO_4-4GalNAcβ1,4GlcNAcβ1,2Manα. *J. Biol. Chem.* 267: 12998–13006.

Smith, P. L., and Baenziger, J. U. (1992). Molecular basis of recognition by the glycoprotein hormone-specific *N*-acetylgalactosamine-transferase. *Proc. Natl. Acad. Sci. USA* 89: 329–333.

Sobel, A. (1991). Stathmin: A relay phosphoprotein for multiple signal transduction? *Trends Biochem. Sci.* 16: 301–305.

Söling, H.-D., Fest, W., Schmidt, T., Esselmann, H., and Bachmann, V. (1989). Signal transmission in exocrine cells is associated with rapid activity changes of acyltransferases and diacylglycerol kinase due to reversible protein phosphorylation. *J. Biol. Chem.* 264: 10643–10648.

Sommer, L., Hagenbüchle, O., Wellauer, P. K., and Strubin, M. (1991). Nuclear targeting of the transcription factor PRF1 is mediated by a protein subunit that does not bind to the PRF1 cognate sequence. *Cell* 67: 987–994.

Spiegel, A. M., Backlund, P. S., Jr., Butrynski, J. E., Jones, T. L. Z., and Simonds, W. F. (1991). The G protein connection: Molecular basis of membrane association. *Trends Genet.* 16: 338–341.

Spiro, R. G., and Bhoyroo, V. D. (1988). Occurrence of sulfate in the asparagine-linked complex carbohydrate units of thyroglobulin. *J. Biol. Chem.* 263: 14351–14358.

Stirling, C. J., Rothblatt, J., Hosobucchi, M., Deshaies, R., and Schekman, R. (1992) Protein translocation mutants defective in the insertion of integral membrane proteins into the endoplasmic reticulum. *Molec. Biol. Cell* 3: 129–142.

Stoller, T., and Shields, D. (1989). The role of paired basic amino acids in mediating proteolytic cleavage of prosomatostatin. *J. Biol. Chem.* 264: 6922–6928.

Stratowa, C., and Rutter, W. J. (1986). Selective regulation of trypsin gene expression by calcium and by glucose starvation in a rat exocrine pancreas cell line. *Proc. Natl. Acad. Sci. USA* 83: 4292–4296.

Strosberg, A. D. (1991). Structure/function relationship of proteins belonging to the family of receptors coupled to GTP-binding proteins. *Eur. J. Biochem.* 196: 1–10.

Symington, B. E., Symington, F. W., and Rohrschneider, L. R. (1989). Phorbol ester induces increased expression, altered glycosylation, and reduced adhesion of K562 erythroleukemia cell fibronectin receptors. *J. Biol. Chem.* 264: 13258–13266.

Tabak, L. A. (1991). Genetic control of salivary mucin formation. In *Aspects of Oral Molecular Biology.* Edited by D. B. Ferguson. Basel, S. Karger, pp. 77–94.

Tabak, L. A., and Levine, M. J. (1981). Characterization of sulphated monosaccharides from stumptail monkey salivary mucin. *Arch. Oral Biol.* 26: 315–317.

Tabak, L. A., Levine, M. J., Mandel, I. D., and Ellison, S. A. (1982). Role of salivary mucins in the protection of the oral cavity. *J. Oral Pathol.* 11: 1–17.

Takuma, T. (1990). Evidence of the involvement of cyclic AMP-dependent protein kinase in the exocytosis of amylase from parotid acinar cells. *J. Biochem.* 108: 99–102.

Tang, W.-J., and Gilman, A. G. (1991). Type-specific regulation of adenylyl cyclase by G protein $\beta\gamma$ subunits. *Science* 254: 1500–1503.

Taylor, C. W., and Richardson, A. (1991). Structure and function of inositol trisphosphate receptors. *Pharmacol. Ther.* 51: 97–137.

Taylor, S. S. (1989). cAMP-dependent protein kinase: Model for an enzyme family. *J. Biol. Chem.* 264: 8443–8446.

Taylor, S. S., Bubis, J., Toner-Webb, J., Saraswat, L. D., First, E. A., Buechler, J. A., Knighton, D. R., and Sowadski, J. (1988). cAMP-dependent protein kinase: Prototype for a family of enzymes. *FASEB J.* 2: 2677–2685.

Tazawa, S., Unuma, M., Tondokoro, N., Asano, Y., Ohsumi, T., Ishimura, T., and Sugano, H. (1991). Identification of a membrane protein responsible for ribosome binding in rough microsomal membranes. *J. Biochem. (Tokyo)* 109: 89–98.

te Heesen, S., Janetzky, B., Lehle, L., and Aebi, M. (1992). The yeast *WBP1* is essential for oligosaccharyl transferase activity in vivo and in vitro *EMBO J.* 11: 2071–2075.

te Heesen, S., Rauhut, R., Aebersold, R., Abelson, J., Aebi, M., and Clark, M. W. (1991). An essential 45 kDa yeast transmembrane protein reacts with anti-nuclear pore antibodies: Purification of the protein immunolocalization and cloning of the gene. *Eur. J. Cell. Biol.* 56: 8–18.

Thomas, R. F., Holt, B. D., Schwinn, D. A., and Liggett, S. B. (1992). Long-term agonist exposure induces upregulation of β_3-adrenergic receptor expression via multiple cAMP response elements. *Proc. Natl. Acad. Sci. USA* 89: 4490–4494.

Tooze, S. A., and Huttner, W. B. (1990). Cell-free protein sorting to the regulated and constitutive secretory pathways. *Cell* 60: 837–847.

van der Krol, A. R., Mol, J. N. M., and Stuitje, A. R. (1988). Modulation of eukaryotic gene expression by complementary RNA or DNA sequences. *BioTechniques* 6: 958–976.

Venter J. C., Fraser, C. M., Kerlavage, A. R., and Buck, M. A. (1989). Molecular biology of adrenergic and muscarinic cholinergic receptors: A perspective. *Biochem. Pharmacol.* 38: 1197–1208.

Volpe, P., Krause, K.-H., Hashimoto, S., Zorzato, F., Pozzan, T., Meldolesi, J., and Lew, D. P. (1988). "Calciosome," a cytoplasmic organelle: The inositol 1,4,5-trisphosphate-sensitive Ca^{2+} store of nonmuscle cells? *Proc. Natl. Acad. Sci. USA* 85: 1091–1095.

von Heijne, G. (1983). Patterns of amino acids near signal–sequence cleavage sites. *Eur. J. Biochem.* 133: 17–21.

von Heijne, G. (1985). Signal sequences: The limits of variation. *J. Mol. Biol.* 184: 99–105.

von Heijne, G. (1986). A new method for predicting signal sequence cleavage sites. *Nucleic Acids Res.* 14: 4683–4690.

von Zastrow, M., Tritton, T. R., and Castle, J. D. (1986). Exocrine secretion granules contain peptide amidation activity. *Proc. Natl. Acad. Sci.* 83: 3297–3301.

von Zastrow, M., and Castle, J. D. (1987). Protein sorting among two distinct export pathways occurs from the content of maturing exocrine storage granules. *J. Cell Biol.* 105: 2675–2684.

Walter, P., and Blobel, G. (1981). Translocation of proteins across the endoplasmic reticulum. III. Signal recognition protein (SRP) causes signal sequence-dependent and site-specific arrest of chain elongation that is released by microsomal membranes. *J. Cell Biol.* 91: 557–561.

Walter, P., Ibrahimi, I., and Blobel, G. (1981). Translocation of proteins across the endoplasmic reticulum. I. Signal recognition protein (SRP) binds to in vitro assembled polysomes synthesizing secretory proteins. *J. Cell Biol.* 91: 545–550.

Walworth, N. C., Brennwald, P., Kabcenell, A. K., Garrett, M., and Novick, P. (1992). Hydrolysis of GTP by Sec4 protein plays an important role in vesicular transport and is stimulated by a GTPase-activating protein in *Saccharomyces cerevisiae*. *Mol. Cell. Biol.* 12: 2017–2028.

Wang, Y., Abernethy, J. L., Eckhardt, A. E., and Hill, R. L. (1992). Purification and characterization of a UDP-GalNAc:polypeptide *N*-acetylgalactosaminyltransferase specific for glycosylation of threonine residues. *J. Biol. Chem.* 267: 12709–12716.

Waters, M. G., Serafini, T., and Rothman, J. E. (1991). "Coatomer": A cytosolic protein complex containing subunits of non-clathrin-coated Golgi transport vesicles. *Nature* 349: 248–251.

Weidman, P. J., Melançon, P., Block, M. R., and Rothman, J. E. (1989). Binding of an *N*-ethylmaleimide-sensitive fusion protein to Golgi membranes requires both a soluble protein(s) and an integral membrane receptor. *J. Cell Biol.* 108: 1589–1596.

Weinrich, S. L., Meister, A., and Rutter, W. J. (1991). Exocrine pancreas transcription factor 1 binds to a bipartite enhancer element and activates transcription of acinar genes. *Molec. Cell. Biol.* 11: 4985–4997.

Wieland, F. T., Gleason, M. L., Serafini, T. A., and Rothman, J. E. (1987). The rate of bulk flow from the endoplasmic reticulum to the cell surface. *Cell* 50: 289–300.

Williams, D., and Schachter, H. (1980). Mucin synthesis. I. Detection in canine submaxillary glands of an *N*-acetylglucosaminyltransferase which acts on mucin substrate. *J. Biol. Chem.* 255: 11247–11252.

Williams, D., Longmore, G., Matta, K. L., and Schachter, H. (1980). Mucin synthesis. II. Substrate specificity and product identification studies on canine submaxillary gland UDP-GlcNac:Gal-β-1-3GalNac(GlcNac-GalNac)-β-6-*N*-acetylglucosaminyltransferase. *J. Biol. Chem.* 255: 11253–11261.

Wilson, D. W., Wilcox, C. A., Flynn, G. C., Chen, E., Kuang, W.-J., Henzel, W. J., Block, M. R., Ulrich, A., and Rothman, J. E. (1989). A fusion protein required for vesicle-mediated transport in both mammalian cells and yeast. *Nature* 339: 355–359.

Wilson, I. B. H., Gavel, Y., and von Heijne, G. (1991). Amino acid distributions around *O*-linked glycosylation sites. *Biochem. J.* 275: 529–534.

Wright, P. S., Lenney, C., and Carlson, D. M. (1990). Regulation of proline-rich protein gene expression by cyclic AMP in primary cultures of hamster parotid glands. *J. Mol. Endocrinol.* 4: 81–87.

Yamashita, S., and Yasuda, K. (1992). Monoclonal antibody to a common antigen of secretory granule membranes: Intracellular localization and recycling of the antigen after secretion. *J. Histochem. Cytochem.* 40: 793–806.

Yatani, A., Mattera, R., Codina, J., Graf, R., Okabe, K., Padrell, E., Iyengar, R., Brown, A. M., and Birnbaumer, L. (1988). The G protein-gated atrial K$^+$ channel is stimulated by three distinct G$_i$ δ-subunits. *Nature* 336: 680–682.

Yeo, K. T., Parent, J. B., Yeo, T.-K., and Olden, K. (1985). Variability in transport rates of secretory glycoproteins through the endoplasmic reticulum and Golgi in human hepatoma cells. *J. Biol. Chem.* 260: 7896–7902.

Yet, M.-G., and Wold, F. (1990). The distribution of glycan structures in individual *N*-glycosylation sites in animal and plant glycoproteins. *Arch. Biochem. Biophys.* 278: 356–364.

Yusuf, H. K. M., Pohlentz, G., Schwarzmann, G., and Sandhoff, K. (1984). Ganglioside biosynthesis in rat liver Golgi apparatus: Stimulation by phosphatidylglycerol and inhibition by tunicamycin. In *Ganglioside Structure, Function and Biomedical Potential*. Edited by R. W. Ledeen, R. K. Yu, M. M. Rapport, and K. Suzuki. New York, Plenum Press, pp. 227–239.

Zhu, X., and Lehrman, M. A. (1990). Cloning, sequence, and expression of a cDNA encoding hamster UDP-GlcNAc:dolichol phosphate *N*-acetylglucosamine-1-phosphate transferase. *J. Biol. Chem.* 265: 14250–14255.

Zhu, X., Zeng, Y., and Lehrman, M. A. (1992). Evidence that the hamster tunicamycin resistance gene encodes UDP-GlcNAc:dolichol phosphate *N*-acetylglucosamine-1-phosphate transferase. *J. Biol. Chem.* 267: 8895–8902.

Ziff, E. B. (1990). Transcription factors: A new family gathers at the cAMP response site. *Trends Genet. 6: 69–72.*

3

Molecular Biophysics of Mucin Secretion

PEDRO VERDUGO

University of Washington
Seattle, Washington

I. Introduction

Our understanding of the early synthetic events in regulated secretion that take place in the endoplasmic reticulum and the Golgi apparatus of the secretory cell has advanced dramatically in the last few years. However, the steps that follow synthesis, namely, the sorting of different secretory products, their concentration and packing in secretory granules, the docking of granules to the plasma membrane, and their release from the cell, still remain very controversial. This review will briefly outline the current and still rudimentary understanding of how mucins, the gigantic polymers of the mucous matrix, are stored in secretory granules and released during exocytosis from the goblet cells of the airway.

The early steps of mucin transcription and glycosylation can be understood within the realm of chemical synthesis. However, the later events of mucin processing, including the condensation of these polymers in the secretory granule, their decondensation upon exocytosis, and their final gelation to form the mucus, are physical rather than chemical in nature and can best be approached and explained by established principles of polymer gel physics.

Mucus is a complex polymer gel. Like other polymer hydrogels, it is composed of a polymer network and a solvent, water. Although the solvent maintains the polymer network's expansion, the network confines the solvent within its own boundaries. A family of highly polyionic polymers of large molecular dimensions composes the mucous network. Among these polymers, mucins are the most ubiquitous; others include proteoglycans and nucleic acids, which are often found in mucus from diseased airways (Potter et al., 1963; Havez and Roussel, 1976; Kaliner et al., 1984; Bhaskar et al., 1985).

We will begin by considering the network–solvent interactions, including the physical properties of the mucins that form the mucous matrix, the topology of interconnections that hold them together, and the interactions of this matrix with water that result in the formation of the mucous gel (Fig. 1). The subsequent sections focus on the condensation of mucins inside the secretory granule, and their decondensation upon exocytosis. The events that follow exocytosis (i.e.,

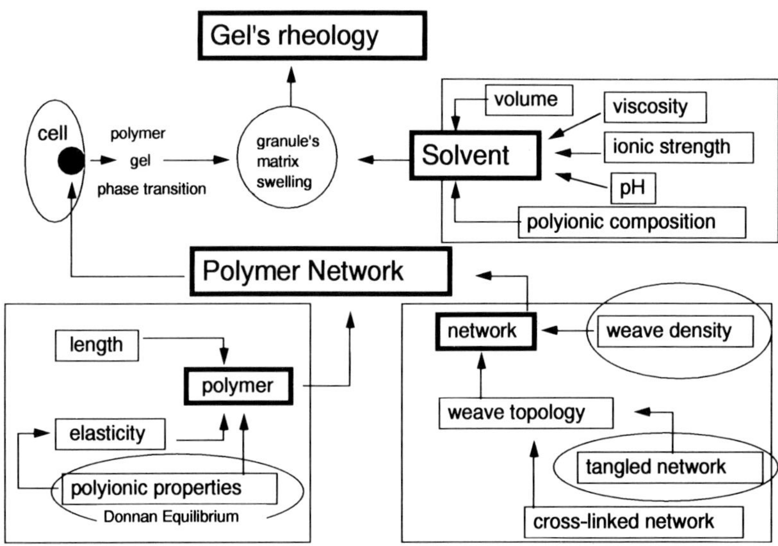

Figure 1   This diagram illustrates the different steps of product release in secretion. It also shows the interrelation of the various physicochemical factors that intervene in secretory product condensation and decondensation. In the particular case of mucin secretion, decondensation leads to the formation of the mucous gel. While stored inside the secretory granule, mucins form a condensed polymer network. During exocytosis the mucin network undergoes a polymer gel-phase transition from condensed to decondensed phase. This transition is accompanied by massive swelling driven by the Donnan potential generated by the polyionic mucin matrix. A detailed description of the interaction of the different factors that intervene in mucin swelling and gelation is in the text. The circles identify those factors that are particularly relevant to mucin condensation, decondensation, and gelation.

mucin gelation and the formation of mucus) have been discussed in previous reviews (Verdugo, 1990, 1991) and will not be covered in detail in this chapter. An elementary knowledge of some fundamental principles of polymer gel physics is necessary to approach the subject of mucous secretion. When pertinent, these principles will be presented briefly at the beginning of each section.

II. Network–Solvent Interactions in Polymer Gels

A. Molecular Topology of the Mucin Network

The rheology of polymer gels can vary widely from a fluid to a solidlike material. The molecular topology of the polymer network plays a critical role in determining the rheological properties of a gel. Both the nature and density of the links among polymers in the matrix are important. The higher the number of interconnections per unit volume, or weave density, the more solid the gel (see Fig. 1). Swelling of the matrix decreases weave density and, therefore, has a strong influence on the rheological properties of gels. In covalently cross-linked gels, swelling is limited to a maximum volume, at which point the interconnections between cross-links are fully extended, restricting further expansion (Flory, 1969). In these gels, the maximum swelling volume decreases as the interchain cross-linking increases. Thus, the rheological properties of cross-linked gels ultimately rely on the degree of covalent bonding in the matrix. Conversely, gels containing a network held together by tangles and low-energy bonds can swell to complete dispersion as the polymers move away from each other by diffusing (reptate) along their longitudinal axis (Edwards and Grant, 1973; Edwards, 1986). As their weave density decreases with the square of increasing volume, swelling becomes the single most important determinant of their rheological properties.

Another significant difference between gels containing tangled, as opposed to covalently cross-linked, polymer matrices, lies in their annealing properties. When two gels come into contact, those having a cross-linked network do not anneal to each other. Conversely, those containing a tangled matrix can easily anneal, because polymers can freely migrate from one gel into another, interpenetrating their polymer networks and forming a single interwoven network.

Cross-Linked Versus Tangled Mucin Matrix

For many years mucus was thought to have a covalently cross-linked mucin polymer matrix. It was believed that mucins were interconnected by cysteine residues of the mucin peptide chains, forming a three-dimensional S:S cross-linked matrix. This idea was based on the observation that cleaving of disulfide bonds results in the dispersion of the mucous gel (Gibbons and Mattner, 1966; Roberts, 1976). As for the regulation of mucus' rheology, in the case of cervical mucus that undergoes broad cyclic variations, it was believed that hormonal or other regulatory messages would modulate the degree of S:S bonding among the mucins produced by secretory cells and, thereby, modulate mucus' rheology (Odeblad, 1976). For respiratory mucus, the picture still found in many textbooks is that mucus results from a mix of a fluid serous secretion with a viscous mucous secretion. Changes in mucus' rheology would result from variations in the proportion of these two secretions.

However, the idea of a covalently bonded mucin matrix cannot explain how mucins released in discrete quantal packages from secretory granules anneal with each other, forming a fully interconnected mucous gel. Nonetheless, the notion of an S:S cross-linked mucin matrix dominated the field of mucus research for many years, and it is still presented in some textbooks.

The application of nondestructive methods to study the conformation of mucus rendered a very different picture of the mucin network's molecular topology. Experiments using laser-scattering spectroscopy to determine the mobility of mucin chains in native undegraded mucus gave the first indications that mucins might not be covalently cross-linked. These measurements reveal that mucins inside the mucous gel exhibit reptative diffusion (Lee et al., 1977; Verdugo et al., 1983). Reptative diffusion, by analogy to a randomly moving snake, refers to the translational diffusional movements that occur along the axis of a polymer chain (Edwards, 1986). Since reptative diffusion does not take place in polymer chains that are covalently cross-linked, these results conflicted with the orthodox idea that mucin chains are interconnected by disulfide bonds. Instead, they provided the first compelling indication that mucins might be loosely held together by tangles and low-energy bonds.

Superficially, the difference between these two conformational models for the mucin network seems insignificant. However, the idea of a tangled network revealed a set of intriguing implications. First, the finding of reptational diffusion in the mucin matrix implied that mucins should be linear, rather than branched, as had been proposed by the disulfide cross-linked model. This subject will be further discussed below. Second, as explained earlier, the rheological properties of a gel containing a tangled matrix depend on tangle density. As the number of tangles decreases with the square of the volume of the gel (Edwards, 1986), swelling becomes the most powerful determinant of mucus' rheology (Wolf et al., 1977). Finally, the notion of a tangled matrix furnished a straightforward explanation for the characteristic annealing properties of the mucous gel.

B. Structure and Functional Properties of the Mucin Polymers

The basic building block of the mucous gel is the mucin polymer. Mucins are glycoproteins containing a long peptide backbone, or apomucin, in which glycosylated (hydrophilic) regions alternate with nonglycosylated (hydrophobic) domains. The glycosylated domains amount to about 75% of the polymer and contain short chains of six to eight sugar monomers. Sugars are connected to the apomucin backbone by *O*-glycosidic bridges between *N*-acetylgalactosamine and either serine or threonine residues of the peptide, forming a bottle-brushlike structure (Boat et al., 1976; Kent, 1978; Carlstedt and Sheehan, 1984; Slayter et al., 1984; Kaliner et al., 1988). For many years mucins were thought to be branched polymers interconnected by disulfide bonds (Gibbons and Mattner, 1966; Roberts, 1976). The finding of reptative diffusion first suggested that mucins might be linear (Lee et al., 1977; Verdugo et al., 1983). Other, more direct and robust lines of structural evidence, including rotary-shadowing electron microscopy, have now demonstrated that mucins form a heterogeneous group of linear polymers of gigantic molecular dimensions, the chain length of which can reach up to several micrometers (Harding et al., 1983; Slayer et al., 1984; Carlstedt and Sheehan, 1984; Sheehan et al., 1986).

Mucin Length

The characteristic size heterogeneity found in mucins had been thought to result from chemical breakdown during preparative procedures. However, the application of molecular cloning to search for the primary structure of epithelial mucins reveals that there are not one, but several, cDNAs that encode for different-sized apomucins (Gendler et al., 1987; Gum et al., 1990; Porchet et al., 1991; see also Chap. 8). The sequence of all these clones contains a characteristic array of tandem repeated nucleotides that encode a correspondingly repeated peptide. However, these tandems exhibit a broad range of variation in both sequence and length between different mucins. The idea of a repeat unit is consistent with the model proposed by Silberberg (1987). His observations indicate that there is a proportional log–log relationship between the radius of gyration and relative molecular mass (M_4) in mucins of different sizes. This is a characteristic feature of a linear random coil. An estimation of the size of the corresponding Kuhn statistical element renders a subunit of 150 nm, with a radius of gyration of about 40 nm, and an M_r of 0.5 MDa. In this model, longer polymer chains would result from the association of subunits.

The finding that secretory cells can produce mucins of different lengths may have important functional significance in explaining how goblet cells can control the swelling properties of the secreted mucin polymer matrix and, thereby, the rheology of the resulting mucus. The swelling of gels is hindered by the mobility or diffusivity of the polymers inside the gel's matrix (Tanaka and Fillmore, 1979). In gels containing a cross-linked matrix, the polymer chains are locked in place by the interchain cross-links, and swelling is limited to a finite maximum volume. However, in gels containing a tangled matrix, such as mucus, the mucin chains can disperse, moving according to their own diffusivities. As the time for chains to diffuse (reptate) away from each other increases with the square of the polymer length (Edwards, 1986), small variations in mucin length can result in drastic changes in the swelling kinetics of the mucin network. This exponential relationship between diffusional time and polymer length also explains why cleaving of the S:S bonds of the apomucin polymer, which shortens the length of the mucin chains, can drastically accelerate the dispersion of the mucous gel.

Thus, if hormones or other transmitters could modulate the expression of mucins of different lengths, they could efficiently control the swelling rate of the mucin matrix and the rheological properties of mucus. Unfortunately, this issue has been ignored and remains a theoretical prediction to be explored in the future.

Mucin Polyionic Properties

Another significant feature of the mucin polymers is their polyanionic properties. Sialic acid and sulfated sugars found in terminal positions in the glycosydic side chains are the moieties that give mucins their remarkably strong polyanionic properties.

The most important consequence of the polyionic character of mucins is in the swelling properties of the networks they form. Although the swelling of neutral gels is driven by concentration gradients and is governed by a simple osmotic mechanism, the swelling of gels containing a polyionic network is driven by charge interactions and is governed by a Donnan equilibrium (Katchalsky et al., 1951).

The finding that desialization has little effect on the rheological properties of mucus brought about the notion that these polyanionic terminals might have little or no significance in the control of mucus rheology (Forstner and Forstner, 1975; Meyer et al., 1975; Crowther and Marriot, 1983). Although sialated and sulfated terminals may have no direct effect on mucus' rheology, these charged moieties can control the rheological properties of mucus insofar as they are the source of the Donnan potential that drives the swelling of mucus (Tam and Verdugo, 1981). The resolution of this apparent controversy is that desialization of a fully swollen mucus should not produce any significant effects on its rheology, since the mucin matrix is already swollen, and tangle density has decreased to a minimum. However, without polyionic terminals, swelling of the mucin network would be driven by simple osmosis. Because of the large size of the mucin polymers, the swelling kinetics of the matrix would be extremely slow, and mucus would remain virtually a highly viscous gel. Thus, the effect of desialization on fully swollen mucus bears little physiological import and can be readily explained by the notion that these moieties have an indirect, rather than a direct, role in mucus' rheology.

Sialation and sulfation of sugar terminals take place in the Golgi and are thought to be highly regulated processes. Although little is known about the signals that modulate sulfation and sialization of mucins in goblet cells, this is another unexplored mechanism whereby hormones or other transmitters could effectively control the swelling properties of the secreted mucins and, thereby, mucus' rheology.

Mucin Polymer Elasticity

The concept of rubber elasticity was introduced by Flory (1969) to characterize the rigidity of polymer chains. When polymer chains are in solution, they adopt a resting equilibrium length. If they are perturbed and displaced from this resting length, the chains will develop a tension that tends to restore the equilibrium length. In polyionic polymers such as mucins, the rubber elasticity of the polymer depends on the charge density of the polymer chain. The higher the charge per unit length, the stiffer the polymer. Since polyionic charges can be screened by counterions, the rubber elasticity of polyionic mucins also depends on the ionic composition of the solvent (Steiner et al., 1984).

When polymers are assembled in a gel matrix, changes in the rubber elasticity of the polymer chains are directly reflected in corresponding changes in the rheological properties of the gel. In mucins, changes in the concentration of Ca^{2+} result in variations in the rheological properties of the mucous gel (Forstner and Forstner, 1975; Marriot et al., 1979). However, desialization of the mucins have had little effect on mucus rheology (Forstner and Forstner, 1975; Meyer et al., 1975; Crowther and Marriot, 1983). In any event, rubber elasticity represents only a small component in the modulation of mucus' rheology, as compared with the effect of changes of hydration of the mucin matrix (Wolf et al., 1977).

Perhaps the most important theoretical implication of changes in rubber elasticity of the mucins is that the high concentrations of Ca^{2+} inside the granule must result in a fairly flexible mucin polymer, lending to its folding and facilitating matrix condensation. Conversely, the shift of shielding cations (Na^+/Ca^{2+}) during exocytosis can result in stiffening of the mucin chains, leading to the unfolding and expansion of the mucin matrix. Unfortunately, none of these alternatives have been experimentally validated, and they remain as homework for future investigations.

C. The Role of the Solvent in Mucin Hydration and Gelation

The most significant consequence from the finding that mucins are held together by tangles and noncovalent bonds is that swelling should be the paramount variable for the control of mucus' rheology. Obviously, the amount of water available can be a limiting factor for hydration of mucus. Other, less obvious, but equally important, factors are the pH and ionic and polyionic composition of the swelling medium. Recent observations suggest that the electrolytic and polyelectrolytic composition of the airway fluid is not constant. The concentration of Na^+, Cl^-, Ca^{2+} (Frizzell, 1988), and albumin (Jacquot et al., 1988), as well as the pH of the airway fluid can vary under the influence of pharmacological mediators. These observations prompted Widdicombe's (1989) idea of a homeostatic mechanism operating in the airway epithelium to control the composition of the airway fluid. Thus, the amount of liquid on the surface of the airway, and especially its composition, plays a most critical function in the regulation of mucus' rheology.

We will examine the importance of the composition of the swelling medium in the following sections.

D. Swelling of Mucus

The early studies of Katchalsky et al. (1951) first indicated that swelling in polyionic gels is governed by a Donnan equilibrium. The polyanionic properties of mucins strongly suggested that swelling of mucus should also be governed by a Donnan equilibrium (Donnan, 1924). The experimental verification that the swelling of mucus is indeed governed by a Donnan principle (Tam and Verdugo, 1981) rendered a solid foundation for understanding the physicochemical mechanisms that control mucus' rheology. It also furnished a powerful predictive paradigm for further investigating the physiology and pathophysiology of respiratory mucus.

According to the Donnan equilibrium, not only the amount, but also the pH and the ionic and polyionic composition of airway surface liquid should be critical determinants of mucus' swelling. In fact, the finding that the swelling of mucus follows a Donnan equilibrium provided one of the first objective indications that defective transepithelial movement of ions, polyions, and water could be the most important factor restricting hydration of mucus in cystic fibrosis (Tam and Verdugo, 1981). The idea that swelling is the main modulator of mucus' rheology also furnished the intriguing implication that mucins might be released in a condensed state, swelling once outside the secretory cell during or after exocytosis (Verdugo, 1984).

In summary, studies by dynamic laser scattering have revealed that mucus is a polymer gel containing a tangled, rather than a covalently cross-linked matrix. These features explain why swelling should be the single most important factor in the control of mucus' rheology. They also emphasize that mucins are linear polymers, and that, according to polymer gel theory, their length and polyionic properties should be the most important determinants of mucous swelling. Owing to the polyionic character of mucins, swelling of mucus is governed by a Donnan equilibrium. Hence, not only the amount, but also the pH and the ionic and polyionic composition of the airway surface liquid should play a critical factor in hydration of mucus in its rheology.

III. Mucin Storage and Release in Goblet Cells

A. Mucin Condensation in the Secretory Granule

For mucins, as for regulated secretion in general, after the secretory material is sorted and segregated into the vesicular compartment, it undergoes variable degrees of condensation (Palade, 1975). That mucins are also condensed in secretory granules is shown indirectly by the high electron density of secretory granules and can also be inferred directly by the dramatic expansion of the mucin–mucin matrix observed during exocytosis (Verdugo, 1984; Verdugo et al., 1987a,b). The nature of molecular mechanisms of condensation of secretory product in goblets, as well as in other secretory cells, remains uncertain. It has been thought that condensation could result from aggregation (Palade, 1975) or from disulfide bonding among intragranular species (Tooze et al., 1989). However, in some mucous granules, the postexocytotic expansion of the mucin network can reach several hundred-fold in just 20–30 ms (Verdugo et al., 1987a,b). These explosive rates of decondensation are not consistent with the idea of protein disaggregation and resolubilization. Neither can they be explained by a covalent bond-breaking mechanism. An alternative explanation can be drawn from the observation that the postexocytotic hydration and expansion of mucins is driven by a Donnan potential (Verdugo et al., 1987a,b; Aitken and Verdugo, 1989). This outcome indicates that decondensation must result from physical charge interactions, rather than from chemical bond breaking. A significant corollary of this argument is that mucin condensation in the granule must require the shielding of the polyionic charges of the mucin matrix.

Charge Shielding in Granule Condensation

Secretory granules of a broad range of secretory cells have two ubiquitous features: they are acidic, and they contain a distinct combination of two counter-charged species: a large polyanionic polymer, which is usually interconnected, forming a polymer matrix, and a small cation or polycation. In most endocrine cells, the polyanion belongs to the chromagranin–secretogranin family of acidic proteins, whereas the polycation is usually the hormonal or transmitter species itself (amines, regulatory peptides, hormones), or else a metallic cation (Ca^{2+}, K^+, Mg^{2+}) (Winkler and Westhead, 1980; Cohen et al., 1981). In mast cells, the polyanion component is heparin, whereas the cation is histamine (Hi^{2+}). In exocrine secretion, as in serous cells of the airway, the polyanion is a proteoglycan, and the polycations are a family of cationic proteins that includes lysozyme, lactoferrin, and antileukoproteinase (Basbaum, 1990).

We have proposed that the interactions between these two countercharged ionic species are of fundamental importance in explaining the condensation of secretory products in the secretory granule. According to this idea, the role of countercations would be to shield the polyanionic charges of the polymer network, screening the strong electrostatic interactions that tend to expand the polymer matrix and prevent its condensation.

In goblet cells, the polyanion is mucin, and the cation is Ca^{2+}. The high amounts of Ca^{2+} found inside the mucin granule can effectively screen the polyanionic charges of the mucins (Isutzu et al., 1985; Roomans et al., 1986; Verdugo et al., 1987b). That charge screening can lead to granule condensation has been shown in both goblet and mast cells. In fact, the small hydrated gels that result from the exocytotic swelling of the granular matrix can be readily recondensed when exposed to conditions that mimic those found inside the granule, namely, low pH (3.5–5) and either 100 mM Ca^{2+} in goblet cells, or 150 mM Hi^{2+} in mast the cells (Verdugo, 1991; Fernandez et al., 1991).

The role of Ca^{2+} and divalent histamine (Hi^{2+}) in the condensation of the mucin and heparin polymer matrices found in goblet and mast cells is now well characterized. We have suggested that they might function as shielding cations in a system that mimics a polymer gel-phase transition. Although some of the main features of this concept have been misinterpreted (Chandler, et al., 1989), the function of cationic shielding in stabilizing the granular matrix in condensed phase is now well supported by experimental evidence (Verdugo, 1991; Fernandez et al., 1991).

B. Polymer Gel-Phase Transition in Granule Condensation–Decondensation

The shielding of polyanionic charges is necessary, yet not sufficient, to explain the physicochemical mechanisms of granule matrix condensation. For instance, polymer networks composed of neutral polymers, like those found in contact lenses, can indeed form fully hydrated gels. The principle that can explain the physicochemistry of condensation–decondensation in polymer gels has emerged only recently in polymer gel physics, and is known as the theory of polymer gel-phase transition (Tanaka, 1981). Tanaka's novel experiments on the swelling behavior of synthetic polymer gels led to the discovery of one of the most revealing observations in modern polymer physics, namely, that polymer gels can undergo discrete reversible transitions of state or phase, from an expanded hydrated phase to a condensed phase, or vice versa. These transitions result from changes in the molecular configuration of the polymer matrix, which depends on temperature, pH, and the composition of the solvent. As observed in other phase transition phenomena, such as the transition to gas in a boiling liquid, the phase transition of polymer gels is also reversible and has the characteristic discontinuity of a critical phenomenon (i.e., the volume of the gel can remain virtually unchanged over a broad range of solvent temperature, pH, or ionic composition). However, at a critical temperature, pH, or ionic concentration of the solvent, the gel undergoes a phase transition, and its volume changes in a characteristically discontinuous manner. The smallest change in the solvent parameters can again discontinuously reverse the gel to its initial phase. Depending on the amount and nature of the interconnections among polymer chains in the matrix of the gel, the change in gel volume associated with the transition from condensed to hydrated phase, or vice versa, can reach up to several hundred-fold (Tanaka, 1981).

Results obtained from the isolated giant mucin granules of the slug *Arioli-*

max columbianus (Verdugo, 1992), and in granules of mammalian mast and respiratory goblet cells (Verdugo, 1990; Fernandez et al., 1991), indicate that the polymer matrix of these granules can indeed undergo phase transitions that resemble those observed in synthetic polymer gels (Tanaka, 1981).

Image processing of videorecorded microscopic observations reveals that during exocytosis the cross-linked heparin matrix of mast cells expands two- to four-fold (Fernandez et al., 1991). Similar expansions have been recorded in isolated secretory granules of mast cells, in which release is triggered by electroporation (Fernandez et al., 1991). The tangled polymer matrix of mucin granules also swells on exocytosis. However, in these granules the volumetric expansion is much broader, reaching up to 300-fold in goblet cell granules, and as much as 600-fold in the isolated giant granule of the terrestrial slug (Verdugo, 1986; Verdugo et al., 1992).

Depending on the composition of the medium, these secretory matrices can be recondensed and forced through several cycles of condensation–decondensation. In goblet and mast cells, recondensation is induced by solutions with compositions that mimic the intragranular environment, whereas decondensation is induced by solutions that mimic the extracellular fluid (Verdugo, 1991; Fernandez et al., 1991). In all these cases, the changes of matrix volume are reversible and demonstrate the characteristic all-or-nothing discontinuity found in polymer gel-phase transition.

A significant thermodynamic constraint in secretory cells is the osmotic work required to keep secretory material stored at high concentration inside membrane-bound secretory granules. Polymer gel-phase transition offers unique advantages to maintain the highly condensed secretory material, with minimum osmotic work. For instance, the recondensed heparin network of the mast cell granule can be exposed to distilled water and will still remain condensed (Fernandez et al., 1991). No osmotic work is required to keep the gel collapsed for as long as it remains in condensed phase.

Another interesting feature of polymer gel-phase transition is that it is a critical phenomenon (i.e., changes in the gel volume are discontinuous). The characteristic all-or-nothing property of polymer gel-phase transition makes it an ideal mechanism for product release in secretion, and it is the basis of what we have called the Jack-in-the-box mechanism in exocytosis (Verdugo, 1990, 1991).

In summary, mucins are stored in high concentration inside secretory granules, forming a condensed polymer network. Their polyanionic charges are shielded by high concentrations of intragranular Ca^{2+}. During exocytosis, the mucin matrix swells, undergoing extensive changes in volume. However, the mucin network can readily be recondensed by equilibration in solutions that imitate the intragranular environment. Condensation–decondensation is reversible and exhibits the typical discontinuity that characterizes a polymer gel-phase transition.

C. Mucin Exocytosis

In regard to regulated exocytosis it is convenient to distinguish the stimulus-coupling step from the product-release step (Fig. 2). The stimulus-coupling step includes the events that start with the binding of an agonist to a membrane receptor. This binding results in the activation of an intracellular information cascade that leads to docking the secretory granule to the plasma membrane and the formation of a secretory pore. Product-release is initiated by switching this pore from low- to high-ionic conductance. The establishment of a high-conductance water bridge leads to the subsequent exchange of ions and water between the intragranular compartment and the extracellular space. This exchange triggers the phase transition of the secretory matrix from a condensed to a hydrated phase, resulting in the massive swelling of the secretory matrix and the final release of the secretory material.

Stimulus–Secretion Coupling

Although a purinergic receptor has been recently identified in goblet cells, the stimulus-secretion coupling cascade that relays the stimulus signal inside these

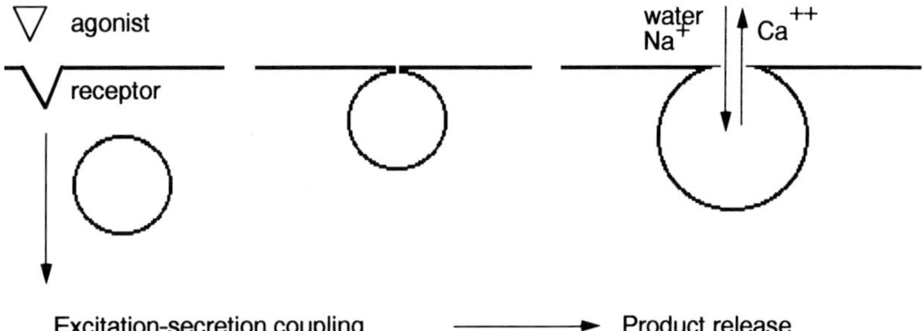

Figure 2 Mechanisms of mucin exocytosis. The final events in regulated secretion encompass two processes that are sequentially aligned, but very different in nature: stimulus–secretion coupling, and product release. The stimulus-coupling step is a biochemical information transfer event. It starts with the excitation of a membrane receptor that leads to the activation of an intracellular information cascade and results in the docking of the granule to the cell membrane and the formation of a fusion pore. The product release step is a mechanochemical transduction process. In this event, the electrochemical energy stored in the condensed polymer network of the granule is dissipated as mechanical energy, driving the release of the secretory products. Product release begins with the switching of the secretory pore from low- to high-ionic conductance. For mucin, the establishment of a high-ionic conductance water bridge between the intragranular and extracellular compartment leads to Na^+–Ca^{2+} exchange, triggering a phase transition phenomenon and the rapid swelling of the mucin matrix that is subsequently released from the cell.

cells has not been clearly delineated. A more detailed discussion of purinergic stimulation and stimulus-secretion coupling in goblet cells can be found in Davis et al. (1992) (see also Chap. 11). In this section we will focus exclusively on the product release step in mucin secretion.

Secretory Pore Formation

Because nothing is known about the formation of the secretory pore in goblet cells, we will briefly review the progress on this controversial subject in other secretory cells. The application of the patch–clamp method to measure membrane capacitance (Neher and Marty, 1982; Fernandez et al., 1984) has furnished a powerful tool for studying the formation and switching of the fusion pore in secretory cells.

Fusion between plasma and granular membranes in both secretory cells and model systems of lipid vesicles has been studied by several groups. It still remains a very controversial subject. For instance, swelling of the granule had been thought to start before the formation of a fusion pore and to be responsible for pore formation (Hampton and Holtz, 1983; Pollard et al., 1984; Zimmerberg and Whitaker, 1985; Zimmerberg et al., 1985; Hermans and Henquin, 1986). However, several lines of evidence indicate that this is unlikely (Zimmerberg et al., 1987; Breckenridge and Almers, 1987; Holz and Senter, 1986). New observations of mast cells show that pore formation and the widening of the secretory pore can be completely uncoupled from granular swelling and product release (Monck et al., 1991). The recent finding that the granular membrane is under tension before docking (Monck et al., 1990) suggests the appealing prospect that the tension of the granular membrane might facilitate not only membrane fusion and pore formation, but also the widening and switching of the secretory pore to high-ionic conductance.

More recently, the controversy has focused on the nature of the secretory pore. Almers (1990) proposed that this pore could be a protein, with conductance properties analogous to those of an ion channel. However, later studies in mast cells have led to the intriguing prospect that the fusion pore might be a lipidic channel (Monck and Fernandez, 1992). The implications of this divergence are too many to describe here. For a comprehensive discussion of the subject, see the aforementioned reviews.

In summary, it is improbable that preexocytic swelling of the granule might promote the formation and widening of the secretory pore, but the chemical nature of the secretory pore still remains controversial.

Product Release in Mucin Exocytosis

Secretory products undergo variable degrees of swelling on decondensation and release from the cell (Verdugo, 1984; Curran and Brodwick, 1984; Breckenridge and Almers, 1987; Fernandez et al., 1991). It has been proposed that swelling is responsible for product release in exocytosis (Verdugo, 1984; Pollard et al., 1984; Holz, 1986; Whitaker and Zimmerberg, 1987). However, the mechanisms of hydration of the secretory product during exocytosis have not been clearly defined, and they still remain controversial. One line of thought proposes that exocytotic swelling could be explained as a simple osmotic process (Pollard et al., 1984; Holz, 1986; Whitaker and Zimmerberg, 1987). There is some compelling evidence to support this idea, as hyperosmotic solutions can inhibit exocytosis in a variety of cells, including chromaffins, sea urchin eggs, mast cells, and neutrophils (Hampton and Holz, 1983; Pollard et al., 1984; Whitaker and Zimmerberg, 1987; Zimmerberg et al., 1985; Zimmerberg and Whitaker, 1985; Hermans and Henquin, 1986).

The other line of thought (Verdugo, 1990; Fernandez et al., 1991) proposes a two-step process in decondensation. The first step is a polymer gel-phase transition that is triggered by a shift of shielding cations, resulting in the decondensation of the secretory matrix. Once phase transition is triggered, the secretory matrix changes from a condensed to a hydrated phase, undergoing rapid swelling. Swelling here is not driven by simple concentration gradients, but by charge interaction; therefore, it is not a simple Einsteinian diffusional process, but a Langevinian convectional–diffusional process. In fact, the evaluation of swelling kinetics of the granular matrix indicates that the diffusivities of the secretory matrix are much too high to be accounted for by a simple concentration gradient-driven osmotic process. By measuring the rate of swelling of the granular matrix, it is possible to calculate the diffusivity of the exocytosed mucin network (Verdugo, 1984; Aitken and Verdugo, 1989). The increase of the radius of the exocytosed mucin network (or of the heparin network in the mast cell), follows a characteristic first-order kinetics, from which it is possible to estimate the diffusivity of the granular matrix. Results of these studies indicate that the diffusivity of the mucin network on exocytosis is about 6×10^{-7} cm²/s, whereas the corresponding reptational diffusion measured by dynamic laser scattering in the fully swollen mucous gel is about 8×10^{-8} cm²/s (Lee et al., 1977; Verdugo et al., 1983; Verdugo, 1984). This discrepancy, together with the demonstration that mucin swelling is governed by a Donnan potential (Tam and Verdugo, 1981), strongly suggest that the swelling of mucins upon exocytosis must be driven by charge interaction, rather than by simple osmotic gradients. In the particular instance of the giant granule of the slug, the mucin network can expand up to 600-fold in 20–30 ms (Verdugo et al., 1987). This explosive rate of swelling can hardly be explained on the basis of simple diffusional motions, as expected in a conventional osmotic process. It must result from convectional forces produced by charge interaction in the polymer matrix. Furthermore, the observation that membrane-free recondensed heparin matrices of mast cells can remain condensed in distilled water (Fernandez et al., 1991) virtually rules out that decondensation of the secretory matrix is governed by a simple osmotic process. This two-step mechanism of product release is also consistent with the observation that hyperosmotic solutions inhibit exocytosis, because very high osmotic pressure could outweigh the Donnan potential that drives swelling in exocytosis.

The Jack-in-the-Box Mechanism of Exocytosis

This hypothesis proposes that the force driving the final product release in exocytosis derives from charge interactions. The driving force for exocytosis is stored as potential energy in a charge-shielded, condensed, polyionic polymer network. Exocytosis begins by the formation of a secretory pore, and subsequent switching of this pore to a high-conductance state (see Fig. 2). Increased pore conductance leads to free ion flow between the intragranular and the extracellular compartments. The shielding species—Ca^{2+} for mucins or Hi^{2+} for mast cells— are exchanged by Na^+ from the extracellular space. Ion exchange triggers a phase transition whereby the polymer network turns from a condensed to a hydrated phase. The secretory matrix undergoes rapid swelling, driven by a Donnan potential (Donnan, 1924). Swelling leads to the unfolding of the matrix, its release to the extracellular space, and the eventual formation of the mucous gel. The Na^+–Ca^{2+} exchange is promoted by the ion-exchange properties of the mucin matrix. That Na^+ can indeed decrease Ca^{2+} binding to mucins has been elegantly demonstrated (Forstner and Forstner, 1975; Crowther and Marriot, 1983), but the import of this finding remains elusive. Similar Na^+–Hi^{2+} ion-exchange properties have been found in the heparin matrix of mast cells (Uvnas and Aborg, 1977). The importance of ion exchange in product release in exocytosis can be readily illustrated by the work of Tanaka on the effect of salts on polymer gel-phase transition. These studies demonstrate that the strength of cations to support condensation in polymer gel is much weaker for the monovalent cations than for divalent cations. For instance, the concentration required to maintain a polyionic polyacrylamide gel condensed is about 4000 times lower for divalent cations than for monovalent cations (Ohmine and Tanaka, 1982). A rigorous evaluation of the effect of Na^+–Ca^{2+} exchange in phase transition of mucin networks has not yet been investigated. However, the ion-exchange properties of the mucin polymer network strongly support the idea that Na^+–Ca^{2+} exchange could be a key element in triggering phase transition in exocytosis. The role of ion exchange in phase transition and exocytosis is further emphasized by the observation that recondensed heparin networks of exocytosed mast cell granules can remain recondensed even in distilled water. However, trace amounts of Na^+ in the water can trigger their decondensation (Fernandez et al., 1991).

A phase transition mechanism, such as the one just described, might well explain exocytosis in secretory cells other than just goblet and mast cells. The paramount feature of this spring-loaded product-release mechanism is the existence inside the secretory granule of both a condensed polyionic polymer network and a corresponding shielding counterion. As a secretory pore is formed and switched to high-ionic conductance, the shielding species is exchanged by Na^+ from the extracellular space, triggering the transition of the granular polymer matrix from a condensed to a decondensed phase. Notice that in this scheme the secretory pore should conduct both mono- as well as divalent cations in both directions. The Donnan-driven swelling of the granular matrix that follows ion exchange results in the final release of the secretory material. Although mucin is the polyionic polymer and Ca^{2+} is the shielding cation in the goblet cell granules (Sasaki et al., 1983; Isutzu et al., 1985; Roomans et al., 1986; Verdugo et al., 1987b), in mast cells, heparin is the polyanion and divalent histamine the cation (Uvnas and Aborg, 1977). The equivalent pair in chromaffin granules would be chromogranin and catecholamine (Winkler and Westhead, 1980), whereas in the parathyroid, the condensed polyion is protein I (SP-I), and the shielding cation is Ca^{2+} (Cohen et al., 1981). The presence of cations has been investigated in only a few secretory granules. However, acidic proteins similar to SP-I have been found in granules of pancreatic islets, the thyroid, anterior pituitary, celiac and mesenteric ganglia, and the gastric antrum. The idea that these polyanion–cation pairs might promote the formation of macromolecular aggregates and decrease osmotic activity of the granule was first suggested by Palade (1975). However, a physical paradigm to explain their condensation had not then been identified. Also, the proposed role of this group of polyanions as molecular springs to drive product release in exocytosis unveils a novel and important functional assignment for the polyionic networks found in secretory granules.

In summary, the structural and functional components of a spring-loaded molecular system to drive exocytosis are present in the secretory granule of a broad spectrum of secretory cells, including mucin-secreting cells. The principle of polymer gel-phase transition provides a novel conceptual paradigm to explain both condensation and decondensation in secretion. It ascribes testable functional roles to polyanionic polymer networks and to the shielding cations ubiquitously found in secretory granules, and it furnishes testable predictions to further investigate the molecular mechanisms of storage and release in secretion.

IV. Concluding Remarks

We are now witnessing a most remarkable revolution in biology, and the plunder is so rich and powerful that it is easy to lose perspective. Molecular biology is winning from Mother Nature some of her most difficult riddles, namely, the blueprints of an ever-increasing number of the fundamental building blocks of the cell. Yet the understanding of how the structures of these molecules relate to their corresponding functions still remains elusive. This quest rests on one of the most intricate, less well-known, and most challenging fields of physicochemistry.

Indeed, the physics of low-energy interactions (molecular interactions not involving the exchange of electrons) that furnishes the paradigms to explain polymer structure–function relationships is now still being discovered. Within this framework, the understanding of the structural basis of the complex function of mucus is no exception. The detailed knowledge of mucin primary structure is certainly not sufficient to give a correspondingly precise understanding of mucin condensation, decondensation, and final gelation to form the mucus. At present, it is presumptuous to pretend that a formal relation between mucin structure and function can be explicitly derived from first principles. Thus, we cannot unequivocally rule out or include, without further experimental testing, the many alternatives that remain open to explain the complex chain of events that start with mucin condensation and end in the formation of respiratory mucus. The safest alternative is to draft ideas, like those presented here, that, conforming with physical laws and experimental results, may serve to guide our quest for a more rigorous understanding of this interesting and most challenging problem.

Acknowledgments

Research presented in this paper was supported in part by grant Nos. NAG-9-604 from the NASA Space Biology Program and HL-38494 from the National Institutes of Health.

References

Aitken, M. L., and Verdugo, P. (1989). Donnan mechanism of mucin release and conditioning in goblet cells: The role of polyions. In *Mucus and Related Topics*. Edited by E. N. Chantler. New York, Plenum Press, pp. 73–80.

Almers, W. (1990). Exocytosis. *Annu. Rev. Physiol.* 52: 607–624.

Basbaum, C. B., Berthold, J., and Kinkbeiner, W. E. (1990). The serous cell. *Annu. Rev. Physiol.* 52: 97–114.

Bhaskar, K. R., O'Sullivan, D. D., Seltzer, J., Rossing, T. H., Drazen, J. M., and Reid, L. M. (1985). Density gradient study of bronchial mucus aspirates from healthy volunteers (smokers and nonsmokers) and from patients with tracheostomy. *Exp. Lung Res.* 9: 289–308.

Boat, T. F., and Cheng, P. W. (1980). Biochemistry of airway mucus secretions. *Fed. Proc.* 39: 3067–3073.

Boat, T. F., Cheng, P. W., Iyer, R. N., Carlson, D. M., and Polony, I. (1976). Human respiratory tract secretions. *Arch. Biochem. Biophys.* 177: 95–104.

Breckenridge, L. J., and Almers, W. (1987). Final steps in exocytosis observed in cells with giant secretory granules. *Proc. Natl. Acad. Sci. USA* 84: 1945–1949.

Carlstedt, I., and Sheehan, J. K. (1984). Macromolecular properties and polymeric structure of mucus glycoproteins. In *Mucus and Mucosa* (Ciba Foundation Symposium). Edited by J. Nugent and M. O'Connor. London, Pitman.

Chandler, D. E., Whitaker, E. M., and Zimmerberg, J. (1989). High molecular weight polymers block cortical granule exocytosis in sea urchin eggs at the level of granule matrix disassembly. *J. Cell Biol.* 109: 1269–1278.

Cohen, F. S., Akabas, M. H., and Finkelstein, A. (1982). Osmotic swelling of phospholipid vesicles causes them to fuse with a planar phospholipid bilayer membrane. *Science* 217: 458–460.

Cohen, D. V., Morrissey, J. J., Hamilton, J. W., Shofstall, R. E., Smardo, F. L., and Chu, L. H. (1981). Isolation and partial characterization of secretory protein I from bovine parathyroid glands. *Biochemistry* 20: 4135–4140.

Crowther, R. S., and Marriot, C. (1983). Counter-ion binding to mucus glycoproteins. *J. Pharm. Pharmacol.* 36: 21–26.

Curran, M., and Brodwick, M. S. (1984). Final steps in exocytosis observed in a cell with giant secretory granules. *Proc. Natl. Acad. Sci. USA* 84: 1945–1949.

Davis, C. W., Dowell, M. L., Lethem, M., and Van Scott, M. (1992). Goblet cell degranulation in isolated canine tracheal epithelium: Response to exogenous ATP, ADP, and adenosine. *Am. J. Physiol.* 262: C1313–C1323.

Donnan F. G. (1924). The theory of membrane equilibria. *Chem. Rev.* 1: 73–90.

Edwards, S. F. (1986). The theory of macromolecular networks. *Biorheology* 23: 589–603.

Edwards, S. F., and Grant, J. W. V. (1973). The effect of entanglements on viscosity of a polymer melt. *J. Phys. A.* 6: 1171–1180.

Fernandez, J. M., Villalon, M., and Verdugo, P. (1991). Reversible condensation of mast cell secretory products in vitro. *Biophys. J.* 59: 1022–1027.

Fernandez, J. M., Neher, E., and Gomperts, B. D. (1984). Capacitance measurements reveal stepwise fusion events in degranulating mast cells. *Nature* 312: 453–455.

Flory, P. J. (1969). Rubber elasticity. In *Principles of Polymer Chemistry*. Edited by P. J. Flory. Ithaca, Cornell University Press, pp. 432–493.

Forstner, J. F., and Forstner, G. G. (1975). Calcium binding to intestinal goblet cell mucin. *Biochim. Biophys. Acta* 386: 283–292.

Frizzell, R. A. (1988). Role of absorptive and secretory processes in hydration of the airway surface. *Am. Rev. Respir. Dis.* 138: S3–S6.

Gendler, S. J., Burchell, J. M., Duhig, T., Lamport, D., White, R., Parker, M., and Taylor-Papadimitriou, J. (1987). *Proc. Natl. Acad. Sci. USA* 84: 6060–6064.

Gibbons, R. A., and Mattner, P. E. (1966). Some aspects of the chemistry of cervical mucus. *Int. J. Fertil.* 11: 366–379.

Gum, J. R., Hicks, J. W., Swallow, D. M., Lagace, R. L., Byrd, J. C., Lamport, D., Siddiki, B., and Kim, Y. S. (1990). *Biochem. Biophys. Res. Commun.* 171: 407–415.

Hampton, R. I., and Holz, R. W. (1983). Effects of change in the osmolality on the stability and function of cultured chromaffin cells and the possible role of osmotic forces in exocytosis. *J. Cell Biol.* 96: 1082–1088.

Harding, S. E., Rowe, A. J., and Creeth, J. M. (1983). Further evidence for a flexible and highly expanded spheroidal model for mucus glycoproteins in solution. *Biochem. J.* 209: 893–896.

Havez, R., and Roussel, P. (1976). Bronchial mucus: Physical and biochemical features. In *Bronchial Asthma: Mechanisms and Therapeutics*. Edited by E. B. Weiss and M. S. Sega. Boston, Little, Brown & Co., pp. 409–422.

Hermans, M. P., and Henquin, J. C. (1986). Is there a role for osmotic events in exocytotic release of insulin? *Endocrinology* 119: 105–111.

Holz, R. W. (1986). The role of osmotic forces in exocytosis from adrenal chromaffin cells. *Annu. Rev. Physiol.* 48: 175–189.

Holz, R. W., and Senter, R. A. (1986). Effect of osmolality and ionic strength on secretion from adrenal chromaffin cells permeabilized with digitonin. *J. Neurochem.* 46: 1835–1842.

Izutsu, K., Johnson, D., Schubert M. et al. (1985). Electron microprobe analysis of human labial gland secretory granules in cystic fibrosis. *J. Clin. Invest.* 75: 1951–1956.

Jacquot, J., Goldstein, G., Sommerhoff, C. P., Benali, R., Puchell, E., and Basbaum, C. B. (1988). Synthesis and secretion of an albumin-like protein by cultured bronchial tracheal serous cells. *Biophys. Biochem. Res. Commun.* 155: 857–862.

Kaliner, M. A., Borson, D. B., Nadel, J. A., Shelhamer, J. H., Patow, C. A., and Marom, Z. (1988). Respiratory mucus. In *The Airways. Neural Control in Health and Disease.* Edited by M. A. Kaliner, and P. J. Barnes. New York, Marcel Dekker, pp. 575–593.

Kaliner, M., Marom, Z., Patow, C., and Shelhamer, J. (1984). Human respiratory mucus. *J. Allergy Clin. Immunol.* 73: 318–323.

Katchalsky, A., Lifson, S., and Eisenberg, H. J. (1951). Equation of swelling for polyelectrolyte gels. *J. Polymer Sci.* 7: 571–574.

Kent, P. W. (1978). Chemical aspects of tracheal glycoproteins. In *Symposium on Respiratory Tract Mucus.* Edited by J. Nuget and M. O'Connor. *Ciba Found. Symp.* 54: 155.

Lee, W. I., Verdugo, P., and Blandau, R. J. (1977). Molecular arrangement of cervical mucus: A re-evaluation based on laser scattering spectroscopy. *Gynecol. Invest.* 8: 254–266.

Marriott, C., Shih, C. K., and Litt, M. (1979). Changes in the gel properties of tracheal mucus induced by divalent cations. *Biorheology* 16: 331–337.

Meyer, F. A., King, M., and Gelman, R. A. (1975). On the role of sialic acid in the rheological properties of mucus. *Biochim. Biophys. Acta* 392: 223–232.

Monck, J. R., Alvarez de Toledo, G., and Fernandez, J. M. (1990). Tension in secretory granule membranes causes extensive membrane transfer through the exocytotic fusion pore. *Proc. Natl. Acad. Sci. USA* 87: 7804–7808.

Monck, J. R., and Fernandez, J. M. (1992). The exocytotic fusion pore. *J. Cell Biol.* 119(6): 1395–1404.

Monck, J. R., Oberhauser, A. F., Alvarez de Toledo G., and Fernandez J. M. (1991). Is swelling of the secretory granule matrix the force that dilates the exocytotic fusion pore? *Biophys. J.* 59: 39–47.

Neher, E., and Marty, A. (1982). Discrete changes of cell membrane capacitance observed under conditions of enhanced secretion in bovine chromaffin cells. *Proc. Natl. Acad. Sci. USA* 79: 6712–6716.

Odeblad, E. (1976). The biophysical aspects of cervical mucus. In *The Cervix.* Edited by J. A. Jordan and A. Singer. London, W. B. Saunders, pp. 155–163.

Ohmine, I., and Tanaka, T. (1982). Salt effects on the phase transition of ionic gels. *J. Chem. Phys.* 77: 5725–5729.

Palade, H. (1975). Intracellular aspects of the process of protein synthesis. *Science* 189: 347–358.

Pollard, H. B., Pazoles, C. J., Creutz, C. E., Scott, H. J., Zinder, O., and Hotchkiss, A. (1984). An osmotic mechanism for exocytosis from dissociated chromaffin cells. *J. Biol. Chem.* 259: 1114–1121.

Porchet, N., Van Cong, N., Dufosse, J., Audie, J. P., Guyonnet-Duperat, V., Gross, M. S., Denis, C., Degand, P., Bernheim, A., and Aupert, J. P. (1991). *Biochem. Biophys. Res. Commun.* 175: 414–422.

Potter, J. L., Matthews, L. W., Lemm, J., and Spector, S. (1963). Human pulmonary secretions in health and disease. *Ann. N. Y. Acad. Sci.* 106: 692–708.

Roberts, G. P. (1976). The role of disulfate bonds in maintaining the gel structure of bronchial mucus. *Arch. Biochem. Biophys.* 173: 528–537.

Roberts, G. P. (1978). Chemical aspects of respiratory mucus. *Br. Med. Bull.* 34: 39–41.

Roomans, G. M., von Euler, A. M., Muller, R. M., and Gilljman, H. (1986). X-ray microanalysis of goblet cells in bronchial epithelium of patients with cystic fibrosis. *J. Submicrosc. Cytol.* 18: 613–615.

Sasaki, S., Nakagaki, I., Mori, H., and Imai, Y. (1983). Intracellular calcium store and transport of elements in acinar cells of the salivary gland determined by electron probe x-ray microanalysis. *Jpn. J. Physiol.* 33: 69–83.

Sheehan, J. K., Oates, K., and Carlstedt, I. (1986). Electron microscopy of cervical, gastric, and bronchial mucus glycoproteins. *Biochem. J.* 239: 147–153.

Silberberg, A. (1987). A model for mucus glycoprotein structure. *Biorheology* 24: 605–614.

Slayter, H. S., Lamblin, G., Le Treut, A., et al. (1984). Complex structure of human bronchial mucus glycoprotein. *Eur. J. Biochem.* 142: 209–218.

Steiner, C. A., Litt, M., and Nossal, R. (1984). Effect of Ca^{2+} on the structure and rheology of canine tracheal mucin. *Biorheology* 21: 235–252.

Tam, P. Y., and Verdugo, P. (1981). Control of mucus hydration as a Donnan equilibrium process. *Nature* 292: 340–342.

Tanaka, T. (1981). Gels. *Sci. Am.* 244(1): 124–138.

Tanaka, T., and Fillmore, D. J. (1979). Kinetic of swelling of gel. *J. Chem. Phys.* 70: 1214–1218.

Tooze, J., Kern, H. F., Fuller, S. D., and Howell, K. E. (1989). Condensation-sorting events in rough endoplasmic reticulum of exocrine pancreatic cells. *J. Cell Biol.* 109: 35–50.

Uvnas, B., and Aborg, C. H. (1977). On the cation exchanger properties of rat mast cell granule and their storage of histamine. *Acta Physiol. Scand.* 100: 309–314.

Verdugo, P. (1984). Hydration kinetics of exocytosed mucins in cultured secretory cells of the rabbit trachea: A new model. In *Mucus and Mucosa.* Edited by J. Nuget and M. O'Connor. *Ciba Found. Symp.* 109: 212–234.

Verdugo, P. (1986). Polymer gel phase transition: A novel mechanism of product storage and release in mucin secretion. *Biophys. J.* 49: 231a.

Verdugo, P. (1990). Goblet cells secretion and mucogenesis. *Annu. Rev. Physiol.* 52: 157–176.

Verdugo, P. (1991). Mucin exocytosis. *Am. Rev. Respir. Dis.* 144: S33–S37.

Verdugo, P., Tam, P. Y., and Butler, J. (1983). Conformational structure of respiratory mucus studied by laser correlation spectroscopy. *Biorheology* 20: 223–230.

Verdugo, P., Deyrup-Olsen, L., Aitken, M., Villalon, M. J., and Johnson, D. (1987b). Molecular mechanism of mucin secretion: The role of intragranular charge shielding. *J. Dent. Res.* 66: 506–508.

Verdugo, P., Aitken, M., Langley, L., and Villalon, M. J. (1987a). Molecular mechanism of product storage and release in mucin secretion. II. The role of extracellular Ca^{2+}. *Biorheology* 24: 625–633.

Verdugo, P., Deyrup-Olsen, I., Martin, A. W., and Luchtel, D. L. (1992). Polymer gel phase transition: The molecular mechanism of product release in mucin secretion. In *Swelling of Polymer Networks*. Edited by E. Karalis. Heidelberg, Springer-Verlag. *NATO ASI Series H* 64: 671–681.

Whitaker, M., and Zimmerberg, J. (1987). Inhibition of secretory granule discharge during exocytosis in sea urchin eggs by polymer solutions. *J. Physiol.* 389: 527–539.

Widdicombe, J. G. (1989). Airway mucus. *Eur. Respir.* 2: 107–115.

Winkler, H., and Westhead, E. (1980). The molecular organization of adrenal chromaffin granules. *Neuroscience* 5: 1803–1924.

Wolf, D. P., Blasco, L., Khan, M. A., and Litt, M. (1977). Human cervical mucus. I. Rheological properties; II. Changes in viscoelasticity during ovulatory menstrual cycle; III. Isolation and characterization of rheologically active mucin. *Fertil. Steril.* 28: 41–58.

Zimmerberg, J., Curran, M., Cohen, F. S., and Brodwick, M. (1987). Simultaneous electrical and optical measurements show that membrane fusion precedes secretory granule during exocytosis of beige mouse mast cells. *Proc. Natl. Acad. Sci. USA* 84: 1585–1589.

Zimmerberg, J., Sardet, C., and Epel, D. (1985). Exocytosis of sea urchin egg cortical vesicles in vitro is retarded by hyperosmotic sucrose: Kinetics of fusion monitored by quantitative light-scattering microscopy. *J. Cell Biol.* 101: 2398–2410.

Zimmerberg, J., and Whitaker, M. (1985). Calcium causes irreversible swelling of secretory granules during exocytosis. *Nature* 315: 581–584.

4

Development of the Airway Secretory Apparatus
Patterns of Mucous Cell Differentiation

JUDITH A. ST. GEORGE

Genzyme Corporation
Framingham, Massachusetts

SHIPING WANG

Huazhong Agricultural University
Wuhan, People's Republic of China

CHARLES G. PLOPPER

University of California
Davis, California

I. Introduction

The secretory cells of the tracheobronchial epithelium and submucosal glands collectively produce the fluid lining of the conducting airways. In fully differentiated airway epithelium, however, there is wide variation from species to species in the type of secretory cell at one airway level to the next, as well as the presence and abundance of submucosal glands. Some species, including rat, mouse, rabbit, hamster, and guinea pig, have few if any glands, whereas, other species, such as human, monkey, dog, cat, sheep, pig, and cow have well-developed glands (for review, see Jeffery, 1983). These differences may affect the amount of mucus available on the epithelial surface for mucociliary clearance. In hypersecretory conditions, such as chronic bronchitis, the increased quantities of airway mucus are thought to compromise the protective function of the mucociliary apparatus (Reid et al., 1983). The sources of the fluid lining include mucous and serous cells of both the epithelial surface and submucosal glands. In some species, the Clara cell may also contribute to the mucous layer (Plopper et al., 1984). These variations in sources of mucus suggests differences in the composition of mucus.

Just as variations exist in the fully differentiated airway epithelium, differences exist in the developmental patterns observed in the secretory apparatus in airways of different species. In some species, including rabbit (Leeson, 1961) and monkey (Plopper et al., 1986a), proximal airway epithelial differentiation is largely prenatal, whereas in other species, such as hamster (Emura and Mohr, 1975; McDowell et al., 1985), rat (Jeffery and Reid, 1977), mouse (Kawamata and Fujita, 1983), and ferret (Leigh et al., 1986), this development continues post-natally. In addition, several changes in the secretory apparatus occur at or near birth, including rapid increase in quantities and content of intracellular secretory glycoconjugates (Mills et al., 1986; Leigh et al., 1986). With the assumption that the adult airway epithelium is at an endpoint for comparison, we will consider information about the secretory apparatus in the following sequence: Characterization of the adult airway secretory apparatus, development of surface mucous cell cytodifferentiation, submucosal gland development, and regulation of airway secretory apparatus development.

II. Adult

A. Histochemistry and Cytochemistry

Carbohydrate histochemistry and cytochemistry have been used to identify carbohydrates containing *vicinal* hydroxyl groups, carboxyl groups, and sulfate esters. Tables 1 and 2 summarize the histochemically defined content of the

Table 1 Carbohydrate Content of Tracheal Epithelium

Ref.	Species	Cell type	Abundance	Carbohydrate content PAS	AB	HID
Emura and Mohr, 1975	Hamster	Clara	+++	+	−	−
		Mucous	+	+	+	−
McCarthy and Reid, 1964a	Rat	Serous	+++	+	−	−
		Mucous	+	+	+	−
McCarthy and Reid, 1964a	Mouse	Mucous	+	+	+	−
Plopper et al., 1984	Rabbit	Mucous	+	+	+	+
		Clara	+++	±	−	−
Scott and Dorling, 1965	Canine	Mucous	++	+	+	+
Jeffery, 1977	Cat	Mucous	++	+	+	+ and −
		Serous	+	ND	ND	ND
Jones et al., 1975	Pig	Mucous	++	+	+	+ and −
Mariassy et al., 1988b	Sheep	Mucous	++	+	+	+ and −
St. George et al., 1984a	Rhesus	Mucous	++	+	+	+
McCarthy and Reid, 1964b	Human	Mucous	+++	+	+	+ and −

Table 2 Carbohydrate Content of Tracheal Submucosal Glands

Ref.	Species	Abundance	Secretory cell	Carbohydrate content		
				PAS	AB	HID
Emura and Mohr, 1975	Hamster	±	Mucous	+	+	−
McCarthy and Reid, 1964a	Rat	+	Serous	+	−	−
			Mucous	+	+	+ and −
McCarthy and Reid, 1964a	Mouse	±	Serous	+	−	−
			Mucous	+	+	+ and −
Plopper et al., 1984	Rabbit	±	Mucous	+	+	+
Spicer et al., 1971	Canine	+ +	Serous	+	−	−
			Mucous	+	+	+ and −
Jeffery, 1977	Cat	+ + + +	Serous	+	+	+ and −
			Mucous	+	+	+
Jones et al., 1975	Pig	+ +	Serous	+	−	−
			Mucous	+	+	+ and −
Mariassy et al., 1988b	Sheep	+ +	Serous	+	−	−
			Mucous	+	+	+
St. George et al., 1984a	Rhesus	+ +	Serous	+	−	−
			Mucous	+	+	+
Lamb and Reid, 1969	Human	+ + +	Serous	+	−	−
			Mucous	+	+	+ and −

secretory cells of the epithelial surface (Table 1) and submucosal glands (Table 2). Human respiratory mucous cells of both the epithelial surface and glands were shown to contain acidic glycoconjugates by the presence of sulfate or sialic acid, whereas neutral glycoconjugates were localized in serous cells of submucosal glands (Lamb and Reid, 1969; McCarthy and Reid, 1964b). With the examination of additional species, it was found that although mucous cells generally contain acidic mucins, the preponderance of either sulfo- or sialomucin varies with species. For example, sulfomucins are preponderant in the mucous cells of surface epithelium in dog (Scott and Dorling, 1965), cat (Jeffery, 1977), rabbit (Plopper et al., 1984), and macaque monkey (St. George et al., 1984a). In the epithelial surface of sheep (Mariassy et al., 1988b) and human (Lamb and Reid, 1969), either sulfo- or sialomucins are preponderant, but this varies according to airway level. In sheep, mucous cells of airway generations greater than 14 in the left cranial lobe or 22 in the left caudal lobe contain sulfomucin (Mariassy et al., 1988b). More proximal generations are lined by mucous cells with either sialo- or sulfomucins. The nasal cavity and distal bronchioles of humans (Thaete et al., 1981) and nasal cavity of macaque monkey (Harkema et al., 1987a) contain preponderantly sulfomucins. By contrast, in both rat and mouse (McCarthy and Reid, 1964a), sialomucins are preponderant in epithelial mucous cells of airway surfaces when mucous cells are found. The preponderant secretory cell of rat tracheobronchial epithelium, however, is a serous cell containing a neutral glycoconjugate (Spicer et al., 1980).

Acidic mucins are found in the mucous cells of submucosal glands as well. Sulfomucins are contained in glandular mucous cells of most species, including rat, mouse (McCarthy and Reid, 1964a), dog (Spicer et al., 1971), sheep (Mariassy et al., 1988b), pig (Jones et al., 1975), and rhesus monkey (St. George et al., 1986b). In rat, the distribution of acidic mucins varies with location within the gland, with mucous tubules containing sulfomucins and mucous ducts containing sialomucins (Mochizuki et al., 1982). In submucosal glands of humans, sialo- and sulfomucins are present in roughly equal proportions (Spicer et al., 1983).

Ultrastructural studies have confirmed and extended the observations made at the light microscopic level. Differences in carbohydrate content have been demonstrated within individual granules of serous and mucous cells. Both cell types may contain monophasic, biphasic, or triphasic granules. Mucous granules of rabbit trachea are biphasic, with an outer cortex at which the sulfated glycoconjugate is concentrated (Plopper et al., 1984). By contrast, in rhesus tracheal mucous cells, the sulfated material is concentrated within the inner one or two core regions (St. George et al., 1984a). In human epithelial mucous cells the cores have been described as invariably negative for carbohydrate (Spicer et al., 1983).

B. Lectin Histochemistry and Cytochemistry

More specific information on the composition of the glycoconjugates contained within the mucous and serous cells of the respiratory system was provided with the use of lectins. Lectins, with specificity for sugars, primarily in the terminal position, were used to localize these sugars in complex carbohydrates. A summary of the lectin reactivity is presented in Table 3. Most of the work in this area was done by Spicer and colleagues and was reviewed for human, rat, and mouse in 1983 (Spicer et al., 1983). The results from the lectin studies provided additional information and further complicated the interpretation of secretory cell content. For example, histochemical analysis had not indicated the heterogeneity of content of both serous and mucous cells that became apparent with lectin application. An important result not reflected in Table 3 is that whereas some cells of a specific type may contain a sugar, not all will, nor will they contain it in the same concentration.

Lectins applied at the level of the electron microscope further elucidated the nature of the airway secretory product(s). Wasano and colleagues (1988) examined mucous cells in hamster trachea and demonstrated that glycoconjugates with discrete terminal sugars are localized within distinct regions of the Golgi apparatus. Sugars appeared in a sequential fashion from *cis-* to *trans-*cisternae.

Table 3 Lectin Reactivity

		Lectin							
		LCA	WGA	BSA$_1$	DBA	SBA Gal−GalNAc	PNA	RCA	UEA$_1$
Species/cell type	Sugar specificity	Man Glc GlcNAc	NANA GlcNAc	Gal	GalNAc	Gal GalNAc	Gal GalNAc	Gal GalNAc	Fuc
In airway surface epithelium									
Human bronchi[a]	Mucous	−	+ + + +	+	+	+ + +	+ + + +	+ + + +	+ + + +
Sheep trachea–	Mucous M1			−	+ + +	+ +	+ + +		+ + + +
bronchiole[b]	Mucous M2			−	+ + +	+ +	+ + +		+ + + +
	Mucous M3			+ + +	+ + +	−	−		−
Rat trachea[a]	Mucous	−		−	+	+	−(+ + +)	+	+ + +
Rhesus trachea	Mucous	+ + + +	+ + + +	+ + + +	+ + + +	−	−(+ + +)[c]	−(+ + +)	+
Of airway submucosal glands									
Human bronchi	Mucous	−	+	+	+	+ + +	+ + + +	+ + +	+ + + +
	Serous	+ + +	+ + +	−	−	+ +	+	+ +	−
Sheep	Mucous M4			−	+ + + +	+ +	−		+ +
	Serous			−	+ + +	+ +	−		+ +
Mouse trachea[a]	Mucous	−		−	−	+	−(+ + +)	−	+ + +
	Serous			−	+ + + +	+ + + +	+ + + +	+ + + +	−
Rat trachea	Mucous	+ +		−	+ +	+ +	−(+ + +)	−	+ + +
	Serous			−	−	−	−(+ + + +)	−	−
Rhesus trachea	Mucous	+ + + +	+ + + +	+ + +	−	−(+ + + +)	−(+ + + +)		+ + +
	Serous	+ +	+ +	+	−	−(+ +)	−(+ +)		+

Abbreviations: LCA, *Lotus tetragonolobus*; WGA, wheat germ agglutinin; SBA, *Glycine max*; BSA I, *Bandeirea simplicifolia* I; DBA, *Dolichos biflorus*; PNA, *Arachis hypogea*; RCA, *Ricinus communis*; UEA, *Ulex europeus*; Man, mannose; Glc, galactose; GalNAc, *N*-acetylgalactosamine; NANA, *N*-acetylneuraminic acid (sialic acid); Gal, galactose; Fuc, fucose.

[a]Spicer et al., 1983

[b]Mariassy et al., 1988a

[c]Reaction in parenthesis is after neuraminidase treatment.

N-acetylgalactosamine was the only sugar detected in the *cis*-cisternae, then *N*-acetylglucosamine and galactose, and lastly, fucose and sialic acid were detected in the *trans*-cisternae. This sequence of sugars coincides with the order of glycosylation of *O*-linked respiratory mucins demonstrated by biochemical methods (Rana et al., 1986).

C. Immunohistochemistry

Immunohistochemical methods can be used to define more precisely the variations in content within cells or granules. For example, the enzyme lysozyme (Bowes et al., 1981) and lactoferrin (Bowes and Corrin, 1977) have been localized within secretory cells of the respiratory tract. Lysozyme, which does not contain carbohydrate, has been detected within serous cells of submucosal glands, leading Spicer and colleagues to suggest that the carbohydrate-negative portion of serous granules is lysozyme (Spicer et al., 1980).

More recent immunohistochemical studies using monoclonal antibodies against respiratory secretory products have expanded the previously discussed heterogeneity (St. George et al., 1984b, 1985; Basbaum et al., 1984). We have used monoclonal antibodies against rhesus or rabbit tracheal secretions to show several antigenically distinct subpopulations of mucous cells (St. George et al., 1984b, 1985). When serial sections of histochemically and immunohistochemically stained samples are compared, secretory cells are found that do not vary histochemically, but do vary immunohistochemically (St. George et al., 1984b). Application of monoclonal antibodies to four airway levels distal to the trachea in rhesus monkey indicates that the more distal the airway, the less the secretory content resembles that in trachea (St. George et al., 1986a). This variation in content suggests variations in biophysical properties of secretion at different airway levels.

D. Quantification

With certain toxicological insults or respiratory diseases, profound changes occur in the volume of secretion produced and stored in the airways. Therefore, it has been important to develop accurate methods to quantify the volume of stored secretory products under normal as well as abnormal conditions. Previous methods have included determining the mean gland/wall ratio (Reid Index; Reid, 1960) or point counting to quantify submucosal glands (Bedrossian et al., 1971). We have used a computerized morphometric method to assess the volume of the secretory product per unit surface area and demonstrated that there is considerable variation at different airway levels in the amount of glycoconjugate stored in airway epithelium of the rhesus monkey (Heidsiek et al., 1987; Plopper et al., 1989). The product of tracheal surface was mainly acidic, whereas that in submucosal glands was neutral. The trachea stored at least twice as much per unit of surface area as did distal airways (generation 11). Additionally, a change in secretory product from preponderantly sulfomucin to increased sialomucin was detected distally. One surprising feature of these studies was the contribution to the total secretory product by submucosal glands versus surface epithelium, as suggested by the amount of stored product in either surface epithelium or submucosal glands. Several investigators have indicated that the overwhelming amount of secretion is from submucosal glands (Reid, 1960). However, morphometric analysis of stored product in rhesus trachea demonstrated that the contribution by the submucosal glands was less than 50% of the total product (Heidsiek et al., 1987).

The same automated morphometric methods were used to detect regional differences in the quantities of secretory glycoconjugates in the nasal cavity of a nonhuman primate (Harkema et al., 1987a). This study defined the normal distribution of epithelial mucosubstance and was used to determine the effects of ozone on primate nasal cavity. After 6 days of exposure to ambient concentrations of ozone, there was a significant increase in stored glycoconjugates, followed by a significant decrease after 90 days exposure (Harkema et al., 1987b).

III. Surface Mucous Cell Cytodifferentiation

Development of the respiratory system is based on the time course of changes that occur in the development of the gas-exchange area. In humans, for example, following the embryonic period, the stages of lung development are pseudoglandular (7–16 weeks), canalicular (17–24 weeks), and terminal sac (24–term) (Boyden, 1972). In different species, the length of gestation and the length of each phase of lung development is variable (Jeffery and Reid, 1977). The secretory elements develop early in gestation, with the appearance of mucous cells preceding the development of submucosal glands. Differentiation of mucous cells and submucosal glands occurs first in the trachea then progresses distally in the airways (for review see Shimura et al., 1990). In the trachea of species for which the mucous goblet cell is the preponderant secretory cell, there is a clear transition from a single undifferentiated cell to the four major cell types observed in the adult. All four cells types, including ciliated, mucous goblet, small mucous granule (SMG), and basal cell, are present by the end of the canalicular phase (Plopper et al., 1986a). The sequence of appearance of these cell types is ciliated cell, mucous cell, SMG, and basal. In primates mucous cells appear early in the pseudoglandular phase, and most of their maturation occurs before birth (Plopper et al., 1986a).

A. Ultrastructure

The ultrastructural features of overall tracheal epithelial differentiation in developing fetuses have been described in the rabbit (Leeson, 1961), mouse (Kawamata and Fujita, 1983), hamster (Emura and Mohr, 1975; McDowell et al., 1985), and rat

(Jeffery and Reid, 1977). In view of the diversity in the airways in different species, small laboratory mammals may not be adequate models for the study of human tracheobronchial epithelium (Jeffery and Reid, 1977). The most extensive study on the development of the mucous cell was performed on the trachea of the rhesus monkey (Plopper et al., 1986a) and will be reviewed here. Gestation for the rhesus averages 168 days, with the stages of lung development as follows: embryonic period 21–55 days gestational age (DGA); pseudoglandular, 56–80 DGA; canalicular, 80–130 DGA; and terminal sac, 131–term (Boyden, 1976).

In the youngest fetuses, all cells appeared as illustrated in Figure 1. The cells were columnar and the apices of most of the cells reached the luminal surface. Nuclei had little heterochromatin and the cytoplasm was filled from base to apex with glycogen. The few organelles present were located in the apex of the cell and included short narrow strands of granular endoplasmic reticulum (GER), small, spherical mitochondria, and a small Golgi apparatus located adjacent to the lateral

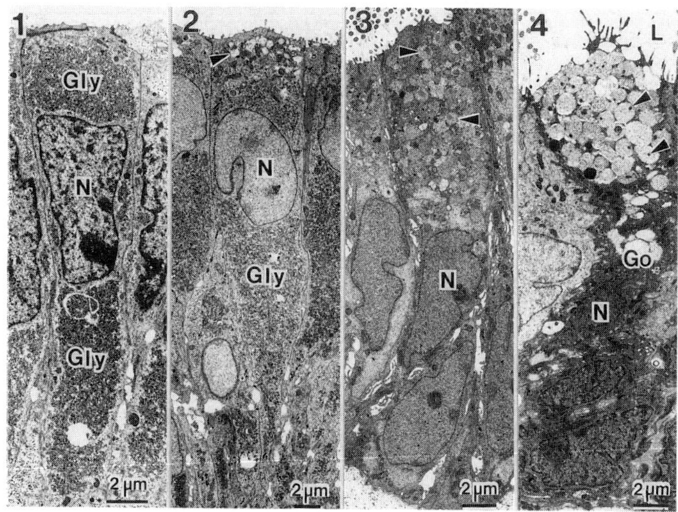

Figures 1–4   Summary of mucous cell differentiation and maturation during gestation in tracheas of fetal rhesus monkeys. Figure 1. Columnar cell containing glycogen (Gly) and a central nucleus (N); 46 days gestational age (GA). Figure 2. Columnar cell with tapered base, containing glycogen (Gly), a central nucleus (N) and apical accumulations of secretory granules (arrowhead) and organelles, 62 day GA. Figure 3. Columnar cell with tapered base, containing numerous apical secretory granules (arrowheads) and little glycogen; 90 days GA. Figure 4. Columnar cell with tapered base and basal nucleus (N), containing abundant apical secretory granules with dense cores (arrowheads and a large Golgi apparatus (Go); airway lumen (L), 141 days GA.

surface of the cell (see Fig. 1). These cells were present in the epithelial lining in the youngest animal in the embryonic stage to the middle of the canalicular phase.

In fetuses near the end of the embryonic period, many cells similar to those at younger ages (see Fig. 1), but containing larger numbers of apical organelles, were observed. These organelles included spherical mitochondria and increased amounts of GER with dilated cisternae. The cisternae of the Golgi apparatus were dilated and surrounded by enlarged membrane-bound vacuoles, and glycogen was concentrated near the nucleus and intermixed with the organelles. These cells were observed in fetuses up to early in the canalicular stage.

Through most of the pseudoglandular stage, most nonciliated cells had increased numbers of apical membrane-bound secretory granules containing a flocculent matrix, with a small electron-dense spherical core (see Fig. 2). Most of the remaining cytoplasm was still filled with glycogen. The cytoplasm surrounding the glycogen was more electron dense than in younger ages and occupied more of the apical portion of the cell. The nuclei exhibited prominent nucleoli and small patches of heterochromatin. The mitochondria exhibited noncircular profiles and appeared to be tubular. The amount of GER appeared to be the same as in younger ages, but the cisternae were no longer dilated. The Golgi apparatus was surrounded by vacuoles of various sizes. The luminal surface of these cells was covered by long, regular microvilli. In somewhat older animals (late pseudoglandular), the apices of a large proportion of the secretory cells were filled with spherical granules (see Fig. 3). Most of these cells had abundant cytoplasmic glycogen, most of which was basal to the nucleus. Apical to the nucleus, glycogen was interspersed among organelles and granules. The cells appeared more fusiform than at younger ages, being wide at the luminal side and narrow at the base (see Fig. 3). Secretory granules in these cells had a flocculent matrix and dense single cores (see Fig. 3). In fetuses from midcanalicular stage and older, secretory cells containing cytoplasmic glycogen were rare, and when observed, the glycogen content was minimal. From this time to parturition, only two forms of secretory cells were observed. Both cells had little cytoplasmic glycogen, and the cytoplasm was condensed. There was a distinct variation in the abundance of apical secretory granules in these cells, ranging from very few, in cells with a narrow cytoplasm and few organelles, to cells with an abundance of these granules (see Fig. 4). The cytoplasm of these cells contained small mitochondria and varying amounts of GER. The Golgi apparatus was located on the apical side of the nucleus and showed variable degrees of activity. In cells with more granules (see Fig. 4), the Golgi apparatus was larger, had more cisternal stacks, and larger and more numerous adjacent vesicles. Long, regular microvilli were a characteristic feature of the surface of the secretory cells. There was considerable variability in the abundance of these cellular forms between 105 days and parturition. In the earlier ages, they were of approximately equal abundance. Near parturition, most of the secretory cells resembled that in Figure 4. Some of the cells had an even larger percentage of their cytoplasm occupied by granules than illustrated in Figure 4.

In the postnatal period, most of the secretory cells had an abundance of electron-lucent granules filling their apical cytoplasm. The majority of these granules had small electron-dense cores. A few had large electron-dense biphasic cores (Fig. 5), as was observed in the adult (Fig. 6). In general, the nucleus and its surrounding cytoplasm were restricted to the basal portion of the cell and the Golgi apparatus, and other organelles occupied a small percentage of the cytoplasm. Up through 134 days postparturition there were, however, a few secretory cells the cytoplasm of which contained abundant organelles and a variable number of secretory granules, as was observed in the late fetal period (see Fig. 4). By 134 days postnatal age, nearly all of the secretory cells had a configuration similar to that observed in adults (see Fig. 6). The cytoplasm was filled with electron-lucent secretory granules that appeared to distend the cell's cytoplasm. The nucleus was compressed at the basal portion of the cell and organelles were minimal. In most cases, the cytoplasmic granules contained a biphasic core. The central part of the core was the most electron-dense portion of the granules (see Fig. 6).

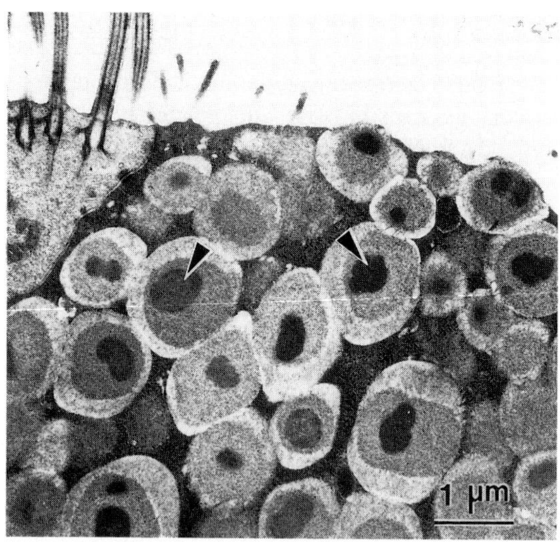

Figure 5   Apex of nonciliated tracheal epithelial cell filled with large triphasic granules. The central cores (arrowheads) are the most electron-dense; 18 days postnatal.

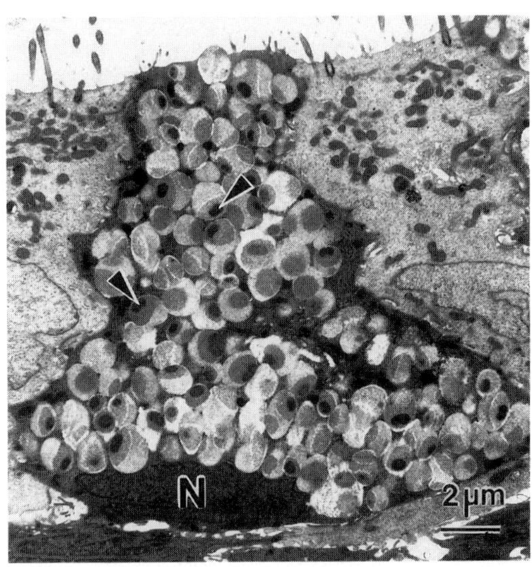

Figure 6   Mucous goblet cell from trachea of adult rhesus monkey. The nucleus (N) is compressed to the base of the cell by the abundant triphasic granules with dense central cores (arrowheads); 11 years 11 months of age.

B.   Carbohydrate Histochemistry and Cytochemistry

Early in the pseudoglandular stage, numerous cells contained periodic acid–Schiff (PAS) stain that was distributed in clumps apical and basal to the nucleus. Cells that were PAS-positive were alcian blue (AB)- and high iron diamine (HID)-negative. Granules were difficult to differentiate from glycogen in cells at this stage. However, at the electron microscopic (EM) level, PAS reactivity was confirmed where granules in the apex of the cells contained periodic acid thiocarbohydrazide (PATCH) reaction product only within the matrix and not within granule cores (Fig. 7). Glycogen was also stained in the basal region of most cells with PATCH (see Fig. 7). Most of these earliest secretory cells that were PAS-positive were AB-positive, but HID-negative in the apex (Fig. 8). Low iron diamine (LID) staining at the EM level was restricted to the matrix around the periphery of the granules if no core was present (Fig. 9). When a core was present, the core was LID-positive (Fig. 10). By ultrastructure, the LID and HID reaction product was restricted to the periphery of granules in cells with uncored granules, whereas in cells with cored granules the cores were HID-positive (Fig. 11). There were more cells that were AB-positive and HID-negative up to early in the canalicular stage. After this age, as in the adult, all of the PAS-positive cells were

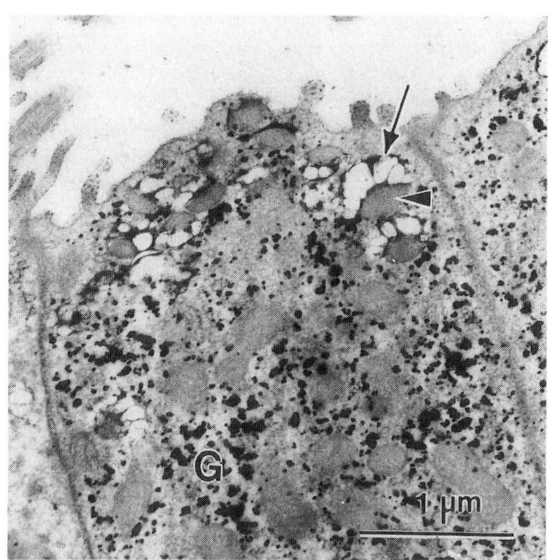

Figure 7 Developing secretory cell with granules in which the matrix is reactive with the stain periodic acid thiocarbohydrazide (PATCH) (arrow). The more electron-dense core is not PATCH-positive (arrowhead). The glycogen surrounding the mitochondria is strongly positive (G); 62 days GA.

also both AB- and HID-positive. Reaction product from all three stains was restricted to the apex. This staining pattern was true, regardless of the amount of reaction product, indicating that even cells with few secretory granules contained periodate reactive glycoconjugates that were acidic owing to sulfate esters.

C. Lectin Histochemistry

Lectins were applied to fetal rhesus trachea to detect terminal sugars in the carbohydrates of secretory granules (Table 4). The specificity of the lectins is provided in Table 3. Two lectins, SWGA and PNA, stained the earliest tracheal secretory cells. Three weeks later in gestation two more lectins, LCA and UEA I reacted with secretory cells. This pattern of reactivity continued through the beginning of the terminal sac stage, when PNA ceased to react with cells. Late in gestation, BSA I was the final lectin to positively stain secretory cells. The pattern of lectin staining seen at 155 DGA, LCA, UEA I, SWGA, and BSA I-positive, was observed through parturition into the postnatal period. At this point in gestation, although the tracheal reactivity of the lectins was the same as adults, the pattern of staining and number of positive cells was not. DBA, specific for

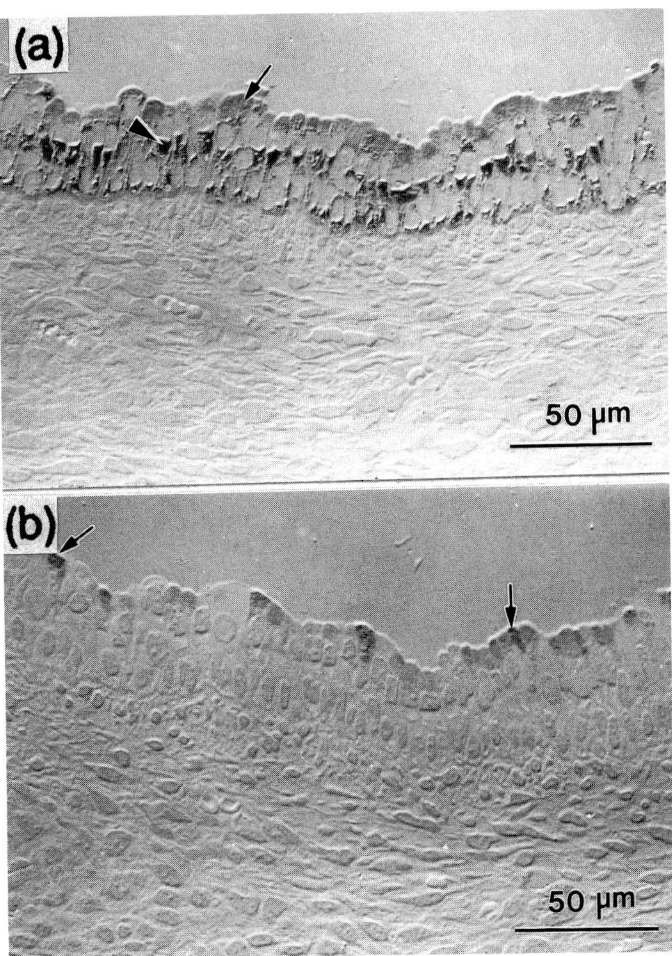

Figure 8 Light micrographs of fetal rhesus tracheal epithelium. (a) Stained with alcian blue/periodic acid–Schiff (AB/PAS). The apical regions of most cells are AB/PAS-positive (arrow). The region just apical of the nucleus contained the darkest PAS reaction product (arrowhead). This area corresponds to dense glycogen deposits. (b) Section serial to that seen in (a), but stained with alcian blue/high iron diamine (AB/HID). All cells stained with AB/PAS were AB-positive, but only of few of these were HID-positive. The HID-positive cells are slightly darker in this light micrograph (arrows); 62 days GA.

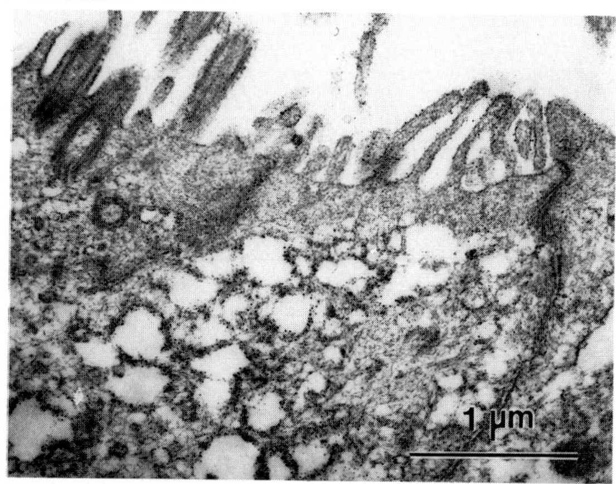

Figure 9   Apical region of a developing secretory cell stained at the EM level with low iron diamine (LID). Only the periphery of these uncored granules contains reaction product with this stain; 62 days GA.

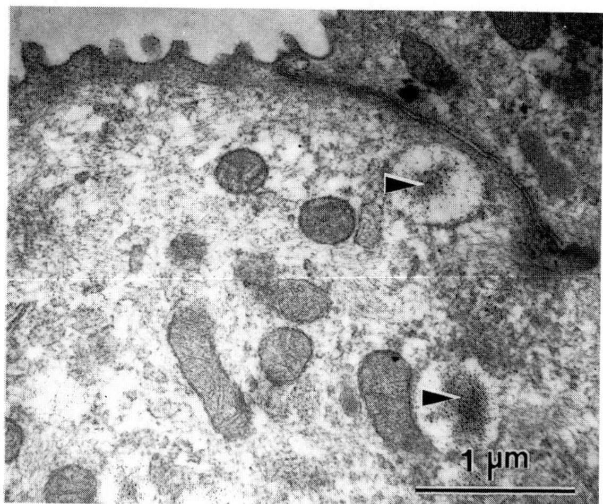

Figure 10   Secretory cell with cored granules. In these granules the LID reaction product is located over the cores (arrowheads); 62 days GA.

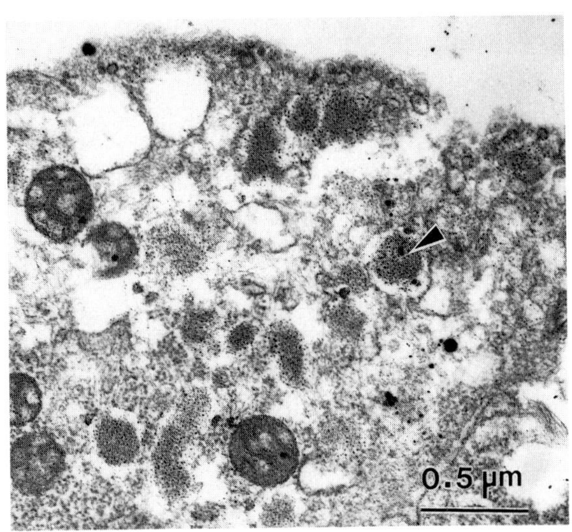

Figure 11　Apical region of a fetal tracheal secretory cell that has been stained with high iron diamine (HID). The reaction product is localized over the cores (arrowhead); 62 days GA.

Table 4　Lectin Reactivity in Developing Rhesus Monkey Trachea

Lectin								

	Days gestational age							
Lectin	50	60	70	80	90	135	155	18 d PN
LCA	−	−	−	+	+	+	+	+
UEA 1	−	−	−	+	+	+	+	+
SWGA	−	+	+	+	+	+	+	+
BSA 1	−	−	−	−	−	−	+	+
PNA	−	+	+	+	+	−	−	−
DBA	−	−	−	−	−	−	−	−

Abbrev: see Table 3.

N-acetylgalactosamine did not react with tracheal cells at any point examined, including adult.

D. Glycoconjugate Immunohistochemistry

We have also used a panel of monoclonal antibodies that react with adult tracheal mucins (St. George et al., 1985) to examine the appearance of secretory products in the airways of developing fetal monkey lungs. From that study, we have concluded that the antigens of adult trachea are present in neonatal trachea at birth, but that the antigens appear sequentially, rather than simultaneously. The results of this and other studies using monoclonal antibodies are probably detecting differences in glycosylation of mucous glycoconjugates, since characterization of the epitopes of our antibodies (Lin et al., 1989) and those of other's (Basbaum et al., 1986) have indicated a carbohydrate specificity.

Two monoclonal antibodies reacted with some nonciliated tracheal cells of a fetal monkey early in the pseudoglandular stage. The cells containing reaction product were located primarily in the cartilaginous region. The reaction product was observed in the middle of the cell cytoplasm (Fig. 12a) and not in the apical region where granules are first observed. When compared with the AB/PAS-staining pattern (see Fig. 12b), the monoclonal antibody staining occurred in areas within the region that contained PAS-positive, AB-negative material. To determine if the antibody reactivity was associated with glycogen deposits, sections were treated with α-amylase before immunohistochemical staining. The PAS reactivity was removed, but the antibody staining remained unaffected. Other monoclonal antibodies the reactivity of which patterns were indistinguishable in the adult trachea from these two antibodies did not stain any cells at this age.

In trachea of slightly older fetal monkeys almost all cells in the cartilaginous region contained granules that were PAS- and AB-positive (Fig. 13a). A few of these secretory cells were recognized by these two antibodies (see Fig. 13c). An even smaller proportion of these cells contained product recognized by an additional four antibodies (see Fig. 13b). These four antibodies reacted with granules, but not regions of the cytoplasm stained by the first two antibodies. The reactivity of the first two antibodies now localized material in granules as well as in the lower three-fourths of the cytoplasm until early in the canalicular stage, at which point stain was seen only in granules. With increasing gestational age, more secretory granules stained HID. With the shift from blue (AB+) to brown (HID+) granules, four antibodies reacted exclusively with granules, but later in gestation stained even more secretory cells, and by the end of the pseudoglandular stage, most of the secretory cells present were HID-positive and antibody reactive. However, there was not a one-to-one correlation of brown HID/AB staining and reactivity with antibody.

Two antibodies that localize secretory product in a subpopulation of adult

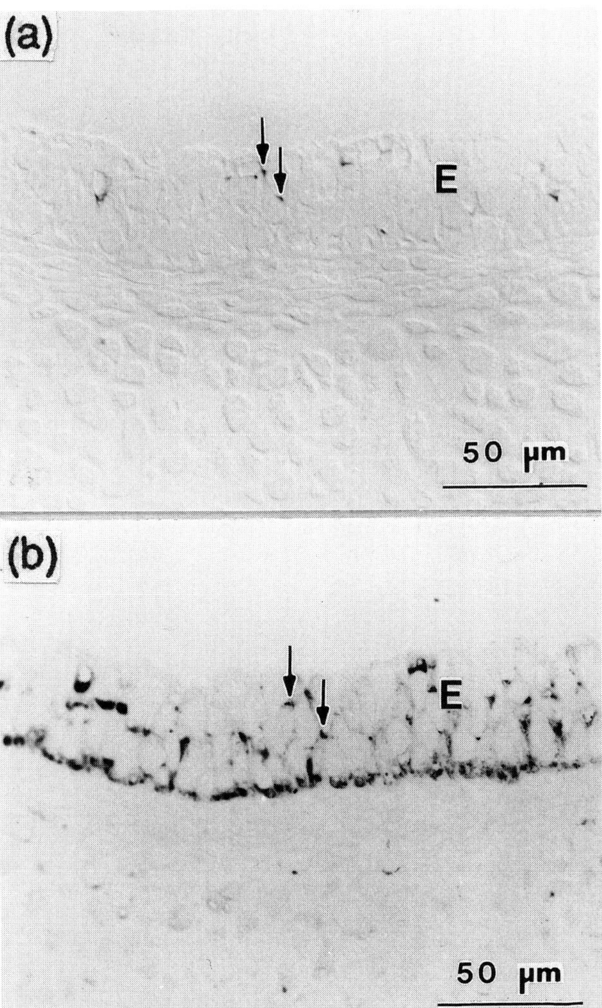

Figure 12 Tracheal epithelium (E) from a fetal rhesus monkey at 50 days GA. (a) A tracheal section that has been immunohistochemically stained with a monoclonal antibody that reacts with all mucous cells in adult trachea. There is light, focal reaction product in a subset of developing secretory cells (arrow). This site does not correspond to the apical region where granules are located. (b) An AB/PAS-stained section serial to panel (a). There is PAS stain in regions that correspond to the immunohistochemically stained regions (arrows) as well as some apical and strong basal and supranuclear stain.

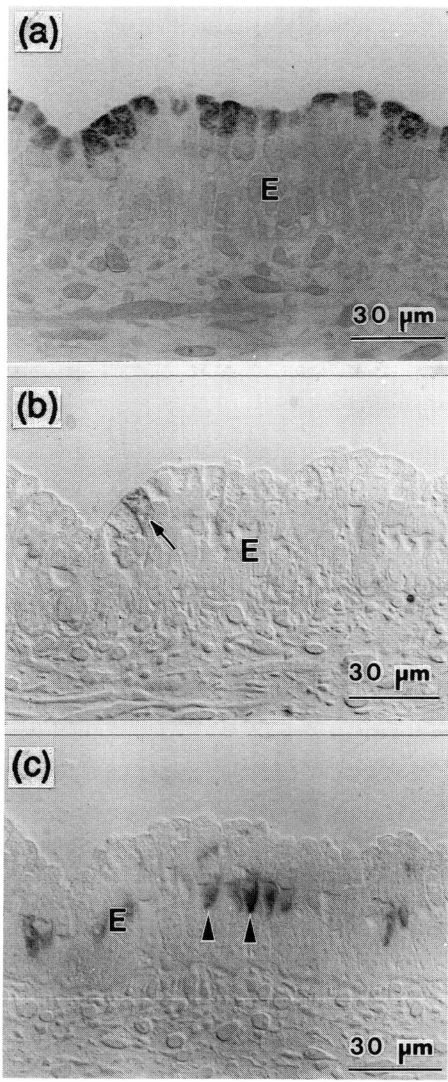

Figure 13 Serial sections of tracheal epithelium (E) of a fetal rhesus monkey at 62 days GA. (a) HID/AB-stained section where most cells are stained either blue or brown in the apex at which granules are located. (b) Immunostained section using an antibody that stains all mucous cells in the adult trachea. A single cell contains reaction product in the region at which granules are located (arrow). (c) Another immunostained section stained with an antibody that reacts with all mucous cells in adult trachea, identical with the antibody used in panel (b). However, this antibody localizes antigen not in the region of granules as in (b), but in a more basal region of the cytoplasm (arrowheads).

tracheal mucous cells, reacted with very few secretory cells in developing trachea midway through the pseudoglandular stage. The proportion of cells recognized by these two antibodies increased with gestational age to peak in late canalicular stage, after which the proportion decreased to the adult levels. It was at this stage in development (midpseudoglandular) that all of the antigens detected by the monoclonal antibodies in adult trachea were present in the surface epithelium of the developing trachea.

IV. Submucosal Gland Development

The development of submucosal glands has been described in a variety of species, including rat (Smolich et al., 1978), opossum (Krause and Leeson, 1973), ferret (Leigh et al., 1986), rhesus monkey (Plopper et al., 1986b), and humans (Thurlbeck et al., 1961; Bucher and Reid, 1961). The sequence of events in humans has been characterized subgrossly (Tos, 1966, 1968) and histologically (Bucher and Reid, 1961; Thurlbeck et al., 1961; Lamb and Reid, 1972; Bucher and Reid, 1961; Jeffery and Reid, 1977). The ultrastructure and histochemistry of gland development has been characterized in the most detail in the rhesus monkey (Plopper et al., 1986b). In the rhesus, most of the process occurs in the fetus between the end of the pseudoglandular stage and the beginning of the terminal sac stage of development. Gland development implies four phases: (1) the formation of buds by projections of undifferentiated cells from the maturing surface epithelium; (2) the outgrowth and branching of these buds into cylinders of undifferentiated cells; (3) the differentiation of mucous cells in proximal tubules associated with proliferation of tubules and acini and with undifferentiated cells distally; and (4) differentiation of serous cells in peripheral tubules and acini, with continued proliferation in most distal areas. The cells forming gland buds are not basal cells, as first thought, but rather, an undifferentiated cell similar to the surface epithelium (see Fig. 1) (Plopper et al., 1986b). Connective tissue appears to play a role in this process, as evidenced primarily through the presence of cartilage plates in the areas of initial bud formation. Glands appear first at the junction of cartilage plate and smooth muscle, followed by areas over cartilage plates, and then in the area over smooth muscle. The secretory cell population differentiates in a centrifugal pattern, with nearly mature cells lining proximal tubules and immature cells in more distal portions. The development of mucous cells in the proximal portion of the gland occurs before that of serous cells. Glandular mucous cells and serous cells differentiate at different times during development and through a different sequence of events (Plopper et al., 1986b).

As an example of gland development, a review of tracheal submucosal gland development in rhesus monkey is provided (Plopper et al., 1986b). Gland buds were first observed in the fetal rhesus monkey at 70-days gestational age. From the beginning of the canalicular stage, the buds grew into cylinders with lumina, and secretory granules were observed in the cells of the cylinders shortly after the formation of the cylinders. In fetuses at the end of the canalicular stage and older, the developing glands included a proximal tubule or duct and a number of alveoli. Ciliated cells were present in proximal ducts at 120-days gestational age. The distal portion of tracheal submucosal glands continued to mature postnatally, primarily with the maturation of the serous cells.

A. Carbohydrate Histochemistry

Early buds and cylinders were PAS-, AB-, and HID-negative, except some tubule cells that were PAS-positive in the basal region. Granules appeared first in proximal tubule cells and were PAS- and AB-positive. Only a few AB-positive cells were HID-positive. The distal portions of proliferating tubules were negative for all stains at this time. When serous acini were proliferating, the epithelial cells lining proximal ducts were strongly PAS-, AB-, and HID-positive, whereas more distal tubules and acini reacted variably. Distal acini and tubules with large lumina contained some cells that were strongly AB-positive, but HID-negative. However, most of the cells in the peripheral portions of the glands were slightly PAS-positive or were negative and did not react with AB or HID. In mature glands, most acinar cells were strongly PAS-positive, but HID- and AB-negative.

B. Carbohydrate Immunohistochemistry

In contrast to surface epithelium, glandular immunostaining was not observed until the end of the pseudoglandular stage, at which time the antibodies reactive to all adult tracheal mucous cells reacted with the cells containing acidic products that were located in the proximal glandular ducts. Antibody specific for the distal portions of adult tracheal glands remained unreactive until midcanalicular stage, when it was found in some PAS-positive cells of the still forming gland. By late in gestation, the distal portion of submucosal glands was PAS-positive, lightly AB- and HID-positive, and stained by the gland-specific antibody.

V. Control of Differentiation

Regulation of the maturation of the fetal airway secretory apparatus has not been well examined; therefore, the factors that control development and the mechanisms of these controls are poorly understood. We have conducted a study to examine the effects of epidermal growth factor (EGF) on lung development in the rhesus monkey. In that study, we demonstrated that EGF treatment in utero markedly stimulates the maturation of the tracheal secretory apparatus, including both the tracheal surface and submucosal glands (St. George et al., 1991). The secretory apparatus was more differentiated in that there were more mucous cells, increased secretory product stored in the epithelium and glands, and increased quantities of secretory product in lavage and amniotic fluid. In contrast, treatment with triamicinalone, a glucocorticoid, induced maturation of the gas exchange area (Bunton and Plopper, 1984), but did not affect the maturation of the secretory apparatus (Table 5).

VI. Summary

Several methods including morphological, histochemical, and immunohisto-chemical have been used to define the maturation and content of secretory apparatus in developing as well as fully differentiated airway epithelium. Application of these methods has demonstrated extensive heterogeneity in content when comparing secretory cells from epithelial surface with those in submucosal glands, in the same cell type at the same airway level in different species, and in secretory cells from different airway levels in the same species. Full understanding of the secretory response and the airway secretory products requires further characterization, especially of the protein portion of this complex secretory glycoconjugate. The influence of secretion by different sites (surface versus glands) on the properties of the mucous blanket and the importance in differences in control in these regions remains to be elucidated. It will be of interest to learn whether the same secretory cell types from different airway levels are controlled differently. Extrapolation of results from one species to another should be done bearing in mind that the aforementioned differences may dictate a very different secretory response to a given stimulus.

Developmental studies of the tracheal surface (Plopper et al., 1986b) and submucosal glands (Plopper et al., 1986a) of nonhuman primates have shown that

Table 5 Effect of EGF and Triamcinalone Acetonide (TAC) on Total Glycoconjugate Detectable in the Trachea of Fetal Rhesus Monkeys

Days gestational age	Treatment	Total secretory product $(mm^3 \times 10^3/mm^2)$ $(\bar{x} \pm 1\ SD)$
128	None	0.48 ± 0.37
150	None	$1.36^a \pm 0.33$
128	EGF	$1.77^a \pm 0.28$
150	TAC (1 mg/day)	1.27 ± 1.35
150	TAC (10 mg/day)	0.75 ± 0.34

[a]$p < 0.05$ compared with 128 DGA control.

mucous cell differentiation in these regions is similar and follows the same three-phase sequence of differentiation. These phases are (1) formation of apical granules containing acid glycoconjugates in cells, with large amounts of glycogen; (2) increase in the numbers of granules and formation of abundant Golgi apparatus; and (3) maturation and filling of cells with secretory granules. Analysis of the content of developing secretory granules has demonstrated that their composition differs from adult airway secretory cells and that the content of surface cells matured differently than that in submucosal glands. In the developing tracheal surface, cells with periodate-reactive granules contain sialic acid, but sulfation follows, appearing before the cells are fully mature. These studies have been performed only in species in which the mucous cell content is sulfated. When terminal sugars were evaluated, they also demonstrated a developmental-dependent expression. In fetal rhesus trachea, N-acetylglucosamine and β-galactose linked to N-acetylgalactosamine were detected in the first secretory cells, followed by the appearance of fucose and mannose or glucose. Finally, α-galactose appeared, with the disappearance or masking of β-galactose-N-acetylgalactosamine. Mucous antigens, some of which have been shown to be carbohydrates (Lin et al., 1989), also appeared in a sequential fashion. The appearance of mucous antigens and terminal sugars were in parallel. The carbohydrate content of secretory granules changes with mucous cell differentiation, possibly owing to the expression of additional glycosyltransferases as maturation progresses. The control of these developmental patterns and the effect of these changes in the fetal or the neonatal lung remains to be defined.

References

Basbaum, C. B., Mann, J. K., Chow, A. W., and Finkbeiner, W. E. (1984). Monoclonal antibodies as probes for unique antigens in secretory cells of mixed exocrine organs. *Proc. Natl. Acad. Sci. USA* 81: 4419–4423.

Basbaum, C. B., Chow, A., Macher, B. A., Finkbeiner, W. E., Veissiere, D., and Forsberg, L. S. (1986). Tracheal carbohydrate antigens identified by monoclonal antibodies. *Arch. Biochem. Biophys.* 249: 363–373.

Bedrossian, C. W. M., Anderson, A. E., and Foraker, A. G. (1971). Comparison of methods for quantitating bronchial morphology. *Thorax* 26: 406–408.

Bowes, D., Clark, A. E., and Corrin, B. (1981). Ultrastructural localization of lactoferrin and glycoprotein in human bronchial glands. *Thorax* 36: 108–115.

Bowes, D., and Corrin, B. (1977). Ultrastructural immunocytochemical localization of lysozyme in human bronchial glands. *Thorax* 32: 163–170.

Boyden, E. A. (1972). Development of the human lung. In *Brennermann's Practice of Pediatrics*, Vol. 4. Hagerstown, Harper & Row.

Boyden, E. A. (1976). The development of the lung in the pig-tail monkey (*Macaca nemestrina*, L.). *Anat. Rec.* 186: 15–38.

Bucher, U., and Reid, L. (1961). Development of the mucus-secreting elements in human lung. *Thorax* 16: 219–225.

Bunton, T. E., and Plopper, C. G. (1984). Triamcinolone-induced structural alterations in the development of the lung of the fetal rhesus macaque. *Am. J. Obstet. Gynecol.* 148: 203–215.

Emura, M., and Mohr, U. (1975). Morphological studies on the development of tracheal epithelium in the Syrian golden hamster. *Z. Versuchstierk de.* 17: 14–26.

Harkema, J. R., Plopper, C. G., Hyde, D. M., and St. George, J. A. (1987a). Regional differences in quantities of histochemically detectable mucosubstances in nasal, paranasal, and nasopharyngeal epithelium of the bonnet monkey. *J. Histochem. Cytochem.* 35: 279–286.

Harkema, J. R., Plopper, C. G., Hyde, D. M., St. George, J. A., and Dungworth, D. L. (1987b). Effects of an ambient level of ozone on primate nasal epithelial mucosubstances: Quantitative histochemistry. *Am. J. Pathol.* 127: 90–96.

Heidsiek, J. G., Hyde, D. M., Plopper, C. G., and St. George, J. A. (1987). Quantitative histochemistry of mucosubstance in tracheal epithelium of the macaque monkey. *J. Histochem. Cytochem.* 35: 435–442.

Jeffery, P. K. (1977). Structure and function of mucus-secreting cells of cat and goose airway epithelium. In *Respiratory Tract Mucus*. New York, Elsevier–North Holland, pp. 5–19.

Jeffery, P. K. (1983). Morphologic features of airway surface epithelial cells and glands. *Am. Rev. Respir. Dis.* 128: S14–S20.

Jeffery, P. K., and Reid, L. M. (1977). Ultrastructure of airway epithelium and submucosal gland during development. In *Development of the Lung*. Edited by W. A. Hodson. New York, Marcel Dekker, pp. 87–134.

Jones, R. A., Baskerville, A., and Reid, L. M. (1975). Histochemical identification of glycoproteins in pig bronchial epithelium: (a) Normal and (b) hypertrophied from enzootic pneumonia. *J. Pathol.* 116: 1–11.

Kawamata, S., and Fujita, H. (1983). Fine structural aspects of the development and aging of the tracheal epithelium of mice. *Arch. Histol. Jpn.* 46: 355–372.

Krause, W. J., and Leeson, C. R. (1973). The postnatal development of the respiratory system of the opossum. I. Light and scanning electron microscopy. *Am. J. Anat.* 137: 337–354.

Lamb, D., and Reid, L. (1969). Histochemical types of acidic glycoprotein produced by mucous cells of the tracheobronchial glands in man. *J. Pathol.* 98: 213–229.

Lamb, D., and Reid, L. (1972). Acidic glycoproteins produced by the mucous cells of the bronchial submucosal glands in the fetus and child: A histochemical autoradiographic study. *Br. J. Dis. Chest* 66: 248–253.

Leeson, T. S. (1961). The development of the trachea in the rabbit, with particular reference to its fine structure. *Anat. Anz.* 110: S214–223.

Leigh, M. W., Gambling, T. M., Carson, J. L., Collier, A. M., Wood, R. E., and Boat, T. F. (1986). Postnatal development of tracheal surface epithelium and submucosal glands in the ferret. *Exp. Lung Res.* 10: 153–169.

Lin, H., Carlson, D. M., St. George, J. A., Plopper, C. G., and Wu, R. (1989). An ELISA method for the quantitation of tracheal mucins from human and nonhuman primates. *Am. J. Respir. Cell Mol. Biol.* 1: 41–48.

Mariassy, A. T., Plopper, C. G., St. George, J. A., and Wilson, D. W. (1988a). Tracheobronchial epithelium of the sheep: IV. Lectin histochemical characterization of secretory epithelial cells. *Anat. Rec.* 222: 49–59.

Mariassy, A. T., St. George, J. A., Nishio, S. J., and Plopper, C. G. (1988b). Tracheobronchial epithelium of the sheep: III. Carbohydrate histochemical and cytochemical characterization of secretory epithelial cells. *Anat. Rec.* 221: 540–549.

McCarthy, C., and Reid, L. M. (1964a). Acid mucopolysaccharides in the bronchial tree in the mouse and rat (sialomucins and sulphate). *Q. J. Exp. Physiol.* 49: 81–84.

McCarthy, C., and Reid, L. M. (1964b). Intracellular mucopolysaccharides in the normal human bronchial tree. *Q. J. Exp. Physiol.* 49: 85–94.

McDowell, E. M., Newkirk, C., and Coleman, B. (1985). Development of hamster tracheal epithelium: I. A quantitative morphologic study in the fetus. *Anat. Rec.* 213: 429–447.

Mills, A. N., Lopez-Vidriero, M. T., and Haworth, S. G. (1986). Development of the airway epithelium and submucosal glands in the pig lung: Changes in epithelial glycoprotein profiles. *Br. J. Exp. Pathol.* 67: 821–829.

Mochizuki, I., Setser, M. E., Martinez, J. R., and Spicer, S. S. (1982). Carbohydrate histochemistry of rat respiratory glands. *Anat. Rec.* 202: 45–59.

Plopper, C. G., St. George, J. A., Nishio, S. J., Etchison, J. R., and Nettesheim, P. (1984). Carbohydrate cytochemistry of tracheobronchial airway epithelium of the rabbit. *J. Histochem. Cytochem.* 32: 209–218.

Plopper, C. G. Alley, J. L., and Weir, A. L. (1986a). Differentiation of tracheal epithelium during fetal lung maturation in the rhesus monkey *Macaca mulatta. Am. J. Anat.* 175: 59–71.

Plopper, C. G., Weir, A. J., Nishio, S. J., Cranz, D. L., and St. George, J. A. (1986b). Tracheal submucosal gland development in the rhesus monkey, *Macaca mulatta*: Ultrastructure and histochemistry. *Anat. Embryol.* 174: 167–178.

Plopper, C. G., Heidsiek, J. G., Weir, A. J., St. George, J. A., and Hyde, D. M. (1989). Tracheobronchial epithelium in the adult rhesus monkey: A quantitative histochemical and ultrastructural study. *Am. J. Anat.* 184: 31–40.

Rana, S. S., Chandrasekaran, E. V., and Mendicino, J. (1986). Structures of the sialylated oligosaccharide chains in swine trachea mucin glycoproteins. *J. Biol. Chem.* 262: 3654–3659.

Reid, L. M. (1960). Measurement of the bronchial mucous gland layer: A diagnostic yardstick in chronic bronchitis. *Thorax* 15: 132–141.

Reid, L. M. Bhaskar, K. R., and Coles, S. (1983). Control and modulation of airway epithelial cells and their secretions. *Exp. Lung Res.* 4: 157–170.

Shimura, S., Sasaki, T., Ikeda, K., Yamauchi, K., Sasaki, H., and Takishima, T. (1990). Direct inhibitory action of glucocorticoid on glycoconjugate secretion from airway submucosal glands. *Am. Rev. Respir. Dis.* 141: 1044–1049.

Smolich, J. J., Stratford, B. F., Maloney, J. E., and Ritchie, B. C. (1978). New features in the development of the submucosal gland of the respiratory tract. *J. Anat.* 127: 223–238.

Spicer, S. S., Chakrin, L. W., Wardell, J. R., and Kendrick, W. (1971). Histochemistry of mucosubstances in the canine and human respiratory tract. *Lab. Invest.* 25: 483–489.

Spicer, S. S., Mochizuki, I., Setser, M. E., and Martinez, J. R. (1980). Complex carbohydrates of rat tracheobronchial surface epithelium visualized ultrastructurally. *Am. J. Anat.* 158: 93–109.

Spicer, S. S., Schulte, B. A., and Thomopoulos, G. N. (1983). Histochemical properties of the respiratory tract in different species. *Am. Rev. Respir. Dis.* 128: S20–S26.

St. George, J. A., Nishio, S. J., and Plopper, C. G. (1984a). Carbohydrate cytochemistry of the rhesus monkey tracheal epithelium. *Anat. Rec.* 210: 293–302.

St. George, J. A., Plopper, C. G., Etchison, J. R., and Dungworth, D. L. (1984b). An immunocytochemical/histochemical approach to tracheobronchial mucus characterization in the rabbit. *Am. Rev. Respir. Dis.* 130: 124–127.

St. George, J. A., Cranz, D. L., Zicker, S., Etchison, J. R., Dungworth, D. L., and Plopper, C. G. (1985). An immunohistochemical characterization of rhesus monkey respiratory secretions using monoclonal antibodies. *Am. Rev. Respir. Dis.* 132: 556–563.

St. George, J. A., Cranz, D. L., Etchison, J. R., and Plopper, C. G. (1986a). Variation of respiratory mucins with airway level in rhesus monkey. *A. Rev. Respir. Dis.* 133: A294.

St. George, J. A., Nishio, S. J., Cranz, D. L., and Plopper, C. G. (1986b). Carbohydrate cytochemistry of rhesus monkey tracheal submucosal glands. *Anat. Rec.* 216: 60–67.

St. George, J. A., Read, L. C., Cranz, D. L., Tarantal, A. F., George-Nasimento, C., and Plopper, C. G. (1991). Effect of epidermal growth factor on the fetal development of the tracheobronchial secretory apparatus in rhesus monkey. *Am. J. Respir. Cell Mol. Biol.* 4: 95–101.

Thaete, L. C., Spicer, S. S., and Spock, A. (1981). Histology, ultrastructure, and carbohydrate cytochemistry of surface and glandular epithelium of human nasal mucosa. *Am. J. Anat.* 162: 243–263.

Thurlbeck, W. M., Benjamin, B., and Reid, L. (1961). Development and distribution of mucous glands in the foetal human trachea. *Br. J. Dis. Chest* 55: 54–64.

Tos, M. (1966). Development of the tracheal glands in man. *Acta Pathol. Microbiol. Scand.* 185(Suppl): 1–30.

Tos, M. (1968). Distribution and situation of the mucous glands in the main bronchus of human foetuses. *Anat. Anz.* 123: S481–495.

Wasano, K., Nakamura, K., and Yamamoto, T. (1988). Lectin-gold cytochemistry of mucin oligosaccharide biosynthesis in Golgi apparatus of airway secretory cells of the hamster. *Anat. Rec.* 221: 635–644.

5

Microscopic Structure of Airway Secretory Cells
Variation in Hypersecretory Disease and Effects of Drugs

PETER K. JEFFERY

Royal Brompton Hospital
National Heart and Lung Institute
London, England

I. Introduction

Normally, the volume of bronchial secretions is not sufficient to cause expectoration, any secretion being imperceptibly swallowed. In hypersecretory diseases, such as chronic bronchitis and cystic fibrosis, and in many cases of asthma, bronchial secretions are increased to a level at which they are coughed up and expectorated as sputum. The observed increase in bronchial secretion is usually mirrored anatomically by an enlargement of the mass of tracheobronchial submucosal gland and by an increased number of surface epithelial goblet (mucous) cells in large bronchi and, in small airways disease, by their appearance and subsequent increase in bronchioli where they are normally absent or sparse. Historical aspects of the first descriptions of airway secretory cells, their fetal development, microscopic structure, and variation in disease and with treatment, are the subject matter of the present chapter.

II. Historical Aspects

In 1602, Laurentius (Rhodin and Dalhamn, 1956) first described a membranous lining to the walls of the airways that, in today's terms, would have included both the mucosa and submucosa. The subsequent development and application of the light microscope and the observations of Malpighi, von Leeuwenhoek, and Bichat culminated in the theory that all physiological and pathological processes depended on changes within biological units they called cells. The theory, postulated by Schleiden (1838) and Schwann (1839) and generally accepted after the publication of Virchow's *cellularpathologie* in 1858 (Cameron, 1952) initiated much research into the microscopic anatomy of the lung, its airways, and the secretion of its moist lining mucosa.

In 1834, Purkinje and Valentin (Sharpey, 1836) published one of the first descriptions of the lining mucosa of airways from several species of birds, reptiles, and mammals, including that of humans. After discovering the cilia, they proceeded to describe their movements in the trachea and bronchial tubes ". . . extending to their smallest divisions capable of examination." In 1836, Sharpey published an extensive review of cilia in the animal kingdom and, in the mammalian respiratory system, traced the direction of beat, observing the movement of charcoal powder entangled in secretion on a strip of dog airway placed in tepid water. He found the movement resulted in successive waves, which he likened to wind in a cornfield, and that it was clearly directed toward the trachea and larynx. He further suggested that ". . . whatever may be its other uses, it at least serves to convey the secretions along the membranes together with foreign matters if any are present." In 1837, Henle and, 10 years later, Bowman (1847) reported that the mucous membrane was lined by a "pavement" (epithelium) resting on a basement membrane and composed of nucleated "particles" (cells) adhering together and of various size, form, and number. Henle described a secretion from the mucous membrane, the "principles" (precursors) of which Bowman regarded as being lodged in the epithelial cells. To these mucus-secreting cells, and by virtue of their shape, the term goblet cell was later, in 1867, applied by Schulze. He showed that goblet cells have a theca ". . . filled with a mucous mass through which numerous highly refractile granules are distributed, and which projects from the upper rounded opening of the cell in the form of a small ball, that sometimes becomes altogether detached" (Schulze, 1872). In 1881, Kolliker (Azzopardi and Thurlbeck, 1969) examined human distal airways and found that the epithelium of the terminal bronchioli lacked goblet cells. In these small airways, ciliated cells were interspersed with nonciliated cells, later to be known as Clara cells.

In the latter part of the 19th century, improvements were made to microscopes and, with the development of achromatic lenses and the use of improved embedding media, thinner sections of tissue could be cut, stained by mono- or polychromatic stains, and viewed to advantage. Distinct cell types and organelles could now be visualized and magnified some 1000 times. By 1932, the reviews of Miller and of Lucas (Miller, 1932) show that the description of human airway epithelium remained essentially that of earlier workers: a pseudostratified epithelium, with ciliated, goblet, intermediate, and basal cells, the thickness diminishing in bronchioli of 1 mm, goblet cells absent and basal cells rare in terminal bronchioli, and cilia absent (now known to be present) from the respiratory bronchiolus, where the nonciliated cuboidal epithelium gradually became flattened, giving way to the simple squamous epithelial lining of the alveoli. Lucas and Douglas (1934) found that the frequency of ciliary motion was unaltered when the flow of overlying mucus was stopped and suggested that the mucous "blanket" must be of two layers, an upper highly viscous layer resting on the tips of the cilia, and a lower, less viscous (periciliary) layer surrounding the cilia: only the tips of the cilia touched the mucus. The existence and nature of the periciliary layer still remains a controversial area and requires much research. Clara (1937) published the results of a histological study that concentrated on the terminal bronchioli of humans and rabbits and described in great detail the nonciliated cells that have since come to be known as "Clara" cells. The distinguishing features of the bronchiolar region were the sparcity of goblet cells and the presence of bulging nonciliated cells that secreted, in a putative apocrine manner, granules that did not stain for mucus. The goblet cells of the larger airways were also described, the ratio of goblet to ciliated cells varied among individuals, and goblet cell numbers markedly increased in certain pathological diseases. Macklin (1949) immersed the living bronchiolar cells of mouse and hamster in an ammoniacal silver solution and observed them with the light microscope. Whereas ciliated cells were "dark" with a cuticle, nonciliated cells (which he considered to be Clara cells) were "light" with protruding egg-shaped ends containing "small silverized particles" and, surmounting this, discoid areas with numerous granules. For the nonciliated bronchiolar cells, two forms were described that he regarded to be different functional states of the same cell type: (1) "club-cells" with protoplasmic processes projecting into the lumen and resembling those described by Clara and (2) "nonciliated cells" that did not project beyond the apex of ciliated cells. von Hayek (1962) agreed with Clara that the club-cell processes could be "broken off" and then "dissolved" into the secretion (i.e., apocrine secretion). Lamb (1968) distinguished by light microscopy three shapes of bronchial secretory cell: (1) medium-sized cells, in which the maximum cell width was half to one-quarter the cell height; (2) thin cells with only a narrow line of secretory product; and (3) nearly spherical or flask-shaped cells, the width being more than half the height. These differences related to the volume of intracellular stainable secretion and, hence, the term goblet cell could strictly be applied to only the last mentioned.

Initiated by the pioneering electron microscopic studies of rat airways by Rhodin and Dalhamn (1956) and of human airways by Rhodin (1966) several researchers have now completed detailed ultrastructural analyses of mammalian airways (Jeffery and Reid, 1975, 1977a; McDowell et al., 1978a; Jeffery, 1983, 1987a, 1990c; Jeffery and Corrin, 1984; Breeze and Wheeldon, 1977; Plopper et al., 1980, 1990; Plopper, 1983).

We now know that the secretory cells that line the conducting airways of adult humans are varied in type and have a multiplicity of function (Table 1). Their combined secretions serve to keep the lining mucosa moist, to humidify inhaled air and, in concert with beating cilia, to clean the air by removal of potentially harmful dust particles, organisms, and adsorbed gases, to the throat, where they are normally swallowed. Their secretions also contain substances, such as lacto-ferrin and lysozyme, that discourage bacterial colonization and growth or make them susceptible to neutralization by the hosts immune system. Apart from their protective role mucus-secreting cells may also act as stem cells, not only in the adult during repair following injury to the mucosa, but also during fetal develop-ment.

III. Histochemical and Ultrastructural Techniques

The epithelial mucins of the respiratory tract are polydisperse, high-molecular-mass glycoproteins. They consist of a filamentous protein core to which oligosac-charide side chains are attached. The core protein contains regions that are densely glycosylated (50–80%), and there are also naked regions rich in serine and threonine residues (Lamblin et al., 1992), such that the structure of the mucin may be likened to that of a bottle brush. According to the distinct chemical composition of the oligosaccharide side chains, the mucins may be acidic or neutral, whereas the naked regions of the peptide are of fairly constant amino acid composition (Bhattacharya et al., 1990). Acidic mucins appear to have a higher molar ratio of threonine, serine, sialic acid, and sulfate. The sugar residues (usually fucose, galactose, N-acetylglucosamine, N-acetylgalactosamine, and sialic acid) appear to play a role in determining the physical and flow properties of the mucus and may also affect bacterial adherence (see Lamblin et al., 1992). Lectins, which have an affinity for specific carbohydrate residues, have been used widely for the ultrastructural localization of the specific carbohydrates (Mazzuca et al., 1977, 1982; Schulte and Spicer, 1983; Plotowski et al., 1990; Frisch and Phillips, 1990). The heterogeneity of mucin types has been demonstrated in primate airway epithelia with several monoclonal antibodies (St. George et al., 1985; Lamblin et al., 1992; Basbaum, 1984). Histochemical methods have been applied at the light microscopic level to identify those cells secreting either acidic or neutral mucins, or both, in combination. Alcian blue (AB; pH 2.5) and periodic acid–Schiff (PAS) used in combination distinguish between the acidic and neutral mucins, respectively. The combined high iron diamine (HID)–AB (pH 2.5) method demonstrates the two main types of acidic glycoprotein, those with sulfomucins that stain brown and those containing sialomucins that stain blue (Spicer et al., 1971; Lamb, 1968). These lectins, antibodies, and histochemical stains demonstrate the translated end product of a gene-controlled secretory process that culminates in exocytotic discharge or intracellular storage, or a combination of both processes. The methods described thus far demonstrate only those cells with stored (intracellular) product, the amount of which is the balance of uptake of glycoconjugate precursors, synthesis, and discharge (Fig. 1). Electron microscopic methods applied to ultrathin sections (Schraufnagel, 1990), freeze-fracture (Robards and Sleytr, 1985), or scanning to show surface topography of previously fixed or frozen tissues (Postek et al., 1980) may demonstrate cells with or without their intracellular secretion (Fig. 2a–c). As with other biological systems, development of a particular secretory cell phenotype is the result of expression of a particular set of genes (Maniatis et al., 1987; Blau, 1989; Mitchell and Tijian, 1989). A common approach to monitoring gene expression in cells is by measurement of the level of mRNA transcription (Darnell, 1982), and cloned cDNA has been recently used to monitor, by northern blotting, mucin mRNA levels in experimental studies of mucus hypersecretion (Jany and Basbaum, 1991). Molecular techniques, in combination with the technique of in situ hybridization (Hamid et al., 1991), now offer viable methods to explore the cellular origins of newly acquired mucus-secreting cells in human hypersecretory disease and a possible novel approach to therapy.

IV. Airway Development

The airways of the lung begin their development 22–26 days postfertilization as a central diverticulum budding from the foregut and lined by epithelium of endodermal origin. In humans, the diverticulum forms two small ventrolateral buds (lung primordia) during the following 4 weeks. As the two ventrolateral buds grow, they become invested by mesenchyme derived from splanchnic mesoderm. This later condenses and differentiates around the growing bronchial tree to form cartilage, muscle, blood vessels, lymphatics, and other connective tissue elements. The diverticula and their surrounding mesenchyme divide, first to form two branches on the left and three on the right (i.e., the five-lobed pattern typical of the human lung). As the hollow bronchial tubes branch again and again, now *within* their respective mesenchymal coats, the numerous blind-ending tubules give the lung the pseudoglandular appearance characteristic of the first postembryonic phase (Fig. 3) (Jeffery, 1990a).

Gestation time varies in different species, as does the length of each developmental phase (i.e., pseudoglandular, canalicular, and terminal sac or alveolar), and the proportion of gestation that it occupies (see, e.g., Jeffery and Reid, 1977b). The human fetal airway mucosa is functional, with many examples of mature cells, by 24 weeks of gestation. In contrast, most of the animals, used to model fetal development, have an immature mucosa, even at birth, with undifferentiated cells, secretory cells, and a few ciliated cells (Jeffery and Reid,

Table 1 Summary of Epithelial Cells and Their Putative Functions

Epithelium	Function/s	Submucosal glands	Function/s	Nerve	Function/s
Ciliated	Moves mucus Secretes mucosubstance Controls periciliary fluid and ions	Serous	Mucus-secreting (neutral) Secretion of ions and fluid Secretory piece (component)	NEB	Chemo/mechanoreceptor Modulation of Growth Vessel and bronchial tone Mucous secretion
Mucous	Mucus-secreting (acidic) Absorptive Proliferative		Lactoferrin Lysozyme Small MW antiproteinase	Nerve terminals	Sensory Bronchoconstrictor Cough Secretion Hyperpnea
Serous	Mucus-secreting (neutral) Secretory piece (component) Lipid Periciliary fluid Proliferative	Mucous	Mucus-secreting (acidic) Proliferative		Motor Secretion Ciliary rate Modifies endocrine response
Clara	Surfactant-hypophase Secretes ions Small MW antiprotease	Oncocyte	Ionic + water modulation Degenerate acinar cell		

DCG/endocrine	Secretes amines (5-HT) Peptides (bombesin)	Myoepithelial	Expulsion of mucus
Basal	Proliferative	Endocrine	Secretoregulatory Vasoregulatory
Lymphocyte	Immunoresponsive	Intra-acinar nerve	Secretoregulatory
		Lymphocyte	Immunoresponsive
Mast cell/globular leukocyte	Releases inflammatory mediators Transports immunoglobulins		
Special-type indeterminate	Function(s) unknown		
Brush (airway and alveolus)	Function unknown		
Type I alveolar	Protective		
Type II alveolar	Secretes surfactant, ions, and fluid Proliferative		

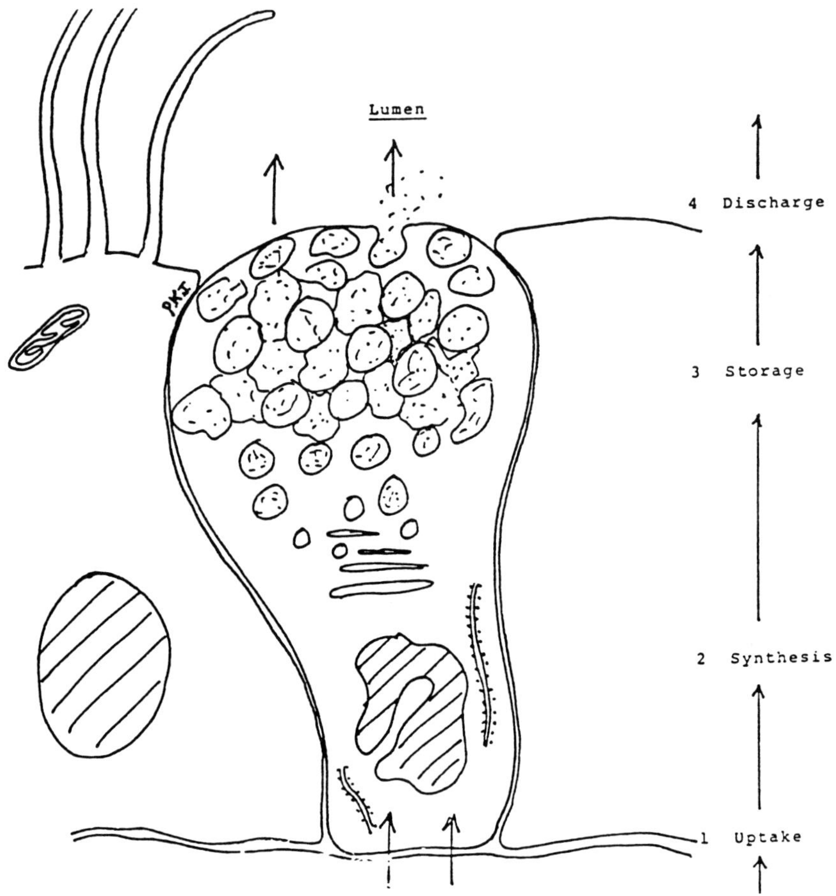

Figure 1   The amount of intracellular secretion detectable by histochemical stains is dependent on the balance of the rate of precursor uptake and glycoprotein synthesis and the rate of discharge from the cell.

1977b; Jeffery, 1990a; Gaillard et al., 1989; McDowell et al., 1985). The species that most approximates the human in the development of its airway mucosa appears to be the monkey (Plopper et al., 1986; see Chap. 4). These and other species differences make it difficult to extrapolate the findings from studies of many animal tissues to the human. The adult pattern of airway branching is complete by the 18th week (Hislop et al., 1986). However, after birth, the size of the tracheobronchial tree increases, and the distal (smallest) airways will grow until at least 8 years of life.

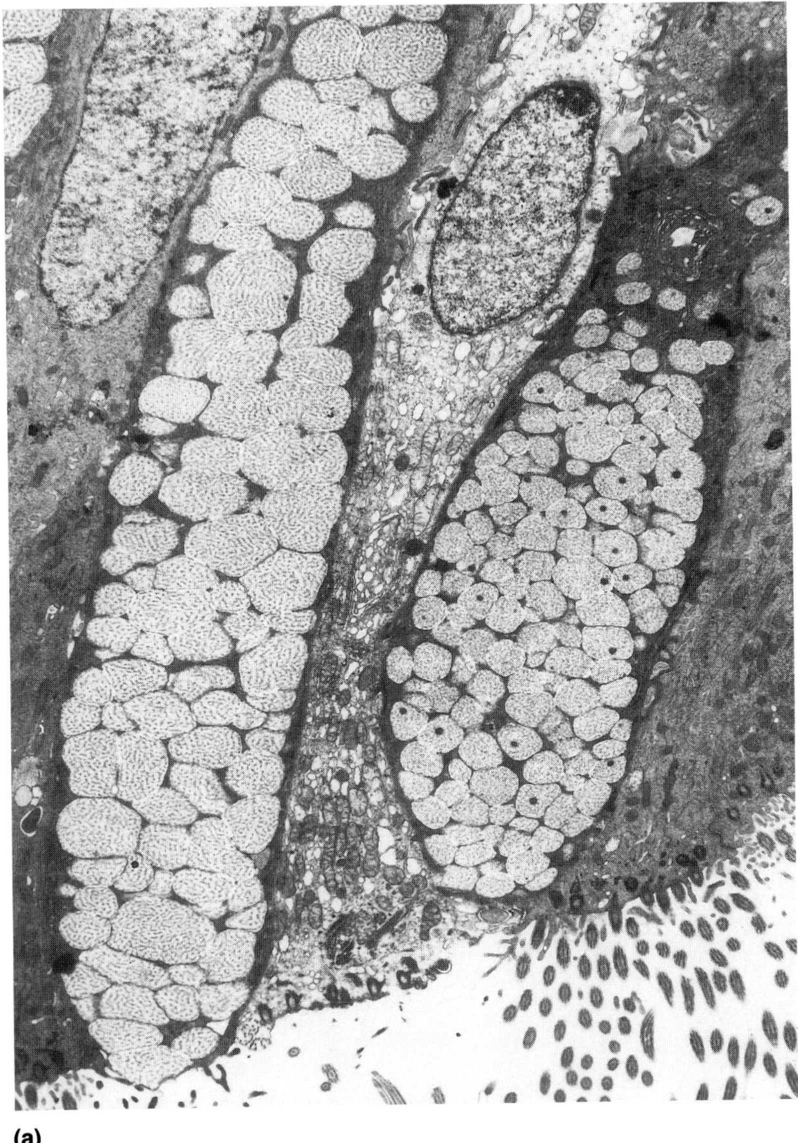

(a)

Figure 2 Electron micrographs of human airway surface secretory cells as they appear using three techniques: (a) transmission (TEM; ×6800); (b) freeze-fracture (FF; ×21,000); and (c) scanning (SEM) microscopy (×8000). All fixed initially in glutaraldehyde: (a, c) secondary fixation in osmium tetroxide; (b) freeze-fracture of original tissue and carbon replica examined by TEM.

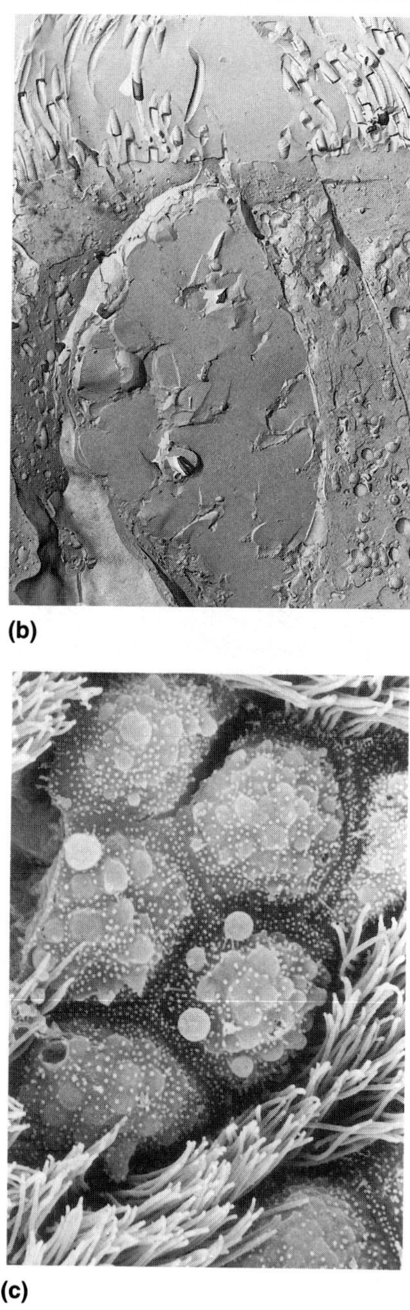

Figure 2 Continued

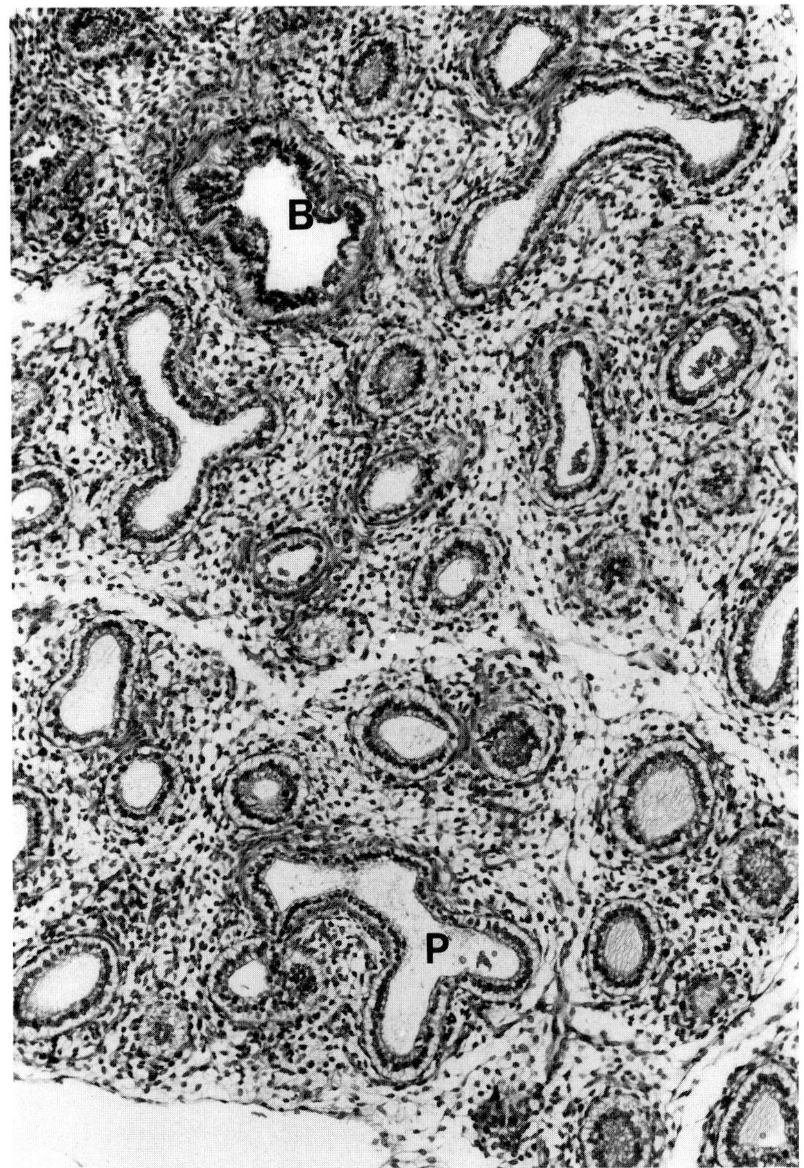

Figure 3 Light microscopic histological section through fetal lung at 16 weeks gestation showing its pseudoglandular appearance at this time. The section illustrates developing bronchi (B) and peripheral airways (P) close to the pleural edge (H&E, ×150).

V. Airway Mucosa

The airway mucosa of the newborn is also not fully developed, as the mucus-secreting cells and connective tissue elements, although present, must still mature. Figure 4a and b shows that the airway wall normally comprises epithelial, lymphoid, muscular, vascular, and nervous elements, in close contact with a pliable connective tissue support, together arranged as (1) a lining mucosa of surface epithelium supported by a reticular basement membrane and (unlike the gut) an ill-defined elastic "lamina propria" in which there are bronchial blood vessels, nerve bundles, and free cells (including fibroblasts and mononuclear cells); (2) a submucosa, in which lie the bulk of the mucus-secreting glands, muscle, and cartilage plates; (3) a relatively thin adventitial coat. The airway epithelium includes the surface epithelium, which lines all airways (nose to alveolus) and is continuous with that forming the tubuloacinar submucosal mucus-secreting glands that develop as an outpushing of the surface epithelium in utero. The stratified squamous epithelium, lining much of the larynx, gives way to one

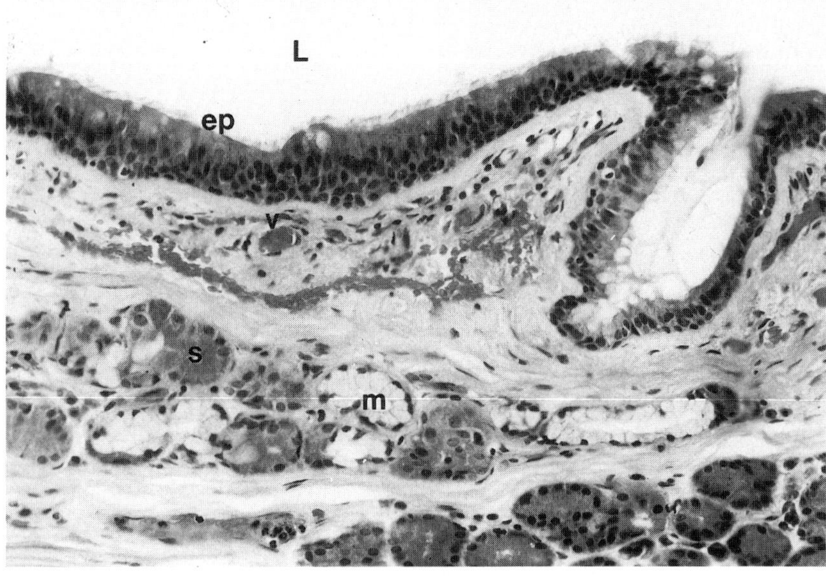

(a)

Figure 4   Human bronchial wall (a) as it appears by light microscopy (×300) and (b) a diagrammatic representation showing airway lumen (L), surface epithelium (ep), bronchial vessels (V) in the ill-defined lamina propria, and mucous (m) and serous (s) acini of the submucosal glands.

that is pseudostratified, ciliated, and columnar, with secretory cells when the trachea is reached. Where it is pseudostratified all cells rest on the basement membrane, but not all reach the airway lumen (Fig. 5a and b). In humans, this type of epithelium persists throughout the major bronchi, becoming simple cuboidal more peripherally within the lungs. Normally, ciliated cells are preponderant, interspersed by mucus-secreting (goblet) cells, which are found regularly in the tracheobronchial tree, but rarely in bronchioles smaller than 1-mm diameter (Jeffery, 1990c; Lumsden et al., 1984).

A variety of cell types are recognized in airway surface epithelium: at least eight different epithelial cell types have now been delineated, depending on species (Jeffery and Reid, 1975; Jeffery, 1983). In addition, cells involved in the immune response and its reactions may migrate through the epithelial basement membrane: some of these remain within the surface epithelium, whereas others are in the process of passing through to the luminal surface (Jeffery and Corrin, 1984). The terminal processes of sensory nerve fibers, the cell bodies of which lie deep to the epithelium, pierce the epithelial basement membrane, lose their myelin coat, and come to lie surrounded closely by epithelial cells (of the surface and gland), where they may initiate airway reflexes, such as bronchoconstriction and cough, and also influence airway secretion (Jeffery, 1982; Barnes, 1986). The origins of secretions and the structure of the secretory cells of both the surface

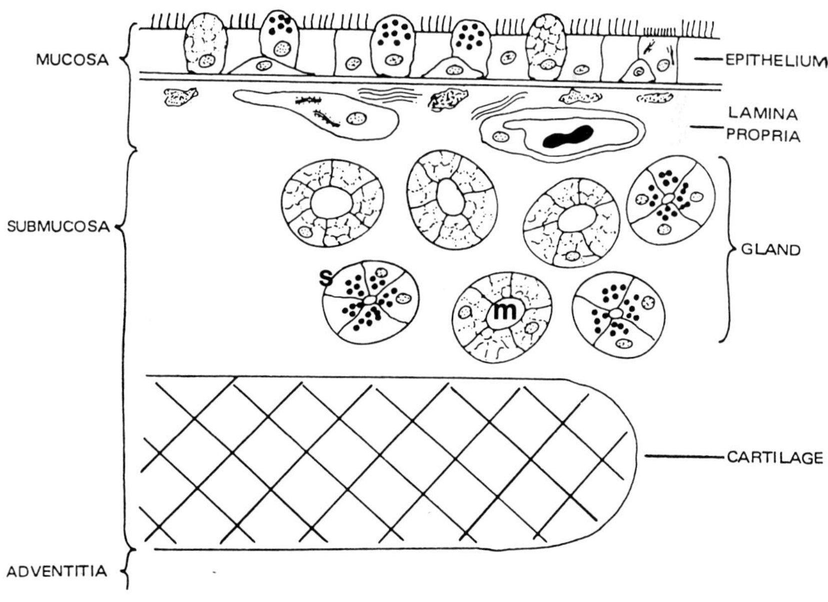

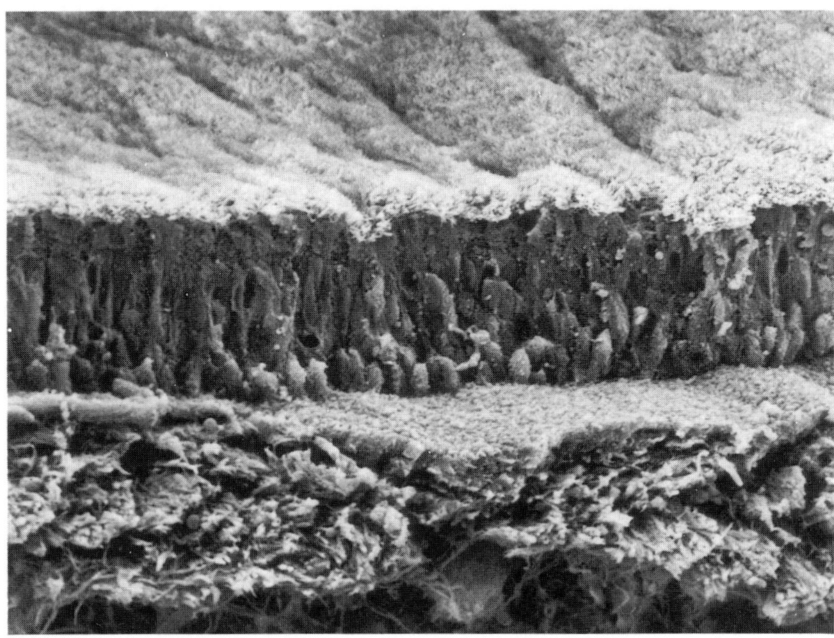

(a)

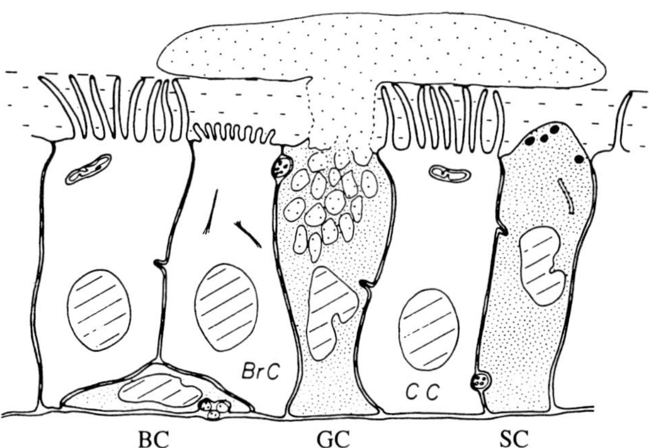

(b)

Figure 5 Human bronchial epithelium (a) as it appears by SEM ($\times 600$) and (b) in diagrammatic form showing the pseudostratified ciliated columnar arrangement, with an abundance of ciliated cells (CC), moderate numbers of surface mucous (goblet) cells (GC) and, rarely, serous cells (SC). Basal cells (BC) are frequent in large bronchi, and brush cells (BrC) are found in many animals, but have not been convincingly demonstrated in human bronchi. Mucus is moved by specific interaction with the ciliary tips.

epithelium and submucosal glands that produce many of them are now considered in further detail.

VI. Surface Epithelium

A. Cell Surface

A surface mucosubstance (SMS) has been described adherent to the luminal surface of airway epithelial cells in the human and several other species (Spicer et al., 1980a, 1983a; Meyer et al., 1971; Jeffery, 1978; Gashi et al., 1987). Two histochemically distinct components are recognized: one associated with the cilia and another with the luminal microvillus border.

The ciliary SMS of rat is acidic, owing to sialic acid, and is unusual in its nonreactivity to PAS (indicating a lack of hexose sugars with adjacent glycol groups). In contrast, the microvillus SMS present at the bases of the cilia shows PAS reactivity. In human, dog, and goose, the microvillus SMS is strongly sulfated (Spicer et al., 1983a; Jeffery, 1978). In humans, [^{35}S]sulfate is avidly incorporated into both SMS and submucosal glands, whereas in the cat, the same label is taken up less readily than is [^{3}H]glucose (Fig. 6). Neither [^{3}H]fucose nor [^{3}H]glucosamine are incorporated into SMS of the cat or goose, and [^{3}H]leucine is not taken into SMS of the goose, yet both leucine and fucose are incorporated into macromolecules within surface mucous and submucosal gland cells (Jeffery, 1978). Therefore, the chemical composition of SMS (polysaccharide or glycolipid) is distinct from that present in the secretory granules of mucus-secreting cells. Studies with monoclonal antibodies show the presence of determinants specific to SMS and of others that are specific for the glycoprotein of mucous or of serous cells, respectively (Basbaum, 1984). Our own studies (Jeffery and Richardson, unpublished data), and those of others (Basbaum, 1984; Gashi et al., 1987; Boat et al., 1976), show that following a pulse label of [^{3}H]glucose (cat), [^{35}S]sulfate (ferret), or of [^{3}H]glucosamine (human), there is initial incorporation into *ciliated* cell macromolecules and migration to the apical membrane, during the first 1–2 h, after which there is gradual loss of the radiolabel from the epithelium. It thus seems likely that many of the glycoconjugates present in respiratory tract secretions originate, at least in part, from ciliated cells.

Cytochemical methods show dialyzed iron (DI) reactivity in ciliated cell Golgi apparatus, apical vesicles, and surfaces of microvilli and cilia of the rat. Whereas the microvilli react with the cytochemical equivalent of a PAS reaction, the cilia do not. The results indicate that the SMS of cilia is composed of glycosaminoglycans (GAG). Spicer et al. (1980) have also shown that the SMS of different cell types is distinct and characteristic and can be presumed to be derived from each cell's own biosynthetic activity (by a route probably different from that for secretory granules) instead of by adsorption of luminal content. A polysaccharide-rich cell coat has also been described attached to the plasma membranes of

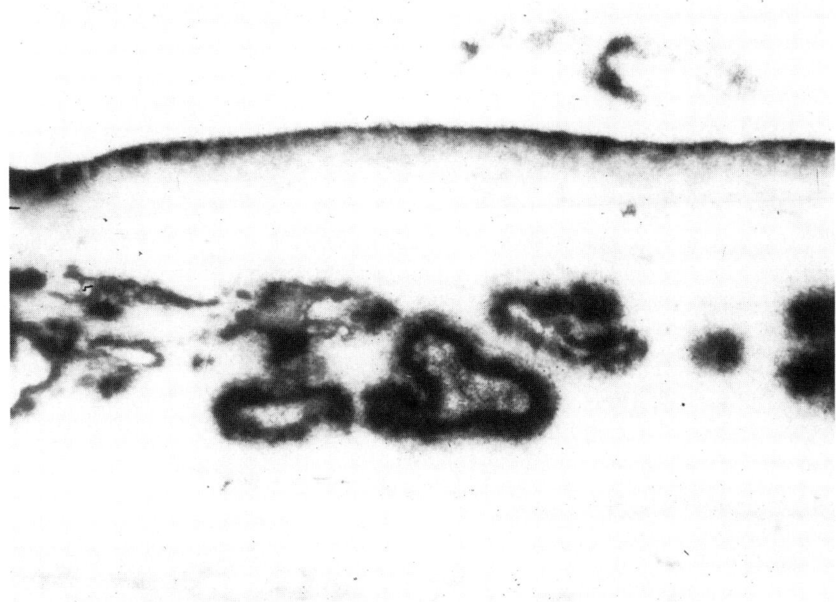

Figure 6 Human bronchial mucosa incubated in vitro with [^{35}S]sulfate and prepared for autoradiography to show localization of the label to both surface epithelium and underlying gland (×49).

alveolar pneumonocytes (Meban, 1984) and the cell surface of Clara cells is also faintly periodate reactive and stains strongly for acidic glycosaminoglycans.

The nature and variety of cell surface GAG–proteoglycans is well reviewed by Hook et al. (1984). Hyaluronate, heparan sulfate, and certain chondroitin sulfates may directly bind to plasma membrane as either an integral or a loosely bound component. They may bind membrane lipid and have a low buoyant density on cesium chloride density-gradient centrifugation. Experimentally, heparan sulfate proteoglycans can be displaced and released by addition of heparin, a finding reminiscent of the loss of [^{3}H]glucose-labeled SMS in the response to irritation by ammonia vapor (Jeffery, 1978). The importance of SMS as a potential contributor of glycoprotein and glycosaminoglycans to airway secretions should not be underestimated, as it constitutes a large surface area from which secretion may originate.

B. Mucus-Secreting Cells

Two types of surface secretory cell are known to secrete mucus: the mucous (goblet) and the, more recently described, epithelial, serous, cell (Jeffery and

Reid, 1975; Jeffery, 1990c; Rogers et al., 1993). Histochemically, the presence of intracellular mucus is seen first in the human fetal trachea from the 13th week of gestation (Bucher and Reid, 1961; De Haller, 1969), when mature ciliated cells are already present. At this time, mucus-secreting cells are sparse or gathered into small groups, each having a centrally placed nucleus and containing sparse apically placed PAS-positive granules. Infrequently, there are goblet-shaped cells distended by their intracellular secretion which, in consequence, compresses the nucleus to its base. Like ciliated cells, mucus-secreting cells appear first in the proximal (central) airways and, then, develop subsequently in the more peripheral airways. Their number increases and peaks in the middle of gestation, when they represent approximately 30–35% of the cells lining the luminal surface (Gaillard et al., 1989). Toward the end of the second term of gestation, there is a relative decrease in the number of mucus-secreting cells, these being replaced by an abundance of ciliated cells. Mucus-secreting cells that are present during the third term and at birth are less frequent than in the adult, but similarly to the adult, they are more numerous in the proximal than in the peripheral airways (Jeffery et al., 1991). At this time, some of the mucus-secreting cell granules contain lysozyme (Gaillard et al., 1990). Both neutral and acidic glycoproteins may be secreted by the same cell, and the acidic component is nearly exclusively sulfomucin until birth (Jeffery et al., 1991). This is retained and exaggerated in airway epithelial cells cultured from patients with cystic fibrosis (Boat et al., 1989).

In the adult human, most surface epithelial cells contain both neutral and acidic glycoproteins, with sialomucins and sulfomucins being represented. By electron microscopy, the fetal mucus-secreting cells have electron-dense cytoplasm and contain glycogen, mitochondria, rough endoplasmic reticulum, and ribosomes and, in addition, a well-developed Golgi apparatus in the supranuclear zone. Most fetal secretory cells of the surface epithelium contain granules that are electron-lucent (Fig. 7a), a few cells contain granules that are heterogeneous in density, and others contain preponderantly electron-dense granules (see Fig. 7b). These last resemble ultrastructurally the epithelial serous cell described in the adult human and specific pathogen-free rat (Jeffery and Reid, 1975), but they do not show immunoreactivity for lysozyme at this time, which contrasts with the findings for the serous cells of the submucosal glands (Gaillard et al., 1990).

The antiproteinase enzyme antileukoproteinase (ALP) has been identified recently in the surface epithelium of the human trachea and bronchi and is present by 20 weeks gestation (Willems et al., 1988). As the submucosal glands of the second term of fetal development are not fully mature until after birth, the fetal surface secretory cells are probably a relatively more abundant source of mucus. In addition to their secretory and protective function, the mucus-secreting cells fulfill a role as progenitors of ciliated and other epithelial cell types (McDowell and Trump, 1983; Ayers and Jeffery, 1988; Gaillard et al., 1989). The progenitor role of surface secretory cells has been realized by studies of the development

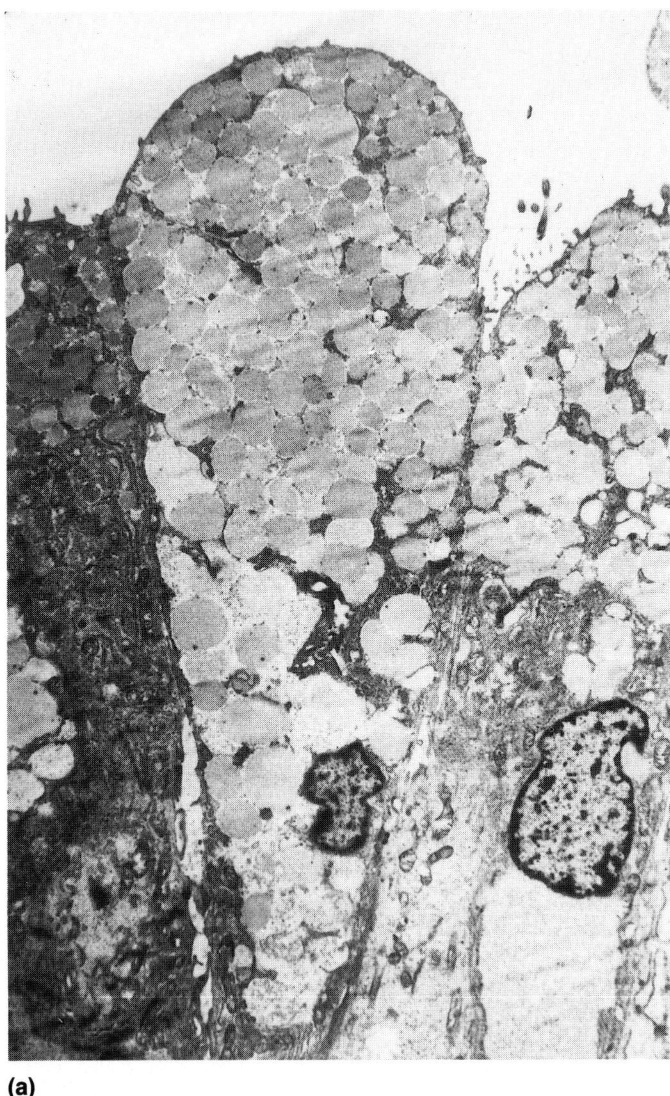

(a)

Figure 7 Human airway epithelium from a fetus of 16 weeks gestation demonstrating the TEM appearance of (a) surface mucous (goblet) cell containing a large mass of electron-lucent confluent secretory granules (×6200) and (b) a surface serous cell with numerous small, discrete electron-dense granules, a well developed Golgi apparatus (Go), and intracytoplasmic glycogen (g) (×20,000). (From Jeffery, 1990b.)

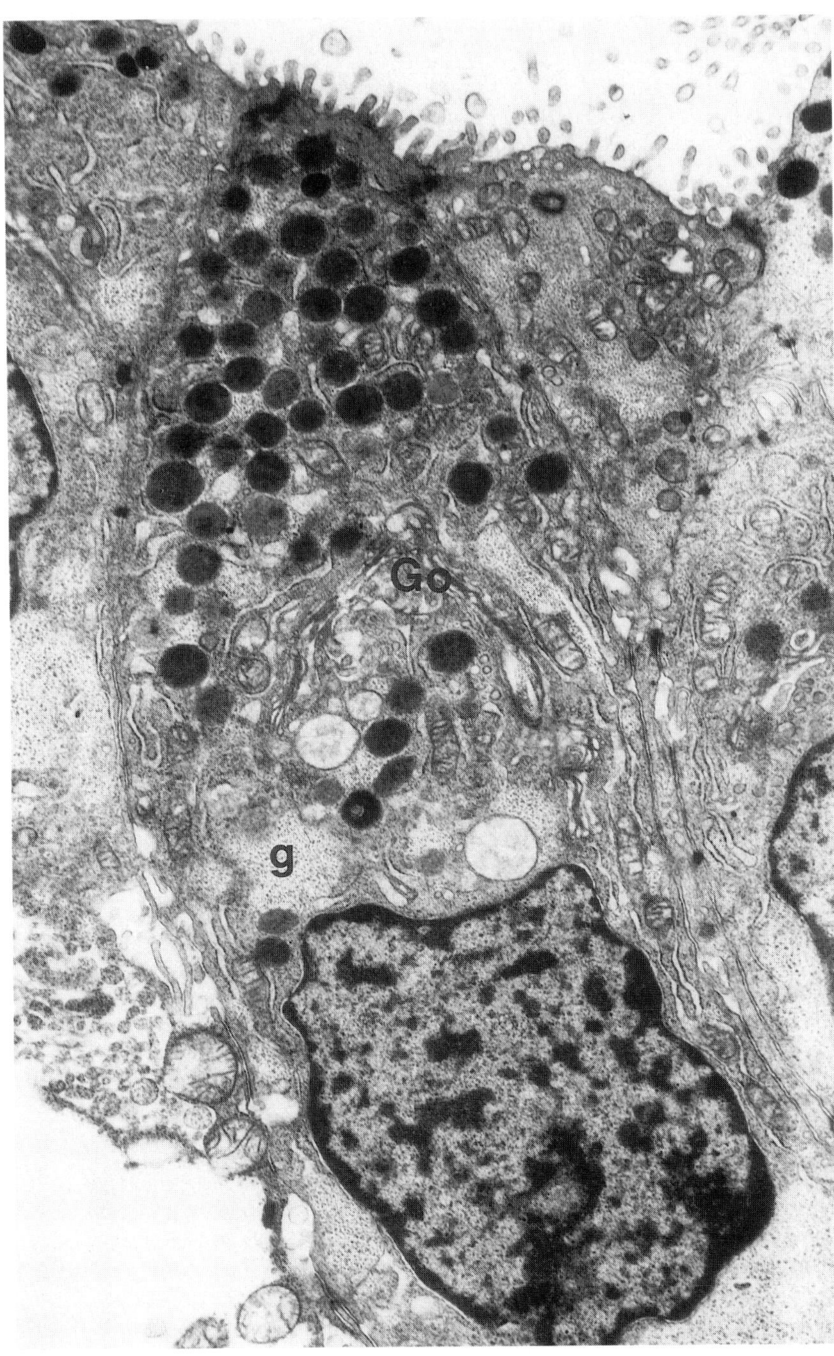

(b)

of the fetal trachea of the hamster (McDowell et al., 1985) and has been described in developing monkey airways (Plopper et al., 1986) and in human fetal trachea (Gaillard et al., 1989). The proliferation potential of surface serous and mucous cells of the rat has been shown both in the normal adult and in response to experimental irritation by cigarette smoke or pharmacological agents (Fig 8a and b). The secretory cell is likely to play a major role in the repair of injured respiratory mucosa in vivo (McDowell et al., 1984) and experimentally in proliferation in vitro (McDowell et al., 1987). Experimental models of airway damage demonstrate the role of both mucous and Clara cells (see following sections) as progenitor cells in response to irritation of the epithelium, and their capacity to proliferate and differentiate into other cell forms is now well recognized (see Ayers and Jeffery, 1982; McDowell and Trump, 1983; McDowell et al., 1987). It has been suggested that mucous cells with relatively few secretory

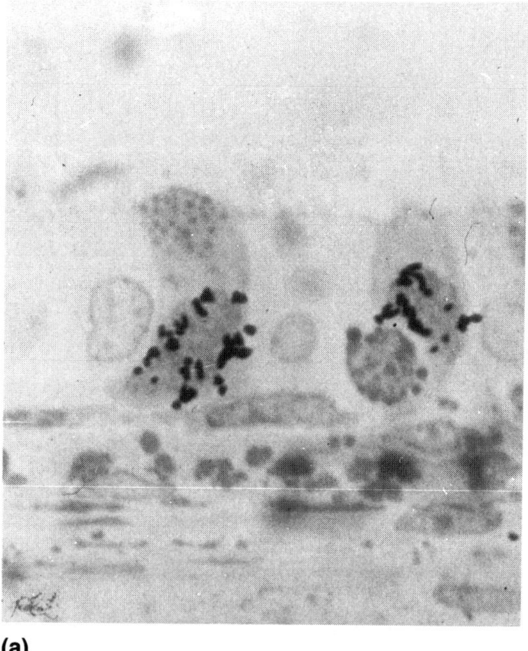

(a)

Figure 8 Dividing surface epithelial secretory cells. (a) Autoradiographic localization of tritiated thymidine incorporation marking rat epithelial serous cells in the S phase of the cell cycle ($\times$2000; 1-μm plastic section) and (b) electron micrograph of surface secretory cell showing pale mucous granules at its apex and the condensation of electron-dense chromosomes and loss of nuclear envelope, characteristic of a dividing cell ($\times$7500).

granules may replicate, in the presence of vitamin A, to provide both new mucous and also ciliated cells (McDowell et al., 1984), whereas those cells distended by secretion may play a relatively more important role as secretors than as progenitors (Breuer et al., 1990). In addition, in the adult, basal cells are present in the proximal airways, and these may divide to replenish both themselves and act as stem cells. In contrast, during early development, where basal cells are sparse and in the regenerating mucosa, the secretory cell may play the pivotal stem cell role.

C. Mucous Cells

In adult human trachea, the normal mean density of surface mucous cells (see Fig. 2) is estimated at between 6000 and 7000/mm^2 surface epithelium (Ellefsen and Tos, 1972). A variety of glycoprotein types may be found in mucous cells, depending on airway level, stage of maturation, and species: a single cell may contain granules of only one type (e.g., either neutral or acidic glycoprotein) or a mixture (Lamb and Reid, 1969a; Reid and Jones, 1979; Spicer et al., 1983a, b; Reid, 1983). Most surface mucous cells contain a glycoprotein with sugar side chains, having terminal sialic acid, penultimate galactose residues, and a variable content of sulfate esters (Lamb and Reid, 1969a; Spicer et al., 1983a; Jones et al.,

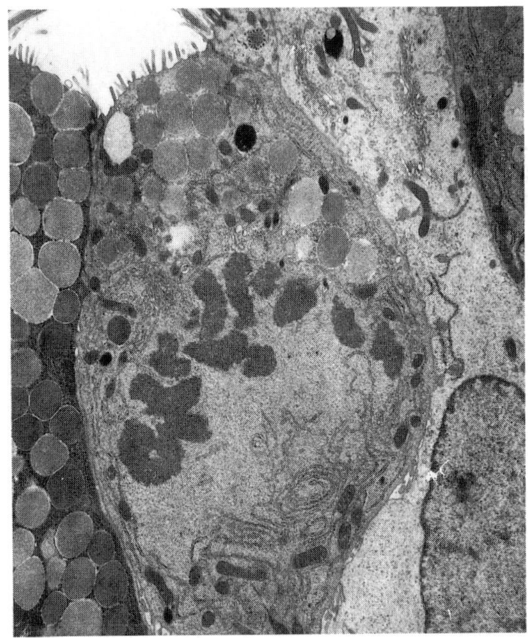

(b)

1973). In humans, sulfomucin predominates in surface mucous cells, and the sulfate/glucosamine uptake ratio may be higher than in mucous cells of submucosal glands (Spicer et al., 1983a). Glycoproteins recovered from cultured human nasal polyps (relatively free of submucosal glands) are highly acidic (Boat et al., 1974, 1976) and, in agreement, secretions recovered from dog trachea, denuded of its epithelium, are less sulfated than those from the whole trachea (Stahl and Ellis, 1973). In contrast, the mucous glycoproteins recovered from cat surface epithelium (physically separated from its underlying mucosa by 20 mM EDTA) appear to be less highly sulfated than those of submucosal glands (Sherman et al., 1981). Earlier studies with [^{35}S]sulfate showed that cat submucosal glands took up sulfate more readily than did surface epithelium (surface mucous cells did not incorporate the label) (Gallagher et al., 1986). The labeling pattern was used to indicate the origin of secretions in response to either pilocarpine or ammonia: the former primarily stimulated secretions rich in [^{35}S]sulfate and the latter released surface glyconjugate as well as that from submucosal glands. In the rat, mucous cells of gland acini contain sulfate esters, whereas in the gland duct and surface they contain sialomucin (Spicer et al., 1980b; Mochizuki et al., 1982). Thus, the source of a particular glycoprotein is likely to vary with species.

As seen with the electron microscope, mucous cells have electron-dense cytoplasm containing electron-lucent granules of about 800 nm in diameter (see Fig. 2a). Tono- or intermediate filament bundles, immunoreactive for keratin, have been described and, infrequently, dense-cored neurosecretory-like granules are also present. Because of their large number, the electron-lucent secretory granules are closely packed, often with incomplete membranes, allowing confluence (Fig. 9a), or have fused (pentalaminar) membranes (Neutra and Schaeffer, 1977); therefore, compound exocytosis or apocrine secretion is likely. The degree of acidity may well determine the extent of postexocytotic hydration and, hence, the gel nature of the mucus (Verdugo, 1990). The secretory granule may show heterogeneity of content, with an electron-dense core reminiscent of the Paneth cells of the gut (see Fig. 9b). Similar to the granules of the Paneth cell, those of the mucous cell may show an outer halo of acidic glycoprotein surrounding a core composed of neutral glycoprotein or of a noncarbohydrate osmiophilic material that may well be lipid (Spicer et al., 1980a, 1983a; Mochizuki et al., 1982). Consequently, exocytosis of a single granule may yield a multiplicity of secretory products.

D. Serous Cells

Serous cells of the surface epithelium have electron-dense cytoplasm, much rough endoplasmic reticulum and, in contrast with mucous cells, fewer discrete electron-dense granules, each of about 600 nm in diameter (Fig. 10a). Little is known of the function of this type of secretory cell. Morphologically, serous cells of the surface epithelium resemble those present in the submucosal glands. They have been described in surface epithelium in the rat, cat, young hamster, and fetal humans (Jeffery and Reid, 1975; Jeffery, 1990a,c). In our experience they are also found normally, but infrequently, in adult human bronchioli (see Fig. 10b) (Rogers et al., 1993). They are thought to contain neutral mucin, and there is evidence that some may also contain a nonmucoid substance, probably lipid (Spicer et al., 1983b).

E. Nonciliated Bronchiolar (Clara) Cells

In spite of much investigation and interest, relatively little is known about the Clara cell, either during development or in the adult. They are thought to develop, during the second half of gestation, from primitive glycogen-containing nonciliated cells of the terminal airways. By 18–19 weeks of gestation, the domelike apical protrusion, characteristic of the mature cell in most species, has formed. Maturation involves gradual loss of cytoplasmic glycogen, increasing ribosomal content, and the appearance of electron-dense secretory granules, which may become numerous by 26 weeks gestation. In the adult human lung, low-molecular-mass antileukoproteinase (ALP) can be localized to nonciliated bronchiolar (Clara) cells and, in addition, is present in serous cells of submucosal glands and surface mucus-secreting cells (Kramps et al., 1981). Recently, ALP has been found in bronchiolar epithelium (presumed to be in Clara cells) by the 38th week of gestation (Willems et al., 1988). These data argue for early appearance of a protective antiproteinase and the maturation of Clara cells at a time before parturition in the human. The timing is in marked contrast to that of the specific pathogen-free laboratory rat, in which Clara cells do not begin to mature until at least 5 days after birth (Jeffery and Reid, 1977b).

Clara cells in the adult human are restricted in location to the terminal bronchioles where they typically bulge into the airway lumen (Fig. 11a and b). They contain electron-dense granules of about 500–600 nm in diameter, ovoid in humans but irregular in most other species (Plopper et al., 1980; Widdicombe and Pack, 1982) (Fig. 12a and b). The apical cytoplasm in most species, with the exception of humans, contains an abundance of smooth endoplasmic reticulum (see Fig. 12c). The function(s) of this cell type is still unclear. It may produce a carbohydrate (hypophase) component of surfactant (Gil and Weibel, 1971) or an antiproteinase (Willems et al., 1988; Kramps et al., 1981) and is known to have ion-absorbing and secreting properties. Furthermore, the Clara cell acts as the stem cell of small airways, in which basal and mucous cells are normally sparse: both ciliated and mucous cells may develop from the Clara cell subsequent to its division and differentiation (see Ayers and Jeffery, 1988).

The Clara cell has a high cytochrome P-450–dependent mixed-function

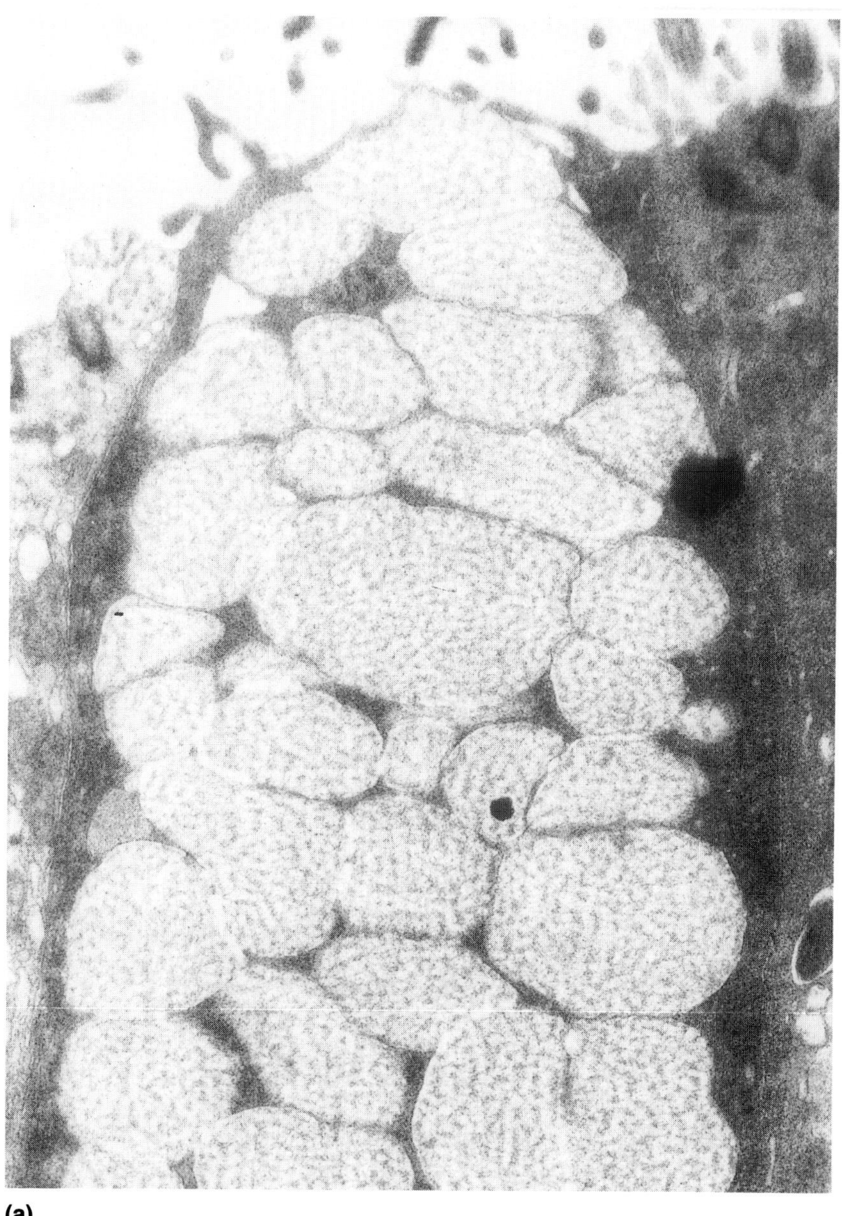

(a)

Figure 9 TEM of human bronchial surface mucous cells to show (a) confluence of electron-lucent secretory granules ($\times$19,000) and (b) granules with electron-dense cores ($\times$13,000). Glutaraldehyde + osmium tetroxide:uranyl acetate + lead citrate.

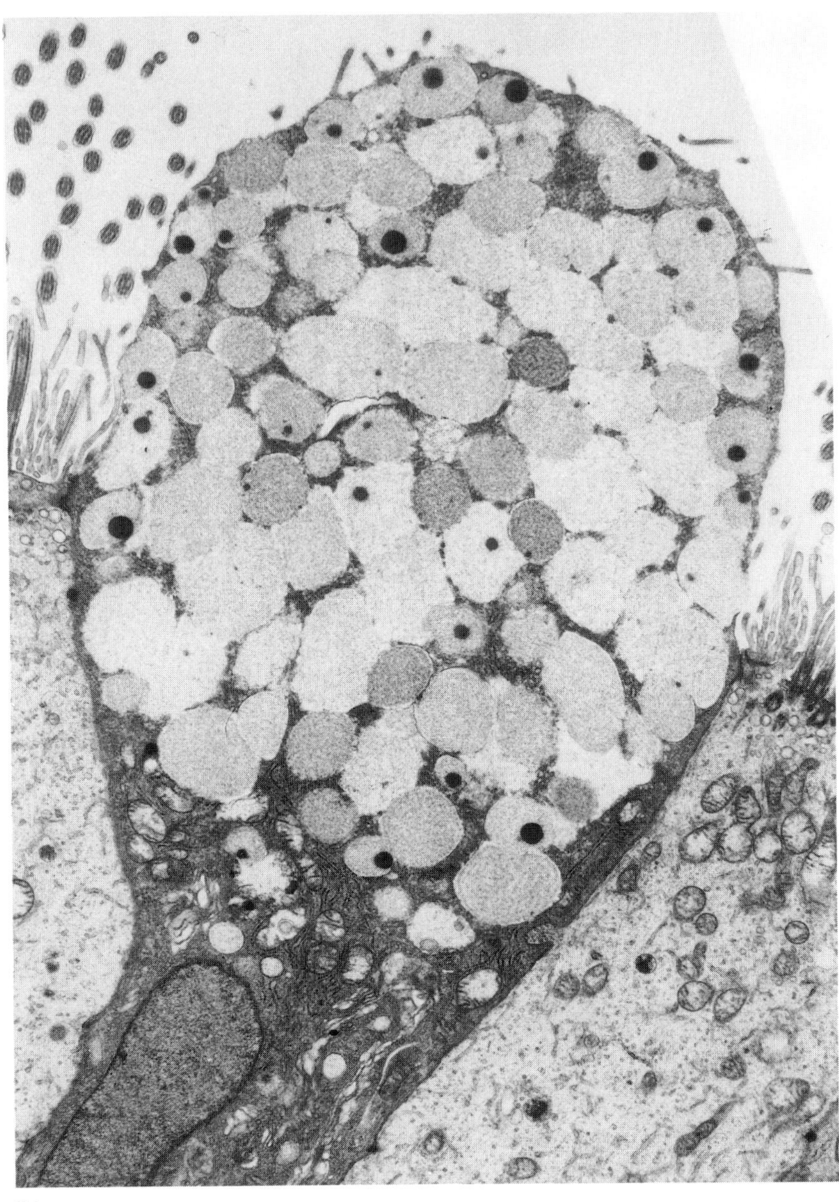

(b)

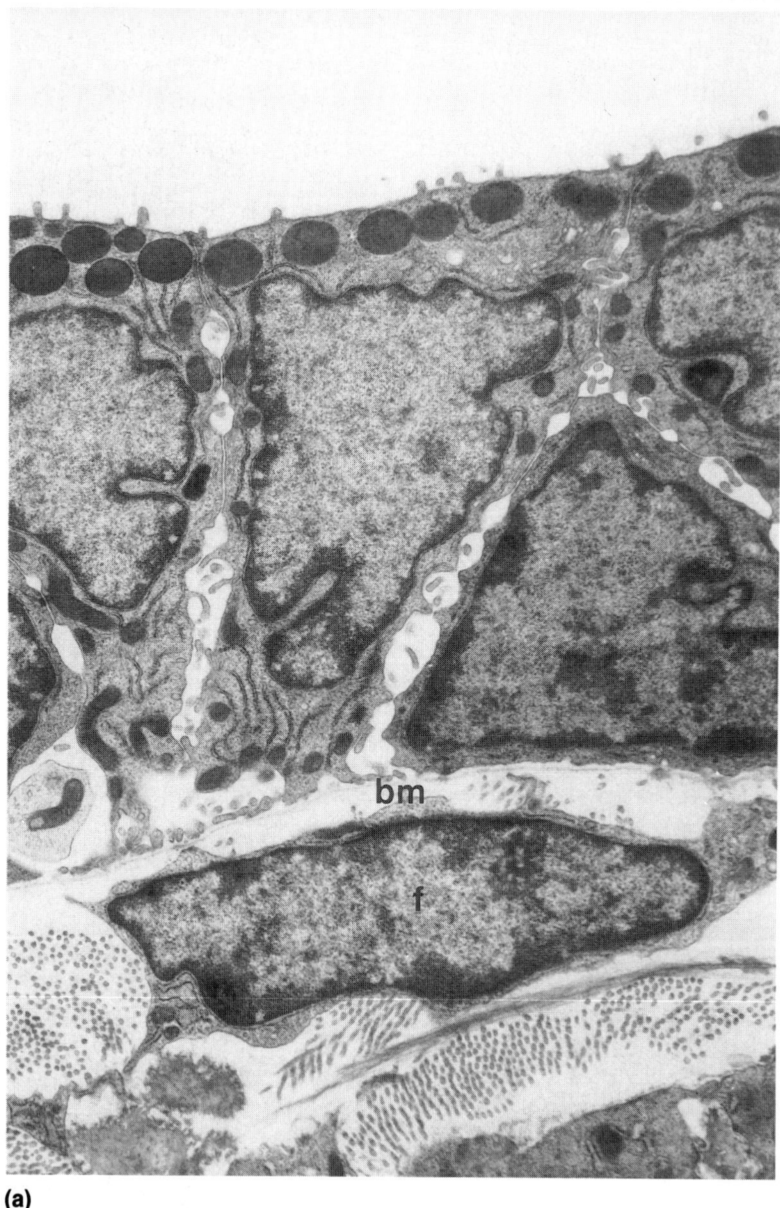

(a)

Figure 10 TEM of epithelial serous cells showing discrete electron-dense secretory granules in (a) bronchus from a specific pathogen-free rat (×11,000) and (b) from a human bronchiolus (×12,000); basement membrane (bm) and fibroblast (f).

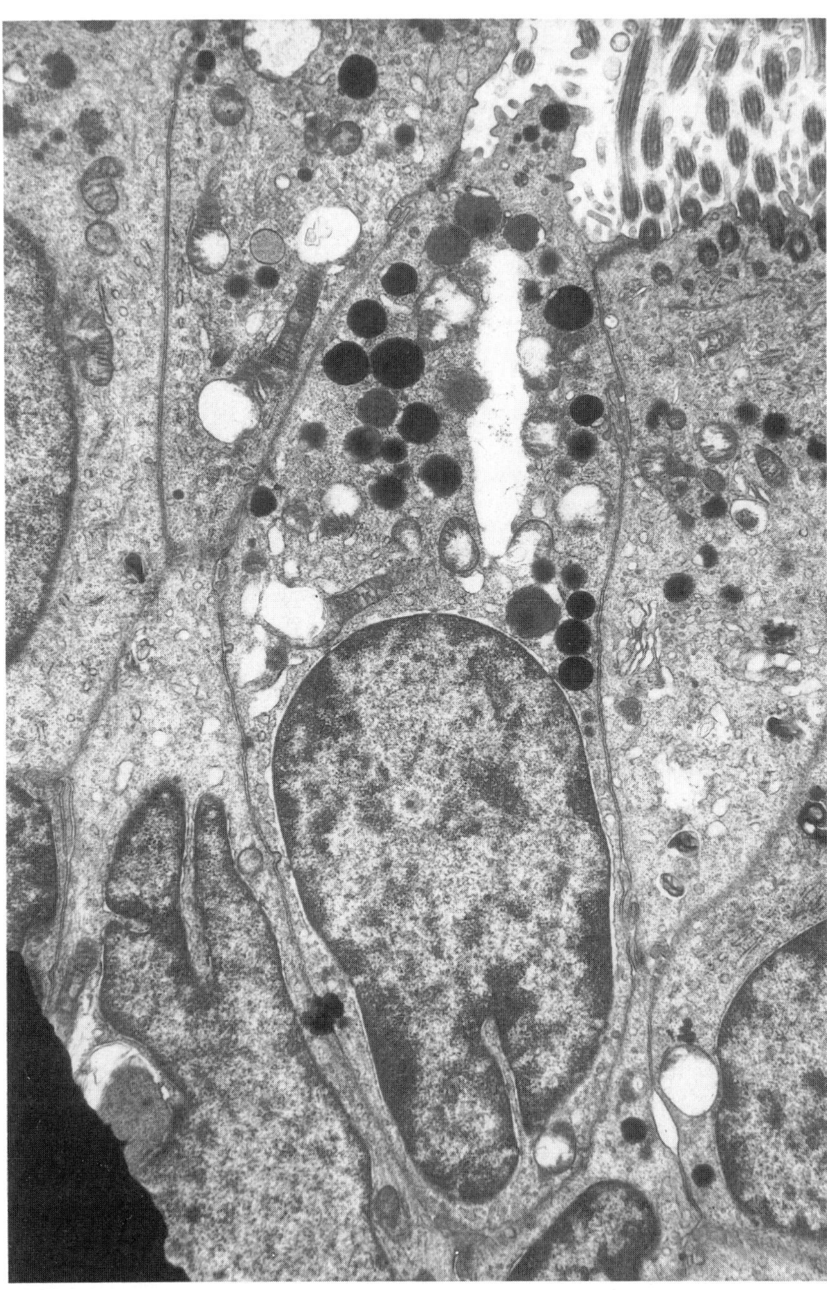

(b)

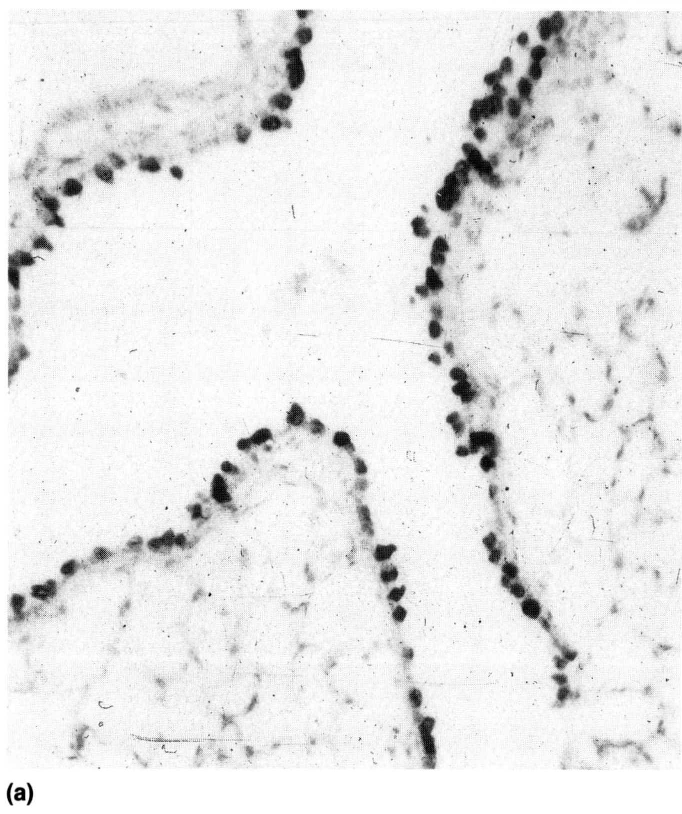

(a)

Figure 11   (a) Light micrograph of rat terminal (TB) and respiratory bronchiole (RB) incubated with an antibody directed against the Clara cell and visualized using the immunogold–silver intensification technique (×200). (b) SEM of human bronchiole showing lumenal aspect of surface epithelium with Clara cells bulging into the airway lumen beyond the ciliary layer (×550).

oxidase activity (Boyd, 1977), which suggests a role for the cell in the processes of detoxification. However, these enzyme systems also make the cell particularly vulnerable to damage and destruction by inappropriate conversion of nonreactive compounds to reactive species. The cell surface is also rich in γ-glutamyltrans-peptidase (Fig. 13), which is involved in the transmembrane transport of gluta-thione (an important antioxidant) from the interior of the cell to and from extracellular fluid (Dinsdale et al., 1992).

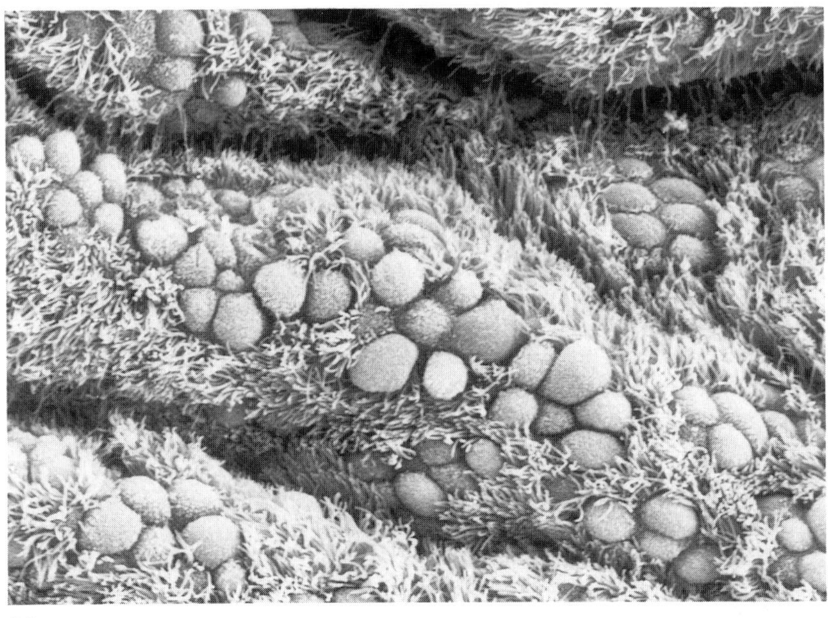

(b)

VII. Transitional Forms

A. Surface Epithelium

Normal or irritated epithelium may comprise secretory cells with morphologies that are transitional (i.e., have features of one or more cell types). The following serve as examples from airway epithelium:

Serous–mucous cells may be found rarely in normal specific pathogen-free (SPF) rats (Jeffery and Reid, 1975), but are frequent in rats that have briefly inhaled cigarette smoke (i.e., for 2 weeks (Fig. 14a) (Jeffery and Reid, 1981) and may be found in epithelium from otherwise grossly and histologically normal airways of lung resected for well-circumscribed carcinoma (see Fig. 9b). The cells have the characteristics of both serous and mucous cells (i.e., secretory granules of the mucous type, with electron-dense cores resembling serous granules).

Clara-mucous cells are rare in SPF rats but may be found after irritation by sulfur dioxide (Jeffery and Reid, 1977a) or multiple injections of isoproterenol (isoprenaline) sulfate (see Fig. 14b). The transitional cell retains the protruding apex, abundance of smooth endoplasmic reticulum, and many of the electron-dense granules of the Clara cell, but has, in addition, many large mucous granules.

Ciliated–mucous cells have been found after injections of isoproterenol

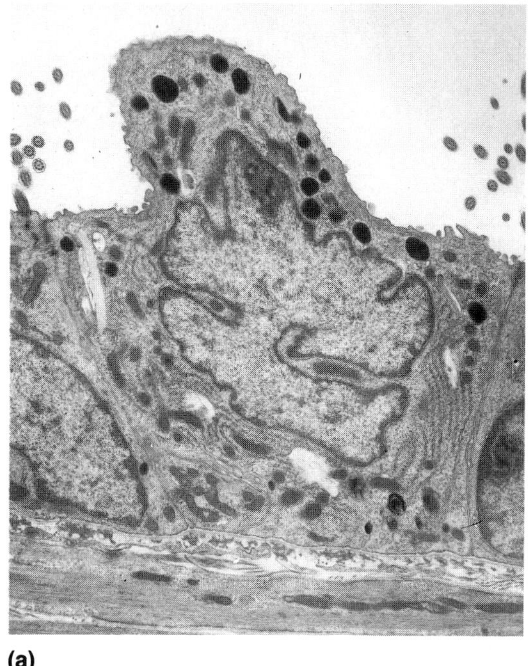

(a)

Figure 12 TEM of Clara cells and their sparse electron-dense granules in the bronchioles of (a) rat (×3000) and (b) human (×10500); and (c) illustrating the abundance of smooth endoplasmic reticulum in the apex of the cell in the rat (×27,500).

sulfate in rats and also occasionally in resected human lung (see Fig. 14c) (Jeffery, 1973; McDowell et al., 1978b). The cell retains the electron-lucent cytoplasm, apical microvilli, and basal bodies of ciliated cells, but also has secretory granules in its cytoplasm.

Neuroendocrine–mucous cell transitional forms have been found by histochemistry in the gut (Popoff, 1939; Schofield, 1953) and described by electron microscopy in both gut and bronchi (Cheng and Leblond, 1974; Hattori et al., 1982; Terzakis et al., 1972).

Basal–mucous–squamous cells. Tracheobronchial epidermoid metaplasia is a change in epithelial structure and function, from one that is pseudostratified, mucus-secreting, and ciliated, to one that is stratified, keratinized, and resembles skin. McDowell and colleagues (McDowell et al., 1978b; McDowell and Trump, 1983) have suggested that such an epidermoid change may arise subsequent to division of mucous cells, rather than by hyperplasia of existing basal cells. The daughter secretory cells then show altered differentiation (cell metaplasia), and

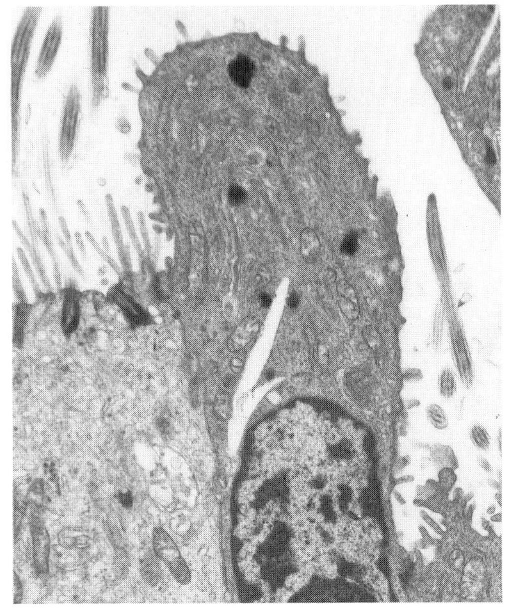

(b)

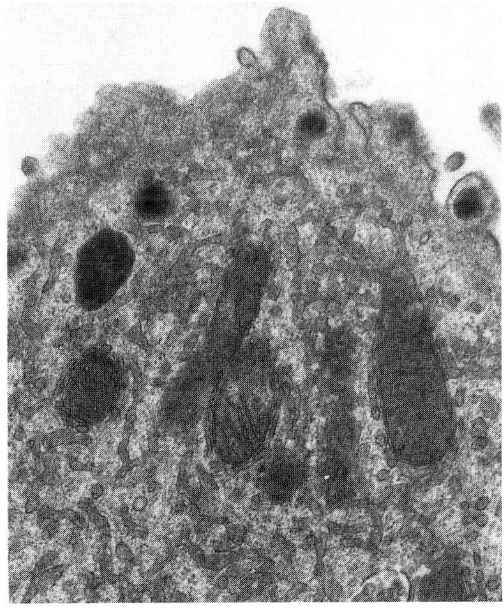

(c)

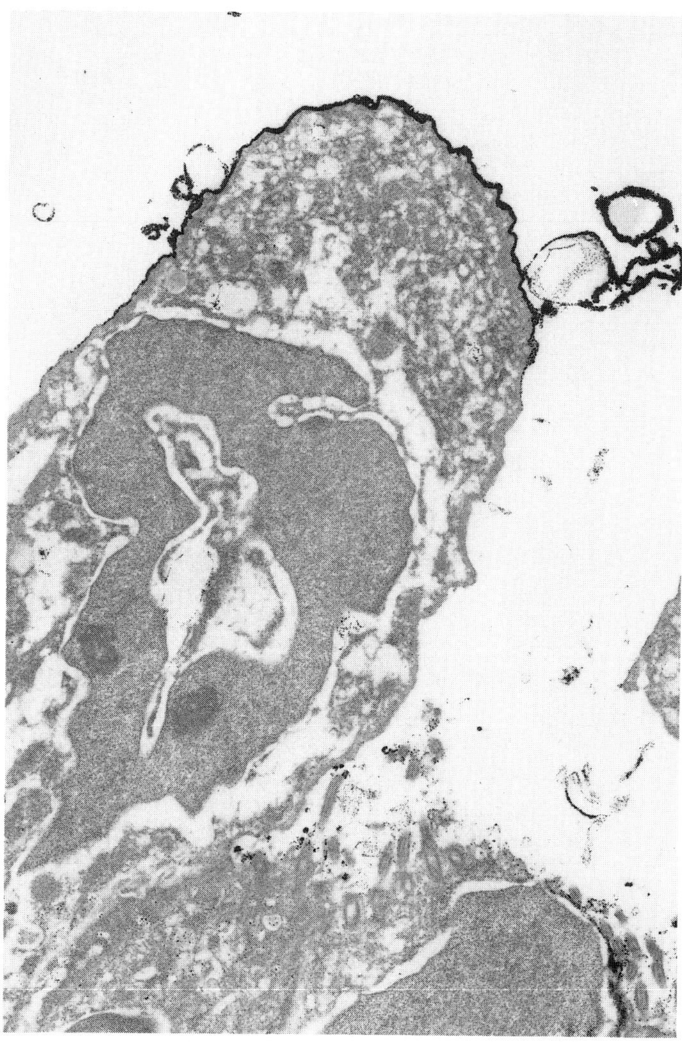

Figure 13 Cytochemical demonstration of the localization of γ-glutamyltranspeptidase to the apical surface of the Clara cell where it is thought to be involved in the transport of the antioxidant, glutathione (×10,000); peroxidase technique. (From Dinsdale et al., 1992.)

any one cell may then show a mixture of both keratin (intermediate) filaments and mucous granules. Experimentally, carcinogens, mechanical trauma, and vitamin A deficiency may each induce changes in mucous cells, leading to squamous cell metaplasia, with or without stratification and keratinization (see Shields and Jeffery, 1987; Zhang and McDowell, 1992).

Dense-Cored Granule or "Neuroendocrine" Cells

Dense-cored granule (DCG) cells (synonyms: neuroendocrine Kultchitsky or Feyrter cell) have been reported to be the first "mature" cell type to differentiate within primitive airway epithelium. Distributed singly or in pairs, they are identified at 10 weeks gestation (Cutz, 1987). They are weakly argyrophilic, show immunoreactivity for serotonin and neuron-specific enolase, but not, at this time, for bombesin and other peptides (see Cutz, 1987; Sheppard et al., 1983; Cutz et al., 1985). The characteristic dense-cored neurosecretory granules are at first sparse and smaller (Fig. 15a) that those seen in the adult: Cutz has suggested they represent granule precursors of the three types of granules found in the adult DCG cell. Bombesin-like immunoreactivity and serotonin positivity is first found at about 12 weeks gestation at a time when submucosal nerves and ganglia show strong immunoreaction for neuron-specific enolase (Cutz et al., 1985). During the alveolar phase of development (i.e., from about 25 weeks gestation), the frequency of bombesin and serotonin immunoreactivity in DCG cells increases significantly toward term primarily from an increase in neuroepithelial bodies in peripheral airways (Sheppard et al., 1983; Track and Cutz, 1982). Associated with this, bombesin-like immunoreactivity in lung tissue extracts is highest during the late fetal–neonatal period and decreases postpartum (Cutz et al., 1981). Calcitonin and leu-enkephalin are detected in DCG cells only late during fetal development and are also identified postnatally (Rosan and Lauweryns, 1972).

Argentaffin-positive and argyrophilic cells can be identified within the surface epithelium of the adult by light microscopy and have been referred to as Feyrter or Kultchitsky cells (Lauweryns et al., 1972; Jeffery and Reid, 1977a). By electron microscopy, they appear as dense-cored granulated cells, infrequently found normally, generally basal in position, but often with a thin cytoplasmic projection reaching the airway lumen (Jeffery and Reid, 1977a; Capella et al., 1987; Lauweryns and Cokelaere, 1973a) (see Fig. 15b). Single cells and clusters of such cells may also be associated with nerve fibers, when they are referred to as neuroepithelial bodies or neurite–receptor complexes (see Jeffery and Reid, 1973; Lauweryns and Cokelaere, 1973a). The cytoplasm of DCG cells usually contains numerous small (70- to 150-nm) spherical granules each with an electron-dense core surrounded by an electron-lucent halo (see Fig. 15b). Granule subtypes have been described (Hage, 1973), and the cells may contain biogenic amines (Lauweryns et al., 1982) or peptides, such as bombesin (Wharton et al., 1978)

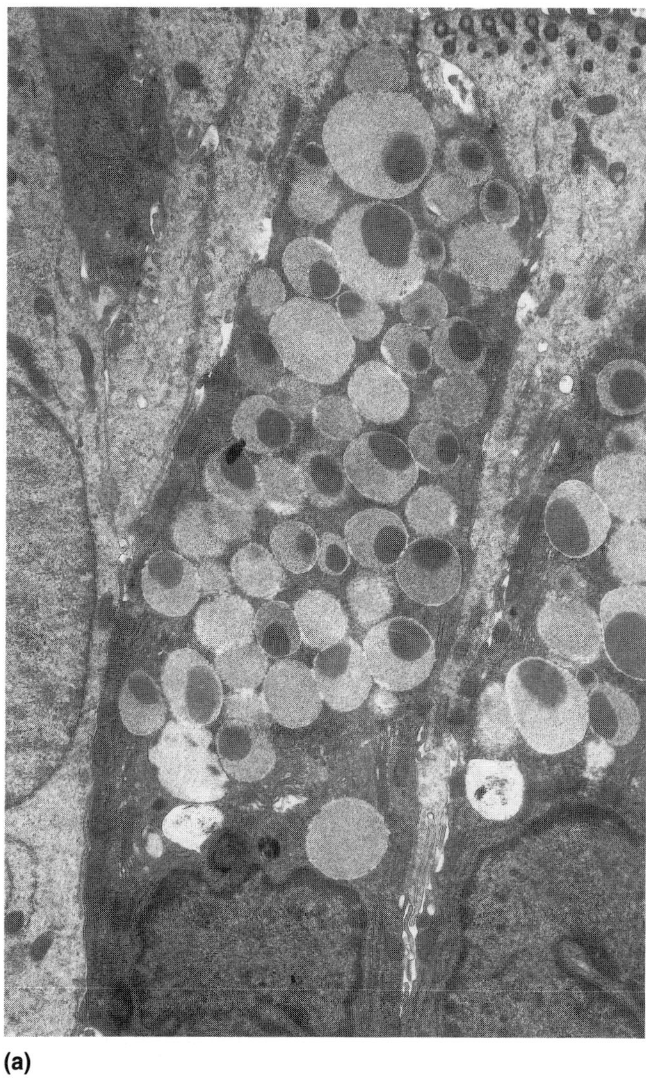

(a)

Figure 14 Transitional forms of secretory cell: (a) serous–mucous cells in the rat following subacute exposure to cigarette smoke (×11,500); (b) Clara–mucous cells with heterogenous granules (arrows) (×9200); and (c) ciliated mucous cells showing mucous granules (g) and basal body formation (arrows) in rat bronchioles after multiple injections of isoproterenol sulfate (×11,500). (From Jeffery, 1987b.)

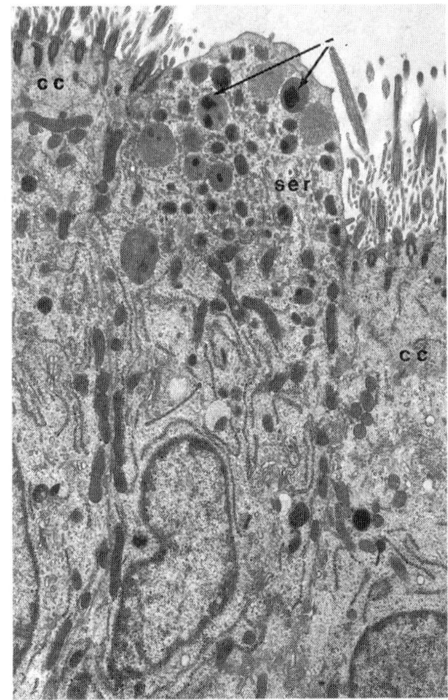

(b)

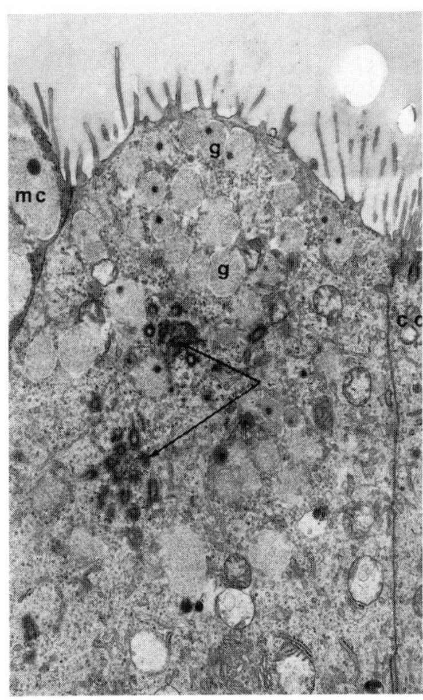

(c)

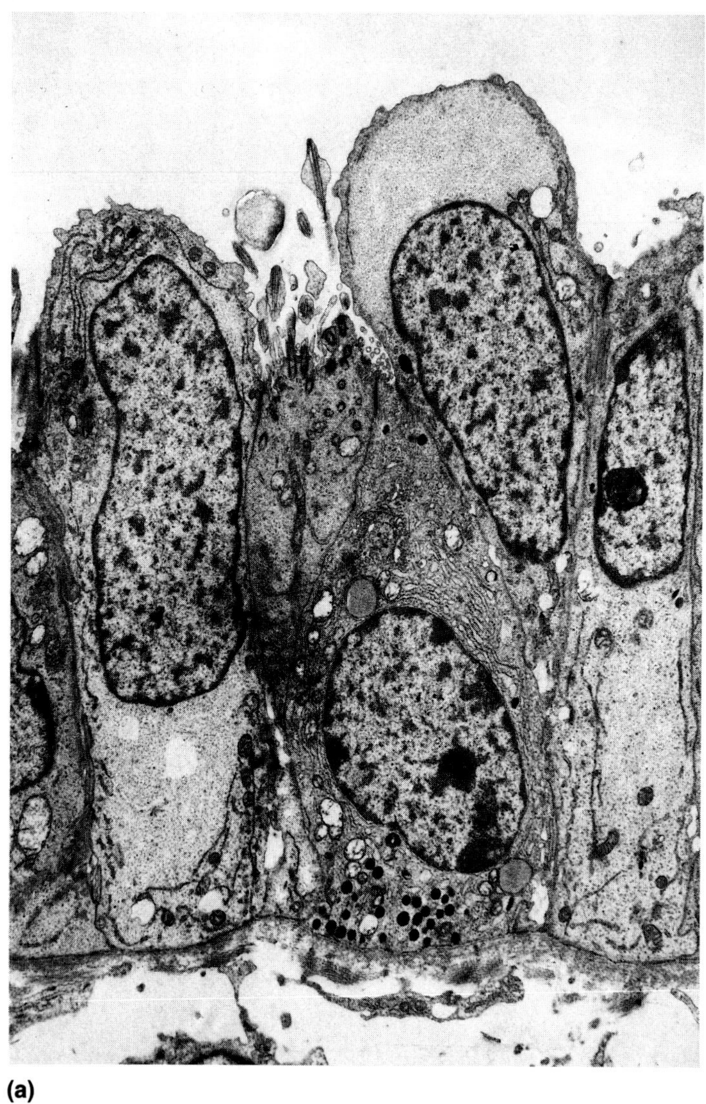

(a)

Figure 15 (a) Dense-cored granule (neuroendocrine) cells in bronchiolar epithelium of a fetus of 16 weeks gestation extending from epithelial basement membrane to the lumen with electron-dense granules in its basal aspect (×9500); (b) base of bronchial epithelium of an adult rat showing a single cell with electron-lucent cytoplasm and an abundance of dense-cored vesicles (×20,000) which are shown at higher magnification (inset ×50,000).

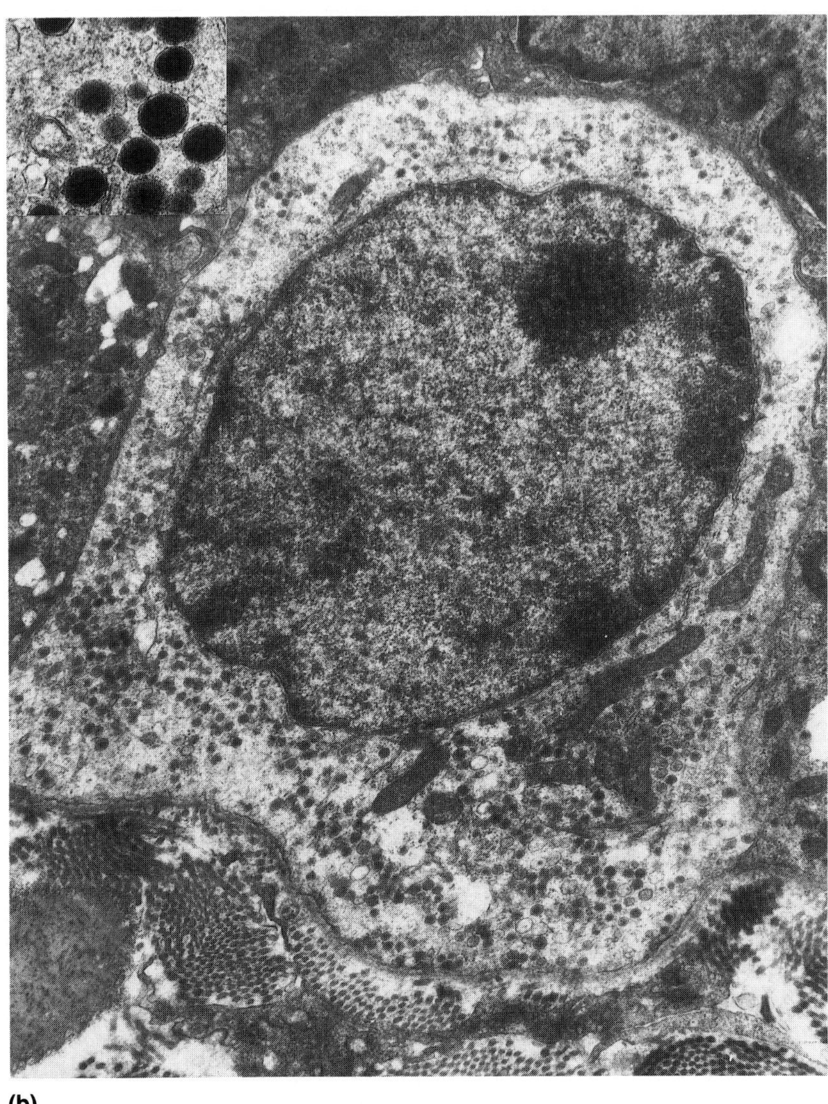

(b)

which, when released, may influence vascular and bronchial smooth-muscle tone, mucous secretion, and ciliary activity.

The function of the DCG cell is controversial. Rosan and Lauweryns (1972) suggest that it may, by its amine secretion, affect lobule growth and differentiation during lung development. With age, there is a decrease in cell number, in the number of granules per cell, and in the electron density of each granule. Moosavi et al. (1973) and Lauweryns and Cokelaere (1973b) have shown that, in hypoxic conditions, there are intracellular changes in the bronchial DCG cell of the young rat, similar to those seen in carotid body chief cells, which suggests that the DCG cell might have a function in the response of the lung to hypoxia.

B. Submucosal Glands

In the adult human trachea and bronchi, glands responsible for producing most of the mucus found in cartilagenous airways are numerous. It is estimated that some 4000 gland units are present in human trachea (Tos, 1968). They are present wherever there is supportive cartilage and are located in the submucosa, the bulk lying between each cartilage plate and the surface epithelium. Each gland unit is tubuloacinar, with a duct opening into the airway lumen (Fig. 16a). In the adult human, each gland may be composed of four regions, the lumina of which are continuous (see Fig. 16b and c): (1) a relatively narrow ciliated duct, the lining cells of which are in continuity with the surface epithelium; (2) an expanded collecting duct lined by cells of indeterminate morphologic structure, or of eosinophilic cells packed with mitochondria (which have also been referred to as "oncocytes") (see Fig. 16c); (3) mucous tubules and acini (see Fig. 16d and e); and (4) serous acini (Meyrick and Reid, 1970; Jeffery and Reid, 1977a) (Fig. 16f).

Airway submucosal glands appear in the human trachea at about 13 weeks gestation. They first appear in the proximal trachea and then progressively more peripherally and reach the main carina some 7 days later (Tos, 1966). In bronchi, they are present by the fourth month of fetal life, in greatest concentration proximally, especially concentrated at airway bifurcations, and the number decreases peripherally (Thurlbeck et al., 1961). Each gland starts its development as part of surface epithelium, by division of its basal cells, to form a sharply defined cluster of cells with dark nuclei (Jeffery and Reid, 1977b; Tos, 1968). Growth then proceeds radially into the lamina propria as a solid cylinder, pushing outward and laying down newly formed basement membrane, which maintains continuity with that of its surface equivalent. Following radial penetration of the muscle layer, there is continued growth and division, but in a tangential or longitudinal direction, either cranially or caudally (Jeffery, 1990a). Tos (1966, 1968) has shown that the appearance of mucus-secreting glands in the membranous wall precedes that in the cartilaginous wall in both bronchus and trachea, and in the trachea by some 9 days. In the bronchus, the rate of gland formation reaches a peak during the 14th–16th fetal week, decreasing after this and terminating during the middle of the 25th week. Tos (1968) reports that there are no sex differences in the gland density during development, whereas Thurlbeck and co-workers (1961) found a male superiority in gland numbers, resulting from a higher concentration of glands, rather than from a difference in absolute size of the trachea. The propor-

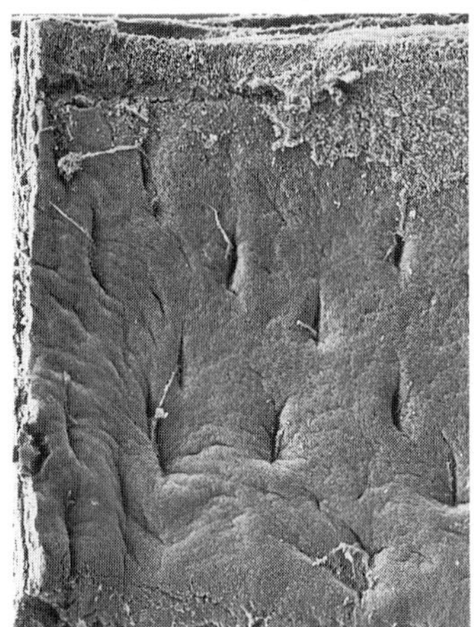

(a)

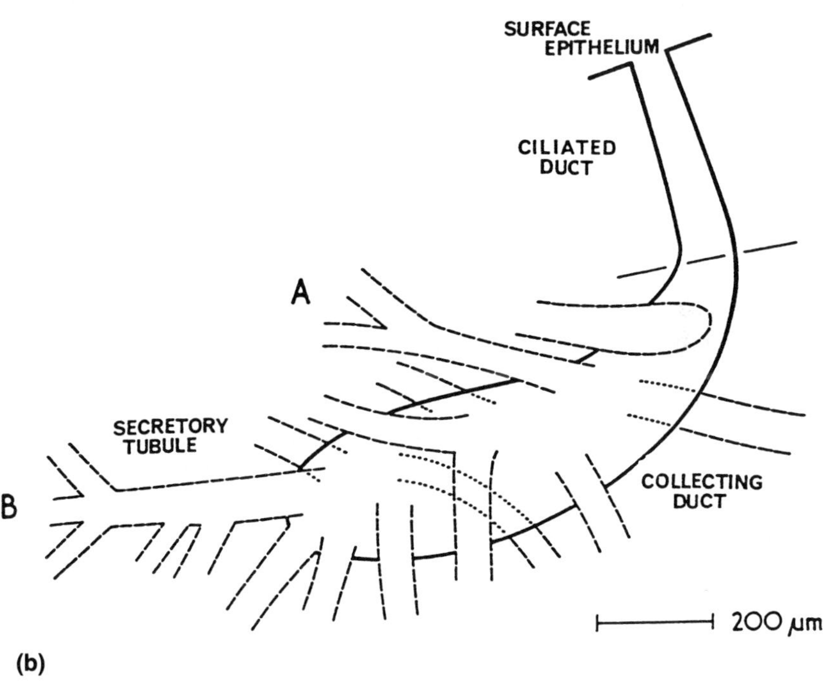

(b)

Figure 16 (a) SEM of human bronchial surface showing slitlike openings of submucosal mucus-secreting glands (×50); (b) diagrammatic representation of reconstruction of a human bronchial gland showing tubular arrangement; (c) SEM of human submucosal gland demonstrating how the surface dips down to form a narrow ciliated duct (arrow), which may

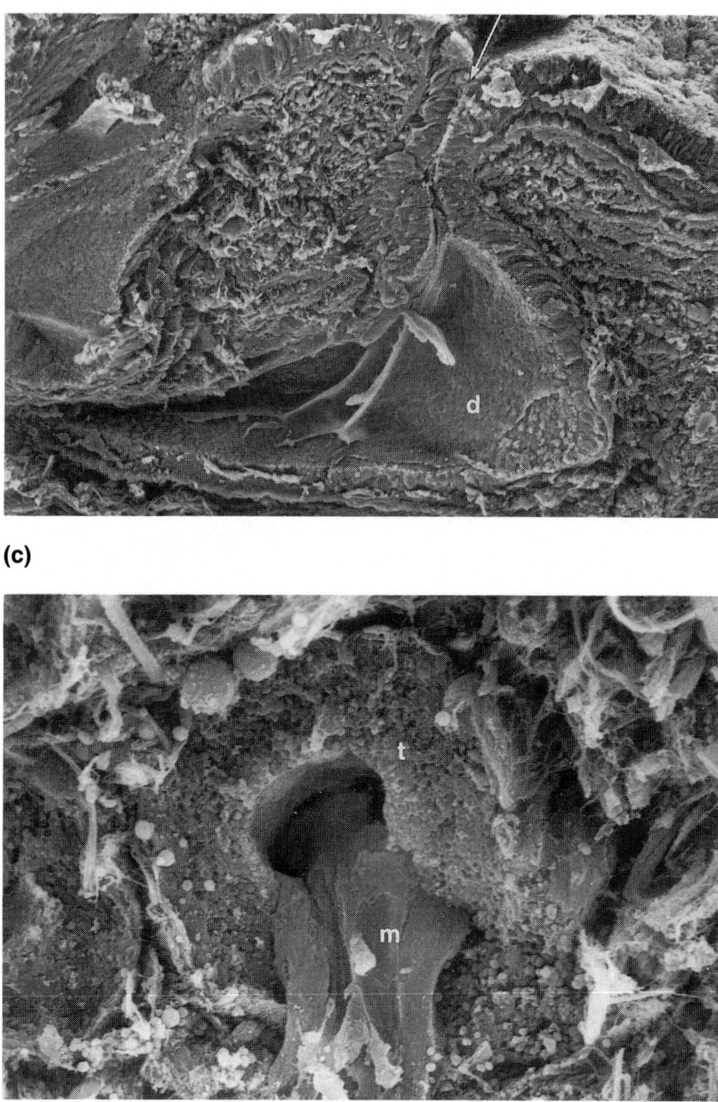

(c)

(d)

Figure 16 (Continued)
expand to form the so-called collecting duct (d) ($\times 200$); (d) SEM to show the cut surface of
a mucous tubule (t) from which mucus (m) is flowing; (e) diagrammatic representation
showing the arrangement of mucous tubules with serous acini located peripherally; and (f)
TEM of a preponderantly serous acinus to show wedge-shaped cells with apically placed
electron-dense secretory granules, round centrally placed nucleus, and small acinar lumen
(1) ($\times$ 4000). (b, From Jeffery and Reid, 1977.)

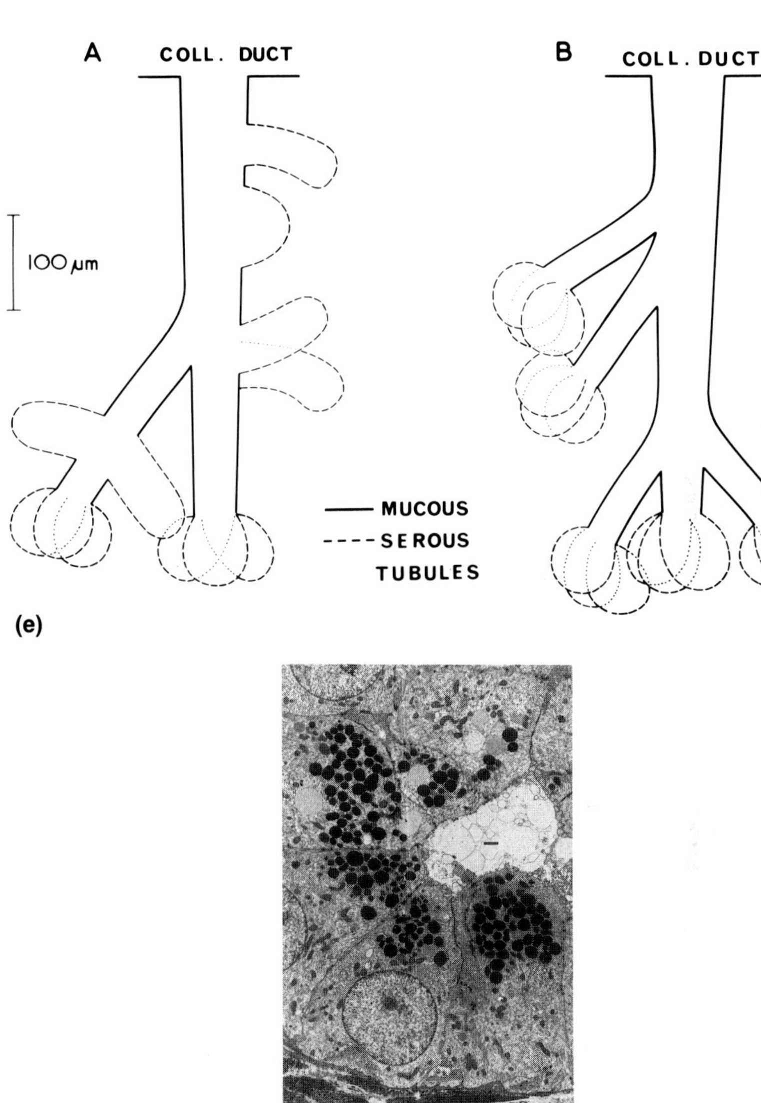

(e)

(f)

tion of the wall occupied by gland (i.e., the gland/wall ratio or Reid index) reaches the adult norm—about one-third the wall—in late fetal life, but during childhood mucous glands form a larger proportion of the walls of major bronchi than in the adult (Tos, 1966; Matsuba and Thurlbeck, 1972). Thus, gland hyperplasia in response to irritation might be a more significant problem in young children than in adults. Few new glands are formed in childhood, the increase in gland area being the result of an increase in gland complexity. The shape of the gland mass varies and is determined by the space available. Not until 13 years of age does the gland approach the form characteristic of the adult and, even then, growth continues up until 28 years of age (see Jeffery and Reid, 1977b).

The solid cylinder of cells originally created is transformed into a tubulo-acinar gland following the initiation of mucus-secretion. Mucus is secreted into the intercellular space, forming a pond that later expands into a canal. Subsequent widening and extension of the canal to the surface pushes the surrounding epithelial cells apart, thereby forming an opening to the airway lumen (Jeffery and Reid, 1977b; Jeffery, 1990a). During early development, the submucosal gland secretory unit consists only of mucous acini, whereas in the adult, serous cells form demilunes around mucous acini or form acini in their own right. Each mucous cell has cytoplasm distended by pale foamy granules, the total volume of which is sufficient to flatten the nucleus by displacing it to the base of the cell (see Fig. 10). By electron microscopy the cytoplasm appears electron-dense and is filled with preponderantly electron-lucent granules (see Fig. 16a).

The glands' serous cells can first be detected by light microscopy as pyramidal-shaped cells, forming crescent shapes about the mucous acini at 25–27 weeks gestation (i.e., before the end of the second term). A weakly eosinophilic ductal region is present by this time. By electron microscopy, between 30 and 33 weeks, there are lysozyme-positive serous cell granules, some of which are electron-dense. Although weak immunoreactivity for lysozyme can also be seen in mucous cells at 16 weeks of gestation, as term approaches, lysozyme becomes confined and acts as a good marker for the serous cell of the glands (Bowes and Corrin, 1977). Low-molecular-mass antileukoproteinase is another marker for maturation of serous cells of the gland and can be detected from 16 weeks gestation in glands of the trachea, and in the main and lobar bronchi (Willems et al., 1988). The relative percentage of serous cells increases during the first 2 years of postnatal life. Histochemical techniques show that serous cells contain glycopro-tein, preponderantly neutral. They differ from mucous cells in producing a secretion with a faster turnover, with less carbohydrate and protein, little or no sialic acid, and no terminal or penultimate galactose (Spicer et al., 1983a; Meyrick and Reid, 1975). However, Lamb and Reid (1970) have shown that carboxyl groups and sulfate esters (the latter confirmed by incorporation of radioactive sulfate) may be present, but their histochemical behavior differs from that of adjacent mucous cells.

By electron microscopy, serous cells have electron-dense secretory granules of about 600-nm diameter (see Fig. 16f). Much, but not all, of the electron-density is lost after fixation with osmium tetroxide alone (which will fix and stain any unsaturated lipid left after processing). The granules are well demarcated by investing membrane and show a greater morphological heterogeneity than those of the mucous cell. The central core may be eccentric and show great variations in cytochemical-staining properties (Spicer et al., 1983a). The heterogeneity is not surprising, as several nonglycoprotein constituents have been identified in this cell type, including lysozyme (used by some investigators as a marker for serous secretions), lactoferrin (Bowes et al., 1981), and low-molecular-mass antiprotein-ase (i.e., bronchial proteinase inhibitor) (Kramps et al., 1981). The last has been detected in sputum (Kramps et al., 1984) and presumably originates from serous cells, if a contribution from saliva can be excluded.

Although the secretory component (piece) of secretory IgA has been identified in submucosal glands of both the upper and lower respiratory tract, the cell type (serous or mucous) most active in its secretion is unclear (Brandtzaeg, 1984). Carbonic anhydrase has also been localized in bronchial serous cells by immunocytochemistry (Spicer et al., 1982). The abundant presence of the enzyme implicates the serous cell in the modulation of ions, pH, and water, which may determine the proportion of respiratory tract fluid that is sol or gel. The presence of albumin-like molecules and a glycosaminoglycans has also been reported (Basbaum et al., 1990).

Thus, serous secretions (from glands or surface) may be normally of low viscosity and contribute to the sol phase (periciliary fluid layer) of airway secretions: additionally, they may regulate the extent of gel formation by altera-tion of its water content as well as by addition of cationic substances that can link mucous molecules by electrostatic interaction. In addition, the proteins secreted by the serous cells may well have an important role in protecting the host against bacterial colonization of the respiratory tract, secretions may be relatively defi-cient early on in life, which may predispose to bacterial colonization and repeated infections. Interaction of bacteria with mucus (Fig. 17a) has been recognized for many years, but has recently received a new focus of attention. The first interaction of inhaled bacteria in the airway mucosa is with mucus (Vishwanath and Ramphal, 1984), which probably contains molecules to which the bacteria bind in a specific manner. This is to the host's advantage in the presence of a normally functioning mucociliary escalator. However, in the presence of bacterial products (e.g., pneumolysin), mucociliary clearance may be delayed (Lourenco et al., 1972; Currie et al., 1987). Such bacterial factors may stimulate production of mucus (Adler et al., 1986) in the presence of the impaired ciliary function (Sykes et al., 1986), and several observations (Mason and Sammons, 1978; Baltimore et al., 1989; Jeffery, 1990b) have suggested that most bacteria in bronchial infections reside in the lumen, associated with bronchial secretions, rather than attached

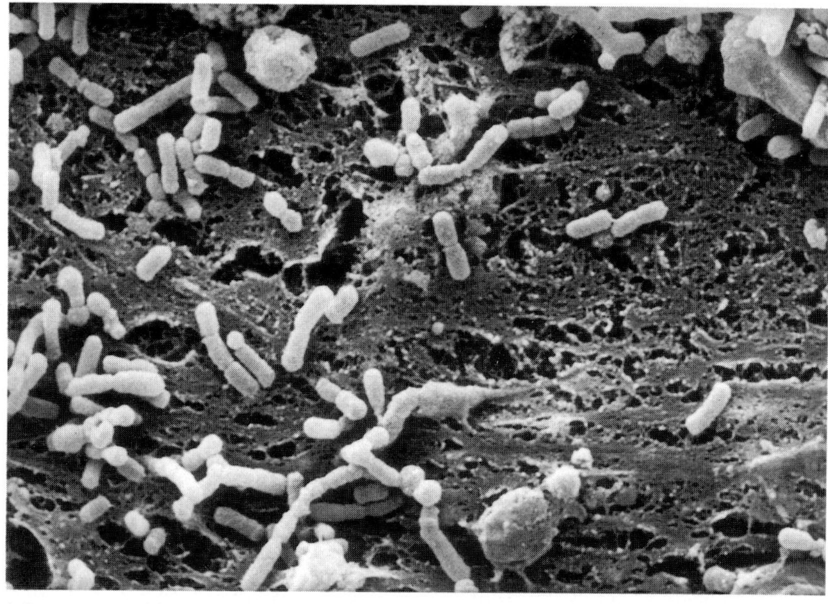

(a)

Figure 17 (a) SEM of human airway mucosal explant which has been experimentally infected with *Haemophilus influenzae*. After 14 h of incubation, there is a thick layer of secretion over the specimen, with a dense concentration of bacteria adhering preferentially to the secretion rather than to the underlying surface cells ($\times$8450). (b) TEM of ciliary fringe of a bronchus from a lung removed at transplant from a patient with cystic fibrosis. The bacteria (arrows) are associated with the overlying secretions, rather than with the apices of the superficial cells ($\times$18,000). (From (a) Read et al., 1991; (b) Jeffery, 1990a).

directly to epithelial cells (see Fig. 17b). Bacterial adherence to the epithelial surface may occur subsequently, permitting a more persistent colonization (Wilson, 1988), and this may particularly occur in areas of epithelial damage (Read et al., 1991).

VIII.   Hypersecretory Disease

A.   Chronic Bronchitis (Mucous Hypersecretion)

Chronic bronchitis (CB) is diagnosed clinically as a persistent cough with the production of sputum (i.e., by convention persisting for more than 3 months of 2 consecutive years) (Medical Research Council, 1965; Thurlbeck et al., 1984). Cough and sputum production are the symptoms most frequently experienced by

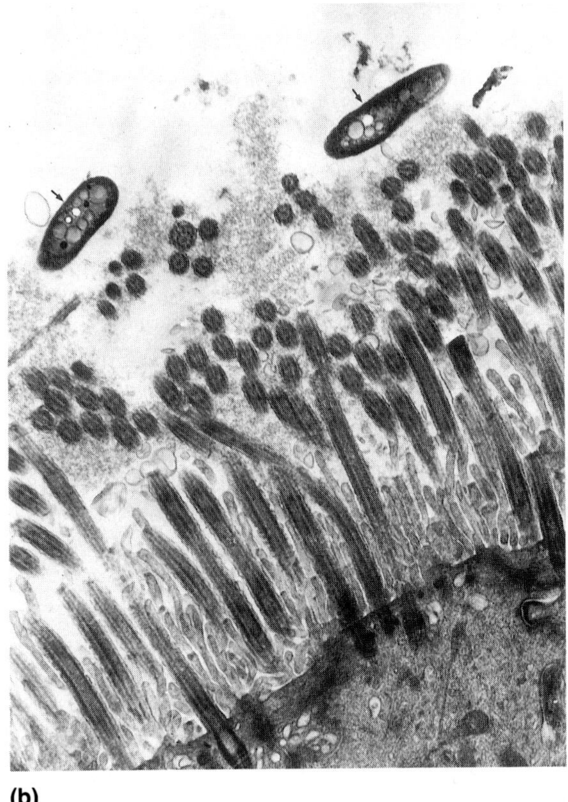

(b)

smokers: both mechanisms are effective in clearing large (proximal) airways (down to about the sixth generation of branching), acting to protect the most distal (peripheral) respiratory portion of the lung from damage. Sputum is, and respiratory tract secretions are, a mixture of constituents comprising glycosaminoglycans, mucus-glycoproteins, proteins and peptides, lipids, antiproteinase and antioxidants, and ions and water (Jeffery, 1987b). Normally, respiratory tract secretions probably amount to less than 100 ml/day (Toremalm, 1960) and have been suggested to consist primarily of glycosaminoglycans (Lopez-Vidriero and Reid, 1985; Coles et al., 1984). Repeated irritation by tobacco smoke (TS) causes an enlargement of submucosal glands (owing to an increase in the number and size of its cells, particularly the mucous cell component), and an increase in the number of secretory cells in the surface epithelium [i.e., hyperplasia (Lamb and Reid, 1969b; Jones et al., 1972; Jeffery and Reid, 1981]. Both mucous gland enlargement and secretory cell hyperplasia are the histological hallmarks of CB and are thought to be the tissue correlate of the associated sputum produced during cough (Reid, 1954). Recent studies have shown that the increase in sputum production may also be related to a TS-induced inflammatory process that occurs in both central and peripheral airways and may relate less to the mass of gland actually present (Mullen et al., 1987).

Also, the *rate* of secretion, rather than gland mass, may contribute relatively more than previously realized. In vitro studies of human mucosa show that enlargement of submucosal glands is associated with more rapid synthesis and discharge of intracellular mucins (Sturgess and Reid, 1972). Parallel animal studies show that, following subacute exposure to TS (2–6 weeks), laryngo-tracheal submucosal glands and surface secretory cells synthesize and discharge epithelial mucins at a faster rate than nonexposed controls (Coles et al., 1979; Rogers et al., 1987b). Experimental exposure of specific pathogen-free rats to an atmosphere of TS increases the number of epithelial secretory cells at all airway levels of the bronchial tree and particularly increases those cells containing acidic glycoprotein (Fig. 18a–c) (Jones et al., 1972; Rogers and Jeffery, 1986a). Increases in acidic mucins are characteristic of the bronchitic patient and smoker also (Kollestrom et al., 1977), and it is thought that the chemical changes may affect the function of mucus by altering its rheological properties (see Chap. 3). The changes just described do not appear to be due to the nicotine content of TS, as experiments show that inhaled or injected nicotine resulting in blood levels far in excess of those achieved by inhalation of TS do not result in mucous cell hyperplasia (Rogers et al., 1986).

Experimental studies in the rat indicate that at least two mechanisms are responsible for the TS-induced increase in surface secretory cell number: (1) mucous transformation of existing serous cells (see Fig. 13a) and (2) cell division (proliferation) of already existing or newly formed mucous cells (Boren, 1970; Jeffery and Reid, 1981; Bolduc et al., 1981; Ayers and Jeffery, 1982) (see Fig. 9a). The stimulus to cell division evokes a rapid response, with a peak of proliferation seen between 1 and 2 days, which then decreases rapidly, in spite of continued exposure, to levels found in unexposed animals (i.e., tolerance develops). If the smoke exposure is interrupted, tolerance is lost and on reexposure there is a further proliferative burst.

Measurements by light and transmission electron microscopy show that epithelial thickening in the experimental animal is an early response to inhaled TS and that the thickening is not due to stratification, but rather, to cell hypertro-phy (Jeffery and Reid, 1981). The defects in mucociliary function in chronic disease could be the result of ciliary malfunction or of alterations to the constituent secretions and their rheology. Experimental results of 2-weeks exposure to TS show that cilia remain normal in both their structure and density, whereas the proportion of all epithelial cells that are ciliated, surprisingly, increases. There is an increase in the maximum length of mitochondria, which provide the major energy for ciliated cells and also of ciliated cell apical microvilli. The increase in surface coverage by cilia and its surface covering of mucus (Fig. 19) is seen clearly when the epithelium is viewed by scanning electron microscopy (Jeffery et al., 1988). In vitro brushings of ciliated cells obtained from bronchitic patients or from the noses of healthy volunteers following exhalation of smoke through the nose show no abnormality of ciliary beat frequency (Yager et al., 1980; Stanley et al., 1986). These results are in contrast with the findings in end-stage disease where atrophy of epithelium (Wright and Stuart, 1965), focal squamous metaplasia, reduction in ciliated cell number and mean ciliary length, and goblet cell hyperplasia are features (Chang, 1957; Wanner, 1977; Misokovitch et al., 1974). Some of the ultrastructural changes in cilia (i.e., appearance of compound cilia) have been directly attributed to the effects of cigarette smoke (Ailsby and Ghadially, 1973), but these changes may be nonspecific and are more likely to be consequences of complicating exacerbations of infection, the bacterial products of which are known to be ciliotoxic (Wilson, 1988).

Impairment of mucociliary transport in the periods between exacerbations of infection is more likely due to alterations in the volume and viscoelastic profile of the secretions, which are known to interact, in a very specific way, with the tips of the cilia (see Figs. 5 and 19). The physical characteristics of the secretions depend on several factors: (1) the constituent glycoproteins are largely responsible for the gellike properties of secretions. Increasing sialylation may contribute to higher viscosity (Lopata et al., 1974; Lopez-Vidriero and Reid, 1978). (2) DNA, either from the host or from invading microorganisms, may contribute significantly to increases in both dry weight and viscosity (Lopez-Vidriero et al., 1977; Lethen et al., 1987). (3) The complexing of mucin with locally produced secretory IgA and electrostatic interaction with cationic proteins, such as lactoferrin and lysozyme, may also contribute to increased viscosity (Lopez-Vidriero et al., 1977; Lamblin et al., 1992; Harbitz et al., 1980). (4) Noncovalently associated neutral, glyco- and phospholipids are found in airway secretions, and these may also interact to affect the viscosity and elasticity of mucus (see Clamp and Creeth, 1984; Jeffery, 1987b). Any one or all of these factors may be important in disease (Lopez-Vidriero and Reid, 1983). There is evidence that once a smoker has developed chronic bronchitis, the impairment of mucociliary function is greater than that seen in smokers without bronchitis and that, in long-standing disease, cessation of smoking does not entirely reverse the impairment of mucociliary transport (Goodman et al., 1978; Agnew et al., 1982). These cigarette smoke-induced effects on the mucociliary system may also contribute to the accumulation and pooling of secretions in the tracheobronchial tree, placing a greater reliance on coughing as a mechanism for maintaining clearance.

Although the volume of sputum produced shows a strong correlation with smoking, the number of infective episodes and individual FEV_1 (forced expiratory volume in 1 s, as a marker of airflow obstruction), it does not correlate with the

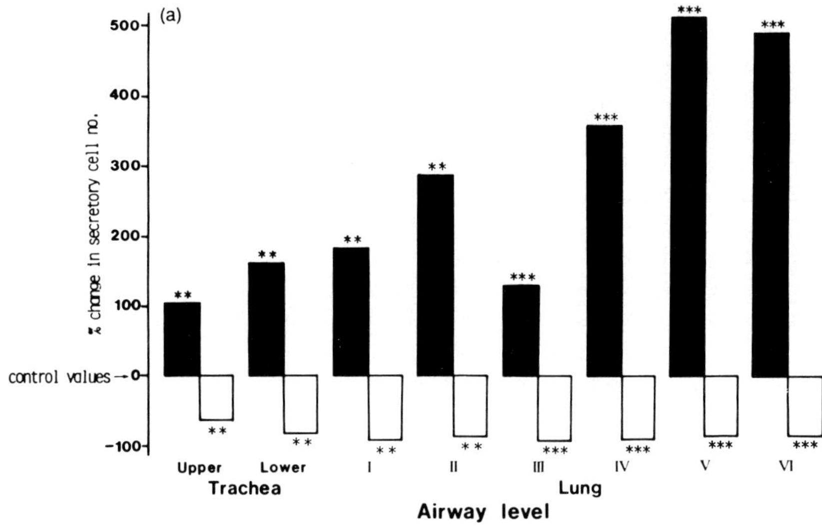

(a)

Figure 18 (a) Effect of cigarette smoke, given by passive inhalation over a period of 2 weeks, on the numbers of secretory cells containing acidic (■) or neutral glycoprotein (□). The bars represent the percentage increase or decrease at each airway level of the rat lung in relation to control values. (**$p < 0.02$; ***$p < 0.001$). (b) TEM of normal (sham-exposed) bronchial epithelium showing surface serous(s), ciliated, and basal cells, and (c) the cigarette smoke-induced increase of epithelial thickness and surface mucous (G) cells following 2 weeks exposure. (b, c, × 3250). Arrow marks position of basement membrane. (From (a) Rogers and Jeffery, 1986b; (b,c) Jeffery and Reid, 1981).

progressive and accelerated decline in FEV_1 seen with age (Fletcher, 1984; Peto et al., 1983). Thus, although excessive secretions in airways may obstruct airflow, they do not result in chronic progressive deterioration of lung function.

B. Chronic Obstructive (Adult) Bronchiolitis: Small Airways Disease

Airflow limitation (as determined by tests of FEV_1) usually occurs late in the course of TS-related events, whereas inflammation in small airways (i.e., bronchioli smaller than 2–3 mm in diameter) occurs relatively early and may be detected physiologically well before the age of 30 years (Buist, 1984; Nemery et al., 1981). The small-airway defect is characterized by persistent airflow limitation, which may show progressive deterioration in the absence of emphysema. Although the site of the lesion and diagnosis is, as yet, difficult to pinpoint

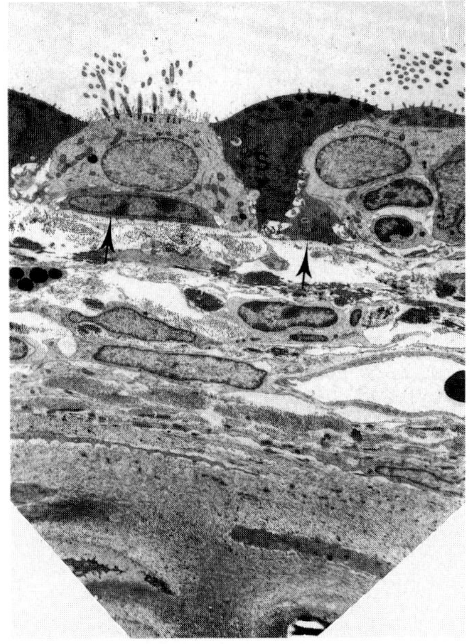

(b)

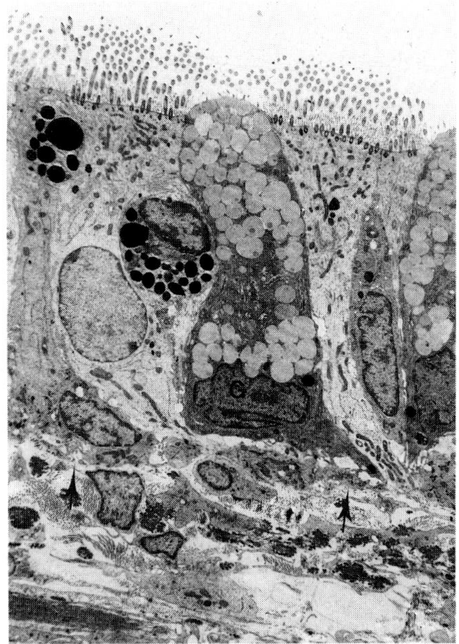

(c)

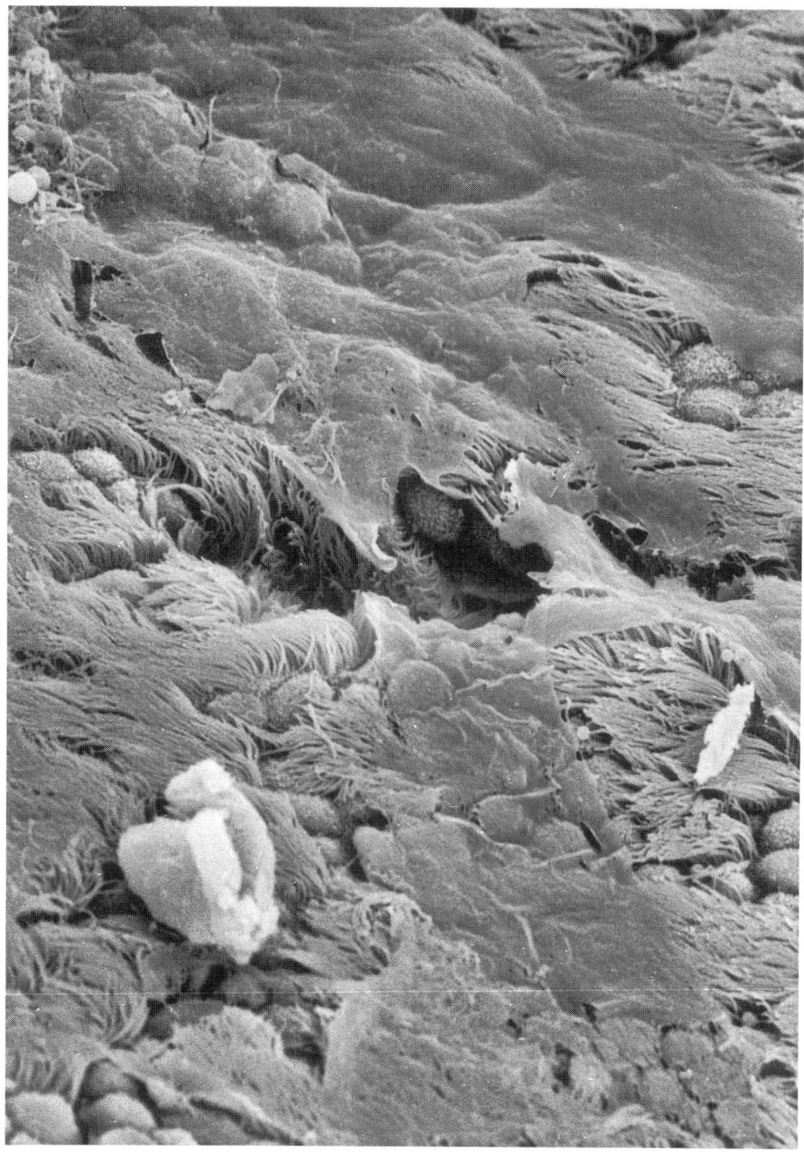

Figure 19   SEM of bronchial surface from a rat exposed to cigarette smoke for 3 months. The surface has a high concentration of cilia, most of which are covered by a layer of mucus (× 2000) (From Jeffery et al., 1988).

by lung function, experimental physiologists (see, e.g., Hogg et al., 1968; van Brabandt et al., 1983) have indicated that the dominant site lies in bronchioli smaller than 3 mm in diameter. Histologically, one of the most consistently observed early effects of smoking is the marked increase in the number of inflammatory cells (macrophages and neutrophils) in humans and also, experimentally, in animal studies. The increase of inflammatory cells is seen within lung interstitium and alveolus and can be detected in bronchoalveolar lavage fluid (see Reynolds 1987). Niewoehner (1974), Mitchell (1976), Cosio (1980), and their colleagues have described early smoking-related changes in studies comparing lungs of young smokers and controls of similar age from a group who had experienced sudden nonhospital deaths. The last-mentioned workers have suggested that the primary lesion is a progressive inflammatory reaction and associated mucous metaplasia leading to peribronchiolar fibrosis, which may predispose to the subsequent development of centrilobular emphysema and may be responsible for the subtle abnormalities detected by lung function. As we have seen, the Clara cell forms the major secretory and progenitor cell of bronchioli and also contains a low-molecular-mass proteinase inhibitor (antileukoproteinase or bronchial mucosal proteinase inhibitor) (Mooren et al., 1983). Scanning electron microscopic studies indicate that Clara cell numbers are reduced in smokers and are replaced by mucous cells (Ebert and Terracio, 1975); indeed, secretion of mucus into terminal bronchioli in incubated tissue from human smokers has been demonstrated (Ebert and Hanks, 1981). Peripheralization of mucous cells is also a histological feature of cigarette smoke-induced experimental bronchitis in the rat (Rogers and Jeffery, 1986a; Jones et al., 1973).

What are the consequences of such a mucous metaplasia in small airways? One mechanism by which smoke may be toxic is by reducing the bronchiolar antiproteinase screen, leading to local proteolytic digestion and tissue damage. Such damage in respiratory bronchioli could predispose to the development of centrilobular emphysema. The extension of mucous cells to a distal site from which they are normally sparse results in secretion of mucus at a site that cannot easily be cleared by cough. Furthermore, replacement of the surfactant lining by mucus is thought to lead to instability of small airways and to early airway closure during expiration (Macklem et al., 1970). However, breathlessness and airflow limitation induced by small-airway changes would be expected to be detectable only as the condition progresses substantially, as the cross-sectional area of the bronchiolar zone of the lung is normally large in relation to the first few bronchial divisions (Horsfield, 1981).

C. Asthma

In asthma, bronchial surface epithelium may show an increase of goblet cell number, which may or may not be paralleled by an increase in their number in small bronchi and bronchioli (Dunnill, 1960; Lamb, 1990; Jeffery, 1991; see Chap. 15). It is as yet unclear how much of the small-airway mucous plugging is due directly to increased secretion by newly acquired goblet cells (in the absence of submucosal glands at this distal site) and how much is due to aspiration of mucus produced in the more proximal airways. In larger bronchi of individuals dying in status asthmaticus, there is a significant enlargement of the mass of mucus-secreting submucosal glands, similar to that seen in chronic bronchitis (Dunnill et al., 1969). In asthma, the normal serous/mucous acinar ratio is reportedly maintained (Glynn and Michaels, 1960), whereas in chronic bronchitis, there is a relative reduction of serous acini, containing the important antibacterial and antiproteolytic substances already discussed (see Sect. VIII.A). Patients with asthma may have intermittent hypersecretion of mucus and cough similar to that of chronic bronchitis. No mucosubstance unique to asthma has been identified, albeit there may be differences in the relative proportion of the constituents that make up respiratory tract fluid. For example, there may be interaction of mucous glyco-proteins with lipid or with serum, which may thicken the secretions and contribute to the marked and characteristic tenacity of airway secretions. The occlusion of medium and small bronchi with viscid gelatinous plugs is seen in most, but not all, asthmatics who die following an acute severe unremitting attack (Fig. 20) (Reid, 1987). Histologically, the lumenal plugs are heterogeneous (as seen by hematoxylin–eosin, H&E stain) with a basophilic component that is mucinous (presumably derived from surface epithelium or submucosal gland) and an eosinophilic component that is likely to be plasma exudate: the last is in keeping with the observed increased contribution to airway fluid by serum proteins, such as albumin. Accordingly, the concentrations of other plasma proteins—α_1-acid glycoprotein, transferrin, haptoglobin, and α_1-antitrypsin—are reported to be significantly higher in asthma than in chronic bronchitis (see Lopez-Vidriero et al., 1977). The contrast of tenacity and viscosity between the airway plugs of asthmatic and bronchitic lungs is amply demonstrated by the observations of Dunnill et al. who reported that, unlike those of bronchitis, the airway plugs of asthmatic subjects require in excess of 1.5-m head (water) pressure to dislodge them during intrabronchial instillation of fixative (Dunnill et al., 1969).

Less is known concerning the structural variation of the secretory apparatus in other airway and lung conditions, such as bronchiectases, bronchorrhea, and pulmonary edema, in which there are also increases in respiratory tract fluid, beyond the normal sufficient to produce sputum. For a review of the associated biochemical alterations, the reader is referred to Lopez-Vidriero et al. (1977).

D. Cystic Fibrosis

Secretion of the correct amount of mucus with an optimal viscoelastic profile is important in the maintenance of normal mucociliary clearance, and this is thought

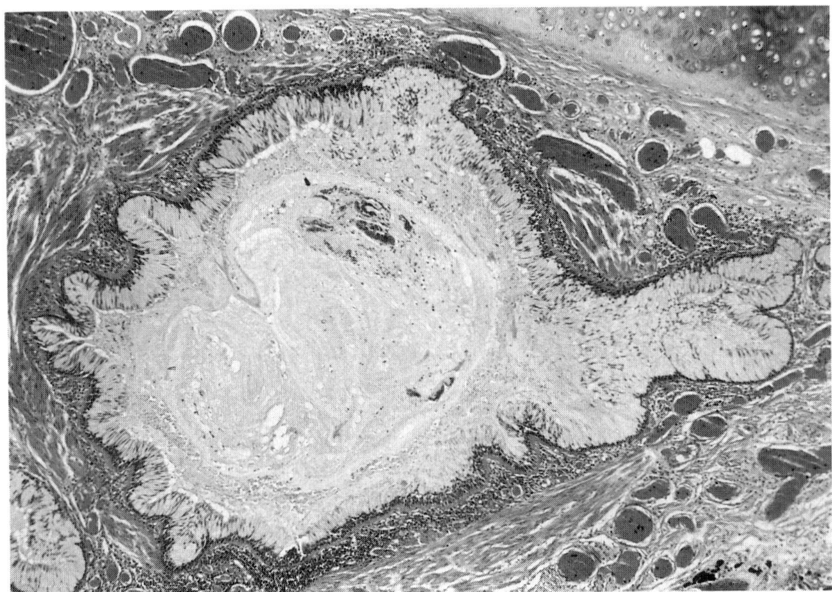

Figure 20 H&E-stained section of a small intrapulmonary bronchus completely blocked by a viscid gelatinous plug of mixed epithelial-derived secretions and inflammatory exudate in a subject who died following an acute attack of severe asthma ($\times$150).

to be defective in cystic fibrosis (CF). Although alterations in the predominant histochemical type of mucus have been associated with airway irritation (Jones et al., 1973) and carcinogenesis (Filipe and Branfoot, 1974), no abnormality specific to CF has been detected (Oppenheimer, 1981). The increase in number and extension to the peripheral bronchioles of goblet cells seen in chronic bronchitis and after cigarette smoke and sulfur dioxide inhalation is also a characteristic of airways in CF (Esterly and Oppenheimer, 1968). The solubility and viscosity of mucus varies considerably with ionic strength. Divalent cations, such as calcium (Ca^{2+}), cause mucus to form a rigid cross-linked gel that may be difficult to clear by mucociliary action or cough (Fig. 21). In biopsy studies, mucous cells from patients with CF have contained substantially raised intracellular Ca^{2+} and sulfate (SO_4^{2-}) levels and lower potassium levels than those of patients with chronic bronchitis: The importance of these results is as yet unclear, but it is in keeping with the reports of high Ca^{2+} and SO_4^{2-} contents of tracheobronchial secretions (Boat et al., 1976, 1989). The *CF* genotype now includes many abnormalities additional to that originally described (Riordan et al., 1989). Physiologically there are abnormalities of transepithelial Cl^- and Na^+ transport, decreased sialylation,

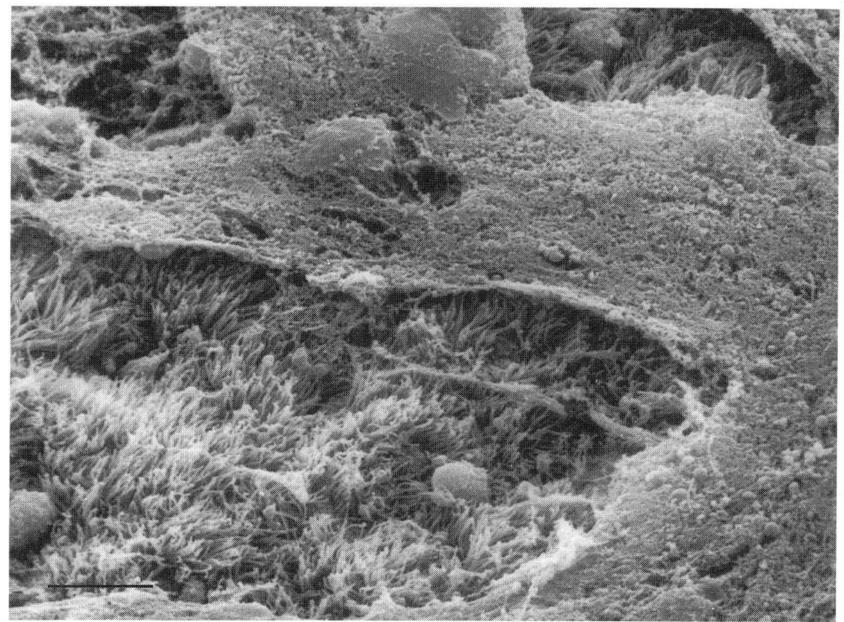

Figure 21 TEM of bronchial surface of a lung freshly removed at transplant for cystic fibrosis. In spite of rigorous flushing with culture medium and tissue processing, the secretions and included cells remain adherent to the epithelium ($\times 2200$).

and increased sulfation and fucosylation of glycoproteins all apparently associated with an increased tendency of the airways to colonization with *Pseudomonas* sp. There is recent evidence (Barasch et al., 1991) that helps to explain the relationships between defects of acidification, diminished Cl^- conductance, and the reduced sialylation of proteins and lipids seen in CF (see Chap. 14).

E. Anti-inflammatory Drugs

Several anti-inflammatory drugs have been explored experimentally relative to their effectiveness in preventing some of the bronchitic changes already outlined (Jeffery, 1986). Phenylmethyloxadiazole (PMO) can inhibit the ciliostatic effect, the mucous metaplasia–hyperplasia, and the epithelial thickening associated with TS inhalation (Dalhamm and Rylander, 1971; Jeffery and Reid, 1981; Jones et al., 1973), and there is evidence that PMO may inhibit the TS-induced mucus hypersecretion seen in rat laryngeal gland (Coles et al., 1979). Inhibitors of the cyclooxygenase pathway of arachidonic acid metabolism prevent the mucous cell hyperplasia, but the mechanism of action may not be their effect on cyclooxygenase. Indomethacin does so in the laboratory rat in a dose-related manner and is particularly effective in bronchioli when given by intraperitoneal injection (Greig et al., 1980; Rogers and Jeffery, 1986b). Selected glucocorticosteroids are effective, albeit at high doses (Rogers and Jeffery, 1986b). A mucoregulatory drug, *N*-acetylcysteine, given orally in the drinking water inhibits the airway mucous cell hyperplasia–metaplasia and epithelial thickening of larger airways (Rogers and Jeffery, 1986a), and attentuates and delays the TS-induced proliferative response (Jeffery et al., 1985), as well as reduces tracheal mucous hypersecretion (Rogers et al., 1989).

In humans, prospective studies in ex-smokers show that symptoms of cough and expectoration usually abate rapidly (Hammond, 1965; Wilhelmsen, 1967; Peterson et al., 1968) and, when young smokers stop smoking, their lung function usually returns to normal (see Fletcher and Horn, 1971). Life expectancy increases with the years of abstinence (Doll and Hill, 1964; Hammond, 1966). In patients with moderately severe airways disease, cessation may result in a dramatic reduction of breathlessness and cough (Fletcher and Horn, 1971), but damage to small airways may already be extensive, with only slight improvement of airflow (Burrows and Earle, 1969).

Some of the milder, acute changes are reversible: permeability changes largely (but not completely) revert to normal after 1-week cessation of smoking (Minty et al., 1981), mucociliary clearance in about 3 months (Camner et al., 1973), and the mucous cell hyperplasia in about 2 years (Betram and Rogers, 1981). Experimentally, mucous cell hyperplasia in the rat recovers in about 3 months after cessation, and its recovery can be accelerated by the inclusion of nonsteroidal anti-inflammatory agents (by injection) or following oral administration of mucoregulatory drugs (Rogers and Jeffery, 1986b; Rogers et al., 1987a).

IX. Conclusion and Future Studies

The variety of epithelial secretory cell types and their various secretions that have been described herein, in the adult, serve to humidify and to protect the more distal respiratory portion of the lung from pollutants and infection. Apart from their protective role, secretory cells play an important role as stem cells from which other cell types may differentiate and mature during development, disease, and the repair that follows irritation and damage of the airway mucosa.

Acknowledgments

My sincere thanks to Jenny Billingham for her help and patience in the preparation of the manuscript and to Andy Rogers for his help in the preparation of the electron micrographs.

References

Adler, K. B., Hendley, D. D., and Davis, G. S. (1986). Bacteria associated with obstructive pulmonary disease elaborate extracellular products that stimulate mucin secretion by explants of guinea pig airways. *Am. J. Pathol.* 125: 501–514.

Agnew, J. E., Little, F., Pavia, D., and Clarke, S. W. (1982). Mucus clearance from the airways in chronic bronchitis: Smokers and ex-smokers. *Bull. Eur. Physiopathol. Respir.* 18: 473–484.

Ailsby, R. L., and Ghadially, F. N. (1973). Atypical cilia in human bronchial mucosa. *J. Pathol.* 109: 75–77.

Ayers, M., and Jeffery, P. K. (1982). Cell division and differentiation in the respiratory tract. In *Cell Biology and the Lung, Vol. 10, Ettore Majoran Intern Life Science Series.* Edited by G. Cumming and G. Bonsignore. New York, Plenum Press, pp. 33–60.

Ayers, M., and Jeffery, P. K. (1988). Proliferation and differentiation in adult mammalian airway epithelium: A review. *Eur. Respir. J.* 1: 58–80.

Azzopardi, A., and Thurlbeck, W. M. (1969). The histochemistry of the nonciliated bronchiolar epithelial cell. *Am. Rev. Respir. Dis.* 99: 516–525.

Baltimore, R. S., Christie, C. D. C., and Walker Smith, G. J. (1989). Immuno-histopathologic localization of *Pseudomonas aeruginosa* in lungs from patients with cystic fibrosis. *Am. Rev. Respir. Dis.* 140: 1650–1661.

Barasch, J., Kiss, B., Prince, A., Saiman, L., Gruenert, D., and Al-Awqati, Q. (1991). Defective acidification of intracellular organelles in cystic fibrosis. *Nature* 352: 70–73.

Barnes, P. J. (1986). State of art: Neural control of human airways in health and disease. *Am. Rev. Respir. Dis.* 134: 1289–1314.

Basbaum, C. (1984). Regulation of secretions from serous and mucous cells in the trachea. In *Mucus and Mucosa. Ciba Found. Symp.* 109: 4–19.

Basbaum, C. B., Jany, B., and Finkbeiner, W. E. (1990). The serous cell. *Annu. Rev. Physiol.* 52: 97–113.

Betram, J. F., and Rogers, A. W. (1981). Recovery of bronchial epithelium on stopping smoking. *Br. Med. J.* 283: 1567–1569.

Bhattacharya, S. N., Veit, B. C., Manna, B., Enriquez, J. I., Walker, M. P., Khorrami, A. M., and Kaufman, B. (1990). Neutral and acidic human tracheobronchial mucin. In New York, Plenum Publishing, pp. 355–373.

Blau, H. M. (1989). How fixed is the differentiated state? *Trends Genet.* 5: 268–272.

Boat, T. F., Kleinerman, J. I., Carlson, D. M., Maloney, W. H., and Matthews, L. W. (1974). Human respiratory tract secretions. I. Mucous glycoproteins secreted by cultured nasal polyp epithelium from subjects with allergic rhinitis and cystic fibrosis. *Am. Rev. Respir. Dis.* 110: 428–441.

Boat, T. F., Cheng, P. W., Iyer, R. N., Carlson, D. M., and Polony, I. (1976). Human respiratory tract secretions: Mucous glycoproteins of non-purulent tracheobronchial secretions, and sputum of patients with bronchitis and cystic fibrosis. *Arch. Biochem. Biophys.* 177: 95–104.

Boat, T. F., Welsh, M. J., and Beaudet, A. L. (1989). Cystic fibrosis. In *The Metabolic Basis of Inherited Disease.* Edited by C. R. Scriver, A. L. Beaudet, W. S. Sly, and D. Valle. New York, McGraw-Hill, pp. 2649–2680.

Bolduc, P., Jones, R., and Reid, L. (1981). Mitotic activity of airway epithelium after short exposure to tobacco smoke and the effect of the anti-inflammatory agent phenylmethyloxadiazole. *Br. J. Exp. Pathol.* 62: 461–468.

Boren, H. G. (1970). Pulmonary cell kinetics after exposure to tobacco smoke. In *Inhalation Carcinogenesis*. Edited by M. G. Harmon. Atomic Energy Commission, Division of Technical Information. Symp. Ser. 18: 229–241.

Bowes, D., Clark, A. E., and Corrin, B. (1981). Ultrastructural localisation of lactoferrin and glycoprotein in human bronchial glands. *Thorax* 36: 108–115.

Bowes, D., and Corrin, B. (1977). Ultrastructural immunocytochemical localization of lysozyme in human bronchial glands. *Thorax* 32: 163–170.

Bowman, W. (1847). Mucous membranes. In *Cyclopaedia of Anatomy and Physiology*, Vol. 3. pp. 484–506.

Boyd, M. R. (1977). Evidence for the Clara cell as a site of cytochrome P450-dependent mixed-function oxidase activity in lung. *Nature* 269: 713–715.

Brandtzaeg, P. (1984). Immune functions of human nasal mucosa and tonsils in health and disease. In *Immunology of the Lung and Upper Respiratory Tract*. Edited by J. Bienenstock. New York, McGraw-Hill, pp. 28–95.

Breeze, R. G., and Wheeldon, E. B. (1977). The cells of the pulmonary airways. State of the art. *Am. Rev. Respir. Dis.* 116: 705–777.

Breuer, R., Zajicek, G., Christensen, J. G., Lucey, E. C., and Snider, G. L. (1990). Cell kinetics of normal adult hamster bronchial epithelium in the steady state. *Am. J. Respir. Cell Mol. Biol.* 2: 51–58.

Bucher, U., and Reid, L. (1961). Development of the mucus secreting elements in human lung. *Thorax* 16: 219–225.

Buist, A. S. (1984). Current status of small airways disease. *Chest* 86: 100–105.

Burrows, B., and Earle, R. H. (1969). Course and prognosis of chronic obstructive lung disease. A prospective study of 200 patients. *N. Engl. J. Med.* 280: 397–404.

Cameron, G. R. (1952). Origins of the cell theory. In *Pathology of the Cell*. Edinburgh & London, Oliver & Boyd, pp. 3–31.

Camner, P., Mossberg, B., and Philipson, K. (1973). Tracheobronchial clearance and chronic obstructive lung disease. *Scand J. Respir. Dis.* 54: 272–281.

Capella, C., Hage, E., Solicia, E., and Usellini, L. (1987). Ultrastructural similarity of endocrine-like cells of the human lung and some related cells of the gut. *Cell Tissue Res.* 186: 25–37.

Chang, S. C. 1957). Microscopic properties of whole mounts and sections of human bronchial epithelium of smokers and non-smokers. *Cancer* 10: 1246–1262.

Cheng, H., and Leblond, C. P. (1974). Origin, differentiation and renewal of the four main epithelial cell types in the mouse small intestine. III. Enteroendocrine cells. *Am. J. Anat.* 14: 132–178.

Clamp, J. R., and Creeth, J. M. (1984). Some non-mucin components of mucus and their possible biological roles. In *Mucus and Mucosa*. Edited by J. Nugent and M. O'Conner. London, Pitman, pp. 121–136.

Clara, M. (1937). Zur Histobiologie des Bronchalepithels. *Z. Mikrobiol. Anat. Forsch.* 41: 321–347.

Coles, S. J., Levine, L. R., and Reid, L. (1979). Hypersecretion of mucus glycoproteins in rat airways induced by tobacco smoke. *Am. J. Pathol.* 94: 459–472.

Coles, S. J., Bhaskar, K. R., O'Sullivan, B. D., Neill, K. H., and Reid, L. M. (1984). Airway mucus: Composition and regulation of its secretion by neuropeptides in vitro. In *Mucus and Mucosa. Ciba Found. Symp.* 109: 40–60.

Cosio, M. G., Hale, K. A., and Niewoehner, D. E. (1980). Morphologic and morphometric effects of prolonged cigarette smoking on the small airways. *Am. Rev. Respir. Dis.* 122: 265–271.

Currie, D. C., Pavia, D., Agnew, J. E., Lopez-Vidriero, M. T., Diamond, P. D., Cole, P. J., and Clarke, S. W. (1987). Impaired tracheobronchial clearance in bronchiectasis. *Thorax* 42: 126–130.

Cutz, E. (1987). Cytomorphology and differentiation of airway epithelium in developing human lung. In *Lung Carcinomas*. Edited by E. M. McDowell. New York, Churchill–Livingstone, pp. 1–41.

Cutz, E., Chan, W., and Track, N. S. (1981). Bombesin, calcistonin and leu-enkephalin immunoreactivity in endocrine cells of human lung. *Experientia* 37: 765–767.

Cutz, E., Gillan, J. E., and Bryan, A. C. (1985). Neuroendocrine cells in the developing human lung: Morphologic and functional considerations. *Paediatr. Pulmonol.* 1: S1–S29.

Dalhamn, T., and Rylander, R. (1971). Reduction of cigarette smoke ciliotoxicity by certain tobacco additives. *Am. Rev. Respir. Dis.* 103: 855–857.

Darnell, J. E. (1982). Variety in the level of gene control in eukaryotic cells. *Nature* 297: 365–371.

De Haller, R. (1969). Development of mucus-secreting elements. In *The Anatomy of the Developing Lung*. London, William Heinemann, pp. 94–115.

Dinsdale, D., Green, J. A., Manson, M. M., and Lee, M. J. (1992). The ultrastructural immunolocalization of gamma-glutamyltranspeptidase in rat lung: Correlation with the histochemical demonstration of enzyme activity. *Histochem. J.* (in press).

Doll, R., and Hill, A. B. (1964). Mortality in relation to smoking: Ten years' observations of British doctors. *Br. Med. J.* 1: 1399–1410.

Dunnill, M. S. (1960). The pathology of asthma, with special reference to changes in the bronchial mucosa. *J. Clin. Pathol.* 13: 27–33.

Dunnill, M. S., Massarella, G. R., and Anderson, J. A. (1969). A comparison of the quantitative anatomy of the bronchi in normal subjects, in status asthmaticus, in chronic bronchitis, and in emphysema. *Thorax* 24: 176–179.

Ebert, R. V., and Hanks, P. B. (1981). Mucus secretion by the epithelium of the bronchioles of cigarette smokers. *Br. J. Dis. Chest* 75: 277–282.

Ebert, R. V., and Terracio, M. J. (1975). The bronchiolar epithelium in cigarette smokers: Observations with the scanning electron microscope. *Am. Rev. Respir. Dis.* 111: 4–11.

Ellefsen, P., and Tos, M. (1972). Goblet cells in the human trachea: Quantitative studies of a pathological biopsy material. *Arch. Otolaryngol.* 95: 547–555.

Esterly, J. R., and Oppenheimer, E. H. (1968). Cystic fibrosis of the pancreas: Structural changes in peripheral airways. *Thorax* 23: 670–675.

Filipe, M. I., and Branfoot, A. C. (1974). Abnormal patterns of mucus secretion in apparently normal mucosa of large intestine with carcinoma. *Cancer* 34: 282–290.

Fletcher, C. M. (1984). Chronic bronchitis and decline in pulmonary function with some suggestions on terminology. In *Smoking and the Lung*, Vol. 17. Edited by G. Cumming and G. Bonsignore. New York, Plenum Press, pp. 397–420.

Fletcher, C. M., and Horn, D. (1971). Smoking and health. World Health Organisation report: Department of Health and Social Security, Scottish Home and Health Department, Welsh Office.

Frisch, E. B., and Phillips, T. (1990). Lectin binding patterns to plasmalemmal glycoconjugates of goblet cells undergoing differentiation in vitro. *J. Elect. Microsc. Technol.* 16: 25–36.

Gaillard, D., Moret, S., Lallemand, A., and Girod, S. (1990). Histochemistry of glycoconjugates and lysozyme in the human fetal trachea. *Eur. Respir. J.* 10: 258.

Gaillard, D. A., Lallemand, A. V., Petit, A. F., and Puchelle, E. S. (1989). In vivo ciliogenesis in human fetal tracheal epithelium. *Am. J. Anat.* 185: 415–418.

Gallagher, J. J., Hall, R. L., Phipps, R. J., et al. (1986). Mucus-glycoproteins (mucins) of the cat trachea—characterization and control of secretion. *Biochim. Biophys. Acta* 886: 243–255.

Gashi, A. A., Nadel, J. A., and Basbaum, C. B. (1987). Autoradiographic studies of the distribution of 35-sulfate label in ferret trachea: effects of stimulation. *Exp. Lung Res.* 12: 83–96.

Gil, J., and Weibel, E. (1971). Extracellular lining of bronchioles after perfusion-fixation of rat lungs for electron microscopy. *Anat. Rec.* 169: 185–200.

Glynn, A. A., and Michaels, L. (1960). Bronchial biopsy in chronic bronchitis and asthma. *Thorax* 15: 142–153.

Goodman, R. M., Bergen, B. M., Lander, J. F., Goinvaux, M. H., and Thackner, M. A. (1978). Relationship of smoking history and pulmonary function tests to tracheal mucus velocity in non-smokers, young smokers, ex-smokers and patients with chronic bronchitis. *Am. Rev. Respir. Dis.* 117: 205–214.

Greig, J., Ayers, M., and Jeffery, P. K. (1980). The effect of indomethacin on the response of rat bronchial epithelium to tobacco smoke. *J. Pathol.* 132: 1–9.

Hage, E. (1973). Electron microscopic identification of several types of endocrine cells in bronchial epithelium of human foetuses. *Z. Zellforsch. Microsk. Anat.* 141: 401–412.

Hamid, Q., Azzawi, M., Ying, S., Mogbel, R., Rance, A. J., Wardlaw, A. J., Corrigan, C. J., Durham, S. R., Jeffery, P. K., and Kay, A. B. (1991). IL-5 mRNA in bronchial biopsies from asthmatic subjects. *J. Clin. Invest.* 87: 1541–1546.

Hammond, E. C. (1965). Evidence on the effects of giving up cigarette smoking. *Am. J. Public Health* 55: 682.

Hammond, E. C. (1966). Smoking in relation to the death rates of one million men and women. *Natl. Cancer Inst. Monogr.* 19: 127–204.

Harbitz, O., Jensson, A. O., and Smidsrod, O. (1980). Quantitation of proteins in sputum from patients with chronic obstructive lung disease: 1. Determination of immunoglobulin A. *Eur. J. Respir. Dis.* 61: 84–94.

Hattori, T., Helpap, B., and Gedigk, P. (1982). Regeneration of endocrine cells of the stomach. *Virchows Arch. [B]* 38: 283–290.

Hislop, A., Wigglesworth, J. S., and Desai, R. (1986). Alveolar development in the human foetus and infant. *Early Hum. Dev.* 13: 1–11.

Hogg, J. C., Macklin, P. T., and Thurlbeck, W. M. (1968). Site and nature of airway obstruction in chronic lung disease. *N. Engl. J. Med.* 278: 1355–1360.

Hook, M., Kjellan, L., Johansson, S., and Robinson, J. (1984). Cell surface glycosamino-glycans. *Annu. Rev. Biochem.* 53: 847–869.

Horsfield, K. (1981). The structure of the tracheobronchial tree. In *The Structure of the Tracheobronchial Tree*. Edited by J. G. Scadding, G. Cumming, and W. M. Thurlbeck. London, William Heinemann, pp. 54–70.

Jany, B., and Basbaum, C. B. (1991). Mucin in disease. Modification of mucin gene expression in airway disease. *Am. Rev. Respir. Dis.* 144: S38–S41.

Jeffery, P. K. (1973). Goblet cell increase in rat bronchial epithelium following irritation and drug administration: An experimental and electron microscopic study. PhD Thesis, London University.

Jeffery, P. K. (1978). The structure and function of the mucus-secreting cells of cat and goose airway epithelium. In *Respiratory Tract Mucus*. Edited by R. Porter, *Ciba Found. Symp.* 56: 5–24.

Jeffery, P. K. (1982). Bronchial mucosa and its innervation. In *Cell Biology and the Lung, Vol. 10. Ettore Majorana Life Sciences Series*. Edited by G. Cumming and G. Bonsignore. New York, Plenum Press, pp. 1–32.

Jeffery, P. K. (1983). Morphology of airway surface epithelial cells and glands. *Am. Rev. Respir. Dis.* 128: S14–S20.

Jeffery, P. K. (1986). Anti-inflammatory drugs and experimental bronchitis. *Eur. J. Dis.* 69 (Suppl 146): 245–257.

Jeffery, P. K. (1987a). The origins of secretions in the lower respiratory tract. *Eur. J. Resp. Dis.* 71: 34–42.

Jeffery, P. K. (1987b). Structure and function of adult tracheobronchial epithelium. In *Lung Carcinomas*. Edited by E. M. McDowell. London, Churchill–Livingstone, pp. 42–73.

Jeffery, P. K. (1990a). Form and function of mammalian airway epithelium. In *Advances in Cell Physiology and Cell Culture*. Edited by C. J. Jones. Lancaster, Kluwer Academic Publishers, pp. 195–220.

Jeffery, P. K. (1990b). Microscopic anatomy. In *Respiratory Medicine*. Edited by R. A. L. Brewis, G. J. Gibson, and G. M. Geddes. London/Toronto, Bailliere Tindall, pp. 57–78.

Jeffery, P. K. (1990c). Embryology and growth. In *Respiratory Medicine*. Edited by R. A. L. Brewis, G. J. Gibson, and D. M. Geddes. Toronto, Bailliere Tindall, pp. 3–20.

Jeffery, P. K. (1991). Morphology of the airway wall in asthma and chronic obstructive pulmonary disease. *Am. Rev. Respir. Dis.* 143: 1152–1158.

Jeffery, P. K., and Corrin, B. (1984). Structural analysis of the respiratory tract. In *Immunology of the Lung*. Edited by J. Bienenstock. New York, McGraw-Hill, pp. 1–27.

Jeffery, P. K., and Reid, L. (1973). Intraepithelial nerves in normal rat airways: A quantitative electron microscopic study. *J. Anat.* 114: 33–45.

Jeffery, P. K., and Reid, L. (1975). New observations of rat airway epithelium: A quantitative electron microscopic study. *J. Anat.* 120: 295–320.

Jeffery, P. K., and Reid, L. (1977a). The respiratory mucous membrane. In *Respiratory Defence Mechanisms*. Edited by J. D. Brain, D. F. Proctor, and L. Reid, New York, Marcel Dekker, pp. 193–246.

Jeffery, P. K., and Reid, L. (1977b). The ultrastructure of the airway lining and its development. In *The Development of the Lung*. Edited by W. A. Hodson. Marcel Dekker, New York, pp. 87–134.

Jeffery, P. K., and Reid, L. (1981). The effect of tobacco smoke with or without phenyl-methyloxadiazole (PMO) on rat bronchial epithelium: A light electron microscopic study. *J. Pathol.* 133: 341–359.

Jeffery, P. K., Rogers, D. F., and Ayers, M. M. (1985). Effect of oral acetylcysteine on tobacco smoke-induced secretory cell hyperplasia. *Eur. J. Respir. Dis.* 139: 117–122.

Jeffery, P. K., Brain, A. P. R., Shields, P. A., Quinn, B. P., and Betts, T. (1988). Response of laryngeal and tracheo-bronchial surface lining to inhaled cigarette smoke in normal and vitamin A-deficient rats: A scanning electron microscopic study. *Scan. Elect. Microsc.* 2: 545–552.

Jeffery, P. K., Gaillard, D., and Moret, T. (1991). Human airway secretory cells during development and in mature epithelium. *Eur. Respir. J.* 5: 93–104.

Jones, R., Bolduc, P., and Reid, L. (1972). Protection of rat bronchial epithelium against tobacco smoke. *Br. Med. J.* 2:142–144.

Jones, R., Bolduc, P., and Reid, L. (1973). Goblet cell glycoprotein and tracheal gland hypertrophy in rat airways: The effect of tobacco smoke with or without the anti-inflammatory agent phenylmethyloxadiazole. *Br. J. Exp. Pathol.* 54: 229–239.

Kollestrom, N., Lord, P. W., and Whimster, W. F. (1977). A difference in the composition of bronchial mucus between smokers and non-smokers. *Thorax* 32: 155–159.

Kramps, J. A., Franken, C., Meijer, C. J. L. M., and Dijkman, J. H. (1981). Localization of low-molecular weight protease inhibitor in serous secretory cells of the respiratory tract. *J. Histochem. Cytochem.* 29: 712–719.

Kramps, J. A., Franken, C., and Dijkman, J. H. (1984). ELISA for quantitative measurement of low-molecular-weight bronchial protease inhibitor in human sputum. *Am. Rev. Respir. Dis.* 129: 959–963.

Lamb, D. (1968). *Intracellular Development and Secretion of Mucus in the Normal and Morbid Bronchial Tree*. Ph.D. Thesis, University of London.

Lamb, D. (1990). Pathology (of asthma). In *Respiratory Medicine*. Edited by R. A. L. Brewis, G. J. Gibson, and G. M. Geddes. London, Bailliere Tindall, pp. 603–609.

Lamb, D., and Reid, L. (1969a). Histochemical types of acidic glycoprotein produced by mucous cells of the tracheobronchial glands in man. *J. Pathol.* 98: 213–229.

Lamb, D., and Reid, L. (1969b). Goblet cell increase in rat bronchial epithelium after exposure to cigarette and cigar tobacco smoke. *Br. Med. J.* 1:33–35.

Lamb, D., and Reid, L. (1970). Histochemical and autoradiographic investigation of the serous cells of the human bronchial glands. *J. Pathol.* 100: 127–138.

Lamblin, G., Aubert, J. P., Perini, J. M., Klein, A., Porchet, N., Degand, P., and Roussel, P. (1992). Human respiratory mucins. *Eur. Respir. J.* 5: 247–256.

Lauweryns, J. M., and Cokelaere, M. (1973a). Hypoxia-sensitive neuro-epithelial bodies: Intrapulmonary secretory neuro-receptors modulated by the CNS. *Z. Zellforsch. Mikrosk. Anat.* 145: 521.

Lauweryns, J. M., and Cokelaere, M. (1973b). Intrapulmonary neuroepithelial bodies hypoxia-sensitive neuro (chemo-) receptors. *Experientia* 29: 1384.

Lauweryns, J. M., Cokelaere, M., and Theunynck, P. (1972). Neuro-epithelial bodies in the respiratory mucosa of various mammals. *Z. Zellforsch. Microsc. Anat.* 135: 569–592.

Lauweryns, J. M., De Bock, V., Verhofstad, A. A. J., and Steinbusch, H. W. M. (1982). Immunohistochemical localization of serotonin in intrapulmonary neuro-epithelial bodies. *Cell Tissue Res.* 226: 215–223.

Lethen, M. I., Smedley, Y., James, S. L., Burke, J., and Marriott, C. (1987). The contribution of non-mucin components to the increased visco-elasticity of cystic fibrosis sputum. *Paediatr. Pulmonol.* 121: 52.

Lopata, M., Barton, A. D., and Lourenco, R. V. (1974). Biochemical characteristics of bronchial secretions in chronic obstructive pulmonary disease. *Am. Rev. Respir. Dis.* 110: 730–739.

Lopez-Vidriero, M. T., and Reid, L. (1978). Chemical markers of mucus and glycosamino-glycans and their relation to viscosity in mucoid and purulent sputum from various hypersecretory diseases. *Am. Rev. Respir. Dis.* 117: 465–477.

Lopez-Vidriero, M. T., and Reid, L. (1985). Bronchial mucus in asthma. In *Bronchial Asthma: Mechanisms and Therapeutics*. Edited by E. B. Weiss, M. S. Segal, and M. Stein. Boston, Little, Brown & Company, pp. 218–235.

Lopez-Vidriero, M. T., and Reid, L. M. (1983). Pathological changes in asthma. In *Asthma*. Edited by T. J. H. Clark and S. Godfrey. London, Chapman & Hall, pp. 79–98.

Lopez-Vidriero, M. T., Das, I., and Reid, L. M. (1977). Airway secretion: Source, biochemical and rheological properties. In *Respiratory Defence Mechanisms*. Edited by J. D. Brain, A. F. Proctor, and L. M. Reid. New York, Marcel Dekker, pp. 289–356.

Lucas, A. M., and Douglas, L. C. (1934). Principles underlying ciliary activity in the respiratory tract. II. Mucous clearance in man, monkey and other mammals. *Arch. Otolaryngol.* 20: 518.

Lumsden, A. B., McLean, A., and Lamb, D. (1984). Goblet and Clara cells of human distal airways: Evidence for smoking-induced changes in numbers. *Thorax* 39: 844–853.

Macklem, P. T., Proctor, D. F., and Hogg, J. C. (1970). The stability of peripheral airways. *Respir. Physiol.* 8: 191–203.

Macklin, C. C. (1949). The two types of epithelium of the finest bronchioles of the albino mouse as revealed by supravital silverization. *Can. J. Res.* 27: 50–58.

Maniatis, T., Goodbourn, S., and Fischer, J. A. (1987). Regulation of inducible and tissue-specific gene expression. *Science* 236: 1237–1245.

Mason, D. Y., and Sammons, R. (1978). Alkaline phosphotase and peroxidase for double immunoenzymatic labelling of cellular constituents. *J. Clin. Pathol.* 31: 454–460.

Matsuba, K., and Thurlbeck, W. M. (1972). A morphometric study of bronchial and bronchiolar walls in children. *Am. Rev. Respir. Dis.* 105: 908.

Mazzuca, M., Roche, A. C., Lhermitte, M., and Roussel, P. (1977). *Limulus polyphemus* lectin sites in human bronchial mucosa. *J. Histochem. Cytochem.* 25: 470–473.

Mazzuca, M., Lhermitte, M., Lafitte, J. J., and Roussel, P. (1982). Use of lectins for detection of glycoconjugates in the glandular cells of the human bronchial mucosa. *J. Histochem. Cytochem.* 36: 337–348.

McDowell, E. M., and Trump, B. F. (1983). Conceptual review: Histogenesis of preneo-plastic and neoplastic lesions in tracheobronchial epithelium. *Surv. Synth. Pathol. Res.* 2: 235–279.

McDowell, E. M., Barratt, L. A., Harris, C. C., and Trump, B. F. (1978a). The respiratory epithelium I: Human bronchus. *JNCI* 61: 539–549.

McDowell, E. M., Becci, P. J., Barrett, L. A., and Trump, C. F. (1978b). Morphogenesis and classification of lung cancer. In *Pathogenesis and Therapy of Lung Cancer*. Edited by C. C. Harris. New York, Marcel Dekker, pp. 445–519.

McDowell, E. M., Keenan, K. P., and Huang, M. (1984). Restoration of mucociliary tracheal epithelium following deprivation of vitamin A: A quantitative morphologic study. *Virchows Arch. [B]* 45: 221–240.

McDowell, E. M., Newkirk, C., and Coleman, B. (1985). Development of hamster tracheal epithelium. I. Quantitative morphologic study in the fetus. II. Cell proliferation in fetus. *Anat. Rec.* 213: 429–456.

McDowell, E. M., Ben, T., Carnell Newkirk, T. B., Chang, S., and De Luca, L. M. (1987). Differentiation of tracheal mucociliary epithelium in primary cell culture recapitulates normal fetal development and regeneration following injury in hamster. *Am. J. Pathol.* 129: 511–522.

Meban, C. (1984). The surface coating of the pneumonocytes in human neonatal lung. *J. Anat.* 139: 371–385.

Medical Research Council (1965). Definition and classification of chronic bronchitis for clinical and epidemiological purposes. A report to the Medical Research Council by their committee on the etiology of chronic bronchitis. *Lancet* 1: 775–780.

Meyer, C., Christner, A., Linss, W., Quade, R., and Geyer, G. (1971). Ultrahistochemical demonstration of the glycocalyx on the surface of tracheal epithelium by means of the colloidal iron method. *Acta Histochem.* 39: 176–178.

Meyrick, B., Sturgess, J., and Reid, L. (1969). Reconstruction of the duct system and secretory tubules of the human bronchial submucosal gland. *Thorax* 24: 729–739.

Meyrick, B., and Reid, L. (1970). Ultrastructure of cells in the human bronchial submucosal glands. *J. Anat.* 107: 201.

Meyrick, B., and Reid, L. (1975). In vitro incorporation of (^{3}H) threonine and (^{3}H) glucose by the mucous and serous cells of the human bronchial submucosal gland: A quantitative electron microscope study. *J. Cell Biol.* 67: 320.

Miller, W. S. (1932). The epithelium of the lower respiratory tract. In *Special Cytology*. Edited by E. V. Cowdry. New York, Hafner, pp. 133–150.

Minty, A. D., Royston, D., Jones, J. G., and Hulands, G. H. (1981). Rapid improvement in abnormal pulmonary epithelial permeability after stopping cigarettes. *Br. Med. J.* 282: 1183–1186.

Misokovitch, G., Appel, J., and Szule, J. (1974). Ultrastructural changes of ciliated columnar epithelium and goblet cells in chronic bronchitis biopsy material. *Acta Morphol. (Hung.)* 22: 91–103.

Mitchell, P., and Tijian, R. (1989). Transcriptional regulation in mammalian cells by sequence-specific DNA binding proteins. *Science* 245: 371–378.

Mitchell, R. F., Stanford, R. E., Johnson, J. M., Silvers, G. W., Dart, G., and George, M. S. (1976). The morphologic features of the bronchi, bronchioles and alveoli in chronic airway obstruction: A clinicopathologic study. *Am. Rev. Respir. Dis.* 114: 137–145.

Mochizuki, I., Setser, M. E., Martinez, J. R., and Spicer, S. S. (1982). Carbohydrate histochemistry of rat respiratory glands. *Anat. Rec.* 202: 45–59.

Mooren, H. W. D., Kramps, J. A., Franken, C., Meijer, C. J. L. M., and Dijkman, J. A. (1983). Localisation of a low-molecular weight bronchial protease inhibitor in the peripheral human lung. *Thorax* 38: 180–183.

Moosavi, H., Smith, P., and Heath, D. (1973). The Feyrter cell in hypoxia. *Thorax* 28: 729–741.

Mullen, J. B. M., Wright, J. L., Wiggs, B. R., Pare, P. D., and Hogg, J. C. (1987). Structure of central airways in current smokers and ex-smokers with and without mucus hypersecretion. *Thorax* 42: 843–846.

Nemery, B., Moavero, N. E., Brasseur, L., and Stanescu, D. C. (1981). Significance of small airways test in middle-aged smokers. *Am. Rev. Respir. Dis.* 124: 232–238.

Neutra, M. R., and Schaeffer, S. F. (1977). Membrane interactions between adjacent mucous secretion granules. *J. Cell Biol.* 74: 983–991.

Niewoehner, D. E., Klienerman, J., and Rice, D. (1974). Pathologic changes in the peripheral airways of young cigarette smokers. *N. Engl. J. Med.* 291: 755–758.

Oppenheimer, E. H. (1981). Similarity of the tracheobronchial mucous glands and epithelium in infants with and without cystic fibrosis. *Hum. Pathol.* 12: 36–48.

Peterson, D. I., Lonergan, L. H., and Hardinge, M. G. (1968). Smoking and pulmonary function. *Arch. Environ. Health* 16: 215–218.

Peto, R., Speitzer, F. E., Cochrane, A. L., Moore, F., Fletcher, C. M., Tinker, C. M., Higgins, I. T. T., Gray, R. G., Richards, S. M., Gilliland, J., and Norman-Smith, B. (1983). The relevance in adults of airflow obstruction, but not of mucus hypersecretion, to mortality from chronic lung disease. *Am. Rev. Respir. Dis.* 128: 491–500.

Plopper, C. G. (1983). Comparative morphologic features of bronchiolar epithelial cells. *Am. Rev. Respir. Dis.* 128: S37–S41.

Plopper, C. G., Mariassy, A. T., and Hill, L. H. (1980). Ultra-structure of the non-ciliated bronchiolar epithelial (Clara) cell of mammalian lung. III. A study of man with comparison with 15 mammalian species. *Exp. Lung Res.* 1: 171–180.

Plopper, C. G., Alley, J. L., and Weir, A. J. (1986). Differentiation of tracheal epithelium during fetal lung maturations in the rhesus monkey *Macaca mulatta*. *Am. J. Anat.* 175: 59–71.

Plopper, C. G., St. George, J., Pinkerton, K. E., Tyler, N., Mariassy, A., Wilson, D., Wu, R., Hyde, D. M., and Evans, M. J. (1990). Tracheobronchial epithelium in vivo: Composition, differentiation and response to hormones. In *Respiratory Epithelium*. Edited by D. G. Thomassen and P. Netteshiem. New York, Hemisphere Publishing, pp. 6–23.

Plotowski, M. C., Girod-Vaquez, S., Hinnrasky, J., Fuchey, C., Ploton, D., and Puchelle, E. (1990). Ultrastructural comparative distribution of carbohydrates in human tracheal and frog palate mucosa using neuraminidase and lectin–colloidal gold complexes. *J. Submicrosc. Cytol. Pathol.* 22: 79–90.

Popoff, N. W. (1939). Epithelial functional rejuvenation observed in the mucous cells of the gastro-intestinal tract and the parietal cells of the stomach. *Arch. Pathol.* 27: 841–887.

Postek, M. T., Howard, K. S., Johnson, A. H., and McMichael, K. L. (1980). *Scanning Electron Microscopy. A Student's Handbook*. Ladd Research Industries.

Read, R. C., Wilson, R., Rutman, A., Lund, V., Todd, H. C., Brain, A. P. R., Jeffery, P. K., and Cole, P. J. (1991). Interaction of nontypable *Haemophilus influenzae* with human respiratory mucosa in vitro. *J. Infect. Dis.* 163: 549–558.

Reid, L. (1954). Pathology of chronic bronchitis. *Lancet* 1: 275–279.

Reid, L. (1983). Experimental bronchitis. *Int. Rev. Exp. Pathol.* 24: 335–382.

Reid, L. M. (1987). The presence or absence of bronchial mucus in fatal asthma. *J. Allergy Clin. Immunol.* 80: 415–416.

Reid, L., and Jones, R. (1979). Bronchial mucosal cells. *Fed. Proc.* 38: 191–196.

Reynolds, H Y. (1987). Bronchoalveolar lavage. *Am. Rev. Respir. Dis.* 135: 250–263.

Rhodin, J. (1966). Ultrastructure and function of the human tracheal mucosa. *Am. Rev. Respir. Dis.* 93: 1.

Rhodin, J., and Dalhamn, T. (1956). Electron microscopy of the tracheal ciliated mucosa in rat. *Z. Zellforsch.* 44: 345–412.

Riordan, J. R., Rommens, J. M., Kerem, B.-S., Alon, N., Rozmahel, R., Grzelczak, Z., Zielenski, J., Lok, S., Plavic, N., Chou, J.-L., Drumm, M. L., Iannuzzi, M. C., Collins, F. S., and Tsui, L.-C. (1989). Identification of the cystic fibrosis gene: Cloning and characterisation of complementary DNA. *Science* 245: 1066–1072.

Robards, A. W., and Sleytr, U. B. (1985). *Low Temperature Methods in Biological Electron Microscopy*, Vol. 10. Oxford, Elsevier.

Rogers, A. V., Dewar, A., Corrin, B., and Jeffery, P. K. (1993). Identification of serous-like cells in the surface epithelium of human bronchioles. *Eur. Respir. J.* 6 (in press).

Rogers, D. F., and Jeffery, P. K. (1986a). Inhibition of cigarette smoke-induced airway secretory cell hyperplasia by indomethacin, dexamethasone, prednisolone or hydrocortisone in the rat. *Exp. Lung Res.* 10: 285–298.

Rogers, D. F., and Jeffery, P. K. (1986b). Inhibition by oral *N*-acetylcysteine of cigarette smoke-induced "bronchitis" in the rat. *Exp. Lung Res.* 10: 267–283.

Rogers, D. F., Williams, D. A., and Jeffery, P. K. (1986). Nicotine does not cause "bronchitis" in the rat. *Clin. Sci.* 70: 427–433.

Rogers, D. F., Godfrey, R. W. A., Majumdar, S., and Jeffery, P. K. (1987a). Oral *N*-acetylcysteine speeds reversal of cigarette smoke-induced mucous cell hyperplasia in the rat. *Exp. Lung Res.* 14: 19–35.

Rogers, D. F., Turner, N. C., Marriott, C., and Jeffery, P. K. (1987b). Cigarette smoke-induced "chronic bronchitis": A study in situ of laryngo-tracheal hypersecretion in the rat. *Clin. Sci.* 72: 629–637.

Rogers, D. F., Turner, N. C., Marriott, C., and Jeffery, P. K. (1989). Oral *N*-acetylcysteine or *S*-carboxymethylcysteine inhibit cigarette smoke-induced hypersecretion of mucus in rat larynx and trachea in situ. *Eur. Respir. J.* 2: 955–960.

Rosan, R. C., and Lauweryns, J. M. (1972). Mucosal cells of the small bronchioles of prematurely born human infants. *Beitr. Pathol.* 147: 145–174.

Schofield, G. (1953). The argentaffin and mucous cells of the small and large intestines of the mouse. *Acta Anat.* 18: 256–272.

Schraufnagel, D. E. (1990). *Electron Microscopy of the Lung*. New York, Marcel Dekker.

Schulte, B. A., and Spicer, S. S. (1983). Light microscopic histochemical detection of sugar residues in secretory glycoproteins of rodent and human tracheal glands with lectin–horseradish peroxidase conjugates and the galactose oxidase–Schiff sequence. *J. Histochem. Cytochem.* 31: 391–403.

Schulze, F. E. (1972). The lungs. I. The lungs of mammals. In *Human and Comparative Histology*. Edited by S. Stricker. London, New Sydenham Society, pp. 49–68.

Sharpey, W. (1836). Cilia. In *The Cyclopaedia of Anatomy and Physiology*, Vol. 1. Edited by R. B. Todd. London, Sherwood, Gilbert & Piper, pp. 606–638.

Sheppard, M. N., Kurian, S. S., Henzen-Logmans, S. C., Michetti, F., Cocchia, D., Cole, P., Rush, R. A., Marangos, P. J., Bloom, S. R., and Polak, J. M. (1983). Neurone-specific enolase and S-100: New markers for delineating the innervation of the respiratory tract in man and other mammals. *Thorax* 38: 333–340.

Sherman, J. M., Cheng, P., Tandler, B., and Boat, T. F. (1981). Mucous glycoproteins from cat tracheal goblet cells and mucous glands separated with EDTA. *Am. Rev. Respir. Dis.* 124: 476–479.

Shields, P. A., and Jeffery, P. K. (1987). The combined effects of vitamin A deficiency and cigarette smoke on rat tracheal epithelium. *Br. J. Exp. Pathol.* 68: 705–717.

Spicer, S. S., Charkin, L. W., Wardel, J. R., and Kendrick, W. (1971). Histochemistry of mucosubstances in the canine and human respiratory tract. *Lab. Invest.* 25: 483–490.

Spicer, S. S., Mochizuki, I., Setser, M. E., et al. (1980a). Complex carbohydrates of rat tracheo-bronchial surface epithelium visualized ultrastructurally. *Am. J. Anat.* 158: 93.

Spicer, S. S., Mochizuki, I., Setser, M. E., and Martinez, J. R. (1980b). Complex carbohydrates of rat tracheobronchial surface epithelium visualized ultrastructurally. *Am. J. Anat.* 158: 93–109.

Spicer, S. S., Sens, M. A., and Tashian, R. E. (1982). Immunocytochemical chemical demonstration of carbonic anhydrase in human epithelial cells. *J. Histochem. Cytochem.* 30: 864–873.

Spicer, S. S., Schulte, B. A., and Chakrin, L. W. (1983a). Ultra-structural and histochemical observations of respiratory epithelium and gland. *Lung Res.* 4: 137–156.

Spicer, S. S., Schulte, B. A., and Thomopoulos, G. N. (1983b). Histochemical properties of the respiratory tract epithelium in different species. *Am. Rev. Respir. Dis.* 128: S20–S26.

St. George, J. A., Cranz, D. L., Zicker, S. C., Etchison, J. R., Dungworth, O. L., and Plopper, C. G. (1985). An immunohistochemical characterization of rhesus monkey respiratory secretions using monoclonal antibodies. *Am. Rev. Respir. Dis.* 132: 556–563.

Stahl, G. H., and Ellis, D. B. (1973). Biosynthesis of respiratory tract mucins: A comparison of canine goblet-cell and submucosal-gland secretions. *Biochem. J.* 136: 845–850.

Stanley, P. J., Wilson, R., Greenstone, M. A., MacWilliam, L., and Cole, P. J. (1986). Effect of cigarette smoking on nasal mucociliary clearance and ciliary beat frequency. *Thorax* 41: 519–523.

Sturgess, J., and Reid, L. (1972). An organ culture study of the effects of drugs on the secretory activity of the human bronchial submucosal gland. *Clin. Sci.* 43: 533–543.

Sykes, D. A., Wilson, R., Watson, D., Taylor, G., MacDermot, J., and Cole, P. J. (1986). *Pseudomonas aeruginosa* phenazine pigments in the sputum in chronic bronchial sepsis (CBS) inhibit human ciliary beat frequency in vitro. *Thorax* 41: 729.

Terzakis, J. A., Sommers, S. C., and Anderson, B. (1973). Neuro-secretory appearing cells of human segmental bronchi. *Lab. Invest.* 26: 127–132.

Thurlbeck, W. M., Benjamin, B., and Reid, L. M. (1961). Development and distribution of mucous glands in the fetal human trachea. *Br. J. Dis. Chest* 55: 54–64.

Thurlbeck, W. M., Fletcher, C. M., and Pride, M. B. (1984). Definitions of emphysema, chronic bronchitis, asthma and airflow obstruction: 25 years on from the Ciba symposium. *Thorax* 39: 81–85.

Toremalm, N. H. (1960). The daily amount of tracheobronchial secretions in man: A method for continuous tracheal aspiration in laryngectomized and tracheostimized patients. *Acta Otolaryngol.* 158: 43–53.

Tos, M. (1966). Development of the tracheal glands in man. *Acta Pathol. Microbiol. Scand.* 185: 1–130.

Tos, M. (1968). Development of the mucous glands in the human main bronchus. *Anat. Anz.* 123: 376–389.

Track, N. S., and Cutz, E. (1982). Bombesin-like immunoreactivity in developing human lung. *Life Sci.* 30: 1553–1556.

Van Brabandt, H., Cauberghs, M., Verbeken, E., Moerman, P. H., Lauweryns, J. M., and Van de Woestijne, K. P. (1983). Partitioning of pulmonary impedance in excised human and canine lungs. *J. Appl. Physiol. Respir. Environ. Exer. Physiol.* 55: 1733–1742.

Van Scott, M. R., Hester, S., and Boucher, R. C. (1987). Ion transport by rabbit nonciliated bronchiolar epithelial cells (Clara cells) in culture. *Proc. Natl. Acad. Sci.* 84: 5496–5500.

Verdugo, P. (1990). Goblet-cells secretion and mucogenesis. *Annu. Rev. Physiol.* 52: 157–176.

Vishwanath, S., and Ramphal, R. (1984). Adherence of *Pseudomonas aeruginosa* to human tracheobronchial mucin. *Infect. Immun.* 85: 197–202.

Von Hayek, H. (1962). Cellular structure and mucus activity in the bronchial tree and alveoli. In *Pulmonary Structure and Function. Ciba Foundation Symposium.* Edited by A. V. S. de Reuck and M. O'Connor. London, Churchill, pp. 99–102.

Wanner, A. (1977). Clinical aspects of muco-ciliary transport. *Am. Rev. Respir. Dis.* 116: 73–125.

Wharton, J., Polak, J. M., Bloom, S. R., et al. (1978). Bombesin-like immunoreactivity in the lung. *Nature* 273: 769–770.

Widdicombe, J. G., and Pack, R. J. (1982). The Clara cell. *Eur. J. Respir. Dis.* 63: 202–220.

Wilhelmsen, L. (1967). Effects on bronchopulmonary system, ventilation, and lung mechanics of abstinence from tobacco smoking. *Scand. J. Respir. Dis.* 48: 407–414.

Willems, L. N. A., Kramps, J. A., Jeffery, P. K., and Dijkman, J. A. (1988). Antileucoprotease in the developing fetal lung. *Thorax* 43: 784–786.

Wilson, R. (1988). Secondary ciliary dysfunction. *Clin. Sci.* 75: 113–120.

Wright, R. R., and Stuart, C. M. (1965). Chronic bronchitis with emphysema: A pathological study of the bronchi. *Med. Thorac.* 22: 210.

Yager, J. A., Ellmann, H., and Dulfano, M. J. (1980). Human ciliary beat frequency at three levels of the tracheobronchial tree. *Am. Rev. Respir. Dis.* 121: 661–665.

Zhang X.-M., McDowell, E. M. (1992). Vitamin A deficiency and inflammation: The pivotal role of secretory cells in the development of atrophic, hyperplastic and metaplastic change in the tracheal epithelium in vivo. *Virchows Arch. [B]* 61: 375–387.

6

Biochemistry of Mucus

THOMAS F. BOAT

University of Cincinnati School of Medicine
Cincinnati, Ohio

**PI-WAN CHENG and
MARGARET WARREN LEIGH**

University of North Carolina School
of Medicine
Chapel Hill, North Carolina

I. Introduction

Airway mucus is a biochemically complex liquid that is capable of forming gels (1). Its complexity reflects that it is a mixture of products from several sources: (1) alveolar liquid, (2) secretory products from a variety of cells along the surface of conducting airways, (3) submucosal gland secretory cell products, and (4) serum transudate. Epithelial cell turnover may also contribute membrane and cytoplasmic components to these secretions. The variable composition of airway mucus also reflects developmental differences in the types and properties of secretory products and variation in secretory cell populations and their products induced by airway stimulation or injury. To further complicate biochemical analyses of these secretions, substantial species differences have been observed. A lack of universally adopted criteria for defining the various glycoconjugate components also has created confusion and has hampered progress in this field. This chapter will describe major components in airway secretions, placing particular emphasis on the high relative molecular mass (M_r) glycoconjugates that appear to play an important role in determining the physical properties of mucus. Considerable attention will be given to methods for collecting, purifying, and analyzing these important secretory products.

II. Hypothesis

High M_r glycoconjugates are complex polyanionic substances that display extensive molecular heterogeneity. They play important roles in establishing the functional properties of airway mucus, including gel formation, clearance of particles deposited on the airway's surface, and protection of underlying epithelial cells. Properties of these glycoconjugates and the mucus in which they reside are determined by their composition and structure, by water content of the mucus, and by interactions with other components present in mucus.

III. Methods

Considerable uncertainty and confusion in the literature has arisen because biochemical studies have been performed on secretions that were gathered by diverse methods, solubilized by a variety of approaches, and fractionated using several different schemes. In most instances, recoveries of major components have not been rigorously documented, and reports are notable as much for what is not analyzed as for what is analyzed and reported. Analyses of high M_r glycoconjugates are, at best, difficult because there is no simple biochemical definition for the specific glycoconjugate components, chiefly because these substances display considerable microheterogeneity. Therefore, adoption of rigorous approaches to analytical biochemistry will be particularly important for additional advances in this area.

A. Collection

Samples of human airway mucus are easily acquired by collecting sputum (Table 1). By definition, sputum production represents a pathological state and, at a minimum, equates with hypersecretion of mucus. Most sputum is an outcome of airways inflammation; inflammation has considerable potential for changing the amounts and distribution of secretory products released, for altering secretory products after release, and for contributing exogenous components to the surface liquids in airways. Sputum also contains variable amounts of saliva. Airway mucus has been characterized by inspection as mucoid (clear) or purulent (opaque), purulent mucus being considered a product of inflamed airways (2). Purulence does not distinguish between infected and noninfected, but inflamed, airways. For example, uninfected mucus from asthmatic subjects may be mucoid or purulent. More precise methods for assessing the inflammatory state of the airways include measurements of lactate dehydrogenase, γ-glutamyltranspeptidase, and DNA in sputum (3,4). These measures reflect cell breakdown and serve to standardize comparisons of sputum from different sources. However, they do not obviate all inflammation-introduced biochemical variables. Alternative collection

Table 1 Approaches to Collection of Airway Secretions

A. In vivo
1. Sputum
    Spontaneous
    Induced (hypertonic saline, $PGF_{2\alpha}$)
2. Expectoration by tracheostomy
3. Aspiration by tracheostomy or endotracheal tube
4. Bronchoscopy
    Aspiration
    Lavage
    Brush
    Filter paper pledgets
5. Perfusion of isolated intact tracheal segments (laboratory animals)
6. Tracheal pouch (laboratory animals)

B. In vitro
1. Tracheal or bronchial explants
    Full thickness
    Mucosal
    Surface epithelium
    Glands
2. Primary cell cultures
    Outgrowth from explants
    Surface epithelial cells
    Gland cells
3. Transformed surface epithelial cell cutures

measures include the induction of sputum by aerosolization of hypertonic saline or by substances such as prostaglandin (PG)$F_{2\alpha}$ (5). These methods are useful in that they avoid inflammatory contributions to mucous content, but much smaller amounts are collected, and the secretions induced are likely to differ in composition from unstimulated native mucus.

Matthews and colleagues collected secretions from laryngectomized subjects for extensive analytical studies (6) and, more recently, secretions from tracheotomized or intubated patients have been assessed (7). The presence of an artificial airway is, in itself, a stimulus to secretion, as is inspiration of incompletely humidified air that is unavoidable for tracheotomized subjects. Many individuals hypersecrete for weeks or months after tracheostomy. This information must be factored into the interpretation of analysis of secretions from these sources.

With the advent of fiber-optic bronchoscopy and bronchoalveolar lavage (BAL), access to airway secretions has improved. Although precise concentrations of mucous components in BAL cannot be determined directly, these techniques facilitate sampling of normal, as well as diseased, airway secretion components. However, the distribution of secretory components collected may be altered by direct or reflex influences on secretory cells induced by airway instrumentation, saline instillation, or pharmacological agents employed in the course of the procedure, such as local anesthetics or cholinergic antagonists (e.g., atropine). Recently, urea dilution has been used to estimate the volume of surface secretions recovered by BAL and to calculate the concentration of specific components in airway mucus (8). Care must be exercised to limit or account for urea diffusion across the epithelium during the time that lavage fluid dwells in the airways (9). Bronchoalveolar lavage can be used primarily to sample conducting airway secretions by instilling small volumes, but some sampling of alveolar lining fluid probably occurs, even with limited lavage techniques (10). Direct aspiration of secretions (mucus) in hypersecretory states can also be accomplished by fiber-optic bronchoscopy. King et al. have introduced a brush (11), and Boucher et al. have placed filter paper pledgets on tracheal or bronchial surfaces (12) through a bronchoscope to collect surface liquids from healthy airways. The small amounts of secretions collected by these techniques allow only limited analysis.

Isolated intact tracheal segments have permitted the recovery of airway mucus in a controlled fashion from laboratory animals. The dog tracheal pouch (13) facilitates recovery of relatively large amounts of mucus, but retention for days in the pouch lumen introduces opportunity for postsecretion modification (e.g., by proteolytic enzymes). Perfused cat tracheas (14) have been used extensively and offer several experimental advantages for studies of modulation of secretory component release.

In vitro techniques also have been very important for collection of mucous components released by airway epithelial tissues from humans and a range of animals. Initial efforts used organ culture of conducting airway tissues, particularly trachea (15–18). These methods have the advantage that the inflammatory response and its effects on secretion can be excluded. In vitro systems have also been very useful for assessing macromolecular secretory responses to putative agonists and antagonists. Potential disadvantages include release of secretory products from nonepithelial cells (e.g., proteoglycans from connective tissue or cartilage cells), which can be mistaken for mucin-type glycoprotein or proteoglycan secretory products of epithelial cells. This obstacle can be overcome by culturing sheets of surface epithelium, separated from the lamina propria by chelating agents (19,20), or by epithelial cell culture (21). Secretory products from primary cultured cells vary extensively as a function of substratum or medium supplements (22). Transformed cells in culture may not generate a secretory cell phenotype (23). Glands, microdissected from surrounding connective tissue, also have served as sources of secretory tissue in organ culture (24).

An extensive literature has been compiled on analyses of macromolecules secreted into culture medium by tracheal or nasal epithelial cells in primary culture systems. When grown on plastic surfaces, these cells reach confluence and secrete glycosaminoglycan components, but little or no mucin-type glycoproteins. If grown on collagen substrata and supplied with certain hormones and nutritional supplements, nontransformed tracheal cells from human (25) and several laboratory animals (26–28) are capable of releasing at least small amounts of mucin-type glycoproteins into bathing medium. Transformed human airway epithelial cells (BEAS) secrete high M_r glycoconjugates but no detectable mucin (29).

B. Solubilization

Native mucous gels are not amenable to the usual biochemical fractionation procedures; the gel structure must be broken down before further processing is carried out. High-speed centrifugation compacts the gel and releases much of the water and the soluble components (30). It is unlikely that this method cleanly separates soluble and gel matrix components. Homogenization, ultrasound, or proteinase treatments disperse, but do not completely solubilize, secretions, and are likely to fragment large (high M_r) proteins and glycoproteins (31). DNase treatment of purulent airway mucus degrades one component contributing to the mucous gel and is a useful adjunct to solubilization procedures aimed at recovery of high M_r glycoconjugates (32). Dilution with water and mechanical agitation have been employed to solubilize mucus from the airways of individuals with asthma (33). Reducing agents, such as 2-mercaptoethanol or dithiothreitol, have been used successfully, often in the presence of 6–8 M urea, to disrupt gel structure (32). Prolonged incubation with reducing agents, especially at room temperature or above, may induce proteolytic enzyme activities (34) and foster cleavage of protein or glycoprotein components. Therefore, reduction in the cold and in the presence of concentrated urea or guanidine hydrochloride is preferred. Treatment with these agents can be followed by carboxymethylation of sulhydryl groups [e.g., with iodoacetamide (32)] to prevent re-formation of disulfide bonds. Mucous gels can also be dispersed with chaotropic agents, such as KSCN (35), before chromatographic fractionation. Choice of the solubilization method is dependent on the analytical goals of the study. For example, if the M_r of native mucins is to be measured, reduction and carboxymethylation or proteinase treatment would not be desirable.

C. Fractionation

Dialysis was perhaps the first fractionation step introduced for airway secretions. Although cumbersome, it does effectively remove unbound low M_r components. Gel filtration chromatography has become the initial fractionation step for most analytical efforts with airway mucus (32). Porous gels are used to separate high M_r glycoconjugates in the void or near void volume fractions from smaller compo-

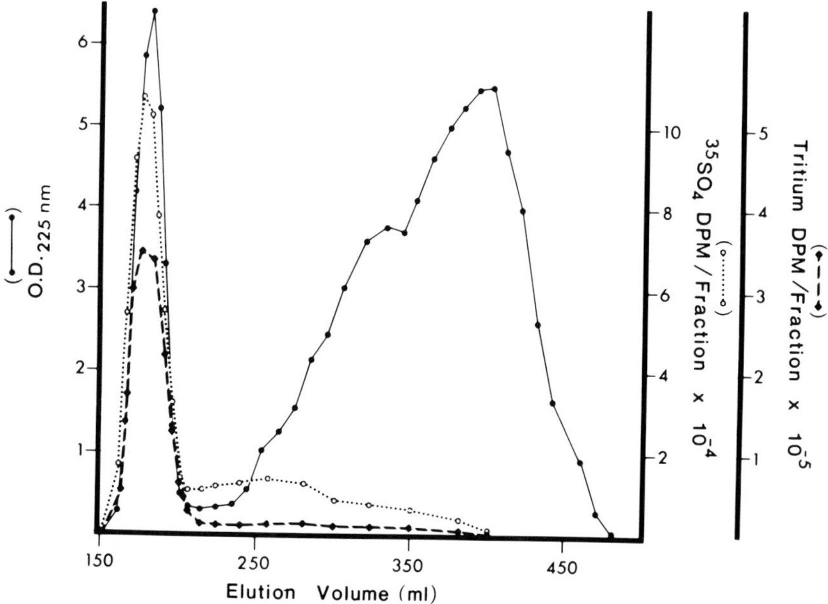

Figure 1 Gel permeation chromatography of reduced and carboxymethylated rabbit tracheal explant secretions on Bio Gel A-5m. Explants were incubated for 24 h in medium 199 containing [^{35}S]sulfate and D-[6-^{3}H]glucosamine. Secretions were collected by harvesting bathing medium followed by reduction, carboxymethylation, and concentration. The column was 2.5×80 cm and was eluted with 0.1 M NaCl, 10 mM Tris-HCl (pH 7.0); $V_0 = $ 175 ml. Recovery of counts applied to the column exceeded 90%. Note that most radiolabeled macromolecules (glycoconjugates) are eluted in the near-void volume fractions.

nents that are retained on these columns (Fig. 1). Mucin and proteoglycan-type glycoconjugates can be separated by density gradient centrifugation (25,27,36). In general, mucins sediment at a density of 1.40–1.60 g/ml and proteoglycans at a density greater than 1.60 g/ml (Fig. 2). High M_r fractions can be further analyzed on the basis of charge by ion-exchange chromatography (Fig. 3). This method is useful, for example, for isolating highly sulfated glycoconjugates, but has the disadvantage of relatively poor yields (32). Absorption to hydroxylapatite also has been employed for purification of tracheobronchial mucins (37). Affinity chromatography using immobilized lectins or antibodies has not been widely applicable, largely because the numbers and types of carbohydrate-binding sites vary from one molecule to the next. Because of extensive microheterogeneity, gel electrophoresis also has limited usefulness for purification of high M_r glycoconjugates or for analytical efforts. Loosely cross-linked acrylamide (3.3%), agarose (1%), or

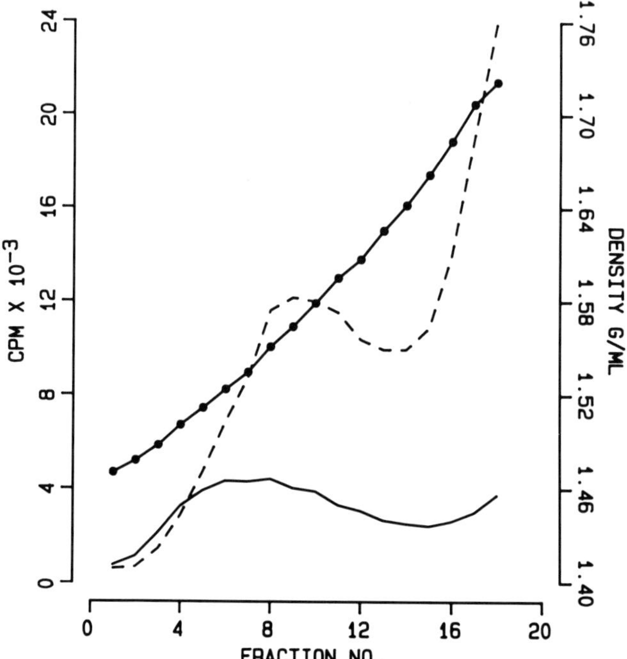

Figure 2 Density-gradient centrifugation of radiolabeled glycoconjugates released by 28-day-old ferret tracheal explants. Explants were incubated for 6 days in 199 medium containing antimicrobials, D-[6-^{3}H]glucosamine and [^{35}S]sulfate. Secretions were harvested daily, pooled, and fractionated on Sepharose CL-6B. Near-void volume fractions were concentrated over a Diaflo membrane, and cesium chloride was added to attain a starting density of 1.58 g/ml. Samples were centrifuged at 130,000 g and 5°C for 40 h. Fractions were removed sequentially from the top of each tube with a Densiflow pump and the density of each fraction determined from the refractive index: ^{3}H counts (——), ^{35}S counts (––––), and buoyant density (●) are shown for each fraction. Fractions through number 11 (density ≤ 1.60) were mucin-containing; those with higher densities contained material with properties of proteoglycans.

combination agarose–acrylamide gels provide the most useful electrophoresis medium (32,38), but glycoconjugates migrate as broad bands (Fig. 4).

Isolation of airway mucous components also has suffered from a lack of definitive and facile assays for the glycoconjugate components. Assay systems based on highly specific lectins or antibodies to defined components is obviously desirable, and some progress toward this goal has been achieved. This problem will be addressed in depth in Section V of this chapter.

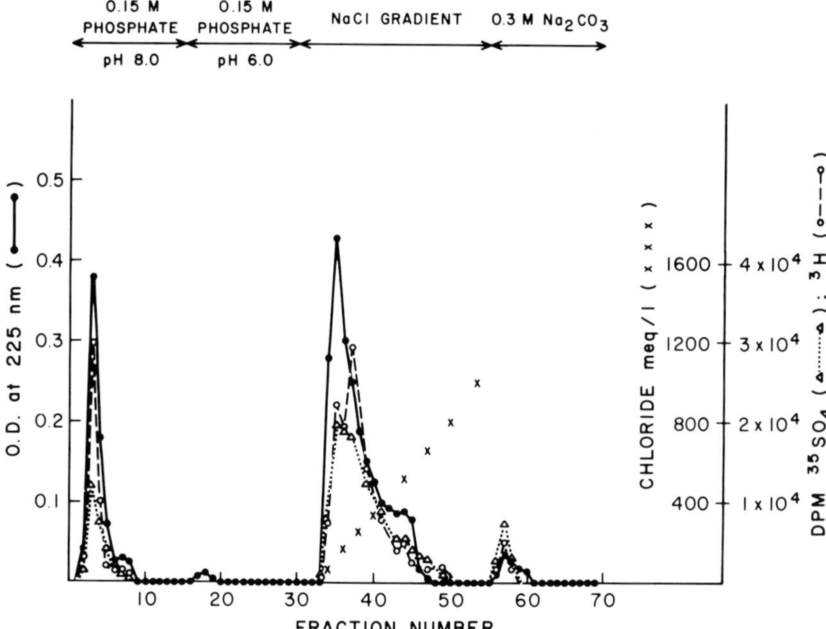

Figure 3 Fractionation of radiolabeled, reduced, and carboxymethylated glycoconjugates secreted by human tracheal explants on DEAE cellulose. Near-void volume material from Bio Gel A-5m chromatography was loaded onto the ion-exchange column in 0.005 M phosphate buffer (pH 8.0) and eluted sequentially with 0.15 M phosphate (pH 8.0), 0.15 M phosphate (pH 6.0), a 0–1 M NaCl gradient, and 0.3 M Na_2CO_3. Three major fractions were recovered, characterized by increasingly greater ratios of $^{35}S/[^3H]$.

IV. Composition

A. General

Airway surface liquid is a complex secretory product that is thought to have an aqueous or periciliary phase and a mucous gel phase. The relations between these phases remain vague, largely because it has not been technically possible to recover aqueous-phase secretions alone in amounts that permit quantitative analyses.

Expectorated human airway mucus contains approximately 95% water and 5% solids, whether from otherwise healthy laryngectomized subjects or from patients with chronic bronchitis (6). The water content of airway surface liquids from entirely healthy human subjects and healthy animals has not been reported. The solids content of expectorated human airway mucus includes 2–3% proteins and glycoproteins, 1% lipids, and 1% minerals (6). Secretions collected from

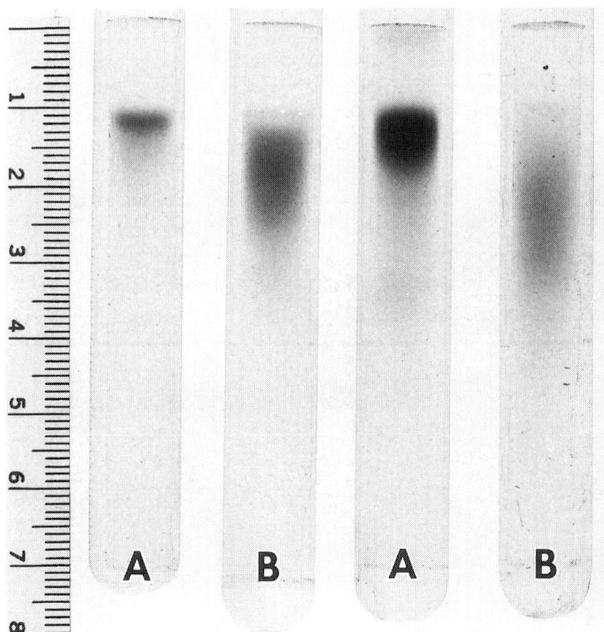

Figure 4 Polyacrylamide gel (3.3%) electrophoresis of mucins purified from sputum of two patients with cystic fibrosis. Samples from two subjects were purified by Bio Gel A-5m chromatography (see Fig. 1) to obtain a high M_r fraction and were fractionated further by DEAE cellulose chromatography (see Fig. 3) to obtain (A) sparsely sulfated (eluant: 0.15 M phosphate, pH 8.0) and (B) highly sulfated (eluant: NaCl) fractions. Highly sulfated mucin has greater electrophoretic mobility and displays greater polydispersity than its less-sulfated counterpart.

healthy dogs by insertion of a screen into the upper trachea contain 4% protein (39). Proteins identified in airway secretions of humans and laboratory animals and thought to be secretory products of epithelial tissues are listed in Table 2. Many additional proteins are present as transudates of serum or products of airway cell breakdown.

Secretions recovered from the large airways of laryngectomized subjects are somewhat hypertonic (Table 3). Compared with serum, sodium levels are isotonic or slightly increased, potassium levels are much lower, and chloride levels appreciably higher (40). Secretions collected directly from submucosal glands of cats are nearly isotonic for sodium and chloride, but lower than serum in potassium content (41). Calcium levels are generally below those in serum (40), even though large amounts of calcium are associated with high M_r glycoconjugates in storage granules of secretory cells (42). There is little doubt that water exchange

Table 2 Proteins Secreted By Airway Cells

Component	Cell source	Animal	Ref.
Mucins	Surface secretory cells Mucous gland cells	All	20,27,28
Proteoglycans			
Chondroitin sulfates	Surface cells	Hamster, ferret	61,63
	Serous gland cells	Cow	60,62
Keratan sulfate	Surface cells	Ferret	63,64
Heparan sulfate	Surface cells	Hamster	61
Hyaluronic acid	Surface cells	Hamster	61
	Serous gland cells	Cow	60,62
Lysozyme	Serous gland cells	Human, ferret	66,67
	Surface cells	Human	71
	Clara cells	Human	69,70
Lactoferrin	Serous gland cells	Human	74
Secretory leukocyte proteinase inhibitor	Serous glands cells Clara cells	Human Human	60 70
Proline-rich proteins	Serous gland cells	Human	84
Clara cell 10-kd protein (CC-10)	Clara cells	Rabbit, dog, human	88
Uteroglobin	Clara cells	Rabbit	89
Surfactant-associated protein A (SPA)	Serous gland cells	Human	91
Surfactant-associated protein B (SPB)	Surface secretory cells Clara cells	Human Human	91a 91a
Surfactant-associated protein C (SPC)	Clara cells	Human	91a
Peroxidase	Surface secretory cells	Hamster	78
	Serous gland cells	Human	60
Secretory IgA	IgA plasma cells	Human	79
Secretory component	Ciliated surface cells	Human	79,81
	Serous gland cells	Human	79
Lipocortin-like proteins	Gland cells	Human	94
β-Galactosidase-binding lectin	Clara cells	Rat	93

between surface liquids and inspired air may change the osmolality and ion concentrations of liquids in the large airways, even on a breath-to-breath basis. Therefore, static measurements may not be entirely informative. Furthermore, laryngectomized subjects do not have full capacity to humidify inspired air; therefore, values derived from the secretions of these subjects may be somewhat misleading because of evaporation. Analysis of osmolality and mineral content of airway surface liquids from entirely healthy subjects has not been performed. The

Table 3 Composition of Airway Secretions

Substance	Laryngectomy	Bronchiectasis (g/100 g wet wt)	Cystic fibrosis
Water	95 ± 2	95 ± 1	89 ± 2
Protein	1.0 ± 0.3	2.0 ± 0.5	5.6 ± 2.0
Carbohydrate	1.0 ± 0.2	1.1 ± 0.1	1.1 ± 0.2
DNA	0.03	0.08	0.41
Lipid	0.8 ± 0.3	1.2 ± 0.4	3.1 ± 1.0
		(mM/1000 g wet wt)	
Sodium	165 ± 42	116 ± 15	101 ± 27
Chloride	162 ± 60	97 ± 14	75 ± 12
Potassium	13 ± 5	19 ± 3	28 ± 8
Calcium	3.1 ± 1.0	4.7 ± 1.3	3.7 ± 1.0

Source: Ref. 40.

differences between secretions collected from isolated cat tracheal submucosal glands in vitro and expectorated secretions can also be attributed to postsecretory modification by absorptive or secretory processes of the surface epithelium (43). Up to 15% of monovalent ions and 30% of calcium are not removed from human airway secretions by dialysis (40). Bound mono- and divalent cations undoubtedly serve, at least in part, as counterions for the sialic acid and sulfate groups of high M_r glycoconjugates.

The pH of rat and rabbit airway mucus in situ is reported to be 7.52 ± 0.05 and 7.70 ± 0.002 (44,45), respectively. In both animals, cholinomimetic stimulation decreased surface liquid pH by 0.07–0.15 pH units, an effect that could be blocked with atropine. Reports of human airway mucus pH values range from 5.4 to 8.15 (31). The variability may be related to purulence, duration of air exposure and, perhaps, other factors. Airways liquid pH reportedly can influence gelation, pHs below 7.5 favoring gel formation of nasal mucus (45). However, elasticity decreases with increasing pH (46). Whether these effects are operative at the airway's surface is currently a matter of conjecture. The influence of factors that may modulate pH, such as a H^+ or HCO_3^- secretion and the presence of other buffering systems, including secreted acidic glycoconjugates or basic macromolecules, such as lysozyme, have not been systematically assessed.

B. Specific Components

Mucins

Mucins, also called mucous glycoproteins or epithelial glycoproteins, are high M_r glycoconjugates characterized by numerous oligosaccharide side chains *O*-glycosidically linked to threonine or serine of a peptide core by *N*-acetylgalactosamine. Mucins are characterized by large size, high content of hydroxyamino acids (>30%), a large carbohydrate content (>70%), and a buoyant density less than 1.60 g/ml (1). They are released onto the airway surface from goblet cells of the surface epithelium and from mucous cells of submucosal glands. In fact, current evidence suggests that only small amounts of these substances are synthesized and released into the lumen of healthy airways. Bronchoalveolar lavage of healthy adult volunteers yields only scant quantities of material that have mucinlike properties (7,47). Similar results have been reported for lavage fluid of dog airways (48). Human and dog airway explants secrete variable amounts of mucinlike material (49). Airway surface cells harvested by proteinase treatment secrete little if any mucin when grown in primary culture on plastic surfaces, but recent data now confirm that if these cells are grown on collagen substrata in the presence of enriched media, they secrete appreciable amounts of mucin (22). Bronchoalveolar lavage of bronchitic airways yields large amounts of typical mucins (7,48). Final verification of capacity for mucin synthesis by airways epithelial cells has come from demonstration of the mRNA for the mucin core peptide in some of these cells by in situ hybridization techniques (see Chap. 8). In summary, it appears that both surface epithelial and gland cells have the capacity to secrete mucins, and that synthesis and release of these substances is proportional to the intensity of previous stimuli or injury (acute or chronic) to the airways. The latter point will be discussed in more detail in Section V.

Mucins display amazing heterogeneity (see Sec. V). This heterogeneity in considerable part reflects variation in peptide chain length as well as in numbers and sizes of oligosaccharide units, their structure, and the density of acidic charges contributed by sialic acid and sulfated sugars present in these saccharide units. Largely from histochemical-staining properties of mucous cells in airways, use of the terms neutral mucins and acidic mucins, the latter including both sialomucins and sulfomucins, became fashionable. Indeed, fractionation of airway mucins by ion-exchange chromatography can segregate mucins on the basis of acidic properties. However, these mucins are eluted as a continuum, and all fractions appear to contain some sialic acid and sulfate (32), there being no true neutral mucin or no mucin containing only sialic acid, but not sulfated sugars, and vice versa. Therefore, these terms should be used with the recognition that they denote relative, not absolute, content of acidic components. Acidic properties of mucins secreted in airways vary, based on cell and tissue source (14,50,51), level of airway (52), species (52), age (53), and the presence of disease states (54). Little is known about the relation between acidic properties and the rheology of mucins.

Glycosaminoglycans and Proteoglycans

Glycosaminoglycans (GAGs), including hyaluronic acid; the chondroitin sulfates A, B (dermatan sulfate), and C; heparan sulfate; and keratan sulfate, differ from mucins in that the carbohydrate chains are considerably longer and contain uronic acids (with the exception of keratin sulfate). Sugars and uronic acids are often sulfated and characteristically form repeating disaccharide units. When GAGs are linked to protein, they are called *proteoglycans*. The linkage sugar to protein is xylose, rather than *N*-acetylgalactosamine, again with the exception of keratan sulfate. Hyaluronic acid–protein linkage has not been demonstrated. Keratan sulfate in many ways has characteristics of both proteoglycans and mucins. Carbohydrate structures of typical GAGs are illustrated in Table 4.

In the past, proteoglycans were thought not to be an epithelial cell product or secreted into the airways lumen. Recent evidence suggests that this may not be true. Sahu and Lynn (55) reported that hyaluronic acid is present in asthmatic sputum in the amount of 2–3 mg/100 mg (dry weight) of delipidated secretions. In addition, they detected this GAG in airway secretions of individuals with cystic fibrosis and alveolar proteinosis. They were unable to ascertain that the hyaluronic acid is a secretory product of intact airway epithelium under these conditions, as it could be released by inflammatory cells (56) or by injured mucosal tissues. Chondroitin sulfate, dermatan sulfate, and hyaluronic acid were detected, but not quantified, in airway mucous aspirates of smokers (7). Healthy dog airway secretions may contain heparan sulfate, whereas SO_2-exposed dogs also have hyaluronic acid and dermatan sulfate in their secretions (49). Chondroitin sulfate was present in 11 of 13 sputum samples from patients with cystic fibrosis but only in 1 of 12 samples from patients with chronic bronchitis (57). In addition, substances with properties of both proteoglycans and mucins have been detected in aspirates of healthy airways from nonsmokers (7). Similar substances with a buoyant density above 1.60 g/dl have been reported in the secretory products of rabbit tracheal mucosal explants (58).

Unfortunately, airway wall explants contain connective tissue elements,

Table 4   Structure of Glycosaminoglycans

Name	Repeating disaccharide	Sulfation
Hyaluronic acid	GlcNAc(β1$\rightarrow$4)GlcAc(β1$\rightarrow$3)	None
Chondroitin	GalNAc(β1$\rightarrow$4)GlcAc(β1$\rightarrow$3)	GalNAc-4-*O*-sulfate, 6-*O*-sulfate
Dermatan sulfate	GalNAc(β1$\rightarrow$4)GlcAc(β1$\rightarrow$3) and GalNAc(β1$\rightarrow$4)L-IdoAc(α1$\rightarrow$3)	GalNAc-4-*O*, or 6-*O*-sulfate; L-iduronic acid may be 2-*O*-sulfated
Heparan sulfate	GlcNR(α1$\rightarrow$4)L-IdoAc(α1$\rightarrow$4)	GlcNAc-6-*O*-sulfate; some of the L-iduronic acid is 2-*O*-sulfated
Keratan sulfate	GlcNAc(β1$\rightarrow$3)Gal(β1$\rightarrow$4)	GlcNAc-6-*O*-sulfate; Gal-6-*O*-sulfate

sometimes including cartilage, that can release GAGs into culture medium. Therefore, primary cultures of epithelial cells may be more useful than explants for discerning whether these substances are epithelial cell secretory products. Fetal rat type II pneumonocytes release substantial amounts of GAGs in vitro, the most abundant being hyaluronic acid (59). Furthermore, serous cells isolated from bovine submucosal glands release chondroitin sulfate and hyaluronic acid into culture medium (60). Cultured surface epithelial cells from the hamster release hyaluronic acid, heparan sulfate, and chondroitin sulfate (mostly 4-sulfated) (61). However, it is not possible to state with certainty that these glycoconjugates were released by exocytosis from apical surface of cultured epithelial cells. Airways and other epithelial cells release proteoglycans onto their basolateral surfaces, where they participate in the process of cell adhesion and formation of the basal lamina. Recovery of these substances from cell culture medium could reflect this process. Therefore, detection of GAGs in secretory granules of airway epithelial cells would give important information about their capacity to secrete these substances onto the airway's surface. Chondoitin sulfate has been identified immunocytochemically in secretory granules of cow and human tracheal epithelial cells. This chondroitin sulfate could be released with cholinergic and β-adrenergic agonists (62). Preliminary immunocytochemical assessment of ferret tracheal surface epithelium with enzyme-linked monoclonal antibodies selective for a panel of proteoglycans has identified chondroitin sulfate and keratan sulfate in a pattern suggestive of secretory granules (63). Varsano and colleagues earlier had reported evidence that keratan sulfate-like glycoconjugates are plasma membrane-associated and are released from the apical surface of confluent dog tracheal epithelial cells (64). Thus "secretion" of glycoconjugates by airway epithelial cells may involve alternative processes.

Quantitation of amounts of GAGs released by airway epithelial cells has not been rigorously attempted. Therefore, amounts of the several GAG species released onto the lumenal surface as a percentage of total high M_r glycoconjugates is unknown. Furthermore, the function of these substances, if present at the surface of healthy airway epithelium, is not known. The GAGs do have the ability to form gels and, therefore, could be important determinants of the physical properties of mucus. This property may be particularly important in healthy airways, which secrete only small amounts of mucins.

Other Secreted Proteins

Lysozyme

Lysozyme is a small (12- to 14-kd) cationic protein that is secreted not only by airway epithelium, but onto most body surfaces and into the circulation by phagocytic cells. Airway lysozyme also is synthesized and released by alveolar macrophages and neutrophils as well as filtered from serum, although most likely in amounts much smaller than that secreted by epithelial cells. Thompson and co-workers estimate lysozyme concentrations in airway secretions by BAL and urea dilution to be 56 ± 14 µg/ml in normal human airways and 390 ± 129 µg/ml in bronchitic subjects (65). Rates of secretion by tracheal epithelial explants from humans and laboratory animals are listed in Table 5.

Immunocytochemical studies have localized lysozyme to serous cells of glands in humans (66) and ferrets (67). Human lysozyme staining is more intense in bronchi than trachea (66). Ferret tracheal submucosal glands secrete more lysozyme from the lower than from the upper trachea (68). Human nonciliated bronchiolar cells and rat type II pneumonocytes also contain lysozyme (69,70). Kinetic studies support the contention that appreciable amounts are secreted by human tracheal surface cells, even though lysozyme is not stored in large amounts by these cells (71). On the other hand, ferret airway lysozyme seems to be exclusively a product of glands (68).

Airways of most laboratory animals, as well as humans, secrete lysozyme (see Table 5). Although human alveolar macrophage, serum, and airway epithelial lysozymes are electrophoretically and immunologically identical (71), lysozyme secreted by the airway epithelium of laboratory animals differs slightly in size or charge (72). Lysozyme hydrolyzes $\beta_{1,4}$-linkages between *N*-acetylmuramic acid and *N*-acety-D-glucosamine in bacterial cell wall glycans. This activity is bacte-

Table 5 Lysozyme Secreted by Tracheal Epithelium: Species Differences

Source	Secretory rate (mg/g tissue per/24 h)	Electrophoretic mobility relative to human
Human	807	100
Baboon	170	79
Ferret	132	106
Dog	88	104
Mouse	64	92
Hamster	47	88
Rat	45	90
Guinea pig	20	90
Chicken	11	96
Sheep	ND	
Rabbit	ND	
Cat	ND	

ND, not detected within limits of the assay (<5).
Source: Ref. 72.

ricidal and is thought to provide nonspecific protection against infection of airways by a variety of inspired bacteria. The basic properties of lysozyme afford opportunities for ionic interactions with the acidic mucins and other glycoconjugates, perhaps influencing the physical properties of mucus (73).

Lactoferrin

Lactoferrin is another cationic serous cell product (74). It is considerably larger than lysozyme, M_r 70–75 kd, and has iron-binding properties. Initially discovered in milk, it is present in a variety of secretions, including bronchial, pancreatic, reproductive tract, lacrimal, salivary, and nasopharyngeal (75). As with lysozyme, lactoferrin is also present in granules of neutrophils (76) and released in the course of their activation. Concentrations have been estimated from lavage fluid to be 122 ± 28 μg/ml in normal airways and 632 ± 156 μg/ml in bronchitic airways (65). Lactoferrin is able to sequester free iron, and this action may provide protection from colonization of airways by iron-dependent bacteria. In addition, lactoferrin-bound iron cannot catalyze hydroxyl radical formation and, therefore, may protect against oxidative injury (65). Some have suggested that lactoferrin also protects against iron-catalyzed degradation of glycoconjugates (77).

Peroxidase

Peroxidase has been detected cytochemically in the airways lumen (epithelial lining fluid) and secretory cells of surface epithelium and glands, but not in ciliated or basal cells (78). It has been reported in submucosal gland serous cells of human airways (60). The staining reaction probably represents a family of enzymes that catalyze the reduction of hydrogen peroxide to water (60). In concert with H_2O_2 and thiocyanate or halide ions, peroxidases provide antimicrobial activity (78). This system is effective against bacteria, viruses, fungi, and mycoplasmas. As with lysozyme and lactoferrin, peroxidases are products of epithelia in most other organs, as well as neutrophils, eosinophils, and macrophages. Whether airway peroxidase is similar to lactoperoxidase or myeloperoxidase is unknown, because chemical or enzymatic characterization is lacking.

Secretory Component and Immunoglobulin A

A complex of these two proteins is secreted by airway epithelium. The complex contains dimeric IgA and a single secretory component molecule. The IgA is synthesized and linked by a small peptide (J-chain) to produce a dimer in plasma cells. This dimer interacts with secretory component, an IgA receptor on the basolateral membrane of airway epithelial cells. The complex is internalized by endocytosis, transported across the epithelial cell in cytoplasmic vesicles, and discharged onto the luminal surface as secretory IgA (sIgA) after proteolytic cleavage of secretory component (79). Secretory component protects sIgA from bacterial and neutrophil proteinases on the epithelial surface. Stockley has estimated that approximately 50% or more of IgA in airway secretions is sIgA, the remainder being the 7S serum IgA (80).

The functions of sIgA in airways include inhibition of microbial adherence and colonization; neutralization of toxins, enzymes, and viruses; and protection against antigen absorption. The sIgA is released by airway cells from the larynx to the respiratory bronchioles. Surface epithelial cells, probably ciliated cells, but not basal cells, stain for secretory component (79,81). Most submucosal gland cells also stain for this component (79). Developmentally, secretory component antedates the appearance of immunoglobulins in human airways (82).

Secretory Leukocyte Proteinase Inhibitor

The secretory leukocyte proteinase inhibitor (SLPI) is a 12-kd, acid-stable protein with cationic properties. It has been localized immunocytochemically to human submucosal gland serous cells (60) and peripheral airway Clara cells (70). This small antiproteinase accounts for most inhibitory activity in airways against neutrophil proteinases, including neutrophil elastase and cathepsin G. The other major antiproteinase is α_1-proteinase inhibitor, a serum protein that is not synthesized by airway cells. The SLPI is present in sputum at levels ranging from 4 to 405 mg/ml (mean, 66 mg/ml) and is also present in nasal secretions and saliva (83). It is concentrated nearly 20-fold in the gel phase of sputum, compared with the sol fraction, suggesting interactions of this cationic protein with acidic glycoconjugates (83).

Proline-Rich Proteins

The proline-rich proteins (PRP) are present in serous cells of human nasal, laryngeal, and tracheobronchial glands and, furthermore, are present in the secretory product of human tracheal explants (84). Detection was carried out with a series of antibodies against both basic and acidic salivary gland PRP. Because antibodies cross-react within this family of small proteins, it is not possible to determine whether one, several, or all ten PRP peptides are synthesized in airway tissues. Pig tracheal epithelial cells in primary culture express an unusual (20-kd) PRP that is not present in intact airway epithelium (85). The function of PRP in airway secretions is unknown, but variation of their concentration influences the airway's mucous viscosity (86). The basic PRPs may interact directly with acidic glycoconjugates; acidic PRPs may act by chelating calcium or other cations that act as counterions for glycoconjugate acidic groups.

Clara Cell 10-Kilodalton Protein

The Clara cell 10-kd protein has been identified in bronchoalveolar lavage of rats, hamsters, mice, rabbits, and humans (87). It can be immunocytochemically detected in secretory granules of nonciliated, nonmucous epithelial cells, consistent with the morphology of Clara cells (88). This protein binds progesterone and inhibits pancreatic phospholipase A_2, the latter perhaps imparting anti-inflammatory properties by down regulating the release of arachidonic acid and production of its inflammatory metabolites (87). A small protein similar in structure and function, *uteroglobin*, is released by Clara cells of the rabbit lung (89).

Surfactant-Associated Proteins

Originally considered to be alveolar type II cell products, four distinct surfactant-associated protein products (SPA, SPB, SPC, SPD) have been described. The SPA, SPB, and SPC also are synthesized by cells of human terminal nonciliated conducting airways (90,91). Occasionally, these proteins may be secreted by large-airway epithelial cells. For example, surfactant-associated protein A (SPA), a 35,000-kd glycoprotein, has been localized to nonmucous submucosal gland cells by immunocytochemistry and in situ hybridization (91). The SPB is present also in gland cells, but not those that contain SPA (91). Dexamethasone is able to stimulate transcription of the SPA gene and increase protein biosynthesis in rat lungs (92). In combination with phospholipids, these proteins enhance the physicochemical properties of extracellular surfactant. Their function at cell sites not associated with surfactant biosynthesis and secretion is unknown.

Several other proteins or small peptides appear to be synthesized by airway mucosa and may be components of airway secretions. A β-*galactosidase-binding lectin* has been recovered from rat BAL and observed immunocytochemically in Clara cells of this species (93). A family of *lipocortin-like proteins* (apparent M_r 33, 35, 37, and 67 kd) are released into the apical culture medium of human tracheal gland cells (94). These proteins may mediate the modulatory effects of corticosteroids on mucin release by airway epithelium (95) and, by inhibiting phospholipase A_2, may dampen the arachidonate cascade contribution to the inflammatory response. A series of small peptides with antimicrobial properties has been described. One of these, a 38-amino acid, cysteine-rich peptide called *tracheal antimicrobial peptide* (TAP), was isolated from bovine tracheal epithelium (96). It inhibits growth of gram-positive and gram-negative organisms as well as *Candida albicans*. Glycosidase activities including β-*glucuronidase* have been detected in lavage fluid of health baboons (97). These activities increase appreciably in lavage fluid of smoking baboons. The source of these enzymes is unknown. Proteinases, including chymotrypsinlike activity, collagenase, and elastolytic activity are present in BAL fluid and sputum of diseased airways (98,99), but only chymotrypsinlike activity could be found in BAL fluid of healthy airways (98). The source of chymotrypsinlike activity (cathepsin B) is alveolar macrophages (99). Most investigators have assumed that small amounts of proteinases are complexed with antiproteinases and inactivated in the airways lumen.

Proteins of Serum Origin

Serum proteins move across the vascular–airway barrier as a transudate. Most proteins in serum can be detected in airway secretions. The process, in general, is thought to be one of physical filtration, the smaller molecules moving more easily through endothelial and epithelial "pores" than the larger molecules (100). The filtration barrier becomes more leaky with airway inflammation (101). Thus, concentrations of these proteins in bronchitic airways (Table 6) are higher than those in healthy airways. Several of these proteins (e.g., IgG, IgA, and lysozyme) are produced locally by airways as well as filtered from serum. Recently, several reports of facilitated albumin transport across intact airway epithelium have been published (102, 103). The extent to which this mechanism contributes to albumin levels in airways is unknown. This observation raises questions of similar processes for movement of other serum proteins onto the airway surfaces.

Serum proteins may play important roles in airway secretions. The immunoglobulins have protective functions, and the antiproteinases are critical for inactivating proteolytic enzymes released by inflammatory cells. Albumin interacts with gastrointestinal mucins to increase their viscosity (104). It may be that this abundant serum protein also contributes to the determination of rheological properties of airway mucus.

Lipids

The lipid composition of airway mucus is highly variable, but apparently appreciable under all circumstances. Sources of lipids may include alveolar surfactant, lipids released (perhaps secreted) by cells along the conducting airways, and membranes of disrupted cells. Amounts of lipid are highest in suppurative airway diseases; for example, mean lipid content of sputum from individuals with cystic fibrosis is 3.1% on a wet weight basis (6). However, mucus from laryngectomized subjects is 1% lipid (6), and similar recoveries can be estimated from analysis of uninfected mucus from quadriplegic patients (105). Bhaskar et al. report that secretions recovered by 10-ml lavages of normal human airways contain less lipid, but amounts were not specified (7).

Compositional analysis of lipids obtained bronchoscopically by small-volume lavage from normal airways of dogs (48) and humans (7) reveals prepon-

Table 6 Serum Proteins in Sol Phase of
Nonpurulent Bronchitic Sputum

Protein	Concentration (mg/100 ml)
Albumin	29.7 ± 8.0
IgG	13.3 ± 8.2
Transferrin	2.9 ± 1.0
α_1-Antitrypsin	2.7 ± 1.6
Haptoglobin	2.2 ± 1.6
α_1-Antichymotrypsin	1.5 ± 1.1
α_1-Acid glycoprotein	1.2 ± 1.0

Source: Ref. 288.

Table 7 Lipid Content of Normal Dog
Tracheobronchial Secretions Collected by Lavage

Lipid	Percentage of total lipids
Neutral lipids[a]	45
Phosphatidylcholine	30
Lysophosphatidylcholine	8
Sphingomyelin	4
Phosphatidylethanolamine	2

[a]Includes triglycerides, free fatty acids, cholesterol and cholesterol ester.
Source: Ref. 48.

derantly neutral lipids and smaller amounts of phospholipids. No glycolipids were detected. The lipid composition of "normal" dog airway mucus, as reported by Bhaskar et al. (48), is given in Table 7. These investigators further demonstrated that glycolipids appear in dog airway secretions following chronic SO_2 exposure (48) or in otherwise healthy human smokers (7). They argue that glycolipids found in quadriplegic or intubated patients (Table 8), and patients with asthma or cystic fibrosis are products of associated, but undefined, pathophysiological processes (105). On the other hand, explants of large-airway mucosa from dogs and humans (49) and primary cultures of hamster tracheal surface epithelial cells (60) release lipids of all three types into culture medium. Some of this lipid may be released as the result of cell death, but current evidence points to the conclusion that epithelial cells release lipid in the course of normal secretory events.

Some of the lipid in airway mucus copurifies with high M_r glycoconjugates (106). However, mucin-associated lipid can be effectively removed by centrifugation in CsCl or guanidinium hydrochloride (107). Similarly, we have been unable to detect appreciable amounts of lipid in human airway mucin prepared by reduction in 8 M urea and carboxymethylation. Claims that mucins contain covalently linked fatty acids (i.e., fatty acids that are not removed by the usual delipidation process, but can be removed by KOH treatment; 108) do not include

Table 8 Lipid Distribution in Noninfected Airways Secretions[a]

Source Ref.	Neutral lipids	Phospholipids	Glycolipids
Intubated patients (160)	40	22	38
Quadriplegic patients (105)	27	22	51

[a]Percentage of total.

tracheobronchial mucins. Houdrel et al. (109) observed that the extent of lipid, including fatty acid binding to airway mucins, is directly related to the purulence of the original secretions. Hansson et al. have also reported that mucins prepared from chronic bronchitic sputum by CsCl density gradient centrifugation contain less than 1 mg lipid per gram of glycoprotein, virtually all of which could be extracted with chloroform/methanol (107).

V. Mucin Structure and Biosynthesis

As described in Section IVB, airway mucus contains several glycoconjugates. Little has been reported about airway epithelial proteoglycans, serum-type glyco-proteins (glycoproteins that contain GlcNAcβAsn linkage), and glycolipids. We have no reason to believe that they differ substantially from their counterparts in other tissues. For those interested in these glycoconjugates, many excellent reviews are available (110–112). In this section, we will focus on the structure and biosynthesis of airway mucins because they have known physiological functions and are extensively characterized.

A. Properties of Airway Mucins

Mucins constitute a subgroup of glycoproteins that contain covalently linked carbohydrates. Although mucins have unique properties, they do share some properties with other glycoconjugates. With the advent of respiratory epithelial cell culture (21,22,25–28,113,114), immortalized epithelial cells (23,24,116,117), and adenocarcinoma cell lines (118), criteria for determining if these cultures secrete mucins are badly needed. In this section, we will define airway mucins by their physicochemical properties and use these properties as a gold standard for the identification of mucins produced by tracheal explants and cultured epithelial cells.

Size, Polydispersity, Microheterogeneity, and Molecular Structure

Size
One feature of a mucin is that it is large. The reported M_r of airway mucins ranges from 1.8×10^6 to 4.4×10^7 Da (115). They have been described as highly expanded macromolecules, behaving as a random coil (122). They aggregate (123) and polymerize (124). Many mucins do not penetrate even low-percentage (1–3%) polyacrylamide gels (125,126) and do not stain with Coomassie Blue. Conse-quently, one purity criterion for mucins is the absence of Coomassie Blue-stained bands on polyacrylamide gel electrophoresis (PAGE). However, mucins can be identified by silver stain. Because of their large size and extended conformation, mucins are excluded by porous gels such as Sepharose 6B (53,127), that has an

exclusion limit of 4×10^6 Da for globular proteins and 1×10^6 Da for polysaccharides. Therefore, Sepharose column chromatography often has been employed as a first step to separate mucins from smaller M_r glycoproteins. However, other large glycoconjugates, such as proteoglycans and nonmucin hyaluronidase-resistant high-M_r glycoconjugates, do not separate from mucins on Sepharose CL-6B (53).

Polydispersity

Airway mucins also display polydispersity. According to Jentoft et al. (119) mucins differ strikingly in peptide length. This finding is supported by the results of scanning electron microscopy and is congruent with the hypothesis of Carlstedt et al. (122) that mucin peptide units are linked head-to-tail. Tandem repeats of amino acid sequences appear to be typical, as shown by the amino acid sequence data obtained from cDNAs of several mucins (120,128–131). For example, tandem repeats of 20, 23, 81, and 16 amino acids have been reported for mucins obtained from adenocarcinomas (120), human intestinal epithelium (129), porcine submaxillary glands (130), and human airway epithelium (199), respectively. Tandem repeats of amino acids for some human airway mucins are not uniform (130,131). Variable numbers of tandem repeats in mucins may, in part, explain their polydispersity. Polydispersity contributes to the typically broad and diffuse mucin bands on gel filtration (119) and PAGE (32,125,126).

Microheterogeneity

Microheterogeneity is also characteristic of mucins and resides in the carbohydrate portion. The number of different oligosaccharide chains of human bronchial mucins has been estimated in the hundreds (115,132). Mucin oligosaccharide chains vary from one to more than 20-sugar residues per chain. Furthermore, oligosaccharides with same composition and chain length may differ greatly in structure (133–139). Respiratory mucins contain sialic acids and sulfate esters that impart acidic properties. Differences in the degree of sialylation or sulfation contribute to a broad distribution of these mucins over a wide range of salt concentrations on DEAE–cellulose columns (32) and over a wide range of isoelectric points on electrofocusing (140). Carbohydrate microheterogeneity also contributes to diffuse bands on gel electrophoresis (32,125,126) and broad peaks on gel permeation (119), anion-exchange chromatography (32), or electrofocusing (140).

Composition

Airway mucins contain 10–20% peptide, 75–85% carbohydrate, and 1–8% sulfate. The amino acid composition of respiratory mucins is similar to that of other mucins (i.e., serine and threonine constitute 30–50 mol% of the total amino acids). Human tracheobronchial mucins have a higher content of threonine than serine (121), although several other mucins have a serine content equal to or higher than threonine (27,28,53) (Table 9). These two amino acids plus glycine, proline, alanine, and glutamic acid make up 70–80% of the peptide. Mucins have a low aromatic amino acid content, resulting in a low extinction coefficient at 280 nm. Therefore, absorbance at 220–230 nm has been employed to monitor mucin purification (32). Respiratory mucins contain trace amounts of cysteine, found primarily in the sparsely glycosylated regions (122). This amino acid may play an important role in mucin polymerization. The amino acid composition of mucins is different from that of keratan sulfate (141). These two glycoconjugates are otherwise difficult to distinguish.

Five sugars, D-*N*-acetylgalactosamine, D-*N*-acetylglucosamine, D-galactose, neuraminic acid (sialic acid), and L-fucose are found in airway mucins. Mucin carbohydrate composition varies from preparation to preparation (microheterogeneity); therefore, one cannot rely solely on carbohydrate composition to assess the purity of mucins. However, the absence of sugars not normally found in

Table 9 Amino Acid Composition of Tracheobronchial Mucins and Keratan Sulfate [a]

Amino acid	Human tracheobronchial secretions (32)	Ferret tracheal explants (53)	Guinea pig tracheal epithelial Cells (27)	Guinea pig tracheal epithelial Explants (27)	Hamster tracheal epithelial cells (28)	Keratan sulfate (141)
Asp	44	30	69	47	88	70
Thr	224	184	140	136	135	58
Ser	134	229	189	178	137	134
Glu	71	87	129	106	122	145
Pro	100	84	31	28	80	109
Gly	91	123	199	256	84	122
Ala	102	48	69	64	80	73
Cys	19	13	4	7	ND[b]	11
Val	19	31	36	30	66	48
Met	19	27	9	6	4	5
Ile	27	26	1	20	36	30
Leu	55	19	21	17	66	72
Tyr	8	11	2	0	3	17
Phe	15	15	41	47	6	35
Lys	29	14	4	23	30	24
His	22	27	35	21	25	13
Arg	21	32	22	15	36	34

[a]Residues per 1000 amino acids.
[b]ND, not determined.

purified mucins is a fairly good criterion for purity; for example, the presence of uronic acid and xylose suggests contamination by proteoglycans. In addition, detection of mannose may indicate contamination by serum-type glycoproteins. However, amino acid sequences deduced from cDNA libraries suggest the presence of some *N*-glycosylation sites (i.e., Asn-X-Thr/Ser) (128,129,131). Therefore, mannose could be a constituent of native mucins.

Respiratory mucins contain various amounts of sulfate, a major determinant of the chromatographic profile of tracheobronchial mucins on anion-exchange chromatography (32,140). The more acidic mucins, eluted with high salt concentrations, have an increased sulfate content (Fig. 5). Sulfate ester is also found in glycosaminoglycans (except hyaluronic acid) and some glycoproteins that contain asparagine-linked carbohydrates (142). Therefore, quantitation of mucins based on [^{35}S]sulfate incorporation without an additional isolation step will overestimate mucin quantities.

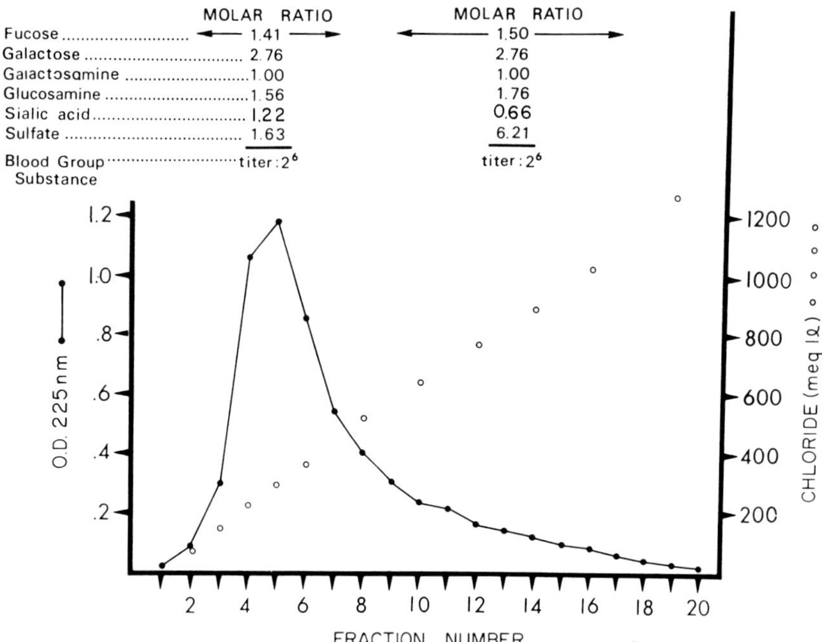

Figure 5 Elution of a highly sulfated human tracheobronchial mucin (component 2, Fig. 3), from DEAE cellulose with a linear chloride gradient. Fractions were combined in two pools as indicated, and each pool was analyzed for sugar, sulfate, and blood group determinant content. Note the decreased sialic acid and markedly increased sulfate content of the second pool.

Carbohydrate-to-Peptide Linkage

Mucin carbohydrate chains are covalently linked to the hydroxyl group of serine or threonine by N-acetylgalactosamine. Demonstration of this linkage is necessary for the identification of mucins and can be accomplished by subjecting purified glycoproteins to mild alkaline (0.05 M) treatment; this removes oligosaccharide chains from the peptide through a β-elimination reaction (143). To prevent further β-elimination (peeling) of the newly eliminated oligosaccharide chains, $NaBH_4$ (1 M) is used to convert the reducing terminal N-acetylgalactosamine to N-acetyl-galactosaminitol. Deglycosylated serine and threonine are converted to alanine and α-aminobutyric acid, respectively (144). The linkage between N-acetyl-glucosamine and serine or threonine, a rare O-glycosidic linkage found in nuclear and some other intracellular membranes (145,146), and the linkage between N-acetylglucosamine and asparagine in serum-type glycoproteins can also be cleaved under mild alkaline-borohydride conditions (147). Therefore, the specific N-acetylhexosaminitol generated must be identified (148). Mucin-type carbohydrate-to-peptide linkage is also found in keratin sulfate (149) and membrane glycopro-teins (150,151). Therefore, demonstration of N-acetylgalactosamine to serine or threonine linkage only indicates the presence of mucin-type carbohydrate, but does not prove that the sample contains mucins.

Buoyant Density

The peak buoyant density of mucin in CsCl varies from 1.43 to 1.60 g/ml (53), depending on the carbohydrate and sulfate contents. Sulfate is heavier than sugar, which in turn is heavier than amino acids (25). Therefore, the buoyant density of mucins is greater when glycosylation and sulfation are increased. In general, buoyant density determination will distinguish mucins from the heavier proteogly-cans. However, keratan sulfate and mucins have similar buoyant densities (53,141).

Other Properties

Blood Group Determinants and Influenza Virus Hemagglutination Inhibition Activity

Mucins secreted by respiratory epithelium carry structures for blood groups A, B, or H(O) if this epithelium contains the GDP-Fuc:β-galactoside $\alpha1\rightarrow2$ fucosyl-transferase, the blood group H(O) enzyme encoded by the secretor gene (152–154). The blood group determinant in these mucins corresponds to the blood type of the donor's red blood cells. If the secretor gene is absent in the tracheal epithelium, secreted mucins will contain Lewis and not A, B, or H(O) blood group structures (153,154).

Influenza virus binding is another property of airway mucins. The type and linkage of the sialic acid determine this binding (155). For example, the wild-type influenza virus binds to $\alpha2\rightarrow6$-linked N-acetylneuraminic acid (156), whereas a receptor variant influenza virus binds to $\alpha 2 \rightarrow 3$ N-acetylneuraminic acid structure (157). Binding of human tracheobronchial mucins to influenza virus is enhanced by higher sulfate content, although sulfated mucins without sialic acid do not bind to influenza virus (32). This binding activity is diminished for mucins containing blood groups A, B, and AB when compared with mucins containing blood group H(O) or Lewis a or b structures (158).

Lipids

Lipids, including phospholipids, neutral lipids, and glycolipids bind noncovalently to mucins (107–109,159,160) and may affect the rheological properties of mucus (159). In addition, mucins are reported to contain covalently bound fatty acids (159,161), formed by fatty acylation, as catalyzed by an acyltransferase (162). However, subsequent analysis by Hanson et al. (109) has questioned whether the covalently linked fatty acid is present in appreciable amounts in airways mucins.

Link Protein

The existence of a link protein associated with epithelial mucins has been debated for several years. Recently, a detailed study of mucins from the gastrointestinal tracts of several mammals has concluded that, in this tissue, there is a common link glycopeptide with an M_r of 118 kd (163). A link protein of similar size (140 kd), dissociable by mercaptoethanol, in pig submaxillary mucin, has also been reported, even though this mucin preparation contains no cysteine (164). Link protein with an M_r of 65–70 kd has also been reported for human (167,208) and canine (165) tracheobronchial mucin. Physicochemical evidence obtained by Carlstedt et al. (122) argues against the presence of a link protein independent of respiratory mucin peptide. Further study is needed to determine whether the putative link protein is part of the mucin peptide or is a nonrelated protein that happens to link to the naked region of mucin molecules by disulfide bonds.

B. Mucin Quantitation

Airway epithelium secretes not only mucins, but other glycoconjugates (53,61). Mucins share some properties with other glycoconjugates. Therefore, investigators need to demonstrate that the method employed for mucin analysis specifically measures mucins. Current criteria for respiratory mucins include exclusion by Sepharose 6B; buoyant density between 1.43 and 1.60 g/ml on CsCl density gradient centrifugation; carbohydrate-to-peptide linkage by GalNAc-serine/threonine; carbohydrate content; GalNAc, GlcNAc, Gal, sialic acid, and Fuc, but no glucuronic or iduronic acid and mannose; predominant amino acids: Ser, Thr, Gly, Ala, Pro, and glutamic acid with Ser + Thr greater than 30 mol%; nonstaining by Coomassie Blue on PAGE and agarose-PAGE analyses.

Mucins have been measured in media bathing respiratory explants (16–18,

20,27,166) and epithelial cells (26–28,61,113,114), sputum (32,48,121), and airway lavage fluid (168). A variety of analytical procedures have been employed, including quantitation of carbohydrate moieties, metabolic labeling (166), and immunoquantitation (168–170). Isolation procedures preceding quantitation have used dialysis (171); precipitation by trichloroacetic acid (TCA; 172), TCA-phosphotungstic acid (173), or ethanol (174); and exclusion by Sepharose (127,166). Clearly, many studies have suffered from a lack of specificity of mucin quantitation methods. The following protocol has been used routinely in our laboratory (127,166) to quantitate metabolically labeled mucins in culture. The procedure entails treatment of the harvested medium with a reducing agent such as dithiothreitol or β-mercaptoethanol to dissociate any glycoconjugates associated with mucins through disulfide bonds. Particulate matter, including cell debris, is removed by low-speed centrifugation. The supernatant is then treated with bovine testicular hyaluronidase to degrade hyaluronic acid, chondroitin sulfates A and C, and dermatan sulfate. Mucins and mucinlike materials are collected semiautomatically in the void volume fraction of Sepharose 6B (1 × 30 cm) using a multichannel pump and quantitated by scintillation counting (127,166). The void volume material is largely mucins for newborn and young ferrets, but mucins represent only a fraction of hyaluronidase-resistant, high M_r glycoconjugates in mature ferrets (53). To quantitate airway mucins in these animals, the mucins are separated from other hyaluronidase-resistant, high M_r glycoconjugates by CsCl density gradient centrifugation performed at a starting density of 1.58 g/ml. If glycolipid is present, it can be dissociated by 0.1% sodium dodecyl sulfate (SDS) added to the chromatographic elution buffer (26,61).

Several radiolabeled precursors have been employed to metabolically label mucins; [³H]glucosamine is the most widely used precursor. Exogenous [³H]glucosamine can label UDP-GlcNAc, UDP-GalNAc, and CMP-sialic acid (Fig. 6), which in turn are substrates for the enzymes that transfer GalNAc, GlcNAc, and NeuAc to newly synthesized mucins. Therefore, when radiolabeled glucosamine is used, these three mucin sugars will be labeled (113,176). Steady-state secretion of radiolabeled glycoconjugates is not reached until 48 h after continuous exposure of tracheal explants to the precursor (166). Other sugars that have been used to label glycoconjugates include glucose (177–179), galactose (113,179–181,183), mannose (113,181–183), fucose (184), galactosamine (177,185), mannosamine (186), *N*-acetylmannosamine (187), and *N*-acetylglucosamine (187). The sugars labeled by these precursors are listed in Table 10. Depending on the sugar used as the radiolabeled precursor and the culture system employed, the efficiency and specificity of the label vary considerably. For example, when glucose is used as the precursor, a much smaller percentage of labeled materials appears in the void volume of Sepharose CL-6B, when compared with radiolabeled glucosamine (178), suggesting that radiolabeled glucose is a relatively nonspecific precursor. Labeled fucose has been proposed as a more specific precursor for mucin labeling,

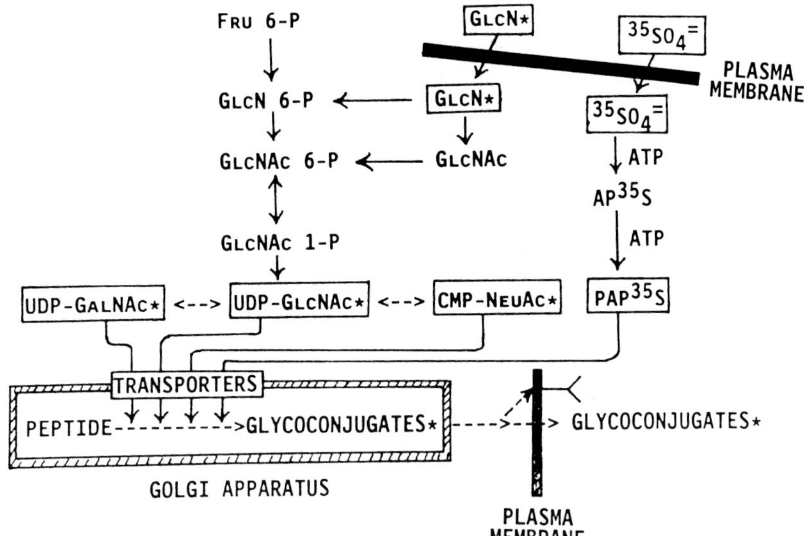

Figure 6 Scheme for incorporation and metabolism of radiolabeled glucosamine and sulfate. Activated sulfate (PAP[35]S) and nucleotide sugars are transported across Golgi membranes and serve as donors for transferase-catalyzed biosynthesis of oligosaccharides. Mature glycoconjugates can be inserted in cell membranes or secreted.

but it also labels *N*-linked glycoproteins and glycolipids. In summary, no sugar precursor labels only mucins, emphasizing the need for isolation steps before quantitation.

Other radiolabeled precursors used for labeling glycoconjugates include [3H]Ser/Thr and [35S]sulfate. [3H]Serine labels peptide, but not nucleic acid, and serine is the only radioactive amino acid detected in labeled high M_r glycoconjugates (25). It has been reported that equilibrium labeling of cell surface glycoconjugates is reached within 2 h using [3H]serine. However, in our experience, steady-

Table 10 Glycoconjugate Sugars Labeled by Sugar Precursors

Precursors	Labeled sugars in glycoconjugates	Ref.
GlcN/GlcNAc	GlcNAc, GalNAc, and sialic acid	113,114,176,187
GalN	GlcNAc and GalNAc	177,185
ManN/ManNAc	Sialic acid	186,187
Glc	Gal, Fuc, hexosamines	177–179
Gal	Gal, Man, hexosamines	113,179–181,183
Man	Man, Gal, Fuc, sialic acid, hexosamines	113,181–183
Fuc	Fuc	184

state secretion of these radiolabeled macromolecules is not reached until 48 h of continuous exposure of airway cells in primary culture to this precursor. Similarly, inconsistent results of kinetic studies for [35S]sulfate labeling have been reported. One report states that equilibrium labeling was achieved within 40 min using [35S]sulfate (188). Another study has claimed steady-state secretion of [35S]sulfate-labeled mucins within 2 h after labeling (175). However, we found that steady-state secretion of 35S-labeled high M_r glycoconjugates was not reached until 24 h and 72 h after continuous exposure of cat and human tracheal explants to this precursor, respectively (Fig. 7). The discrepancy between these reports may be attributed to the measurement of different pools of glycoconjugates. Continuous exposure of glycoconjugates to a radiolabeled precursor labels all glycoconjugates, whereas pulse–chase methods label only a subpopulation of glycoconjugates, presumably a pool with rapid turnover.

Enzyme-linked immunosorbent assays (ELISA; 169,170) and enzyme-linked lectin assays (ELLA; 189) have been used to measure mucins in sputum and airway lavage fluids. Both methods employ a sandwich approach; that is, the plate is coated with monoclonal antibody (or lectin) and then the bound antigen is detected with the same antibody (or lectin) linked with horseradish peroxidase. Monovalent antigen, such as glycolipids, will not be detected, thereby minimizing nonspecific measurement. The sensitivity of the ELISA method (169) for human mucin, reported by Lin et al., is approximately 10 ng, whereas the sensitivity of ELLA for ferret mucin by *Dolichol biflorus* lectin is about 0.1 ng (189). The high

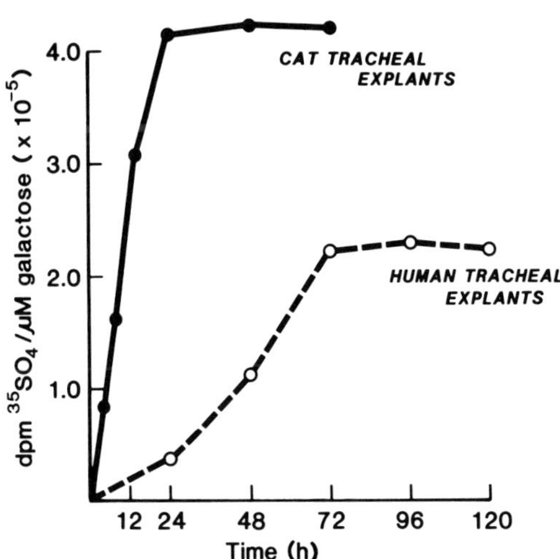

Figure 7 Specific activity of 35SO4-labeled mucins released by tracheal mucosal explants as a function of time in medium 199 containing label precursor. These calculations assume that galactose is the sulfated sugar.

sensitivity of the latter method is due to a high blood group A titer of ferret mucins (53). The advantages of these procedures include rapidity of analysis, capability of simultaneous multiple sample assays, and no need for purification. Potential disadvantages include interference by other glycoconjugates that contain the same carbohydrate epitopes and lower sensitivity when compared with radiolabeling methods. The importance of showing that the compounds measured by monoclonal antibodies and lectins in these assays are mucins should not be underemphasized.

C. Mucin Structure

Peptide Structure

Mucin peptide constitutes only a small portion of the mucin molecule and is largely masked by carbohydrates, hampering the measurement of peptide size and structure. However, chemical deglycosylation procedures (128,190,191), application of physicochemical techniques and electron microscopy to measure mucin size (115), and advances in mucin peptide molecular biology (128–131) have greatly advanced our understanding of mucin peptide structure. As shown in Table 11, with the exception of the reports by Sangadala et al. (193,194) and Bhattacharyya et al. (203), mucin peptides from several animal species display polydispersity, ranging in size from 10 to 2480 kd.

Table 11 Peptide Size of Airway Mucins

Mucin sources	Size (kd)	Methods	Comments	Ref.
Human	100	TFMS[a] and glycosidase	Polydisperse band	191
	97	TFMS	Sharp	203
	67	TFMS	Sharp	193
	67	In vitro translation	Sharp	194
	60–100	TFMS	Polydisperse	204
	100–500	In vitro translation	Polydisperse	205
	10–200	TFMS and immunoprecipitation	Polydisperse	131
	56–833[b]	EM[c]	Polydisperse	206
Canine	100	TFMS and glycosidase	Polydisperse	191
Swine	67	TFMS	Sharp	193
	67	In vitro translation	Sharp	194
Cat	55–2480[b]	EM	Polydisperse	207

[a]TFMS, trifluoromethanesulfonic acid.
[b]The size of the peptide was estimated based on the assumption that a 100-kd peptide measures 363 nm by EM (115).
[c]EM, electron microscopy.

Complete amino acid sequence data for an airway mucin is not yet available. However, partial amino acid sequences of human airway mucins have been determined by sequencing the sparsely glycosylated region released by proteinases (195). These sequences have been matched with the deduced amino acid sequences of cloned human airway mucin cDNAs (131), confirming the authenticity of the cloned genes. Amino acid sequences deduced from cloned human airway mucin cDNAs (131) provide further insight into mucin peptide structure. These data indicate that hydroxyamino acids do not distribute evenly along the peptide chain. In fact, the bulk of these two amino acids is found in a tandem repeat domain of the molecule (130,131). Oligopeptide tandem repeats and their sizes differ among airway mucin genes (130,131,199). Consensus asparagine glycosylation sites are located in the nontandem repeat domain (128,129,131) near the COOH-terminus. Among the human airway mucin genes that have been cloned, one is homologous (130), but not identical with, the rat tracheal mucin (196) and human intestinal mucin (197,128) gene. Genes encoding human airway mucin peptides have been located on several different chromosomes (198), including 3 (199), 11p13-11pTer (130), 11p15 (200), and 13 (200). It is not now known why human airway mucin genes are so diverse. Further studies are needed to resolve this enigma (for more detail, see Chap 8).

Carbohydrate Structure

Mucin carbohydrate chains share one common structure (i.e., reducing terminal GalNAc linked to Ser/Thr). Oligosaccharide size is highly variable and chains can be neutral or acidic, depending on the absence or presence of sialic acid or sulfate ester. In addition, mucin oligosaccharide structures vary greatly in anomeric configuration and linkages. For example, galactose can link to an adjacent sugar as either an α- or β-anomer, and in a 1-3, 1-4, or 1-6 linkage. The composite carbohydrate structure of airway mucins is depicted in Figure 8. Mucin carbohydrate structures can be divided into several distinctive groups: cores, backbones, and peripherals (115,133–139,201,202). Four core structures are found in airway mucins: core 1, Galβ1-3GalNAcα-O-Ser/Thr; core 2, Galβ1-3(GlcNAcβ1-6)-GalNAcα-O-Ser/Thr; core 3, GlcNAcβ1-3GalNAcα-O-Ser/Thr: core 4, GlcNAc-β1-3(GlcNβ1-6)GalNAcα-O-Ser/Thr. There are also four backbone structures; type 1, Galβ1-3GlcNAc; type 2, Galβ1-4GlcNAc; i antigen, GlcNAcβ1-3Gal; and I antigen, GlcNAcβ1-3(GlcNAcβ1-6)Gal. The carbohydrate structures of the peripherals are rather complex. For example, sialic acid can link to C-3 or C-6 of galactose (134,135,192) and C-6 of reducing terminal GalNAc, whereas sulfate has been identified at C-6 of galactose (201,202). Substitutions at the nonreducing terminus of a type 1 chain can form blood group H, Fucα1-2Gal; B, Galα1-3-(Fucα1-2)Gal; A, GalNAcα1-3(Fucα1-2)Gal; Lewis a (Le[a]), Galβ1-3(Fucα1-4)-GlcNAc; Lewis b (Le[b]), Fucα1-2Galβ1-3(Fucα1-4)GlcNAc; and sialyl Le[a],

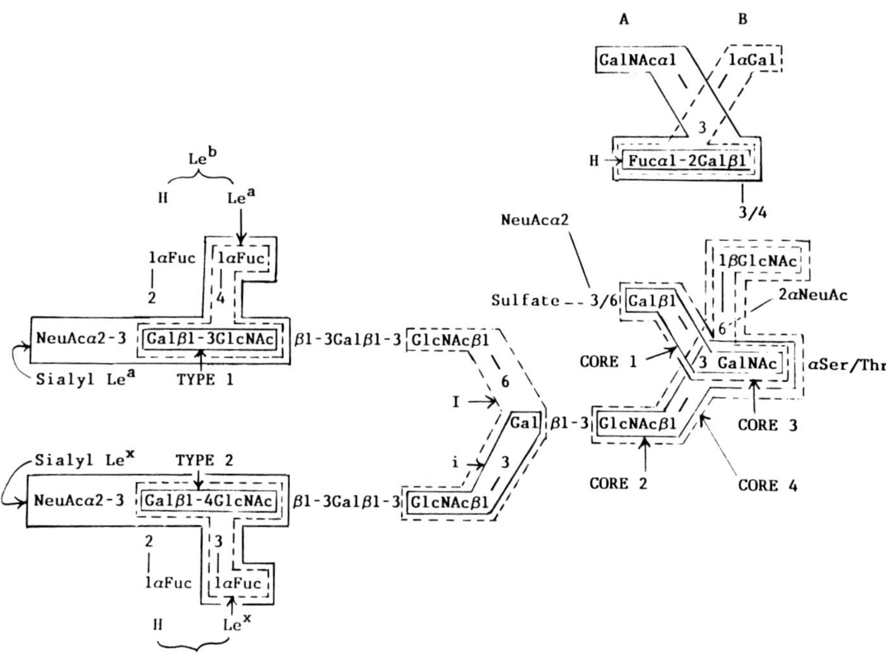

Figure 8 A composite oligosaccharide structure for airway mucin, depicting the four possible core structures (1, 2, 3, 4), the four possible backbone structures (type 1, type 2, I, i) and several peripheral structures, including blood group determinants, sulfated sugars, and sialylation sites.

NeuAcα2-3Galβ1-3(Fucα1-4)GlcNAc. Substitutions at the nonreducing terminus of a type 2 chain can form Lewis x (Le^x), Galβ1-4(Fucα1-3)GlcNAc; Lewis y (Le^y), Fucα1-2Galβ1-4(Fucα1-3)GlcNAc; and sialyl Le^x, NeuAcα2-3Galβ1-4-(Fucα1-3)GlcNAc in addition to blood group H, B, and A determinants. Fucose can also link α1-2 to internal galactose (138), a novel structure recently identified.

Molecular Assembly

Intra- and intermolecular disulfide bonds are thought to play a prominent role in the polymerization of airway mucins (122). However, mucin aggregation is not dependent solely on disulfide linkages, because mucins that do not contain cysteine will aggregate (123). Other forces that contribute to mucin aggregation include interactions between carbohydrates (123), charged groups [e.g., sialic acid or sulfate and cationic compounds, such as lysozyme (209) and Ca^{2+} (210)], and hydrophobic groups (e.g., bound lipids) (159).

The original molecular model proposed for gastrointestinal mucins by Allen (124) depicts a polymer made up of subunits that are joined by a link protein through disulfide bonds. Identification of a putative link protein from intact airway mucins (165,167,208) has lent some support to this model for airway mucins. However, failure to demonstrate a reduction in size following treatment of airway mucins with reducing agents has led Carlstedt et al. (122) to propose a new model. This model depicts a mucin as a molecule containing a linear peptide chain that has alternating heavily glycosylated and sparsely or nonglycosylated ("naked") regions. The naked region is rich in cystine and is susceptible to proteolysis. Establishment of a definitive molecular model for airway mucins awaits identification and characterization of a full-length cDNA encoding airway mucin peptide.

D. Mucin Biosynthesis

Biosynthesis Scheme

Mucin peptide is encoded by an mRNA template at the rough endoplasmic reticulum. Addition of the first sugar, GalNAc, to the nascent peptide occurs at the *cis*-Golgi membranes and is catalyzed by mucin peptide:αGalNAc transferase (211,212). Formation of subsequent carbohydrate structures also takes place in the Golgi. Mucin oligosaccharide synthesis is controlled by many factors, as reviewed elsewhere (213,214), including availability of donor nucleotide sugars, relative activities of glycosyltransferases acting on the same acceptor, and pH in the Golgi lumen (215). The product formed serves as the acceptor for subsequent glycosyltransferase reactions. In other words, the assembly of mucin carbohydrates is not directed by a template, but by various glycosyltransferase-catalyzed reactions. This method of assembly is why mucin carbohydrate structures are very heterogeneous.

Despite the complex process of mucin carbohydrate synthesis, certain guidelines can be followed to qualitatively correlate glycosyltransferase activities with carbohydrate structures formed. Glycosyltransferases involved in the assembly of mucin oligosaccharides can be classified into the chain-elongation and chain-termination groups. Chain-elongation enzymes generate carbohydrate structures that permit continued growth of carbohydrate chains. This group of enzymes includes mucin peptide:α1GalNAc transferase (211,216), βGal transferases (217–219), and βGlcNAc transferases (220–226). On the other hand, the carbohydrate structures generated by the chain-termination enzymes stop or limit further chain growth. These enzymes include sialytransferases (227,231), fucosyltransferases (228), and blood group A (229), B (230), and H (152) enzymes. As indicated in Figure 9, if sialic acid is linked to the first sugar (i.e., GalNAc), the product cannot accept additional sugars. However, if galactose is added, the disaccharide, Gal-GalNAc, will permit additional sugar transfers and form many different carbohydrate structures. The high ratio of sialyl/galactosyl

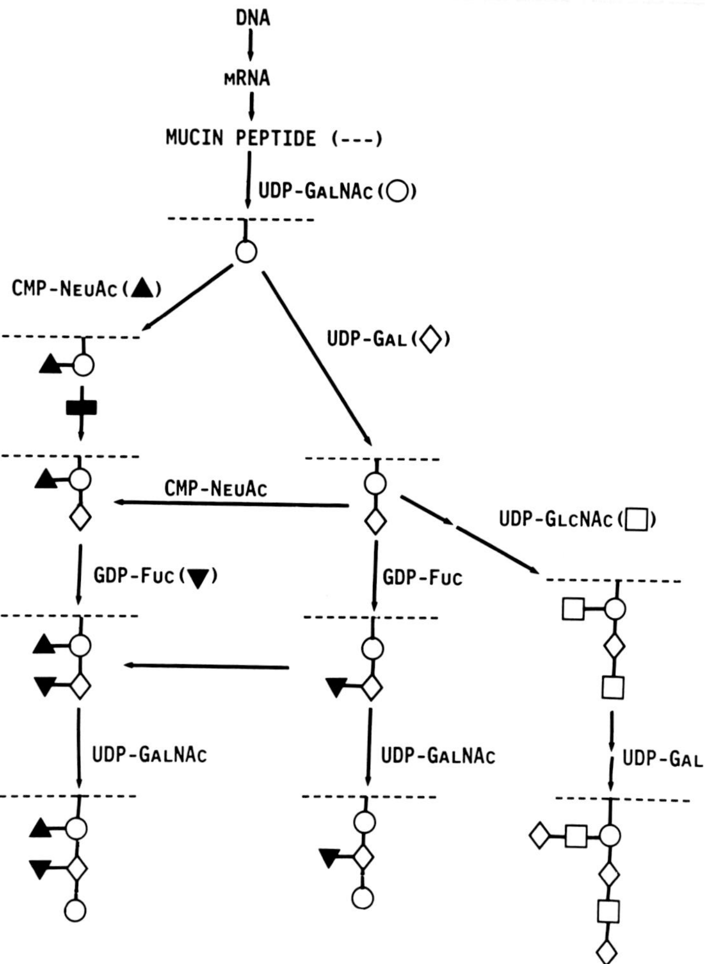

Figure 9 A scheme depicting biosynthesis of mucin oligosaccharides and regulation of this process. Each branch point represents an opportunity for competition between chain elongation and chain termination transferase-catalyzed biosynthetic reactions. Heavy bars represent points at which carbohydrate synthesis cannot proceed.

transferase activity (18:1) found in ovine submaxillary glands (219,242) results in the formation of sialyl-GalNAc, the major oligosaccharide identified in ovine submaxillary mucins (123). When the ratio is 1:1, as is found in porcine submaxillary glands (219,242), eight different mucin oligosaccharides ranging, in size from one to five sugar units per chain are formed (143). When the ratio is even lower (1:2), as is found in human tracheal epithelium (219,231), hundreds of different mucin oligosaccharides are formed (115,132).

When mucin synthesis nears completion, sulfation of oligosaccharides takes place at the *trans*-Golgi membranes (232), before mucin is packaged into the secretory granules and secreted (see Fig. 6). Sulfotransferase-catalyzed reactions use the sulfate donor, 3'-phospho-5'-phosphoadenosylsulfate (PAPS), which is formed from inorganic sulfate, by two reactions that consume two molecules of ATP and are sequentially catalyzed by ATP sulfurylase and adenosine 5'-phosphosulfate kinase (233–235).

Mucin Glycosyltransferases

Glycosyltransferases catalyze the transfer of the donor sugars from nucleotide sugars to the acceptor molecules as shown:

$$\text{Nucleotide-sugar(*)} + \text{Acceptor} \xrightarrow{\text{Glycosyltransferase}} \text{Sugar(*)}-\text{Acceptor} + \text{Nucleotide.}$$

To facilitate the assay of glycosyltransferase activities, the donor sugars are usually radiolabeled (*). The radiolabeled products are then separated from the nucleotide–sugar and quantitated by scintillation counting. Because several glycosyltransferase activities may be assayed simultaneously in a crude enzyme preparation, it is imperative to characterize the product(s) to identify the glycosyltransferase activities being measured.

Several mucin glycosyltransferase activities have been reported in airway epithelium (Table 12). Enzyme 6 has been highly purified (217) and enzymes 2 (240) and 4 (226) have been purified to homogeneity. Ropp et al. (226) have shown that the purified β6GlcNAc-transferase can form all the branched GlcNAc structures found in mucin carbohydrates, including core 2 and 4 structures and I antigen. Therefore, modulation of the activity of this enzyme could have a profound effect on mucin carbohydrate structures, in particular, the formation of branched versus linear chains.

E. Species Differences

Peptide

The amino acid composition of airway mucins varies from species to species (see Table 9). Because compositional data cannot predict the peptide structure, we are now unable to tell how much mucin peptide structure will vary across species. As indicated earlier (see Sec. V.B) an airway mucin peptide gene in rat (196,197) and human (130,197) airway epithelium is homologous to a human intestinal mucin peptide cDNA (129), suggesting that this mucin gene may be expressed in mucus-secreting tissues of several animals. One potential level of complexity is that more than one mucin gene may express in the same tissue, as in human tracheal

Table 12 Mucin Glycosyltransferases in Airway Epithelium

No.	Glycosyltransferases	Tracheal sources	Ref.
1.	UDP-GalNAc:apomucin (GalNAc-ser/thr)α GalNAc TF	Dog, human	236,238,239
2.	UDP-Gal:GalNAcα ser/thr β3 Gal TF	Dog, human, porcine, ferret	219,236,238–240,53
3.	CMP-NeuAc:GalNAcα ser/thr α2,6 NeuAc TF	Dog, human, ferret	231,236,238,239,53
4.	UDP-GlcNAc:Gal β3 GalNAcα ser/thr (GlcNAc-Gal) β6 GlcNAc TF	Bovine, porcine	222,226,241
5.	UDP-GlcNAc:Gal β3 GalNAcα ser/thr (GlcNAc-Gal) β3 GlcNAc TF	Porcine	241
6.	UDP-Gal:GlcNAc β3 Gal TF	Porcine	217
7.	UDP-Gal:GlcNAC β4 Gal TF	Human, porcine	217–219
8.	GDP-Fuc:GalβR α2 Fuc TF	Human, ferret	152,53
9.	UDP-GalNAc:Fucα2 Galβ-R (GalNAc-Gal) α3 GalNAc TF	Dog	237

epithelium (200). More studies are clearly needed to understand mucin structure across species lines.

Carbohydrate

It is not fruitful to try to compare mucin carbohydrate structures between species based on compositional data. Carbohydrate structures from only two airway mucins have been elucidated, human and porcine. The basic mucin carbohydrate structures from these two species are in agreement with known mucin carbohydrate structures. One notable difference is that porcine mucin contains a NeuAcα2-6Gal structure (192), which has not been reported in human airways mucin. On the other hand, many carbohydrate structures found in human mucins are not detected in porcine airway mucins (115,133–139,192,201,202).

Species differences in carbohydrate structure are also suggested by reactivity with monoclonal antibody. For example, monoclonal antibody 17B1 recognizes monkey and human airway mucins, but does not react with ferret tracheal mucins (Cheng, unpublished observation). Characterization of the epitope recognized by this antibody would elucidate mucin carbohydrate structural differences between these species. This approach should have general applicability in future structural analyses of airways mucin carbohydrates.

VI. Developmental Changes in Airway Secretions

Maturation of human surface epithelium and submucosal glands occurs, for the most part, prenatally. Restrictions on fetal studies have precluded systematic or comprehensive investigation of airway secretory products during early maturation in the human. More is known about maturational changes in animal models, although species variation limits our ability to make generalizations. We will address what is known about maturational changes of airways secretory structures and products in humans and then discuss the relevant changes in animal models, such as the ferret (243) and sheep (244), in which substantial airway development occurs postnatally.

A. Developmental Changes in Secretory Structures of Human Airways

As discussed in Chapter 4, the distribution, morphology, and histochemical staining of airway secretory cells change with maturation. In the human fetus, the rudimentary airway appears at 4 weeks of gestation as a diverticulum from the foregut and undergoes serial dichotomous division to form a complete tracheobronchial system, including terminal bronchioles, by 16 weeks gestation (245). The epithelial lining of the developing tracheobronchial tree is of endodermal origin and initially resembles that of the developing esophagus (246–248). At least some of these cells are pluripotential and differentiate into the various cells of the respiratory system, including the secretory cells in the airway epithelium and submucosal glands. In humans, most airway epithelial and glandular development occurs during the second trimester of gestation.

Secretory Cells in the Surface Epithelium

Between 12 and 13 weeks of gestation, two types of secretory cells in the tracheal epithelium can be distinguished by histochemical-staining characteristics. One type contains "neutral" granules (acquiring a magenta color after staining with alcian blue–PAS) typically at the base of the cell; this cell also may contain "acidic" granules (staining purple with alcian blue–PAS) at the apex of the cell (247). The second type of secretory cell is distended by acidic granules, typical of airway goblet cells (247). As the human fetus matures, the first type decreases in number and the second becomes more prominent (247), suggesting that the first cell is a precursor cell and that the secretory product changes with maturation. An increase in acidic staining predicts that the glycoconjugates secreted by mature airways contain more highly sialylated or sulfated glycoconjugates than those secreted by the less mature airways. Differentiation of ciliated cells within the tracheal epithelium (249) coincides with the maturation of secretory cells.

Submucosal Glands

Submucosal glands are compound tubuloacinar structures consisting of a central duct and multiple side tubules that terminate in acinar structures. Mucous cells are located in the proximal tubules and serous cells in the peripheral tubules and acini. Primordial submucosal glands appear in human tracheas at 12–14 weeks of gestation as round intraepithelial buds (246,250,251) that elongate into cylinders, protruding into the submucosal region (250). The submucosal portion of this cylinder divides to form two lateral ducts that then undergo repeated dichotomous division to form acini (250). The glands first appear near the larynx and then increase in number distally until 17 weeks gestation, when there is no difference in gland density in the upper and lower trachea (251). After 23 weeks of gestation, glands increase in size, but not in number (251). Given the assumption that all glands are present at birth, but the airways continue to increase in size postnatally, it has been estimated that gland density decreases from 36 glands per square millimeter at 15 weeks, to 10 glands per square millimeter at birth, to 1 gland per square millimeter in adults (252). Therefore, the relative contribution of gland secretion per unit of airway surface area may decrease with age.

Variation in the distribution of different secretory cell types within the submucosal glands has not been studied in the maturing human airways. In the fetal rhesus monkey, mucous cells in the proximal tubules undergo differentiation before serous cells in the peripheral tubules and acini (253). Dyssynchronous maturation of cell types could result in age-related changes in the relative concentration of secretory products in submucosal gland secretions.

B. Developmental Changes in Secretory Function of Human Airways

Secretory function of human airways has not been evaluated during the early stages of development. The presence of periodic acid–Schiff (PAS) staining material in goblet cells as early as 13 weeks (247) and in the ducts of developing tracheal submucosal glands as early as 16 weeks of gestation (251) suggests the potential for early secretory activity. At 26 weeks gestation, the earliest stage studied, explanted human tracheas secrete mucinlike substances and lysozyme (254). The rates of baseline secretion of mucins tend to decrease with maturation for the three age groups studied: preterm infants at 26–32 weeks of gestation, term newborns, and children 2–6 years old; however, in this study the differences did not reach significance (254). This trend suggests that immature airways may secrete more glycoconjugates than mature airways, as has been observed in animal studies, cited in the next two sections. Increased mucin-type glycoprotein secretion was apparent with methacholine stimulation for both preterm and term explants (254), suggesting that cholinergic responsiveness has been established by 26 weeks of gestation. The chemical composition of glycoconjugates secreted by tracheal explants is similar for preterm infants, term newborns, and young children; however, sialic acid and fucose contents increase and sulfation decreases with age (254). These changes may alter the charge density and, thereby, the histochemical-staining properties as well as the viscoelastic properties of mucous secretions.

Lysozyme secretion changes with maturation of epithelium and submucosal glands. The rate of lysozyme secretion by preterm tracheal explants is one-half that for term explants and close to one-fourth of that for explants from children 2–8 years old (254). The lower concentrations of lysozyme, a bacteriolytic enzyme, suggest increased susceptibility of preterm and young infants to bacterial infections of airways. Methacholine stimulation increased the rate of lysozyme secretion by term, but not preterm explants (254), suggesting that cholinergic responsiveness for lysozyme secretion lags behind that for mucin secretion.

C. Developmental Changes in Airway Secretory Structures and Products in the Ferret

Developmental changes in the tracheas of ferrets between birth and 28 days of age are similar to those that occur in the human fetus between 13 and 20 weeks of gestation (243). In the first 4 weeks, the density of ciliated cells increases from 9 to 54%, the density of secretory cells decreases from 66 to 22%, histochemical staining of the surface epithelial cell changes from predominately nonacidic to acidic, and submucosal glands develop from intraepithelial buds into complex tubuloacinar structures (243).

Newborn ferret tracheal explants secrete hyaluronidase-resistant, high M_r glycoconjugates (presumably mucins) at a rate that is six times greater than that for 28-day-old adult ferrets (Fig. 10) (166). This age-related decrease in the rate of unstimulated hyaluronidase-resistant, high M_r glycoconjugate release parallels a

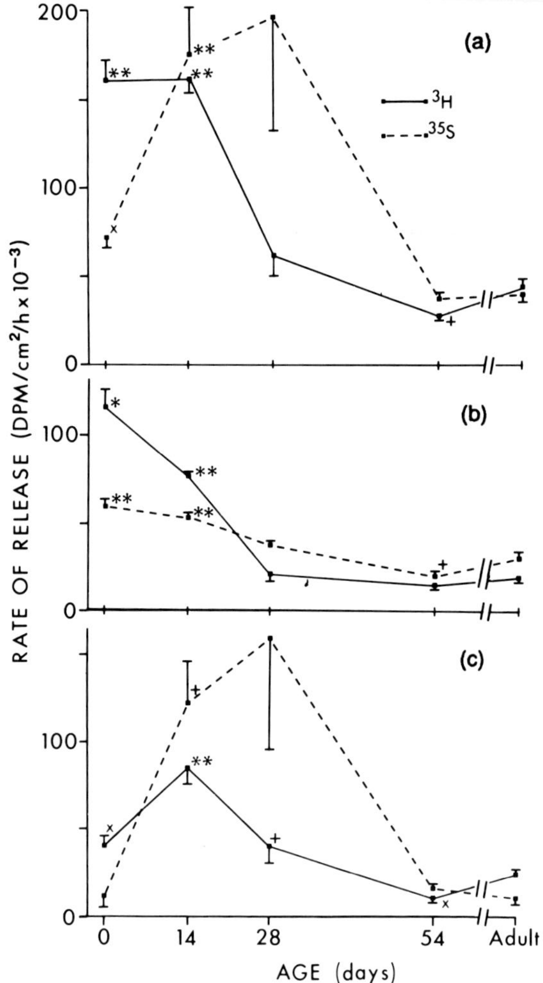

Figure 10 Rate of release of ferret tracheal high M_r (excluded from Sepharose 6B-CL) glycoconjugates labeled with [³H]glucosamine or [³⁵S]sulfate. Data are shown for (a) total high M_r glycoconjugates, (b) hyaluronidase-resistant glycoconjugates, largely mucins, and (c) hyaluronidase-susceptible glycoconjugates. These data demonstrate the high level of secretory activity immediately after birth, followed by declining secretory rates for mucins and the changes in sulfation in the first 28 days of life for all categories of glycoconjugates.

diminishing density of secretory cells in the surface epithelium over the same postnatal period (166). Stimulation of secretion with cholinergic agonists is not demonstrable until 28 days of age (see Fig. 10) (166) suggesting that submucosal glands must attain a mature tubuloacinar structure before their secretion can be modulated.

Mucin-type glycoconjugates are secreted at all ages; however, the proportion of total glycoconjugates secreted as mucins decreases from 36% in newborns to 8% in adults (53). Between zero and 28 days of age, secretion of proteoglycans that are susceptible to hydrolysis by bovine testicular hyaluronidase increases progressively (see Fig. 10) (166). By using immunohistochemical studies, we have observed that the density of several proteoglycans within the secretory cells including keratan sulfate and chondroitin sulfate increases over this same time interval (63), suggesting developmental changes in specific proteoglycan secretion that warrant further investigation.

Mucin amino acid and total carbohydrate contents do not vary with ferret age; however, sialic acid content (53) and sulfation (166) increase with age (Table 13;

Table 13 Age-Related Changes in Mucin Carbohydrate Composition and Glycosyltransferase Activities in Ferret Tracheas

	Newborn	14 days	28 days	Adult
Sugar content[a]				
Galactose	1344	1249	1374	1076
GalNAc	730	649	713	782
GlcNAc	591	536	566	582
Fucose	250	222	224	171
Sialic acid	138	167	310	314
Mannose	≤ 6	<1	<1	<1
Glucuronic acid	<1	<1	<1	<1
Total sugars	3053	2823	3187	2925
Glycosyltransferases[b,c]				
Gal TF	214.5	128.5	124.4	127.0
GlcNAc TF	20.3	6.3	7.3	2.5
Fuc TF	40.3	22.4	14.3	7.4
NeuAc TF	2.3	2.2	2.4	1.8
Relative enzyme activities				
NeuAc TF/GlcNAc TF	0.11	0.35	0.33	0.72

[a]Residues per 1000 amino acids.

[b]nmol sugar transferred per hour per milligram protein.

[c]The four glycosyltransferases are as follows: Gal TF = UDP-Gal:GalNAc αser/thr β3-galactosyltransferase; GlcNAc TF = UDP-GlcNAc:Gal β3GalNAc (GlcNAc-GalNAc) β6-*N*-acetylglucosaminyltransferase; Fuc TF = GDP-Fuc:Gal α2-fucosyltransferase; NeuAc TF = CMP-NeuAc:GalNAc αser/thr α2$\rightarrow$6-neuraminyltransferase.

see Fig. 10), consistent with changes in histochemical staining. An age-related increase in the relative activity of sialytransferase is consistent with the increased content of sialic acid in mature mucin (53).

Lysozyme secretion is not detectable for newborn ferret tracheas, but the lysozyme secretory rate increases progressively from 7 to 28 days, at which time the secretory rate reaches 60% of that in the adult (255). Increase in lysozyme release correlates with the development of submucosal glands and suggests that lysozyme is a marker of submucosal gland secretory activity in the ferret (255). In both human and ferret airways, the capacity to secrete lysozyme lags behind that of mucinlike glycoconjugates.

D. Developmental Changes in Airway Secretory Structures and Products in Sheep

Postnatal maturation of airway epithelium in the sheep differs from that in the ferret. In sheep, the tracheal epithelium is fully ciliated at birth; however, the prevalence of mucous cells decreases with age from 23% in the newborn, to 18% at 8 weeks, to 13% at 5–12 months, to 8% in the adult (>12 months) (244). Likewise, the rate of secretion of nondialyzable macromolecules metabolically labeled with [^{3}H]threonine and ^{35}SO$_4$ decreases with age; secretion rates for newborn tracheal explants are approximately three times greater than those for adult tracheal explants (244). This observation provides further support for the notion that basal secretion is generally greater for immature than for mature airways.

A pattern across species for developmental changes in sulfation of secreted glycoconjugates is not apparent. Sulfation of nondialyzable macromolecules from both human (254) and sheep (244) airways decreases with age. In contrast, sulfation of the hyaluronidase-resistant, high M_r glycoconjugates secreted by ferret tracheal explants increases with age (166). It is unclear whether these differences reflect species variation or differences in purification protocols. Nondialyzable macromolecules isolated in the human and sheep studies may include a larger proportion of highly sulfated glycosaminoglycans than hyaluronidase-resistant, high M_r glycoconjugates.

E. Developmental Changes in Immunoglobulin Production in Airways

In human airways, secretory component appears in bronchial epithelium at 16 weeks and in bronchioles at 22 weeks. The number of immunostained cells increases with age. Immunoglobulin-containing plasma cells appeared after birth; those bearing IgA and IgM cluster around submucosal glands. Apical portions of serous cells in surface epithelium and glands also stain positively for these two immunoglobulins (258). The relationship between immunolocalization studies and capacity to secrete functional antibodies into the airways remains to be determined.

F. Developmental Changes in Serum Protein Concentrations in Lung Secretions

With the exception of albumin and sIgA, serum proteins are thought to move passively into the tracheobronchial secretions. Little is known about transudation of these proteins at different maturational stages. For two serum proteins, α_1-proteinase inhibitor (α_1PI) and α_2-macroglobulin (α_2M), concentrations in serum and lung secretions have been measured in both adults and newborns. In adults, the molar ratio of α_1PI (54,900 Da) to α_2M (725,000 Da) in lung secretions is 20-fold higher than in serum (256), suggesting that transudation of proteins is influenced by their relative sizes. However, in intubated newborns, the molar ratios in serum and lung secretions are similar (257), suggesting that the capillary endothelium in the newborn is a less effective barrier for larger proteins than it is in the adult. Further studies are needed to define relative concentrations of the serum components at different maturational stages. Developmental changes in the concentrations of these serum proteins could influence some of the protective functions of airway secretions. For example, increased concentrations of immunoglobulins and antiproteinases may be important for protecting airways from infectious and inflammatory insults, respectively. Viscoelastic properties of airway secretions may be altered as well. For example, increasing concentrations of serum albumin enhance the viscosity of pig gastric mucin (104) and could have a similar influence on airway mucins.

VII. Disease-Related Changes of Airway Mucus and Its Components

Amounts of mucus secreted onto the airways surface in healthy lungs are small. Pathogen-free rats have serous cells, but very few mucous cells, in their airways (259). Mucus is not visible by fiber-optic bronchoscopy in healthy human airways. Lavage of airways from normal volunteers recovers little mucin and other macromolecules (7,48). Most human airway secretory cells reside in glands (260). However, we postulate that glands act largely as reservoirs of secretory product, releasing large amounts of mucus into the lumen with appropriate stimuli, but contributing little mucus if unprovoked. Thus, normal subjects may secrete substantial amounts of mucus only if they inhale noxious fumes (e.g., ammonia) or irritating substances, such as hypertonic saline, or acquire an acute respiratory tract infection. Unfortunately, there is no known marker that distinguishes gland from surface cell secretions in humans, complicating efforts to determine the source of airways mucus under basal conditions and with provocation.

For laboratory animals as well as humans, chronic irritation or injury induces a state of mucous hypersecretion. Study models include SO_2 inhalation, cigarette smoking, intratracheal elastase, and infection (49,261–263). Both basal and stimulated secretion appear to be enhanced by these substances. Changes include increased numbers of goblet cells in surface epithelium, as well as submucosal gland hypertrophy. It appears that mucin peptide biosynthesis is induced in multipotential cells by these stimuli (196). These changes speak to the striking plasticity of airway epithelial cells (264).

Less is known about alterations of secretory products. Studies of rat airways epithelium by Jany and Basbaum demonstrate no mucin mRNA before, and readily detectable mucin RNA after, 1 week of SO_2 exposure or Sendai virus infection (265). Whatever the mechanism at a cellular level, it is clear that mucin gene expression is one response to chronic injury. Leigh et al. have demonstrated (266) that a single 3-h exposure of weanling ferrets to 500 ppm SO_2 rapidly alters surface cells, decreasing numbers of goblet (glycoconjugate storage) cells, and greatly increasing numbers of small granule secretory cells, similar to those present in immature airways. Mature ferret airways secrete mostly nonmucin high M_r glycoconjugates, but immature ferret airways secrete mucin in preference to other large glycoconjugates (55). Together, these observations suggest that secretory cell populations do have the capacity to alter their secretory product. Mucin biosynthesis may be a response to acute as well as chronic airways injury.

For humans, it is clear that in states of chronic airways inflammation, such as asthma, chronic bronchitis, or cystic fibrosis (32,33,48,49), mucins are the preponderant secreted glycoconjugate. Thus, mucin secretion may well be a protective response of airways that can be turned on as needed. How mucins provide protection has not been precisely determined. Certainly, they have the ability to form gels and provide a physical barrier that may protect against injurious inhalants. In addition, mucins interact with both bacterial (267) and viral (268) pathogens and may prevent many of these organisms from reaching receptor sites on surface epithelial cells (269), an important step in the pathogenesis of infection.

Mechanisms by which induction of mucin biosynthesis and release are achieved in cell injury or inflammatory states are not fully understood. From our current information about the products of inflammation and modulation of glyco-protein secretion, we and others have proposed that reflex release of neurohumoral agonists, a number of proteinases, reactive oxidative products of neutrophils, metabolites of arachidonic acid, and certain neuropeptides (270–272) may play pathophysiological roles by stimulating mucin release. Furthermore, massive release of secretory products could be a stimulus to accelerated biosynthesis of secretory products such as mucins. There is some histochemical evidence that chronic inflammation favors the elaboration of more acidic, especially sulfated, glycoconjugates (56) by airways. The molecular basis for this change and its importance for the final secretory product also remain a mystery.

An array of proteolytic and glycosidic enzymes released by inflammatory cells and microbial agents also have the potential to alter mucous components. As an example, mucins in sputum from patients with cystic fibrosis appear to have undergone proteolytic degradation (273,274). The heavily glycosylated region of these mucins is relatively protected from proteolysis, but the so-called naked region is vulnerable. Convincing evidence for enzymatic modification of saccharide chains on mucins or other glycoconjugates in purulent airway secretions has been difficult to obtain. For example, neuraminidase activity produced by *Pseudomonas aeruginosa* does not desialylate airways mucins (275). Other mucus components are also modified. For example, proteolytic alteration of immunoglobulins in cystic fibrosis airways interferes with their opsonic activity (276) or with their ability to inhibit binding of organisms to epithelial cells (277). Modifications of other secretory proteins are likely. There is no direct evidence that these modifications alter the physical properties of airway mucus, but controlled comparisons are virtually impossible because of the numerous variables introduced by the inflammatory state.

Airway inflammation is also associated with increased lipid, DNA, and serum protein content of airway secretions (see Table 3). The contribution of lipids to mucous obstruction and difficulty clearing secretions in chronic obstructive lung disease has been presumed, but never carefully documented.

A. Diseases for Which Altered Airway Secretion Composition or Components May Play a Primary Pathogenetic Role

Cystic Fibrosis

As suggested by an early designation, mucoviscidosis, for this genetically determined, chronic obstructive lung process, investigators have long suspected that alterations of mucus are responsible for airway obstruction and infection. Observation of dilated airway gland acini and ducts within the first days of life, before the onset of chronic infection, and the occurrence of mucous obstruction in noninfected organs, strongly suggest that mucous obstruction is not secondary to infection. An array of mucous abnormalities have been postulated and experimentally examined (Table 14).

Early studies found an increased fucose and a decreased sialic acid content of CF mucous glycoproteins, especially those from the gastrointestinal tract (278). The CF fibroblast membrane glycoproteins may demonstrate similar glycosylation changes (279). However, CF respiratory tract mucins do not consistently display this alteration (32). On the other hand, a recent report suggests decreased acidification of Golgi components in CF respiratory epithelial cells and consequent decreased sialylation capacity (215). Further pursuit of these findings and their implications for airways pathophysiology are warranted.

In the early 1980s, several observations focused attention on epithelial cell transport dysfunction in CF, and the consequences of this dysfunction for the clearance of airway mucus. Knowles and associates (280) observed that the electrical potential difference across CF epithelia was more negative than that of

Table 14 Alterations of CF Mucus with Potential Significance
for Airways Dysfunction

Secretion of structurally abnormal mucins or other glycoconjugates
    Increased fucose content
    Decreased sialic acid content
    Increased sulfate content
Qualitative or quantitative abnormalities of lipid content
Altered electrolyte content
    Increased calcium concentration
    Decreased sodium, and chloride concentrations
Paucity of water

---

controls, and that this difference could be abolished by inhibiting sodium channel
function with amiloride. Subsequent in vitro studies with intact epithelium, as
well as confluent primary cell cultures, have demonstrated not only excessive
sodium absorption through amiloride-inhibitable channels, but also down regulation of chloride channel function, preventing chloride secretin onto the luminal
surface. These abnormalities appear to be the result of a regulatory defect common
to both the cAMP-dependent and C-kinase systems (281,282). Recent work has
demonstrated that the fundamental lesions occur as the result of a mutation in the
gene for CFTR, a membrane glycoprotein that itself functions as a chloride
channel (283). The consequence of this abnormality appears to be an inability to
secrete salt and, secondarily, water in the face of excessive absorption of these
substances. Indeed, the water, Na^+, and Cl^- contents of CF sputum are all
deficient (6), although direct measurements of these key components in airways
secretions of uninfected CF airways have not been made. The viscoelastic and
gelation properties of mucous secretions are highly dependent on water content
(124); therefore, the transport deficit in CF airway epithelium and consequent
failure of mucous hydration is the best current explanation for failure of clearance
of secretions.

The sulfate content of mucins purified from CF respiratory tract secretions,
collected both in vivo and in vitro, and from gastrointestinal as well as respiratory
sources, also is consistently elevated (25). This change was initially ascribed to the
chronic inflammatory state characteristic of CF airways. However, with the advent
of primary cell culture of airway epithelium, it has been possible to reexamine
sulfation of CF glycoconjugates independent of an inflammatory environment.
Primary cultures of CF tracheal epithelial cells secrete mucins and glycosaminoglycans, both of which are oversulfated. In addition, CF cells oversulfate cell
surface glycoconjugates, which can be removed with trypsin (25). These observations suggest that sulfate metabolism is perturbed in CF cells. However, prelimi-

nary studies in our laboratories (unpublished) appear to exclude alterations of sulfate efflux or increased accumulation of inorganic sulfate in CF respiratory epithelial cells. Whatever the mechanism, it is clear that oversulfation of mucins and other glycoconjugates by CF epithelium is a genetically determined property of CF cells, and that the consequences of this abnormality for the rheological and clearance properties of CF airway mucus deserve careful scrutiny. Of interest, here, is that the rate of propulsion of middle ear mucus on a frog palate system varies with the degree of sulfation, the more highly sulfated product being less briskly transported when reconstituted at physiological concentrations (284).

CF airway mucus also has an increased content of lipids (109). Quantitative changes are reported (285), but all seem to be related to the fatty acid deficiencies common in CF subjects or to chronic infection and injury to the airways (109). There is little to suggest that lipid abnormalities play a primary role in the pathogenesis of CF pulmonary disease. However, the tendency of CF mucins, as compared with those from asthmatic subjects, to aggregate (286) could be the result of higher lipid content, which was not measured in this study.

Fucosidosis

Frequent respiratory tract infections are characteristic of children who have deficient levels of α-L-fucosidase (287). Mucus from the middle ear of these children is watery and has low elasticity, characteristics that are unfavorable for mucociliary clearance. The question raised is whether or not these patients are able to modify fucose-containing glycoconjugates in respiratory secretions. Analytical data pertinent to this question are not available.

References

1. Boat, T. F., and Cheng, P. W. (1980). Biochemistry of airway mucus secretions. *Fed. Proc.* 39: 3067–3074.
2. Miller, D. L., and Jones, R. (1963). A study of techniques for the examination of sputum in a field survey of chronic bronchitis. *Am. Rev. Respir. Dis.* 88: 473–483.
3. Burgi, H., Wiesmann, U., Richterich, R., Regli, J., and Medici, T. (1968). New objective criteria for inflammation in bronchial secretion. *Br. Med. J.* 2: 654–656.
4. Sachdev, G. P., Chace, K. V., Leahy, D. S., and Flux, M. (1982). Studies on the relationship of levels of DNA and gamma-glutamyltranspeptidase activity in bronchial secretions of patients with cystic fibrosis with the degree of severity of disease. *Chest* 81S: 41–43.
5. Lopez-Vidriero, M. T., Das, I., Smith, P., Picot, R., and Reid, L. (1977). Bronchial secretion from normal human airways after inhalation of prostaglandin $F_{2\alpha}$, acetylcholine, histamine, and citric acid. *Thorax* 32: 734–739.
6. Matthews, L. M., Spector, S., Lemm, J., and Potter, J. L. (1963). Studies on pulmonary secretions. *Am. Rev. Respir. Dis.* 88: 199–204.

7. Bhaskar, K. R., O'Sullivan, D. D., Seltzer, J., Rossing, T. H., Drazen, J. M., and Reid, L. M. (1985). Density gradient study of bronchial mucus aspirates from healthy volunteers (smokers and nonsmokers) and from patients with tracheostomy. *Exp. Lung Res.* 9: 289–308.

8. Rennard, S., Basset, G., Lecoissier, D., O'Donnell, K., Martin, P., and Crystal, R. G. (1986). Estimation of volume of epithelial lining fluid recovered by lavage using urea as a marker of dilution. *J. Appl. Physiol.* 60: 532–538.

9. Van de Graaf, E. A., Jansen, H. M., Weber, J. A., Koolen, M. G. J., and Out, T. A. (1991). Influx of urea during bronchoalveolar lavage depends on the permeability of the respiratory membrane. *Clin. Chim. Acta.* 196: 27–40.

10. Rennard, S. I., Ghafouri, M., Thompson, A. B., Linder, J., Vaughan, W., Jones, J., Ertle, R. F., Christensen, K., Prince, A., Stahl, M. G., and Robbins, R. A. (1990). Fractional processing of sequential bronchoalveolar lavage to separate bronchial and alveolar samples. *Am. Rev. Respir. Dis.* 141: 208–217.

11. Jeanneret-Grosjean, A., King, M., Michoud, M. C., Liote, H., and Amyot, R. (1988). Sampling technique and rheology of human tracheobronchial mucus. *Am. Rev. Respir. Dis.* 137: 707–710.

12. Mentz, W. M., Brown, J. B., Friedman, M., Stutts, J., Gatzy, J. T., and Boucher, R. C. (1986). Deposition, clearance and effects of amiloride in sheep airways. *Am. Rev. Respir. Dis.* 134: 938–943.

13. Wardell, J. R., Chakrin, L. W., and Payne, B. J. (1970). The canine tracheal pouch. *Am. Rev. Respir. Dis.* 101: 741–754.

14. Gallagher, J. T., Kent, P. W., Passatore, M., Phipps, R. J., and Richardson, P. S. (1975). The composition of tracheal mucus and the nervous control of its secretion in the cat. *Proc. R. Soc. Lond.* 192: 49–76.

15. Ellis, D. B., and Stahl, G. H. (1973). Biosynthesis of respiratory tract mucins: Incorporation of radioactive precursors into glycoproteins by canine tracheal explants in vitro. *Biochem. J.* 136: 837–844.

16. Boat, T. F., Kleinerman, J. I., Carlson, D. M., Maloney, W. H., and Matthews, L. W. (1974). Human respiratory tract secretions. 1. Mucous glycoproteins secreted by cultured nasal polyp epithelium from subjects with allergic rhinitis and with cystic fibrosis. *Am. Rev. Respir. Dis.* 110: 428–441.

17. Boat, T. F., and Kleinerman, J. I. (1975). Human respiratory tract secretions. 2. Effect of cholinergic and adrenergic agents on in vitro release of protein and mucous glycoprotein. *Chest* 67: 32S–34S.

18. Gallagher, J. T., and Kent, P. W. (1975). Structure and metabolism of glycoproteins and glycosaminoglycans secreted by organ cultures of rabbit trachea. *Biochem. J.* 148: 187–196.

19. Tandler, B., Sherman, J., and Boat, T. F. (1981). EDTA-mediated separation of cat tracheal lining epithelium. *Am. Rev. Respir. Dis.* 124: 469–475.

20. Sherman, J. M., Cheng, P. W., Tandler, B., and Boat, T. F. (1981). Mucous glycoproteins from cat tracheal goblet cells and mucous glands separated with EDTA. *Am. Rev. Respir. Dis.* 124: 476–479.

21. Wu, R., Groekle, J. W., Chang, L. Y., Porter, M. E., Smith, D., and Nettesheim, P. (1982). Effects of hormones on the multiplication and differentiation of tracheal

epithelial cells in culture. In *Cold Spring Harbor Conferences on Cell Proliferation*, Vol. 9. Cold Spring Harbor, N.Y., Cold Spring Harbor Press, p. 641.

22. Wu, R., Nolan, E., and Turner, C. (1985). Expression of tracheal differentiated functions in serum-free hormone supplemented medium. *J. Cell. Physiol.* 125: 167–181.

23. Gruenert, D. C., Basbaum, C. B., Welsh, M. J., Li, M., Finkbeiner, W. E., and Nadel, J. A. (1988). Characterization of human tracheal epithelial cells transformed by an origin-defective simian virus 40. *Proc. Natl. Acad. Sci. USA* 85: 5951–5955.

24. Finkbeiner, W. E., Nadel, J. A., and Basbaum, C. B. (1986). Establishment and characterization of a cell line derived from bovine tracheal glands. *In Vitro* 22: 561–567.

25. Cheng, P. W., Boat, T. F., Cranfill, K., Yankaskas, J. R., and Boucher, R. C. (1989). Increased sulfation of glycoconjugates by cultured nasal epithelial cells from patients with cystic fibrosis. *J. Clin. Invest.* 84: 68–72.

26. Kim, K. C. (1991). Biochemistry and pharmacology of mucin-like glycoproteins produced by cultured airway epithelial cells. *Exp. Lung Res.* 17: 533–545.

27. Adler, K. B., Cheng, P. W., and Kim, K. C. (1990). Characterization of guinea pig tracheal epithelial cells maintained in biphasic organotypic culture: Cellular composition and biochemical analysis of released glycoconjugates. *Am. J. Respir. Cell. Mol. Biol.* 2: 145–154.

28. Wu, R., Plopper, C. G., and Cheng, P. W. (1991). Mucin-like glycoprotein secreted by cultured hamster tracheal epithelial cells. *Biochem. J.* 277: 713–718.

29. Cheng, P. W. (1991). Unpublished observation.

30. Ryley, H. C., and Brogan, T. D. (1968). Variation in the composition of sputum in chronic chest diseases. *J. Exp. Pathol.* 49: 625–633.

31. Boat, T. F., and Matthews, L. W. (1973). Chemical composition of human tracheo-bronchial secretions. In *Sputum*. Edited by M. J. Dulfano. Springfield, Ill., Charles C Thomas, pp. 243–274.

32. Boat, T. F., Cheng, P. W., Iyer, R. N., Carlson, D. M., and Polony, I. (1976). Human respiratory tract secretions: Mucous glycoproteins of nonpurulent tracheobronchial secretions and sputum of patients with bronchitis and cystic fibrosis. *Arch. Biochem. Biophys.* 177: 95–104.

33. Feldhoff, P. A., Bhavanandan, V. P., and Davidson, E. A. (1979). *Biochemistry* 18: 2430–2436.

34. Houdret, N., Lamblin, G., Scharfman, A., Humbert, P., and Roussel, P. (1983). Activation of bronchial mucin proteolysis by 4-aminophenylmercuric acetate and disulfide bond reducing agents. *Biochim. Biophys. Acta* 758: 24–29.

35. Shankar, V., Naziruddin, B., de la Rocha, S. R., and Sachdev, G. (1990). Evidence of hydrophobic domains in human respiratory mucins. Effect of sodium chloride on hydrophobic binding properties. *Biochemistry* 29: 5856–5864.

36. Cheng, P. W., Boucher, R. C., Yankaskas, J. M., and Boat, T. F. (1988). Glycoconjugates secreted by cultured human nasal epithelial cells. In: *Cellular and Molecular Basis of Cystic Fibrosis*. Edited by G. Mastella and P. M. Quinton. San Francisco, San Francisco Press, pp. 233–238.

37. Rose, M. C., Lynn, W. S., and Kaufman, B. (1979). Resolution of the major

components of human lung mucosal gel and their capabilities for reaggregation and gel formation. *Biochemistry* 18: 4030–4037.

38. Peacock, A. C., and Dingman, C. W. (1968). Molecular weight estimation and separation of ribonucleic acid by electrophoresis in agarose-acrylamide composite gels. *Biochemistry* 2: 668–674.

39. Reasor, M. J., Adams, G. K., Proctor, D. F., and Rubin, R. J. (1978). Tracheo-bronchial secretions collected from intact dogs. I. Protein and mucous glycoprotein composition. *J. Appl. Physiol.* 45: 182–189.

40. Potter, J. L., Matthews, L. W., Spector, S., and Lemm, J. (1967). Studies on pulmonary secretions. 2. Osmolality and ionic environment of pulmonary secretions from patients with cystic fibrosis, bronchiectasis, and laryngectomy. *Am. Rev. Respir. Dis.* 96: 83–87.

41. Quinton, P. M. (1979). Composition and control of secretions from tracheobronchial submucosal glands: Implications in cystic fibrosis. *Nature* 279: 551–552.

42. Verdugo, P. (1991). Mucin exocytosis. *Am. Rev. Respir. Dis.* 144: S33–S37.

43. Boucher, R. C., Willumsen, N. J., Knowles, M. R., Yankaskas, J., and Gatzy, J. T. (1988). Na^+ and Cl^- absorption in respiratory epithelia: The role of apical and basolateral membranes. In *Cellular and Molecular Basis of Cystic Fibrosis.* Edited by G. Mastella and P. M. Quinton. San Francisco, San Francisco Press, pp. 107–114.

44. Gatto, L. A. (1981). pH of mucus in rat trachea. *J. Appl. Physiol.* 50: 1224–1226.

45. Gatto, L. A. (1985). pH of mucus in rabbit trachea. Cholinergic stimulation and block. *Lung* 163: 109–115.

46. Lutz, R. J., Litt, M., and Chakrin, L. W. (1973). Physical-chemical factors in mucus rheology. In *Rheology of Biological Systems.* Edited by H. L. Gabelnick. Springfield, Ill., Charles C Thomas, pp. 119–157.

47. Sachdev, G. P., Meyers, F. J., Horton, F. O., Fox, O. F., Wen, G., Rogers, R. M., and Carubelli, R. (1980). Isolation, chemical composition and properties of the major component of normal human tracheobronchial secretions. *Biochem. Med.* 24: 82–94.

48. Bhaskar, K. R., Drazen, J. M., O'Sullivan, D. D., Scanlon, P. M., and Reid, L. M. (1988). Transition from normal to hypersecretory bronchial mucus in a canine model of bronchitis: Changes in yield and composition. *Exp. Lung Res.* 14: 101–120.

49. Bhaskar, K. R., O'Sullivan, D. D., Opaskar-Hincman, H., Reid, L. M., and Coles, S. J. (1986). Density gradient analysis of secretions produced in vitro by human and canine airway mucosa. *Exp. Lung Res.* 10: 401–422.

50. Spicer, S. S., Schulte, B. A., and Chakrin, L. W. (1983). Ultrastructural and histochemical observations of respiratory epithelium and gland. *Exp. Lung Res.* 4: 137–156.

51. Stahl, G. H., and Ellis, D. B. (1973). Biosynthesis of respiratory tract mucins: A comparison of canine epithelial goblet cell and submucosal gland secretions. *Biochem. J.* 163: 845–850.

52. Spicer, S. S., Chakrin, L. W., Wardell, J. R., and Kendrick, W. (1971). Histochemistry of mucosubstances in the canine and human respiratory tract. *Lab. Invest.* 25: 483–490.

53. Leigh, M. W., Cheng, P. W., and Boat, T. F. (1989). Developmental changes of ferret tracheal mucin composition and biosynthesis. *Biochemistry* 28: 9440–9446.

54. Chace, K. V., Leahy, D. S., Martin, R., Carubelli, R., Flux, M., and Sachdev, G. P. (1983). Respiratory mucous secretions in patients with cystic fibrosis: Relationship between levels of highly sulfated mucin component and severity of the disease. *Clin. Chim. Acta* 132: 143–155.

55. Sahu, S., and Lynn, W. S. (1978). Hyaluronic acid in the pulmonary secretions of patients with asthma. *Biochem. J.* 173: 565–568.

56. Lagunoff, D., Phillps, M. T., Iseri, O. A., and Benditt, E. P. (1964). *Lab. Invest.* 13: 1331–1344.

57. Rahmoune, H., Lamblin, G., Lafitte, J., Galabert, C., Filliat, M., and Roussel, P. (1991). Chondroitin sulfate in sputum from patients with cystic fibrosis and chronic bronchitis. *Am. J. Respir. Cell Mol. Biol.* 5: 315–320.

58. Boat, T. F., Boat, A. C., Cheng, P. W., and Leigh, M. W. (1988). Identification of glycoconjugates secreted by rabbit tracheal surface epithelium. *Am. Rev. Respir. Dis.* 137: A8, 1988.

59. Skinner, S. J. M., Post, M., Torday, J. S., Stiles, A. D., and Smith, B. T. (1987). Characterization of proteoglycans synthesized by fetal rat lung type II pneumocytes in vitro and the effects of cortisol. *Exp. Lung Res.* 12: 253–264.

60. Basbaum, C. B., Jany, B., and Finkbeiner, W. E. (1990). The serous cell. *Annu. Rev. Physiol.* 52: 97–113.

61. Kim, K. C., Opaskar-Hincman, H., and Bhaskar, K. R. (1989). Secretions from primary hamster tracheal surface epithelial cells in culture: Mucin-like glycoproteins, proteoglycans and lipids. *Exp. Lung Res.* 15: 299–314, 1989.

62. Escudier, E., Forsberg, L. S., and Basbaum, C. B. (1988). Chondroitin sulfate is a secretory product of tracheal gland serous cells in vivo as well as in culture. *J. Cell Biol.* 105: 330a (Abstr).

63. Boat, T. F., Cheng, P., Caterson, B., Johnstone, B., and Leigh, M. (1992). Proteoglycan secretory components of surface epithelial cells in postnatal ferret trachea. *Chest* 101: 10S (Abstr).

64. Varsano, S., Basbaum, C. B., Forsberg, L. S., Borson, D. B., Caughey, G., and Nadel, J. A. (1987). Dog tracheal epithelial cells in culture synthesize sulfated macromolecular glycoconjugates and release them from the cell surface upon exposure to extracellular proteinases. *Exp. Lung Res.* 13: 157–184.

65. Thompson, A. B., Bohling, T., Payvandi, F., and Rennard, S. I. (1990). Lower respiratory tract lactoferrin and lysozyme arise primarily in the airways and are elevated in associated with chronic bronchitis. *J. Lab. Clin. Med.* 115: 148–158.

66. Hinnrasky, J., Chevillard, M., and Puchelle, E. (1990). Immunocytochemical demonstration of quantitative differences of lysozyme in human airways secretory granule phenotypes. *Biol. Cell* 68: 239–243.

67. Tom-May, M., Basbaum, C. B., and Nadel, J. A. (1983). Localization and release of lysozyme from ferret trachea: Effects of adrenergic and cholinergic drugs. *Cell Tissue Res.* 228: 549–562.

68. Leigh, M. W., Cheng, P. W., and Boat, T. F. (1988). Regional differences in lysozyme and high MW glycoconjugate release by ferret tracheas. *Am. Rev. Respir. Dis.* 137: 8 (Abst.)

69. Singh, G., Katyal, S. L., Brown, W. E., Collins, D. L., and Mason, R. J. (1988).

Pulmonary lysozyme—a secretory protein of type II pneumocytes in the rat. *Am. Rev. Respir. Dis.* 138: 1261–1267.

70. Franklin, C., Meijer, C. J. L. M., and Dijkman, J. H. (1989). Tissue distribution of antileukoprotease and lysozyme in humans. *J. Histochem. Cytochem.* 37: 493–498.

71. Konstan, M. W., Cheng, P. W., Sherman, J. M., Thomassen, M. J., Wood, R. E., and Boat, T. F. (1981). Human lung lysozyme: Sources and properties. *Am. Rev. Respir. Dis.* 123: 120–124.

72. Konstan, M. W., Cheng, P. W., and Boat, T. F. (1982). A comparative study of lysozyme and its secretion by tracheal epithelium. *Exp. Lung Res.* 3: 175–181.

73. Creeth, J. M., Bridge, J. L., and Horton, J. R. (1979). An interaction between lysozyme and mucus glycoproteins. *Biochem. J.* 181: 717–724.

74. Bowes, D., Clark, A. E., and Corrin, B. (1981). Ultrastructural localization of lactoferrin and glycoprotein in human bronchial glands. *Thorax* 36: 108–115.

75. Masson, P. L., and Heremans, J. F. (1966). Studies on lactoferrin, the iron-binding protein of secretions. *Protides Biol. Fluids* 14: 115–124.

76. Briggs, R. C., Glass, W. F., Montiel, M. M., and Hnilica, L. S. (1981). Lactoferrin: Nuclear localization in the human neutrophilic granulocyte. *J. Histochem. Cytochem.* 29: 1128–1136.

77. Clamp, J. R., and Creeth, J. (1984). Some non-mucin components of mucus and their possible biological roles. In *Mucous and Mucosa.* Edited by J. Nugent and M. O'Connor, London, Pitman, pp. 121–136.

78. Christensen, T. G., and Hayes, J. A. (1982). Endogenous peroxidase in the conducting airways of hamsters. *Am. Rev. Respir. Dis.* 125: 341–346.

79. Goodman, M. R., Link, D. W., Brown, W. R., and Nakane, P. K. (1981). Ultrastructural evidence of transport of secretory IgA across bronchial epithelium.

80. Stockley, R. A., Afford, S. C., and Burnett, D. (1980). Assessment of 7S and 11S immunoglobulin A in sputum. *Am. Rev. Respir. Dis.* 22: 959–964.

81. Fiedler, M. A., Kaetzel, C. S., and Davis, P. B. (1991). Sustained production of secretory component by human tracheal epithelial cells in primary culture. *Am. J. Physiol.* 5: L255–L261.

82. Takemura, T., and Eishi, Y. (1985). Distribution of secretory component and immunoglobulins in the developing lung. *Am. Rev. Respir. Dis.* 131: 125–130.

83. Kramps, J. A., Franken, C., and Dijkman, J. H. (1984). ELISA for quantitative measurement of low molecular weight bronchial protease inhibitor in human sputum. *Am. Rev. Respir. Dis.* 129: 959–963.

84. Warner, T. F., and Azen, E. A. (1984). Proline-rich proteins are present in serous cells of submucosal glands in the respiratory tract. *Am. Rev. Respir. Dis.* 130: 115–118.

85. Tesfaigzi, J., An, G., Wu, R., and Carlson, D. M. (1990). Induction in the expression of an unusual proline-rich protein by pig tracheal surface epithelial cells maintained in primary culture. *Biochem. Biophys. Res. Commun.* 172: 1304–1309.

86. Bailleul, V., Richet, C., Hayem, A., and Degand, P. (1977). Properties rheologiques des secretions bronchiques: Mise en evidence et role de polypeptides riches en proline (PRP). *Clin. Chim. Acta* 74: 115–123.

87. Singh, G., and Katyal, S. L. (1991). Pulmonary proteins as cell-specific markers. *Exp. Lung Res.* 17: 245–253.

88. Bedetti, C. D., Singh, J., Singh, G., Katyal, S. L., and Wong-Chong, M. L. (1987). Ultrastructural localization of rat Clara cell 10KD secretory protein by the immunogold technique using polyclonal and monoclonal antibodies. *J. Histochem. Cytochem.* 35: 789–794.

89. Patton, S. E., Gilmore, L. B., Jetten, A. M., Nettesheim, P., and Hook, G. E. R. (1986). Biosynthesis and release of proteins by isolated pulmonary Clara cells. *Exp. Lung Res.* 11: 277–294.

90. Phelps, D. S., and Floros, J. (1988). Localization of surfactant synthesis in human lung by in situ hybridization. *Am. Rev. Respir. Dis.* 137: 939–942.

91. Khoor, A., Gray, M. E., Benn, S., and Stahlman, M. T. (1991). Expression of surfactant protein A (SP-A) gene in the developing human respiratory system as detected by in situ hybridization. *Pediatr. Res.* 29: 322A.

91a. Khoor, A., Gray, M. E., and Stahlman, M. T. (1992). Differential expression of surfactant protein B (SP-B) and C (SP-C) genes in the developing human lung epithelium. *Pediatr. Res.* 31: 312A.

92. Floros, J., Phelps, D. S., Harding, H. P., Church, S., and Ware, J. (1989). Postnatal stimulation of rat surfactant protein A synthesis by dexamethasone. *Am. J. Physiol.* 257: L137–L143.

93. Wasano, K., and Yamamoto, T. (1989). Rat lung 29 kd beta-galactoside-binding lectin is secreted by bronchiolar Clara cells into airways. *Histochemistry* 90: 447–451.

94. Jacquot, J., Dupuit, F., Elbtaouri, H., Hiunrasky, J., Antonicelli, F., Haye, B., and Puchelle, E. (1990). Production of lipocortin-like proteins by cultured human tracheal submucosal gland cells. *FEBS Lett.* 274: 131–135.

95. Lundgren, J. D., Hirata, F., Marom, Z., Logun, C., Steel, L., Kaliner, M., and Shelhamer, J. (1988). Dexamethasone inhibits respiratory glycoconjugate secretion from feline airways in vitro by the induction of lipocortin synthesis. *Am. Rev. Respir. Dis.* 137: 353–357.

96. Diamond, G., Zasloff, M., Eck, H., Brasseur, M., Maloy, W. L., and Bevins, C. L. (1991). Tracheal antimicrobial peptide, a cysteine-rich peptide from mammalian tracheal mucosa. *Proc. Natl. Acad. Sci. USA* 88: 3952–3956.

97. Radhakrishnamurthy, B., Smart, F., Berenson, G. S., and Rogers, W. R. (1983). The composition of glycoproteins and activities of glycosidases in bronchoalveolar lavages from smoking baboons. *Lung* 161: 165–172.

98. Hayem, A., Scharfman, A., Laine, A., Lafitte, J. J., and Sablonniere, B. (1980). Proteases and antiproteases in bronchoalveolar lavage. *Bull. Eur. Physiopathol. Respir.* 16S: 247–258.

99. Burnett, D., Crocker, J., and Stockley, R. A. (1983). Cathepsin B-like cysteine proteinase activity in sputum and immunhistologic identification of cathepsin B in alveolar macrophages. *Am. Rev. Respir. Dis.* 128: 915–919.

100. Stockley, R. A., Mistry, M., Bradwell, A. R., and Burnett, D. A. (1979). A study of plasma proteins in the sol phase of sputum from patients with chronic bronchitis. *Thorax* 34: 777–782.

101. Stockley, R. A. (1984). Measurement of soluble proteins in lung secretions. *Thorax* 39: 241–247.

102. Webber, S. E., and Widdicombe, J. G. (1989). The transport of albumin across the ferret in vitro whole trachea. *J. Physiol.* 408: 457–472.

103. Price, A. M., Webber, S. E., and Widdicombe, J. G. (1990). Transport of albumin by the rabbit trachea in vitro. *J. Appl. Physiol.* 68: 726–730.

104. List, S. J., Findlay, B. P., Forstner, G. G., and Forstner, J. F. (1978). Enhancement of the viscosity of mucin by serum albumin. *Biochem. J.* 175: 565–571.

105. Opaskar-Hineman, H., Bhaskar, K. R., O'Sullivan, D. D., Brown, R., and Reid, L. (1990). Lipids in airway mucus of acute quadriplegic patients. *Exp. Lung Res.* 16: 369–285.

106. Woodward, H., Horsey, B., Bhavanandan, V. P., and Davidson, E. A. (1982). Isolation, purification, and properties of respiratory mucus glycoproteins. *Biochemistry* 21: 694–701.

107. Hansson, G. C., Sheehan, J. K., and Carlstedt, I. (1988). Only trace amounts of fatty acids are found in pure mucus glycoproteins. *Arch. Biochem. Biophys.* 266: 197–200.

108. Slomiany, A., Slomiany, B. L., Witas, H., Aono, M., and Newman, L. J. (1983). Isolation of fatty acids covalently bound to the gastric mucus glycoprotein of normal and cystic fibrosis patients. *Biochem. Biophys. Res. Commun.* 113: 286–293.

109. Houdret, N., Perini, J. M., Galabert, C., Scharfman, A., Humbert, P., Lamblin, G., and Roussel, P. (1986). The high lipid content of respiratory mucins in cystic fibrosis is related to infection. *Biochim. Biophys. Acta* 880: 54–61.

110. Spiro, R. G. (1973). Glycoproteins. *Adv. Protein Chem.* 27: 349–367.

111. Sweeley, C. C., Fung, Y. K., Macher, B. A., Moskal, J. R., and Nenez, H. A. (1978). Structure and metabolism of glycolipids. In *Glycoproteins and Glycolipids in Disease Processes.* Edited by E. J. Walborg, Jr. *ACS Symp. Ser.* 80: 47–85.

112. Kjellen, L., and Lindahl, U. (1991). Proteoglycans: Structures and interactions. *Annu. Rev. Biochem.* 60: 443–475.

113. Kim, K. C., Rearick, J. I., Nettlesheim, P., and Jetten, A. M. (1985). Biochemical characterization of mucous glycoproteins synthesized and secreted by hamster tracheal epithelial cells in primary culture. *J. Biol. Chem.* 260: 4021–4027.

114. Rearick, J. I., Deas, M., and Jetten, A. M. (1987). Synthesis of mucous glycoproteins by rabbit tracheal cells in vitro: Modulation by substratum retinoids and cyclic AMP. *Biochem. J.* 242: 19–25.

115. Roussel, P., Lamblin, G., Lhermitte, M., Houdret, N., Lafitte, J. J., Perini, J. M., Kelin, A., and Scharfman, A. (1988). The complexity of mucins. *Biochimie* 70: 1471–1482.

116. Jetten, A. M., Yankaskas, J. R., Stutts, M. J., Willumsen, N. J., and Boucher, R. C. (1984). Persistence of abnormal chloride conductance regulation in transformed cystic fibrosis epithelia. *Science* 244: 1472–1475.

117. Scholte, B. J., Kansen, M., Hoogeveen, A. T., Willemse, R., Shim, J. S., Tan Der Kamp, A. W. M., and Bigman, J. (1989). Immortalization of nasal polyp epithelial cells from cystic fibrosis patients. *Exp. Cell Res.* 182: 559–571.

118. McCool, D. J., Marcon, M. A., Forstner, J. F., and Forstner, G. G. (1990). The T-84

human colonic adenocarcinoma cell line produces mucin in culture and releases it in response to various secretagogues. *Biochem. J.* 267: 491–500.

119. Jentoft, N., Shogren, R. L., Jamieson, A. M., Blackwell, J., and Jentoft, J. E. (1985). Gel filtration of pig submaxillary mucin. In *Proceedings of the VIIIth International Symposium of Glycoconjugates*. Houston, Texas 1: 55.

120. Genderler, S., Taylor-Papadimitriou, J., Duhig, T., Rothbard, J., and Burchell, J. (1988). A highly immunogenic region of a human polymorphic epithelial mucin expressed by carcinomas is made up of tandem repeats. *J. Biol. Chem.* 263: 12820–12823.

121. Bhaskar, K. R., and Reid, L. (1981). Application of density gradient methods for the study of mucus glycoprotein and other macromolecular components of the sol and gel phase of asthmatic sputa. *J. Biol. Chem.* 256: 7583–7589.

122. Carlstedt, I., Sheehan, J. K., Corfield, A. P., and Gallagher, J. T. (1985). Mucous glycoproteins: A gel of a problem. *Essays Biochem.* 20: 40–76.

123. Hill, H. D., Reynolds, J. A., and Hill, R. L. (1977). Purification, composition, molecular weight, and subunit structure of ovine submaxillary mucin. *J. Biol. Chem.* 252: 3791–3798.

124. Allen, A. (1978). Structure of gastrointestinal mucus glycoproteins and the viscous and gel-forming properties of mucus. In *Mucus*. Edited by J. R. Clamp. *Br. Med. Bull.* 34(1): 28–33.

125. Holden, K. G., Kim, N. C. F., Griggs, L. J., and Weisbach, J. A. (1971). Gel electrophoresis of mucous glycoproteins. I. Effect of gel porosity. *Biochemistry* 10: 3105–3109.

126. Holden, K. G., Kim, N. C. F., Griggs, L. J., and Weisbach, J. A. (1971). Gel electrophoresis of mucous glycoproteins. II. Effect of physical deaggregation and disulfide-bond cleavage. *Biochemistry* 10: 3110–3113.

127. Cheng, P. W., Sherman, J. M., Boat, T. F., and Bruce, M. (1981). Quantitation of radiolabeled mucous glycoproteins secreted by tracheal explants. *Anal. Biochem.* 117: 301–306.

128. Gum, J. R., Byrd, J. C., Hicks, J. W., Toribara, N. W., Lamport, D. T., and Kim, Y. S. (1989). Molecular cloning of human intestinal mucin cDNAs: Sequence analysis and evidence for genetic polymorphism. *J. Biol. Chem.* 264: 6480–6487.

129. Timpte, C. S., Eckhardt, A. E., Abernethy, J. L., and Hill, R. L. (1988). Porcine submaxillary gland apomucin contains tandemly repeated identical sequence of 81 residues. *J. Biol. Chem.* 263: 1081–1088.

130. Gerard, C., Eddy, R. L., Jr., and Shows, T. B. (1990). The core polypeptide of cystic fibrosis tracheal mucin contains a tandem repeat structure: Evidence for a common mucin in airway and gastrointestinal tissue. *J. Clin. Invest.* 86: 1921–1927.

131. Aubert, J. P., Porchet, N., Crepia, M., Duterque-Coquilland, M., Vergnes, G., Mazzuca, M., Dubuine, B., Petitprez, D., and Degand, P. (1991). Evidence for different human tracheobronchial mucin peptides deduced from nucleotide cDNA sequences. *Am. J. Respir. Cell. Mol. Biol.* 5: 178–185.

132. Roussel, P. (1985). Structure and function of lung mucins. In *Proceedings of the VIIIth International Symposium on Glycoconjugates*. Edited by E. A. Davidson, J. C. Williams, and N. M. DiFerrante. 1: 99–100.

133. Lamblin, G., Boersma, A., Lhermitte, M., Rouseel, P., Mutsaers, J. H. G. M., Van Halbeek, H., and Vliegenthart, J. F. G. (1984). Further characterization by a combined high performance liquid chromatography/^{1}H-NMR approach, of heterogeneity displayed by the neutral carbohydrate chains of human bronchial mucins. *Eur. J. Biochem.* 143: 227–236.

134. Lamblin, G., Boersma, A., Klein, A., Roussel, P., van Halbeek, H., and Vliegenhart, J. F. G. (1984). Primary structure determination of five sialylated oligosaccharides derived from bronchial mucous glycoproteins of patients suffering from cystic fibrosis. *J. Biol. Chem.* 259: 9051–9058.

135. Breg, J., VanHalbeek, H., Vliegenhart, J. F. G., Lamblin, G., Houvenaghel, M., and Roussel, P. (1987). Structure of sialyloligosaccharides isolated from bronchial mucus glycoproteins of patients (blood group O) suffering from cystic fibrosis. *Eur. J. Biochem.* 168: 57–68.

136. Klein, A., Lamblin, G., Lhermitte, M., Roussel, P., Breg, J., Van Halbeek, H., and Vliegenhart (1988). Primary structure of neutral oligosaccharides derived from respiratory mucus glycoproteins of a patient suffering from bronchiectasis, determined by a combination of 500-MHz ^{1}H-NMR spectroscopy and quantitative sugar analysis. 1. Structure of 16 oligosaccharides having the Galβ(1–3)GalNAc-ol core (type 1) or the GlcNAcβ(1–3)[ClcNAcβ(1–6)]GalNAc-ol core (type 2). *Eur. J. Biochem.* 171: 631–642.

137. Breg, J., VanHalbeek, H., Vliegenhart, J. F. G., Klein, A., Lamblin, G., and Roussel, P. (1988). Primary structure of neutral oligosaccharides derived from respiratory mucus glycoproteins of a patient suffering from bronchiectasis, determined by combination of 500 MHZ ^{1}H-NMR spectroscopy and quantitative sugar analysis. 2. Structure of 19 oligosaccharides having the GlcNAcβ(1–3)GalNAc-ol core (type 3) or the GlcNAcβ(1–3)[GlcNAcβ(1-6)]GalNAc-ol core (type 4). *Eur. J. Biochem.* 171: 643–654.

138. Klein, A., Carnoy, C., Lambin, G., Roussel, P., VanKuik, J. A., DeWaard, P., and Vliegenhart, J. G. (1991). Isolation and structural characterization of novel neutral oligosaccharide alditols from respiratory mucus glycoproteins of a patient suffering from bronchiectasis. 1. Structure of 11 oligosaccharides having the GlcNAcβ(1-3)-Galβ(1-4)GlcNAcβ(1-6)GalNAc-ol structural element in common. *Eur. J. Biochem.* 198: 151–168.

139. Van Kuik, J. A., DeWaard, P., Vliegenhart, J. F. G., Klein, A., Carnoy, C., Lamblin, G., and Roussel, P. (1991). Isolation and structural characterization of novel neutral oligosaccharide-alditols from respiratory mucus glycoproteins of a patient suffering from bronchiectasis. 2. Structure of twelve hepta-to-nonasaccharides, six of which possess the GlcNAcβ(1-3)[Galβ(1-4GlcNAcβ(1-6)]Galβ(1-3) GalNAc-ol common structural element. *Eur. J. Biochem.* 198: 169–182.

140. Boat, T. F., Cheng, P. W., and Wood, R. E. (1977). Tracheobronchial mucus secretion in vivo and in vitro by epithelial tissues from cystic fibrosis and control subjects. *Mod. Prob. Pediatr.* 19: 141–152.

141. Hascall, T., and Riolo, R. L. (1972). Characteristics of the protein-keratin sulfate prepared from bovine nasal cartilage proteoglycan. *J. Biol. Chem.* 247: 4529–4538.

142. Green, E. D., Boime, I., and Baenziger, J. U. (1986). Differential processing of Asn-linked oligosaccharides on pituitary glycoprotein hormones: Implications for biologic function. *Mol. Cell. Biochem.* 72: 81–100.

143. Carlson, D. M. (1968). Structures and immunochemical properties of oligosaccharides isolated from pig submaxillary mucins. *J. Biol. Chem.* 243: 616–621.

144. Downs, F., Herp, A., Moschera, J., and Pigman, W. (1973). β-Elimination and reduction reactions and some applications of dimethylsulfoxide on submaxillary glycoproteins. *Biochim. Biophys. Acta* 328: 182–192.

145. Torres, C. R., and Hart, G. W. (1984). Topography and polypeptide distribution of terminal *N*-acetylglucosamine residues on the surface of intact lymphocytes: Evidence for *O*-linked GlcNAc. *J. Biol. Chem.* 259: 3308–3317.

146. Hart, G. W., Holt, G. D., and Haltiwanger, R. S. (1986). Nuclear and cytoplasmic glycosylation: Novel saccharide linkages in unexpected places. *TIBS* 13: 380–384.

147. Ogata, S. I., and Lloyd, K. O. (1982). Mild alkaline borohydride treatment of glycoproteins—a method for liberating both *N*- and *O*-linked carbohydrate chains. *Anal. Biochem.* 119: 351–359.

148. Cheng, P. W. (1987). High performance liquid chromatographic analysis of galactosamine, glucosamine, glucosaminitol, and galactosaminitol. *Anal. Biochem.* 167: 256–269.

149. Hascall, V. C. (1983). Structure and biosynthesis of proteoglycans with keratin sulfate. In *Limb Development and Regeneration, Part B*. New York, Alan R. Liss, pp. 3–15.

150. Fukuda, M. (1989). Leukosialin, a major sialoglycoprotein defining leucocyte differentiation. In *Carbohydrate Recognition in Cellular Function. Ciba Found. Symp.* 145: 257–276.

151. Codington, J. F. (1978). Masking of cell surface antigens by ectoglycoproteins. In *Glycoproteins and Glycolipids in Disease Processes*. Edited by E. F. Walborg, Jr. *ACS Symp. Ser.* 80: 277–294.

152. Cheng, P. W., and DeVries, A. (1986). Mucin biosynthesis: Enzymatic properties of human tracheal epithelial GDP-Fuc:β-galactosideα1→2 fucosyltransferase. *Carbohydr. Res.* 149: 253–261.

153. Watkins, W. M. (1980). Biochemistry and genetics of the ABO, Lewis, and P blood group systems. *Adv. Hum. Genet.* 10: 1–136.

154. Watkins, W. M. (1977). The glycosyltransferase products of the A,B,H, and Le genes and their relationship to the structure of the blood group antigens. In *Human Blood Groups*. Edited by J. F. Mohn, R. W. Plunkett, R. K. Cunningham, and R. M. Lambert, Basel, S. Karger, pp. 134–142.

155. Higa, H. H., Rogers, G. N., and Paulson, J. C. (1985). Influenza virus hemagglutins differentiate between receptor determinants bearing *N*-acetyl, *N*-glycolyl, and *N,O*-diacetylneuraminic acid. *Virology* 144: 279–282.

156. Carrol, S. M., Higa, H. H., and Paulson, J. C. (1981). Different cell-surface receptor determinants of antigenically similar influenza virus hemagglutinins. *J. Biol. Chem.* 256: 8357–8363.

157. Rogers, G. N., Daniels, R. S., Skehel, J. J., Wiley, D. C., Wang, X.-F., Higa, H. H.,

and Paulson, J. C. (1985). Host-mediated selection of influenza virus receptor variants: Sialic acid α2,6Gal specific clones of A/Duck/Ukraine/1/63 revert to sialic acid α2,3Gal specific wild type in vivo. *J. Biol. Chem.* 260: 7362–7367.

158. Boat, T. F., Davis, J., Stern, R. C., and Cheng, P. W. (1979). Effect of blood group determinants on binding of human salivary mucous glycoproteins to influenza virus. *Glycoconjugate Res.* 1: 503–505.

159. Slominany, A. L., Nadziejko, C., Mizuta, K., and Slomiany, A. (1988). Role of associated and covalently bound lipids in the physicochemical properties of mucus glycoprotein. In *Cellular and Molecular Basis of Cystic Fibrosis*. Edited by G. Mastella, and P. M. Quinton. San Francisco, San Francisco Press, pp. 263–292.

160. Slomiany, A., Murty, W. L. N., Aono, M., Snyder, C. E., Herp, A., and Slomiany, B. L. (1982). Lipid composition of tracheobronchial secretions from normal individuals and patients with cystic fibrosis. *Biochim. Biophys. Acta* 710: 106–111.

161. Chandrasekaran, E. B., Rana, S. S., Davila, M., and Mendicino, J. (1984). Structures of the oligosaccharide chains in swine trachea mucin glycoproteins. *J. Biol. Chem.* 259: 12908–12914.

162. Slomiany, A., Liau, Y. H., Takagi, A., Laszewicz, W., and Slomiany, B. L. (1984). Characterization of mucus glycoprotein fatty acyltransferase from gastric mucosa. *J. Biol. Chem.* 259: 13304–13308.

163. Robertson, A. M., Mantle, M., Fahim, R. E. F., Specian, R. D., Bennick, A., Kawagishi, S., Sherman, P., and Forstner, J. F. (1989). The putative "link" glycopeptide associated with mucus glycoprotein composition and properties of preparations from the gastrointestinal tract of several animals. *Biochem. J.* 261: 637–647.

164. Gupta, R., and Jentoft, N. (1989). Subunit structure of porcine submaxillary mucin. *Biochemistry* 28: 6114–6121.

165. Ringler, N. J., Selvakumar, R., Woodward, H. D., Simet, I. M., Bhavanandan, V. P., and Davidson, E. A. (1987). Structure of canine tracheobronchial mucin glycoprotein. *Biochemistry* 26: 5322–5328.

166. Leigh, M. W., Cheng, P. W., Carson, J. L., and Boat, T. F. (1986). Developmental changes in glycoconjugate secretion by ferret tracheas. *Am. Rev. Respir. Dis.* 134: 784–790.

167. Tabachnik, N. F., Blackburn, P., and Cerami, A. (1981). Biochemical and rheological characterization of sputum mucins from a patient with cystic fibrosis. *J. Biol. Chem.* 256: 7161–7165.

168. Lethem, M. I., Cheng, P. W., Wood, R. E., and Wu, R. (1990). Infection increases the mucus glycoprotein content of lung surface fluid in cystic fibrosis patients. *Pediatr. Pulmonol.* 5(Suppl.): 233.

169. Lin, H., Carlson, D. M., St. George, J. A., Plopper, C. G., and Wu, R. (1989). An ELISA method for the quantitation of tracheal mucins from human and nonhuman primates. *Am. J. Respir. Cell. Mol. Biol.* 1: 41–48.

170. Roberts, D. D., Rose, M. C., Wang, W., Chernick, M., and Frates, R. C., Jr. (1990). Isolation and characterization of mucin from the serum of cystic fibrosis patients. *Am. J. Respir. Cell Mol. Biol.* 2: 373–379.

171. Phipps, R. J., Nadel, J. A., and Davis, B. (1980). Effect of alpha-adrenergic

stimulation on mucus secretion and on ion transport in cat trachea in vitro. *Am. Rev. Respir. Dis.* 12: 359–365.

172. Mossman, B. T., Adler, K. B., Jean, L., and Craighead, J. E. (1982). Mechanisms of hypersecretion in rodent tracheal explants after exposure to chrysotile asbestos. *Chest* 81: 235–245.

173. Marom, Z., Shelhammer, J. H., and Kaliner, M. (1985). Human monocyte-derived mucus secretogogue. *J. Clin. Invest.* 75: 191–198.

174. Marom, Z., Shelhammer, J. H., Sun, F., and Kaliner, M. (1983). Human airway monohydroxyeicosatetraenoic acid generation and mucus release. *J. Clin. Invest.* 72: 122–127.

175. Estep, J. A., Zorn, J. P., and Marin, M. G. (1981). Kinetics of sulfated mucous glycoprotein secretion in dog trachea in vitro. *J. Appl. Physiol. Respir. Environ. Exer. Physiol.* 50: 383–391.

176. Schachter, H. (1978). Glycoprotein biosynthesis. In *The Glycoconjugates*. Edited by M. Horowitz and W. Pigman. New York, Academic Press, 11: 87–181.

177. Schachter, H., and Roden, L. (1973). The biosynthesis of animal glycoproteins. In *Metabolic Conjugation and Metabolic Hydrolysis*. Edited by W. H. Fishman. New York, Academic press, 3: 1–149.

178. Boat, T. E. (1982). Quantitation of mucous glycoprotein secretion by airways epithelium. *Chest* 81: 29S–31S.

179. Sarcione, E. J. (1964). The initial subcellular site of incorporation of hexose into liver protein. *J. Biol. Chem.* 239: 1686–1689.

180. Richmond, J. E. (1965). Role of sugar nucleotides in the incorporation of sugars into glycoproteins. *Biochemistry* 4: 1834–1839.

181. Moscarello, M. A., Kashupa, L., and Sturgess, J. M. (1972). The incorporation of [^{14}C]galactose and [^{3}H]mannose into Golgi fractions of rat liver and into serum. *FEBS Lett.* 26: 87–91.

182. Mitranic, M., and Moscarello, M. A. (1972). The conversion of mannose-^{3}H to protein bound sialic acid, fucose, galactose and hexosamines in rat serum. *Biochem. Biophys. Res. Commun.* 47: 74–80.

183. Whur, P., Herscovics, A., and Leblond, C. P. (1969). Radiographic visualization of the incorporation of galactose-^{3}H and mannose-^{3}H by rat thyroids in vitro in relation to the stages of thyroglobulin synthesis. *J. Cell Biol.* 43: 289–311.

184. Sturgess, J. M., Minaker, E., Mitranic, M. M., and Moscarello, M. A. (1973). The incorporation of L-fucose into glycoproteins in the Golgi apparatus of rat liver and in serum. *Biochim. Biophys. Acta* 320: 123–132.

185. White, B. N., Shetlar, M. R., Shurley, H. M., and Shilling, J. A. (1965). Incorporation of D-[1-^{14}C]galactosamine into serum proteins and tissues of the rat. *Biochim. Biophys. Acta* 101: 259–266.

186. Gan, J. C. (1975). Metabolism of D-mannosamine in bovine thyroid gland slices. *Biochim. Biophys. Acta* 385: 412–420.

187. Manaco, F., and Robbins, J. (1973). Incorporation of N-acetylmannosamine and N-acetylglucosamine into thyroglobulin in rat thyroid in vitro. *J. Biol. Chem.* 248: 2072–2077.

188. Iwamoto, I., Nadel, J. A., Varsano, S., and Forsberg, L. S. (1988). Turnover of cell-surface macromolecules in cultured dog tracheal epithelial cells. *Biochim. Biophys. Acta* 966: 336–346.

189. Cheng, P. W., Leigh, M. W., Kylander, J., and Boat, T. F. (1992). Mucin quantitation by enzyme-linked lectin assay (ELLA). *Am. Rev. Respir. Dis.* 145: A370.

190. Edge, A. S., Faltynek, C. R., Hof, L., Reichert, L. E., Jr., and Weber, P. (1981). Deglycosylation of glycoproteins by trifluoromethanesulfonic acid. *Anal. Biochem.* 118: 131–137.

191. Woodward, H. D., Ringler, N. J., Selvakumar, R., Simet, I. M., Bhavanandan, V. P., and Davidson, E. A. (1987). Deglycosylation studies on tracheal mucin glycoproteins. *Biochemistry* 26: 5315–5322.

192. Rana, S. S., Chandrasekaran, E. V., and Mendicino, J. (1987). Structures of the sialylated oligosaccharide chains in swine trachea mucin glycoproteins. *J. Biol. Chem.* 262: 3654–3659.

193. Sangadal, S., Kim, D., Brewer, J. M., and Mendicino, J. (1991). Subunit structure of deglycosylated human and swine trachea and Cowper's gland, mucin glycoproteins. *Mol. Cell. Biochem.* 102: 71–93.

194. Sangadal, S., Wallace, P., and Medicino, J. (1991). Characterization of mucin-glycoprotein-specific translation products from swine and human trachea, pancreas and colon. *Mol. Cell. Biochem.* 106: 1–14, p 62.

195. Rose, M. C., Kaufman, B., and Martin, B. M. (1989). Proteolytic fragmentation and peptide mapping of human carboxyamido methylated tracheobronchial mucin. *J. Biol. Chem.* 264: 8193–8199.

196. Jany, B., and Basbaum, C. B. (1991). Mucin in disease: Modification of mucin gene expression in airway disease. *Am. Rev. Respir. Dis.* 144: S38–S41.

197. Jany, B. H., Gallup, M. W., Yan, P. S., Gam, J. R., Kim, Y. S., and Basbaum, C. B. (1991). Human bronchus and intestine express the same mucin gene. *J. Clin. Invest.* 87: 77–82.

198. Prochet, N., Dufosse, J., Audie, J. P., Duperat, V. G., Perini, J. M., Cong, N. W., Degand, P., and Aubert, J. P. (1991). Structural features of the core proteins of human airway mucins ascertained by cDNA cloning. *Am. Rev. Respir. Dis.* 144: S15–S18.

199. Porchet, N., Nguyen, I. C., Dufosse, J., Audie, J. P., Guyonnet-Duperate, V., Gross, M. S., Denis, C., Degand, P., Bernheim, A., and Aubert, J. P. (1991). Molecular cloning and chromosomal localization of a novel human tracheobronchial mucin cDNA containing tandemly repeated sequence of 48 base pairs. *Biochem. Biophys. Res. Commun.* 175: 414–422.

200. Nguyen, V. C., Aubert, J. P., Gross, M. W., Porchet, N., Degand, P., and Frezal, J. (1990). Assignment of human tracheobronchial mucin gene(s) to 11P15 and a tracheobronchial mucin-related sequence to chromosome 13. *Hum. Genet.* 86: 167–172.

201. Mawhinney, T. P., Adelstein, E., Morris, D. A., Mawhinney, A. M., and Barbero, G. J. (1987). Structure determination of five sulfated oligosaccharides derived from tracheobronchial mucus glycoproteins. *J. Biol. Chem.* 262: 2994–3001.

202. Lamblin, G., Rahmoune, H., Wieruszeski, J., Lhermitte, M., Strecker, G., and

Roussel, P. (1991). Structure of two sulfated oligosaccharides from respiratory mucins of a patient suffering from cystic fibrosis. *Biochem. J.* 275: 199–206.

203. Bhattacharyya, S. N., Veit, B C., Manna, B., Enriquez, J. I., Walker, J. P., Khorrami, A. M., and Kaufman, B. (1990). Neutral and acidic human tracheo-bronchial mucin: Isolation and characterization of core protein. *Inflammation* 14: 355–373.

204. Perini, J. M., Marianne, T., Lafitte, J. J., Lamblin, G., Rouseel, P., and Mazzuca, M. (1989). Use of an antiserum against deglycosylated human mucins for cellular localization of their peptide precursors: Antigenic similarities between bronchial and intestinal mucins. *J. Histochem. Cystochem.* 37: 869–875.

205. Perini, J. M., Vandamme-Cubadda, M., Aubert, J. P., Porchet, N., Mazzuca, M., Lamblin, G., Herscovics, A., and Roussel, P. (1991). Multiple apomucin-translation products from human respiratory mucosa mRNA. *Eur. J. Biochem.* 196: 321–328.

206. Thornton, D. J., Davies, J. R., Kraayenbrink, M., Richardson, P. S., Sheehan, J. K., and Carlstedt, I. (1990). Mucus glycoproteins from normal human tracheobronchial secretion. *Biochem. J.* 265: 179–186.

207. Davies, J. R., Gallagher, J. T., Richardson, P. S., Sheehan, J. K., and Carlstedt, I. (1991). Mucins in cat airway secretions. *Biochem. J.* 275: 663–669.

208. Ringler, N. J., Selvakumar, R., Woodward, H. D., Bhavanandan, V. P., and Davidson, E. A. (1988). Protein components of human tracheobronchial mucin: Partial characterization of a closely associated 65-kilodalton protein. *J. Biol. Chem.* 27: 8056–8063.

209. Van-Seuningen, I., Houdret, N., Hayem, A., and Davril, M. (1992). Strong ionic interactions between mucins and two basic proteins, mucus proteinase inhibitor and lysozyme, in human bronchial secretions. *Int. J. Biochem.* 24: 303–311.

210. Forstner, J. F., and Forstner, G. G. (1975). Calcium binding to intestinal goblet cell mucin. *Biochim. Biophys. Acta* 386: 283–292.

211. Abeijon, C., and Hirschberg, C. B. (1987). Subcellular site of synthesis of the N-acetygalactosamine (α1-0) serine (or threonine) linkage in rat liver. *J. Biol. Chem.* 262: 4153–4159.

212. Roth, J. (1984). Cytochemical localization of terminal N-acetyl-D-galactosamine residues in cellular compartments of intestinal goblet cells: Implications for the topology of O-glycosylation. *J. Cell Biol.* 98: 399–406.

213. Schachter, H., Narasimhan, S., Gleeson, P., Vella, G., and Brockhausen, I. (1985). Glycosyltransferases involved in the biosynthesis of protein-bound oligosaccharides of the asparagine-N-acetyl-D-glucosamine and ser(threonine)-N-acetyl-D-galactos-amine types. In *The Enzymes of Biological Membranes*, Vol. 2; *Biosynthesis and Metabolism.* Edited by A. N. Martonosi. New York, Plenum Press, pp. 227–277.

214. Beyer, T. A., Sadler, J. A., Rearick, J. I., Paulson, J. C., and Hill, R. L. (1981). Glycosyltransferases and their use in assessing oligosaccharide structure and structure–function relationships. *Adv. Enzymol. Relat. Areas Mol. Biol.* 52: 22–175.

215. Barasch, J., Kiss, B., Prina, A., Saiman, L., Gruenert, D., and Al-Awqati, Q. (1991). Defective acidification of intracellular organelles in cystic fibrosis. *Nature* 352: 70–73.

216. Elhammer, A., and Kornfeld, S. (1986). Purification and characterization of UDP-N-

acetylgalactosamine: Polypeptide *N*-acetylgalactosaminyl-transferase from bovine colostrum and murine lymphoma BW5147 cells. *J. Biol. Chem.* 261: 5249–5255.

217. Sheares, B. T., and Carlson, D. M. (1983). Characterization of UDP-Gal:GlcNAcβ3-galactosyltransferase from pig trachea. *J. Biol. Chem.* 258: 9893–9898.

218. Sheares, B. T., and Carlson, D. M. (1984). Two distinct UDP-galactose:2-acetamido-2-deoxy-D-glucoseβ₄-galactosyltransferase in swine trachea. *J. Biol. Chem.* 259: 8045–8047.

219. Cheng, P. W., and Bona, S. (1982). Mucin biosynthesis: characterization of UDP-galactose:α-*N*-acetylgalactosaminide β1-3galactosyltransferase from human tracheal epithelium. *J. Biol. Chem.* 257: 6251–6258.

220. Wingert, W. E., and Cheng, P. W. (1984). Mucin biosynthesis: Characterization of rabbit small intestinal UDP-*N*-acetylglucosamine:galactose β3-*N*-acetylgalactosamine (GlcNAc→GalNAc) β6*N*-acetylglucosaminyltransferases. *Biochemistry* 23: 690–697.

221. Brockhausen, I., Williams, D., Matta, K. L., Orr, J., and Schachter, H. (1983). Mucin synthesis. III. UDP-GlcNAc:Galβ1-3 (GlcNAcβ1-6) GalNAc-*R* (GlcNAc to Gal) β3-*N*-acetylglucosaminyltransferase, an enzyme in porcine gastric mucosa involved in the elongation of mucin-type oligosaccharides. *Can. J. Biochem. Cell Biol.* 61: 1322–1333.

222. Cheng, P. W., Wingert, W. E., Little, M. R., and Wei, R. (1985). Mucin biosynthesis: Properties of a bovine tracheal mucin β6-*N*-acetylglucosaminyltransferase. *Biochem. J.* 227: 405–412.

223. Koenderman, A. H. L., Koppen, P. L., and Van den Eijuden, D. H. (1987). Biosynthesis of polylactosamino glycans: Novikoff ascites tumor cells contain two UDP-GlcNAcβ-galactoside β1→6 *N*-acetylglucosaminyltransferase activities. *Eur. J. Biochem.* 166: 199–208.

224. Van den Eijnden, D. H., Koenderman, A. H. L., and Schiphorst, W. E. C. M. (1988). Biosynthesis of blood group i-active polylactosaminoglycans: Partial purification and properties of an UDP-GlcNAc:*N*-acetyllactosaminide β1→3-*N*-acetylglucosaminyltransferase from Novikoff tumor cell ascites fluid. *J. Biol. Chem.* 263: 12461–12471.

225. Leppanen, A., Panttila, L., Niemela, R., and Renkonen, O. (1989). A novel enzyme activity involved in the synthesis of branches within liner chains of *N*-acetyllactosaminoglycans. *Proceedings of the Xth International Symposium on Glycoconjugates.* Jerusalem, Israel, September 10-15, 1989, pp. 144.

226. Ropp, P. A., Little, M. R., and Cheng, P. W. (1991). Mucin biosynthesis: Purification and characterization of a mucin β6 *N*-acetylglucosaminyltransferase. *J. Biol. Chem.* 266: 23863–23871.

227. Sadler, J. E., Rearick, J. I., Paulson, J. C., and Hill, R. L. (1979). Purification to homogeneity of a β-galactoside α2→6 sialytransferase from porcine submaxillary gland. *J. Biol. Chem.* 254: 4434–4443.

228. Sarnesto, A., Khlin, T., Hindsgaul, O., Vogele, K., Blaszcyk-Thurin, M., and Thurin, J. (1992). Purification of the β-*N*-acetylglucosaminide α1-3fucosyltransferase from human serum. *J. Biol. Chem.* 267: 2745–2752.

229. Schwyzer, M., and Hill, R. L. (1977). Porcine A blood group-specific *N*-acetyl-

galactosaminyltransferase: I. Purification from porcine submaxillary glands. *J. Biol. Chem.* 252: 2338–2345.

230. Nagai, M., Dave, W., Muensch, H., and Yoshidi, A. (1978). Human blood group glycosyltransferase: II. Purification of galactosyltransferase. *J. Biol. Chem.* 253: 380–381.

231. Cheng, P. W., Moeller, S. L., and Boat, T. F. (1980). Properties of sialyltransferase(s) in human tracheal epithelium. *Fed. Proc.* 39: 2002.

232. Hirschberg, C. B., and Snider, M. D. (1987). Topography of glycosylation in the rough endoplasmic reticulum and Golgi apparatus. *Annu. Rev. Biochem.* 56: 63–87.

233. Carter, S. R., Slomiany, A., Gwazdzinski, K., Lau, Y. H., and Slomiany, B. L. (1988). Enzymatic sulfation of mucus glycoprotein in gastric mucosa. Effect of ethanol. *J. Biol. Chem.* 263: 11977–11984.

234. Renosto, F., Martin, R. L., and Segel, I. H. (1987). ATP sulfurylase from *Penicillium chrysogenum*. Molecular basis of the sigmoidal velocity curves induced by sulfhydryl group modification. *J. Biol. Chem.* 262: 16279–16288.

235. Renosto, F., Seubert, P. A., and Segel, I. H. (1984). Adenosine 5′-phospho-sulfate from *Penicillium chrysogenum*. Purification and kinetic characterization. *J. Biol. Chem.* 259: 2113–2123.

236. Baker, A. P., Sawyer, J. L., Munro, J. R., Weimer, G. P., and Hillegass, L. M. (1972). Glycosyltransferases of canine respiratory tissue. *J. Biol. Chem.* 247: 5173–5179.

237. Baker, A. P., Griggs, L. J., Munro, J. R., and Finkelstein, J. A. (1973). Blood group A active glycoproteins of respiratory mucus and their synthesis by an N-acetylgalactosaminyltransferase. *J. Biol. Chem.* 248: 880–883.

238. Baker, A. P., Lawrence, W. C., and Wardell, J. R. Jr. (1975). Chronic cholinergic stimulation of canine respiratory tissue: Its effect on the activities of glycosyltransferases and release of macromolecules. *Am. Rev. Respir. Dis.* 111: 423–431.

239. Baker, A. P., and Sawyer, J. L. (1975). Glycosyltransferases in human respiratory tissue: Alterations in subjects with hypersecretion of mucus. *Biochem. Med.* 14: 42–50.

240. Mendicino, J., Sivakami, S., Davila, M., and Chenadrasekaran, E. V. (1982). Purification and properties of UDP-Gal:N-acetylgalactosaminide mucin $\beta1,3$-galactosyltransferase from swine trachea mucosa. *J. Biol. Chem.* 257: 3987–3994.

241. Sangadala, S., Sivakami, S., and Mendicino, J. (1991). UDP-GlcNAc:Gal3GalNAc-mucin:(GlcNAc--GalNAc)$\beta6$-N-acetylglucosaminyltransferase and UDP-GlcNAc:-Gal$\beta3$(GlcNAc$\beta6$)GalNAc-mucin(GlcNAc-Gal)$\beta3$-N-acetylglucosaminyltransferase from swine trachea epithelium. *Mol. Cell. Biochem.* 101: 125–143.

242. McGuire, E. J. (1970). In *Blood and Tissue Antigens*. Edited by D. Aminoff. New York, Academic Press, pp. 461–478.

243. Leigh, M. W., Gambling, T. M., Carson, J. C., et al. (1986). Postnatal development of tracheal surface epithelium and submucosal glands in the ferret. *Exp. Lung Res.* 10: 153–169.

244. Phipps, R. J., Abraham, W. M., Mariassy, A. T., Torrealba, P. J., Sielczak, M. W., Ahmed, A., McCray, M., Stevenson, J. S., and Wanner, A. (1989). Developmental changes in the tracheal mucociliary system in neonatal sheep. *J. Appl. Physiol.* 67: 824–832.

245. Bucher, U., and Reid, L. (1961). Development of the intrasegmental bronchial tree: The pattern of branching and development of cartilage at various stages of intrauterine life. *Thorax* 16: 207–218.

246. Bucher, U., and Reid, L. (1961). Development of the mucus-secreting elements in the human lung. *Thorax* 16: 219–225.

247. deHaller, R. (1969). Development of mucus-secreting elements. In *The Anatomy of the Developing Lung*. Edited by J. Emery. London, Heinneman Medical Books, pp. 94–115.

248. Jeffrey, P. K., and Reid, L. (1977). Ultrastructural features of airway epithelium and submucosal gland during development. In *Development of the Lung*. Edited by W. A. Hodson. New York, Marcel Dekker, Inc., pp. 87–135.

249. Gaillard, D. A., Lallement, A. V., Petit, A. F., and Puchelle, E. S. (1989). In vivo ciliogenesis in human feteal tracheal epithelium. *Am. J. Anat.* 185: 415–428.

250. Tos, M. (1966). Development of the tracheal glands in man. *Act Pathol. Microbiol. Scand.* 68(Suppl. 185): 1–130.

251. Thurlbeck, W. M., Benjamin, B., and Reid, L. (1961). Development and distribution of mucous glands in the foetal human trachea. *Br. J. Dis. Chest* 55: 54–64.

252. Sturgess, J. M. (1985). Ontogeny of the bronchial mucosa. *Am. Rev. Respir. Dis.* 131(Suppl.): S4–S7.

253. Plopper, C. G., Weir, A. J., Nishio, S. J. et al. (1986). Tracheal submucosal gland development in the rhesus monkey, *Macaca mulatta*: Ultrastructure and histochemistry. *Anat. Embryol.* 174: 167–178.

254. Boat, T. F., Kleinerman, J. I., Fanaroff, A. A., and Stern, R. C. (1977). Human tracheobronchial secretions: Development of mucous glycoprotein and lysozyme-secreting systems. *Pediatr. Res.* 11: 977–980.

255. Leigh, M. W., Cheng, P. W., and Boat, T. F. (1987). Developmental changes in lysozyme release by ferret tracheas. *Am. Rev. Respir. Dis.* 135: A35.

256. Gadek, J. E., Fells, G. A., Zimmerman, R. L., Rennard, S. I., and Crystal, R. G. (1981). Antielastases of the human alveolar structures: Implications for the protease–antiprotease theory of emphysema. *J. Clin. Invest.* 68: 889–898.

257. Bruce, M. C., Martin, R. J., and Boat, T. F. (1984). Concentrations of α_2-macroglobulin in serum and lung secretions of intubated infants. *Pediatr. Res.* 18: 35–40.

258. Takemura, T., and Eishi, Y. (1985). Distribution of secretory component and immunoglobulins in the developing lung. *Am. Rev. Respir. Dis.* 131: 125–130.

259. Huang, H., Haskell, A., and McDonald, D. M. (1989). Changes in epithelial secretory cells and potentiation of neurogenic inflammation in the trachea of rats with respiratory tract infections. *Anat. Embryol.* 180: 325–341.

260. Reid, L. (1960). Measurement of the bronchial mucus gland layer: A diagnostic yardstick in chronic bronchitis. *Thorax* 15: 132–141.

261. Koshino, T., Bhaskar, K. R., Reid, L. M., Gerard, C., Warner, A., Shore, S. A., Anderson, K., Butler, G., Iijima, H., and Drazen, J. M. (1990). Recovery of an epitope recognized by a novel monoclonal antibody from airway lavage during experimental induction of chronic bronchitis. *Am. J. Respir. Cell Mol. Biol.* 2: 453–462.

262. Lamb, D., and Reid, L. (1969). Goblet cells increase in rat bronchial epithelium after exposure to cigarette and cigar smoke. *Br. Med. J.* 1: 33–35.

263. Christensen, T. G., Korthy, A. L., Snider, G. L., and Hayes, J. A. (1977). Irreversible bronchial goblet cell metaplasia in hamsters with elastase-induced panacinar emphysema. *J. Clin. Invest.* 59: 397–404.

264. Basbaum, C., and Jany, B. (1990). Plasticity in the airway epithelium. *Am. J. Physiol.* 259: L38–L46.

265. Jany, B., Gallup, M., Tsuda, T., and Basbaum, C. (1991). Mucin gene expression in rat airways following infection and irritation. *Biochem. Biophys. Res. Commun.* 181: 1–8.

266. Leigh, M. W., Carson, J. L., Gambling, T. M., and Boat, T. F. (1992). Loss of cilia and altered phenotypic expression of ciliated cells after acute sulfur dioxide exposure. *Chest* 101: 16S (Abstr.).

267. Ramphal, R., and Pyle, M. (1983). Evidence for mucins and sialic acid as receptors for *Pseudomonas aeruginosa* in the lower respiratory tract. *Infect. Immun.* 41: 339–344.

268. Boat, T. F., Davis, J., Stern, R. C., and Cheng, P. W. (1978). Effect of blood group determinants on binding of human salivary mucous glycoproteins to influenza virus. *Biochim. Biophys. Acta* 540: 127–133.

269. Plotkowski, M. C., Chevillard, M., Pierrot, D., Altemayer, D., Zahm, J. M., Colliot, G., and Puchelle, E. (1991). Differential adhesion of *Pseudomonas aeruginosa* to human respiratory epithelial cells in primary culture. *J. Clin. Invest.* 87: 2018–2028.

270. Lundgren, J. D., and Shelhamer, J. H. (1990). Pathogenesis of airway mucus hypersecretion. *J. Allergy Clin. Immunol.* 85: 399–417.

271. Hiraishi, H., Terano, A., Ola, S., Mutoh, H., Sugimoto, T., Razandi, M., and Ivey, K. J. (1991). Oxygen metabolities stimulate mucous glycoprotein secretion from cultured rat gastric mucous cells.

272. Boat, T. F., Cheng, P. W., Klinger, J. D., Liedtke, C. M., and Tandler, B. (1984). Proteinases release mucin from airways goblet cells. *Ciba Found. Symp.* 109: 72–88.

273. Rose, M. C., Brown, C. F., Jacoby, J. Z., Lynn, W. S., and Kaufman, B. (1987). Biochemical properties of tracheobronchial mucins from cystic fibrosis and non-cystic fibrosis individuals. *Pediatr. Res.* 22: 545–551.

274. Houdret, N., Ramphal, R., Scharfman, A., Perini, J. M., Filliat, M., Lamblin, G., and Roussel, P. (1989). Evidence for the in vivo degradation of human respiratory mucins during *Pseudomonas aeruginosa* infection. *Biochim. Biophys. Acta* 992: 96–105.

275. Scharfman, A., Ramphal, R., Neut, C., Christopher, C., Lamblin, G., and Roussel, P. (1991). Arylneuraminidase activity of *Pseudomonas aeruginosa* does not degrade natural substances such as human respiratory mucins. *Infect. Immun.* 59: 4283–4285.

276. Bainbridge, T., and Fick, R. B. (1989). Functional importance of cystic fibrosis immunoglobulin G fragments generated by *Pseudomonas aeruginosa* elastase. *J. Lab. Clin. Med.* 114: 728–733.

277. Ramphal, R., Houdret, N., Koo, L., Lamblin, G., and Roussel, P. (1989). Differences in adhesion of *Pseudomonas aeruginosa* to mucin glycopeptides from sputa of patients with cystic fibrosis and chronic bronchitis. *Infect. Immun.* 57: 3066–3071.

278. Boat, T. F., and Dearborn, D. G. (1984). Etiology and pathogenesis. In *Cystic Fibrosis*. Edited by L. M. Taussig. New York, Thieme Stratton, pp. 25–84.

279. Wang, Y.-M., Hare, T. R., Won, B., Stowell, C. P., Scanlin, T. F., Glick, M. C., Hard, K., van Kuik, J. A., and Vliegenhart, J. F. G. (1990). Additional fucosyl residues on membrane glycoprotein but not a secreted glycoprotein from cystic fibrosis fibroblasts. *Clin. Chim. Acta* 188: 193–210.

280. Knowles, M., Gatzy, J., and Boucher, R. (1981). Increased bioelectric potential difference across respiratory epithelia in cystic fibrosis. *N. Engl. J. Med.* 305: 1489–1495.

281. Welsh, M. J., and Liedtke, C. M. (1986). Chloride and potassium channels in cystic fibrosis airway epithelia. *Nature* 322: 467–470.

282. Li, M., McCann, J. D., Anderson, M. P., Clancy, J. P., Liedtke, C. M., Nairn, A. C., Greengard, P., and Welsh, M. J. (1989). Regulation of chloride channels by protein kinase C in normal and cystic fibrosis airway epithelia. *Science* 244: 1353–1356.

283. Kartner, N., Hanrahan, J. W., Jensen, T. J., Naismith, A. L., Sun, S., Ackerley, C. A., Reyes, E. F., Tsui, L.-C., Rommens, J. M., Bear, C. E., and Riordan, J. R. (1991). Expression of the cystic fibrosis gene in non-epithelial invertebrate cells produces a regulated anion conductance. *Cell* 64: 681–691.

284. Litt, M. (1984). Comparative studies of mucus and mucin physicochemistry. In *Mucus and Mucosa. Ciba Found. Symp.* 109: 196–206.

285. Galabert, C. G., Jacquot, J., Zahmn, J. M., and Puchelle, E. (1987). Relationships between lipid content and rheological properties of airway secretions in cystic fibrosis. *Clin. Chim. Acta* 164: 139–149.

286. Chace, K. V., Flux, M., and Sachdev, G. P. (1985). Comparison of physicochemical properties of purified mucus glycoproteins isolated from respiratory secretions of cystic fibrosis and asthmatic patients. *Biochemistry* 24: 7334–7341.

287. Rubin, B., MacLeod, P. M., Sturgess, J., and King, M. (1991). Recurrent respiratory infections in a child with fucosidosis: Is the mucus too thin for effective transport? *Pediatr. Pulmonol.* 10: 304–309.

288. Lopez-Vidriero, M. T., Das, I., and Reid, L. M. (1977). Airway secretion: Source, Biochemical and Rheologic Properties. In *Respiratory Defense Mechanisms*. Edited by J. D. Brain, D. F. Proctor, and L. M. Reid. New York, Marcel Dekker, p. 315.

7

Rheology of Airway Mucus
Relationship with Clearance Function

MALCOLM KING

University of Alberta
Edmonton, Alberta, Canada

BRUCE K. RUBIN

St. Louis University School of Medicine
St. Louis, Missouri

I. Introduction

Mucus is a viscoelastic gel consisting of water and high relative molecular mass (M_r), cross-linked glycoproteins mixed with serum and cellular proteins (albumin, enzymes, immunoglobulins), and lipids. There are variable amounts of cell debris and particulate matter in normal mucus. Respiratory mucus is usually cleared by airflow and ciliary interactions. Sputum, which is mucus mixed with inflammatory cells, cellular debris, and bacteria, is generally cleared by cough.

Airway clearance of mucus depends on the physical properties of the mucous gel, serous fluid properties, and ciliary function, as well as interactions between mucus and airflow or mucus and cilia. The *rheology* of mucus is its capacity to undergo flow and deformation. The proper evaluation of the rheology of mucus is essential for a complete understanding of mucociliary and cough clearance, for monitoring the action of medications that might affect its behavior, and for fitting the role of mucus within the larger context of epithelial function. However, the rheological properties of mucus are complex and, as a result, useful parameters that characterize its viscoelastic behavior are not simple to define in mathematical terms, nor are they easy to measure experimentally. Indeed, mucus can be considered one of the most difficult biological materials to deal with from the point of view of biophysical analysis.

In this chapter, methods of collecting, storing, and physical characterization of respiratory tract mucus from both animals and human subjects will be reviewed. Collection methods include ways to minimize contamination of sputum collected from patients, as well as techniques for obtaining mucus from normal humans and experimental animals. Methods for physical characterization of mucus include the measurements of viscosity, viscoelasticity, spinability, and surface wettability and adhesiveness.

II. Mucus Collection

Collection of mucus is the first major problem in any study related to this substance. The collection method chosen depends on both the study population and information sought. If rheological testing is one of the goals (i.e., physical characterization), then the mucus must be collected nondestructively. If normal or quasi-normal human subjects are to be studied, the quantity of mucus available will be severely limited, and access to it will be difficult. Experimental animals may be somewhat easier to study, but the smaller species present particular problems of both access and quantity.

A. Human Respiratory Tract Mucus

Noninvasive Collection of Mucus

For humans with lung diseases characterized by chronic hypersecretion, neither quantity nor access represent any special problem. Expectoration is the logical choice for such studies. Care should be taken to minimize contamination with oral and nasal secretions (i.e., ask the patient to clear the nose and rinse the mouth before expectorating). The use of dental cotton, as introduced by Puchelle and co-workers (1984), to minimize admixture with saliva is useful; however, even with this technique, some contamination is inevitable. In designing studies related to asthma, it should be remembered that production of mucus will be particularly dependent on the degree of exacerbation, and one could find that subjects are unable to produce the necessary sample after a successful treatment.

Sputum samples should be covered and sealed immediately after expectoration to minimize evaporation. If immediate analysis is not practical, samples can be deep-frozen ($-80°C$ freezer or dry ice) for later analysis. This method has proved useful in several recent studies we have undertaken for which samples were collected in a distant center and shipped to our laboratory for analysis (Shim et al., 1987; Paul et al., 1989; Knowles et al., 1990). In our experience, cryopreservation of sputum is not absolute, but sample deterioration is small enough that one can be reasonably confident that comparisons between study groups will remain valid.

Invasive Collection Methods in Humans

For human subjects who do not produce sputum, there are numerous methods to either induce sputum production or to collect mucus invasively. Sputum production can be induced by irritant inhalation, such as with citric acid or hypertonic saline. Some years ago, Lopez-Vidriero and co-workers (1977) used histamine, acetylcholine, and prostaglandin $F_{2\alpha}$ to induce sputum in normal subjects. Although this technique achieved its goal of producing rheologically characterizable sputum, it was clearly unpleasant, and likely resulted in "abnormal" mucus, since these agents alter the rheological properties of tracheal mucus in experimental animals (King et al., 1985a). Sputum induction is clearly of value as a means of harvesting inflammatory cells and may be valid as far as chemical analysis is concerned, but its validity in studying the physical properties of mucus remains to be evaluated.

For chemical analysis of mucins, bronchial lavage methods are an important option. Several studies have used lavage methods to obtain material for biochemical analysis, even from normal healthy volunteers (Williams et al., 1982; Bhaskar et al., 1985). To obtain mucus suitable for physical analysis from subjects who cannot expectorate, one needs to resort to either bronchoscopy or intubation during surgical procedures. During bronchoscopy, mucus can be readily collected from the trachea or mainstem bronchi by carefully placing a cytology brush in contact with the airway epithelium. Sufficient mucus for analysis by magnetic rheometry can be obtained in 20–30 s, even from normal subjects (Jeanneret-Grosjean et al., 1988; Zayas et al., 1990). The collection of mucus should precede other bronchoscopy procedures, such as lavage and biopsy, which could result in sample contamination. If the bronchoscopy is medically indicated, there is little ethical problem—mucus collection adds little extra time and no significant morbidity to the bronchoscopy procedure; if bronchoscopy is not otherwise indicated, its use in collecting mucus from human subjects would have to be fully justified.

An alternative source of mucus is to recover it from the endotracheal tubes normally discarded from patients being extubated after surgical procedures (Rubin et al., 1990a). We have used this technique to characterize mucus from a variety of patients otherwise inaccessible to study—"healthy" smokers (Rubin et al., 1992b), stable asthmatics, and young children, who happen to undergo surgery for nonpulmonary reasons (Rubin et al., 1990c). We have even managed with the use of this novel collecting technique to obtain mucus for rheological analysis from premature infants (Rubin et al., 1992a). This technique is clearly of value in studying the properties of mucus in cross sections of the population, but could not be rationally used in studying the effects of acute pharmacological manipulations, except those of interest in the intensive care unit or surgical suite.

The use of *nasal* mucus as an alternative to lower respiratory tract secretions has largely been ignored. Relatively little information is available on the rheological properties of nasal mucus, but given the common features of the nasal and tracheobronchial epithelial and the parallels between allergic rhinitis and extrinsic asthma, the nasal system could serve as a useful model in the study of experimental asthma therapy. Further developments in this area should be undertaken.

B. Collection Methods for Mucus in Animals

Generally speaking, the invasive methods of mucus collection just referred to are also used in animal studies. Our group uses two main methods for collecting mucus from experimental animals—the cytology brush method or the endotracheal tube method. The cytology brush technique involves placing a soft-bristled cytology brush in contact with the tracheal or bronchial epithelium for a time, and allowing the mucus to collect on the brush by normal mucociliary flow (King et al., 1989a). In dogs and other large animals, the cytology brush is best placed under bronchoscopic guidance. In smaller animals, such as ferrets or rats, one must be prepared to insert the brush blindly. Mucus can also be obtained from the exterior surface of an endotracheal tube (App and King, 1990), just as in humans. Other workers have used a variety of other techniques to collect mucus from experimental animals—collecting from the downstream end of a tracheal segment (Boyd, 1972) or frog palate (Rubin et al., 1990b), trapping the mucus on screen material in contact with the epithelium (Adams et al., 1976), periodic harvesting from a tracheal pouch (Lutz et al., 1973), and the very elegant technique of micropipetting from gland duct openings (Leikauf et al., 1984).

The amount of mucus that can be collected from healthy control animals is very small, even under ideal circumstances. In dogs, we normally collect volumes of 1–10 μl in 5–10 min by the cytology brush collection method, and can recover perhaps 50 μl from the endotracheal tube after 1 h of intubation. In rats or ferrets, it generally takes 20–30 min of collection time to obtain 1–2 μl in the absence of stimulation by a secretagogue. Clearly, microanalytical methods are required to deal with these small sample quantities.

III. Physical Analysis of Mucus

Several physical methods for analysis of mucus are available. Historically, before the mid-1960s, mucus was treated by workers studying its mechanical properties as a simple liquid, characterizable by a viscosity and, as a consequence, methods were applied to it based on conventional viscometry. This was not necessarily out of ignorance; many workers were undoubtedly aware of the complex physical nature of mucus, but preferred an empirical approach designed to achieve the collection of data. Hence, many early studies in respiratory tract mucus focused on its viscosity and pourability. Curiously, cervical mucus, because of its distinct capacity to form threads, characterized by the term *Spinnbarkeit*, was treated not as a simple liquid, but as a simple solid with elastic properties.

Toward the end of the 1960s, the formulation of theory and methodology for characterizing the viscoelastic nature of mucus began to emerge. In 1969, Davis and Dippy, in England, and Hwang et al., in the United States, independently reported on developments designed to explore and interpret the viscoelastic behavior of mucus. Since that time, several different practical approaches to deal with the viscoelastic nature of mucus have been described, and a large body of literature on mucus' viscoelasticity has emerged.

Modern instruments available for studying the bulk viscoelastic properties of mucus include controlled shear rate rheometers (either cone-and-plate or double concentric cylinder geometry), the double-capillary rheometer, the magnetic rheometer, and the Filancemeter. Methods for studying the surface properties or adhesivity are less well developed; these include the platinum ring technique and tack-testing methods.

A. Viscoelasticity of Mucus

Mucus can be considered a viscoelastic fluid, since it exhibits both liquidlike (viscous) and solidlike (elastic) properties (Fig. 1). *Viscosity* is the resistance to flow and represents the capacity of a material to absorb energy as it moves. *Elasticity* is the capacity of a material to store the energy used to move or deform it. As a viscoelastic gel, mucus exhibits a response to stress that is neither solidlike nor liquidlike, but some combination of the two. A true solid (and this includes gels with stable cross-links) responds to a stress with a finite deformation that is totally recovered after the stress is removed. A true liquid responds to the same stress by deforming or flowing continuously for the time that the stress is applied; after the removal of the stress, the flow ceases and there is no recovery of the strain. Mucus can be viewed as deviating from either of these extremes of behavior, and rheological techniques appropriate to the study of either liquids or solids can be applied to it. Our perception of mucus will depend very much on the technique chosen.

B. Mucus as a Viscous Liquid

Simple viscosity is the proportionality constant between the pressure or stress producing flow of a material and the resulting flow rate, as originally described by Newton.

$$\text{Stress} = \text{Viscosity} \times \text{Rate of Strain} \tag{1}$$

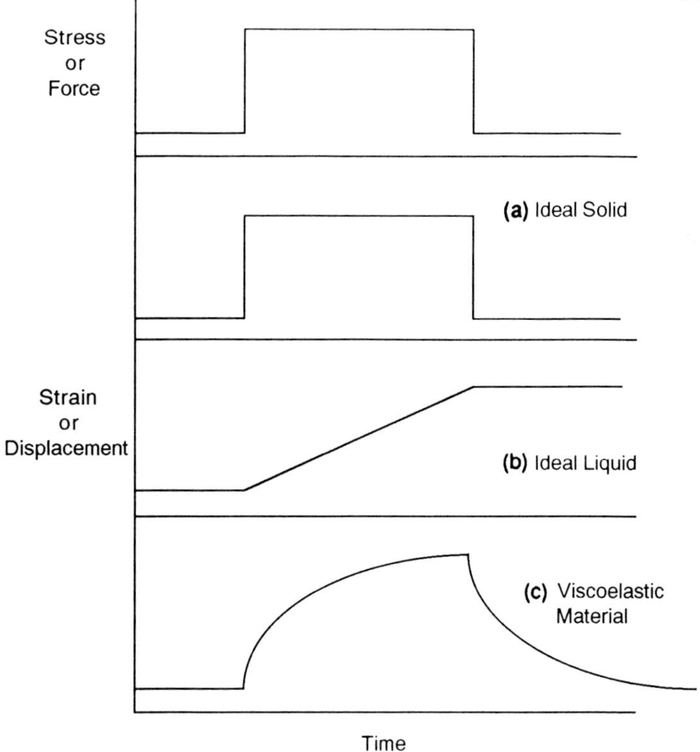

Figure 1   Stress–strain relationships in idealized materials. Mucus is a viscoelastic semisolid.

If stress and rate of strain form a linear relationship, the material is considered to be newtonian in behavior. Water and honey are examples of newtonian liquids. Mucus is far from newtonian, since the ratio of stress to rate of strain is very nonlinear. If anything, mucus can be considered as a pseudoplastic liquid; that is, one the viscous behavior of which changes with strain rate, and that shows elements of solidlike character. When subjected to an accelerated strain, mucus shows the following response (Fig. 2).

At first there is relatively little motion, the mucus exhibiting essentially solidlike behavior. Then with increasing stress, the mucus begins to move, and moves increasingly more readily with each increase in strain rate. (In reality, there is no true yield behavior, because the mucous network is not permanent.) Viscosity can be evaluated at any stress level or at any rate of strain as the ratio between the two. It is easy to see that the result will be highly dependent on the measuring conditions. In practical terms, mucus' viscosity is highly shear-

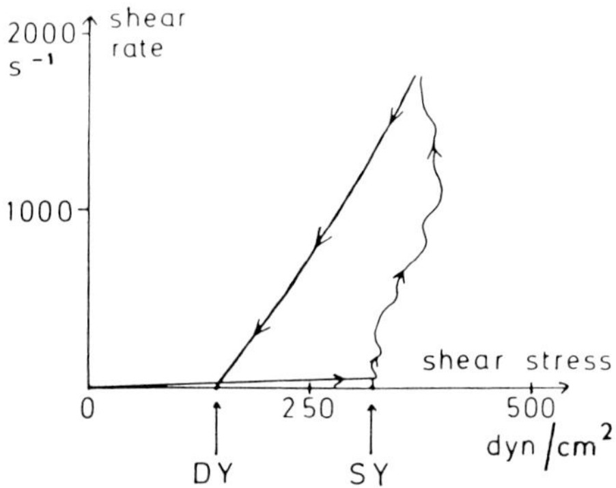

Figure 2 Stress vs rate of strain behavior of mucus when subjected to an experiment in which the rate of strain is cycled from low to high and back again.

dependent, varying by several orders of magnitude over the measurable range. It does appear to exhibit a newtonian region of behavior, however, at very low shear rates. This indicates that its cross-links, or at least the ones holding the larger network together, are not truly permanent, but instead, are based on physical entanglements, which can rearrange, given sufficient time. An infinite network of permanent cross-links would exhibit no limit to viscosity at low shear rates. An additional complication is that with higher rates of strain, disruption of the network (either permanent or temporary) will result, resulting in a different return pathway, and a lower apparent viscosity during the second test. Temporary disruption of the network leads to the phenomenon of thixotropy, which will be discussed later.

The liquidlike character of mucus can be studied in a rheometer designed primarily for studying the viscous properties of liquids. In an experiment of this type, a shear stress is applied to the sample and the resulting rate of strain (flow) is measured. The liquidlike character is quantified by the viscosity, the ratio of the stress to the rate of strain. With mucus, as with any gellike material, the apparent or measured viscosity varies considerably with the applied stress (or with the resultant strain rate). Figure 3 illustrates a typical result for the dependence of apparent viscosity on strain rate for a sample of canine tracheal mucus. The curve exhibits the classic sigmoidal shape of a relaxation process, with a remarkable three orders of magnitude difference between the low- and high-strain rate limits of apparent viscosity.

In addition to the variation illustrated in Figure 5, there is also the phenomenon of shear-thinning. This is commonly observed as a decrease in the apparent viscosity at low-strain rate after the sample has been exposed to a period of high strain. Phenomena of this type have been studied widely with instruments in which the shear stress is cycled from low to high to low (Charman and Reid, 1972;

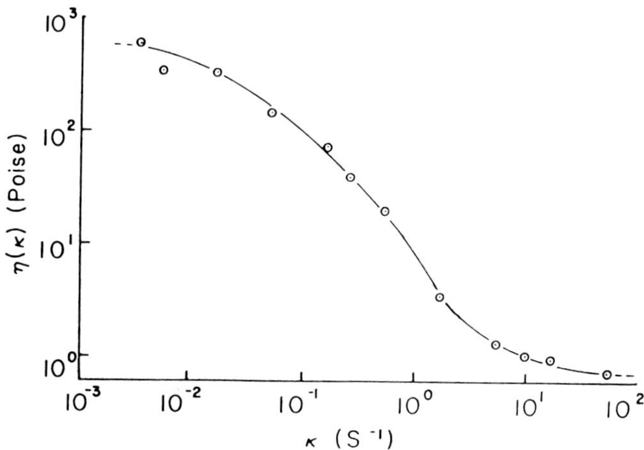

Figure 3 Variation in apparent viscosity of canine tracheal mucus as a function of strain rate. (From Powell et al., 1974.)

Davis, 1973; Marriott and Richards, 1974). The reduction in apparent viscosity can be permanent, consistent with the rupture of the macromolecular chains making up the gel network, or temporary, consistent with the introduction of a strained molecular configuration. The latter phenomenon—reversible shear-thinning—is also termed thixotropy; it has been observed (Sturgess et al., 1970) with exposure of sputum samples to intermediate-shear rates (<10 s^{-1}); with high-shear rate exposure, permanent disruption of the gel network begins to occur.

Since mucus possesses elastic character, in a steady-flow experiment, sudden removal of the stress results in recoil or a partial recovery of the strain. The magnitude of this response can serve as a relative measure of mucous elasticity (Barnett and Dulfano, 1970; Puchelle et al., 1973a). As in apparent viscosity, the measurement of elasticity depends a great deal on the applied stress and the strain history. For a complete description of viscoelasticity, steady-flow and recoil experiments at different levels of applied stress would have to be done.

The liquidlike behavior of mucus is useful in understanding the role in cough in the clearance of secretions. The near-explosive expulsion of air from the lung imparts very high-shearing forces to the mucus that is lining the upper airways. Exposed to high-shear stress, the mucus flows easily forward, since its effective viscosity (flow resistance) in this condition is low. After the cough, exposed only to the modest shear stress of gravity, it does not flow back into the lung because its effective viscosity is high again, although because of shear-thinning, it is perhaps not as high as before the cough. In this respect, tracheobronchial mucus resembles a well-engineered paint which, when brushed rapidly, flows easily, but when the brushing ceases, sticks to the wall.

C. Mucus as an Elastic Solid

Simple elasticity is governed by Hooke's law, which relates the stress producing a deformation to the degree of deformation.

$$\text{Stress} = \text{Elasticity} \times \text{Strain} \tag{2}$$

The simplest elastic material to consider is a rubber band, which elongates under stress and snaps back to its original length when the stress is released. Mucus behaves like an imperfectly cross-linked rubber band; that is, one that elongates and snaps back when stretched rapidly (but only at low amplitude), and that snaps back only partially when stretched more slowly, or if the elongation is maintained (Fig. 4). This deviation from ideal elastic behavior can be considered as partial recoil.

The solidlike character of mucus can be studied in an experimental configuration in which the strain (rather than the rate of strain) resulting from an applied stress is monitored. This mode of deformation is known as *creep*, and is a classic method of studying the mechanical behavior of an imperfectly elastic solid (such as an unvulcanized natural rubber). In a creep experiment, a constant stress is applied to the sample for a period, and then released (see Fig. 4a). A typical result of a creep test on a sample of canine tracheal mucus is shown in Figure 4b. The mucus responds with a rapid deformation (generally termed "instantaneous,"

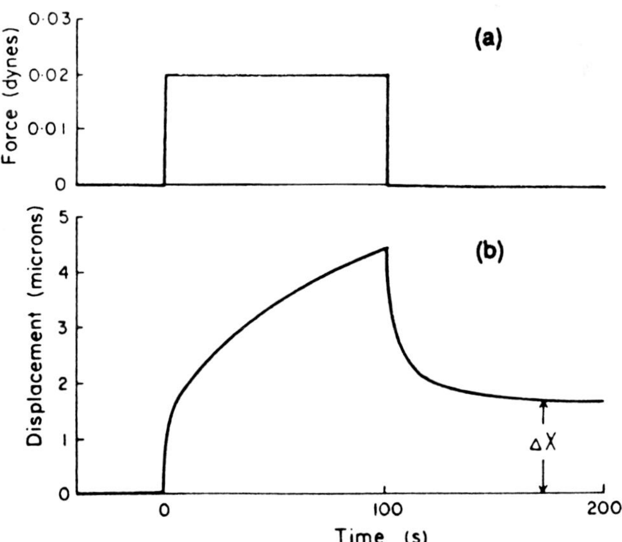

Figure 4 Creep experiment with magnetic rheometer. The steady-shear viscosity is computed from the nonrecoverable displacement, ΔX. (From King, 1988.)

although this is obviously only an approximation); from this an instantaneous elasticity (stress/strain) can be determined. The initial deformation is followed by a period of retarded deformation seen as an approximately logarithmic increase in strain with time, owing to the relaxation of the macromolecular network. Finally, the rate of strain approaches linearity in a terminal region in which the viscouslike behavior of the material is exhibited. Because of the latter, permanent deformation results (i.e., after release of the stress, only a partial recovery of the strain is achieved). The response of the material in the strain recovery period can be divided into an elastic component (stress/recoverable strain) and a viscous component (stress × time of application/nonrecoverable strain).

D. Mucus as a Viscoelastic Solid

Oscillatory Testing

Although the creep experiment provides information about both the solid and the liquid properties of mucus, this information is more directly obtainable from a dynamic experiment. A dynamic viscoelasticity experiment consists essentially of the application of a periodic (generally sinusoidal) stress to the sample and monitoring the resultant strain. In the steady state, the strain will exhibit the same periodicity as the stress, but because mucus is viscoelastic, the strain will lag behind the stress. If the sinusoidal strain is plotted against the sinusoidal stress, an ellipse is described (Fig. 5). The magnitude of phase lag is indicative of the relative proportion of viscous and elastic behavior: a purely elastic material would exhibit no lag in response; for a purely viscous material, the phase lag would be 90°. The viscoelastic properties are computed from the relative amplitudes of stress and strain, the phase between them, and a geometric constant, as indicated in the figure. The viscosity and elasticity are, in general, frequency-dependent.

A variety of geometric configurations have been employed in making dynamic mechanical measurements of mucus. These include cone-and-plate (Davis, 1973; Powell et al., 1974) and concentric cylinder (Eliezer, 1974) geometries, in which the sample is loaded in the gap between a moving element and a fixed element, and oscillating sphere geometry (Lutz et al., 1973; King and Macklem, 1977), in which a ferromagnetic sphere placed within a sample of mucus is oscillated by means of an external magnetic force. All of these instruments provide approximately equivalent information, the only essential difference being the geometric factor relating strain to displacement. As in the previous cases, the rheological information is stress-dependent, strain amplitude in general increasing faster than stress amplitude. However, most dynamic viscoelastic devices operate at low-strain amplitude so that the measured viscoelastic properties depend only on the cycling frequency.

An example of the dynamic viscoelastic properties of mucus is shown in Figure 6, the measurements having been made on canine tracheal mucus using a

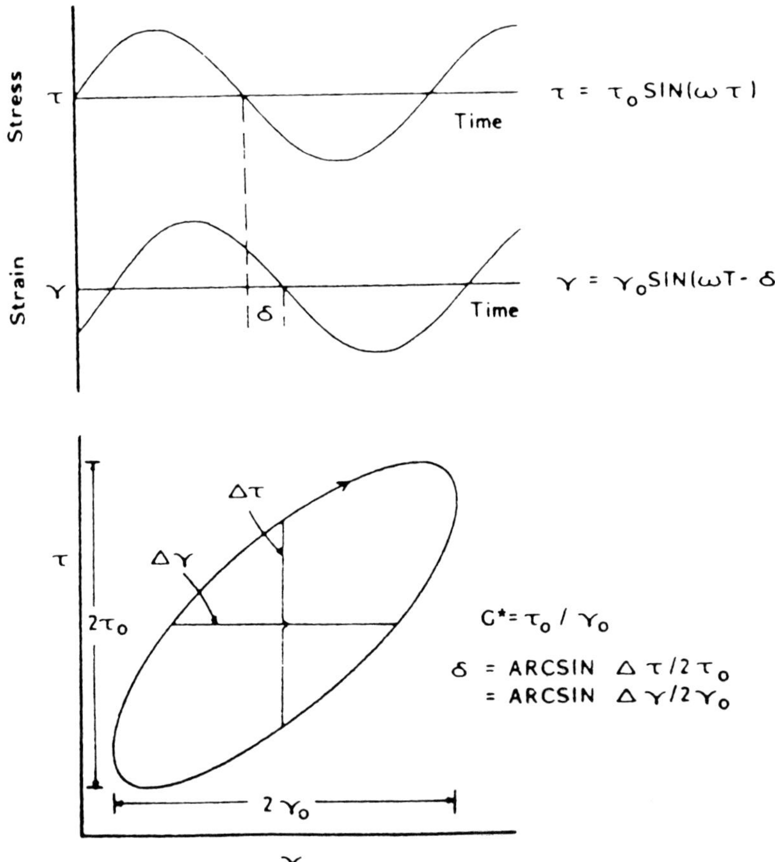

Figure 5 Stress–strain relationships in oscillatory rheological testing. In a viscoelastic material, strain lags behind the applied stress. The in-phase strain gives the elasticity, the out-of-phase component the viscosity.

magnetic microrheometer. The rapid decrease in viscosity accompanied by a moderate increase in elasticity over the intermediate-frequency range is typical of results obtained in various laboratories. Also shown in this figure is the low shear viscosity computed from creep experiments on the same samples, illustrating that considerable relaxation must still occur at frequencies beyond the dynamic range of the instrument. This pattern of frequency response is not unique to mucus; it is possible to duplicate these curves with rheological simulants of mucus, such as cross-linked guaran (King and Macklem, 1977).

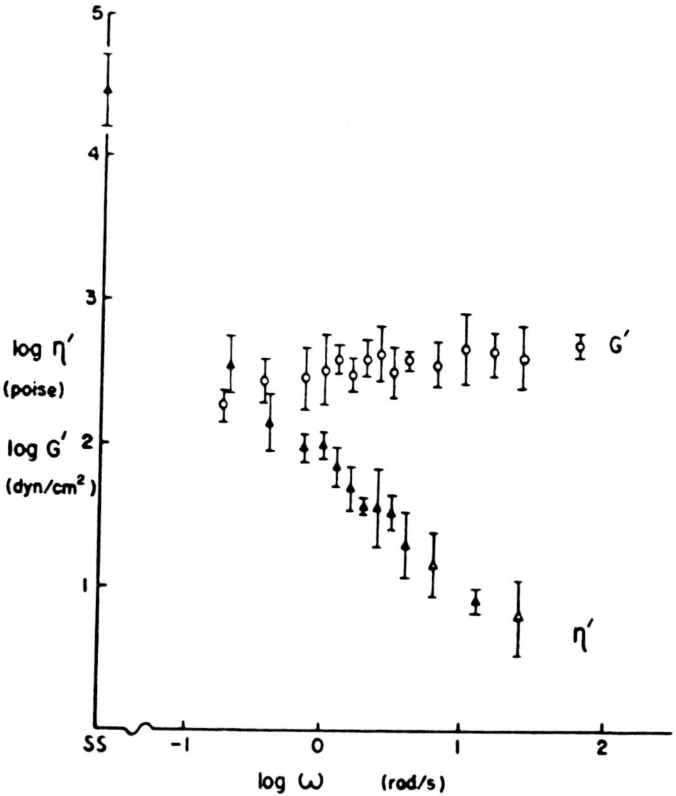

Figure 6 Dynamic viscoelastic response (elasticity G' and viscosity η' vs frequency ω) of canine tracheal mucus. Steady-shear viscosity from creep experiment also shown. (From King and Macklem, 1977.)

The shapes of these curves are a reflection of the gellike nature of mucus. The magnitude of the elastic component in the flat, intermediate-frequency domain serves as an index of the cross-link density of the macromolecular network forming the gel. The reduction in the dynamic viscosity with increasing frequency is quantitatively similar to the reduction in apparent viscosity with strain rate. They both reflect the same processes. At high frequency, the viscosity is low because only local rearrangements between neighboring macromolecular segments have time to occur during any period of stress application; at low frequency, the viscosity is high because the response to the applied stress involves the rearrangement of the whole network.

It should be remembered that all experimental techniques result in some degree of destruction or preshearing of the mucous sample, whether this is through the insertion of a steel ball or the loading of the sample into a gap between concentric cylinders or parallel plates. Expectoration of mucus by coughing is itself a form of preshearing and, although it is as yet untested, it likely leads to some permanent destruction of the gel network. Thus, comparisons of absolute levels of mucous viscoelasticity between different techniques are subject to uncertainties. However, with consistent handling procedures, comparisons between samples are valid, and valuable information on the variation in mucous viscoelasticity can be obtained.

The relative proportions of elasticity and viscosity are as important in describing how a material, such as mucus, behaves when it is subjected to external forces as are the absolute values of either parameter by itself. Because of the viscoelastic nature of mucus, it lends itself well to oscillatory testing, where strain and stress are varied sinusoidally. In dynamic testing, *tangent* δ is the ratio of viscosity to elasticity; this is also known as the loss tangent and can be considered as a recoil factor (see Fig. 5). **G*** is the vector sum of viscosity and elasticity, known as mechanical impedance, which can be termed the rigidity factor.

There are several terms used to designate the properties of viscoelasticity and, unfortunately, there is no uniformity within the field of rheology for their use. As an alternative representation for dynamic viscoelasticity, the properties can be described in terms of G' and G'', the dynamic storage and loss moduli, representing the elastic and viscous components, respectively. The relationship between **G***, tan δ, G' and G'' can be appreciated from Figure 7.

The coordinates of the vector location of **G*** are given either by the cartesian representation G' and G'' or by the polar representation **G*** and δ. G'', the loss modulus, is also directly related to η', the dynamic viscosity through the relationship $G'' = \omega\eta'$, where ω is the measurement frequency in radians per second.

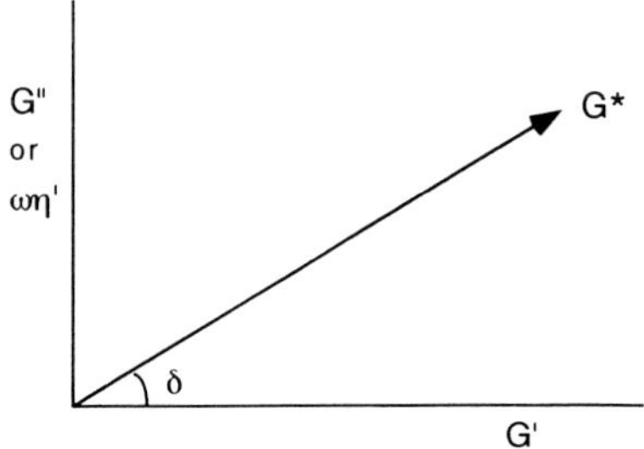

Figure 7 Vector diagram indicating relationship between **G***, tan δ, G', G'', and η'.

IV. Historical Methods for Viscosity

A. Pourability

The pourability of mucus should be considered as a semiquantitative method. Keal and Reid (1970) described a very simple clinical test that required no advance equipment. Pourability represents the capacity of a fluid to adhere to the walls of a container and flow under gravity. Keal and Reid graded sputum into four grades, ranging from those adhering to the container and those that moved instantly when the container was reversed. They observed a significant and inverse correlation between the pourability grade and the viscosity, as measured by conventional viscometry. However, such a semiquantitative test would have to be used with caution, because the pourability clearly also depends on the surface properties of the mucus, which will be very dependent on the degree of contamination with saliva.

B. Simple Capillary Rheometers

The simple capillary rheometers were among the first instruments used to determine the rheological properties of mucus. This type of rheometer generally determines only viscosity, although it can be readily adapted to determine measure recoil or elasticity. The problem is that the viscosity measured depends heavily on the rate of flow and that, even if this is controlled, the variation of shear within the sample is not constant. Often shear rates are high, and the testing itself is destructive of the sample. Nevertheless, studies using such instruments (e.g., Charman and Reid, 1972) have given us a great deal of our early information on properties of mucus and their relationships with chemical makeup and pathophysiological features.

V. Current Methods for Viscoelasticity

A. Controlled Shear Rate Rheometers

Controlled shear rate rheometers are the classic instruments for measuring the bulk viscoelastic properties of biofluids. They are generally based on deformation in the cone-and-plate geometry or between double-concentric cylinders. Both setups provide the advantage that the shear rate in the testing fluid (i.e., the mucus) is definable and uniform. Since the viscoelastic properties of mucus are highly dependent on the rate of shear applied to the sample, this is a clear advantage. Both dynamic testing (oscillatory motion) (Braga, 1988) and transient testing (steady rotation and recoil) (Davis, 1988) can be performed. Both modes of testing yield equivalent information in principle—separate measures of viscosity and elasticity at different rates of shear or at different oscillatory frequencies. The main disadvantage of these instruments is that they are inherently size-limited, because of edge or end effects, to volumes of about 0.5 ml or more. For sputum samples, this is not a serious limitation, but for samples of mucus from humans without hypersecretion or from experimental animals, other rheological testing methods must be used.

B. Double-Capillary Method

When fluid is pulled from a reservoir through a simple capillary tube under vacuum pressure, its rate of progression decreases the farther it enters the tube. Thus, no steady flow rate is reached, and no single value of viscosity (proportional to driving pressure over flow rate) can be defined. This problem can be overcome by the use of a smaller capillary tube segment within the larger tube (Fig. 8). The smaller tube will account for most of the pressure drop, and act essentially as a flow-limiting segment, based on the principle that pressure drop in a tube is inversely proportional to the fourth power of the radius. The viscosity of mucus is then determined directly from the ratio of the pressure drop and the flow rate across the flow-limiting segment. By varying the driving pressure, measurements of viscosity at different shear rates can be determined. By observing the recoil after the pressure is released, one can determine a measure of the elastic modulus.

The double-capillary method is well suited to the study of mucus. It can easily be miniaturized down to the range of 20μl–sample volumes (Kim, 1988). Beyond that, the measurement of elasticity is limited because the meniscus changes shape during the recoil. Further miniaturization (down to the 100-nl range) has been achieved by converting to a plug flow setup (Leikauf et al., 1984), in which the shape changes in the two menisci tend to balance each other. One disadvantage is that with capillary flow, the shear rate within the mucus is not constant, since it varies from a maximum at the wall to zero along the midline of the tube. It is also essential to assure that the no-slip condition is met (i.e., that the mucus adheres firmly to the capillary surface). This could be problematic for mucus mixed with saliva, or containing surfactant or lipidic components, a consideration that also applies to the macroscopic, controlled shear rate viscoelastometers discussed earlier.

C. Magnetic Rheometer

The magnetic microrheometer is another instrument designed to measure the viscoelastic properties of very small quantities of mucus (Fig. 9). A steel ball is positioned in a 1- to 5-μl sample of mucus and oscillated by an electromagnet at different driving frequencies. The magnitude of displacement of the ball and its phase lag relative to the driving force are used to calculate the viscoelasticity of the mucus (King, 1988). The magnetic rheometer works well with microliter quantities of mucus, in fact, better than it does with larger quantities, since it depends

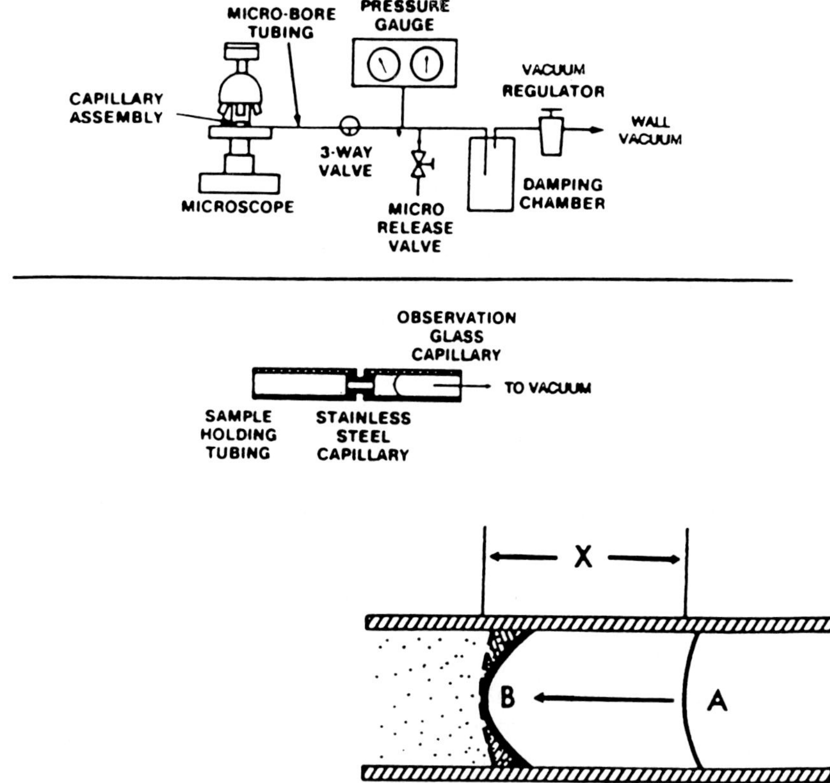

Figure 8 Schematic diagram of double-capillary rheometer. Inset shows the meniscus shape change that can occur during the elastic recoil phase. (Adapted from Kim, 1988.)

on an optical detection system, and mucus is semiopaque. In principle, it is not size-limited, but miniaturization much beyond its present microliter range would require the development of a more potent magnet and much stronger light source or better optical detection system. Its limitations, besides the need for a minimum of optical clarity, are that the shear rate in the mucus is also not well defined, and that it is difficult to work with samples that are too watery because the steel ball becomes nonbuoyant and sinks to the bottom of the container. This latter problem was overcome in a modification in which the rheometer was turned on its side, and a bias current was applied to the magnet to balance the pull of gravity on the ball (Majima et al., 1990).

The magnetic rheometer is probably insensitive to the presence of surfac-

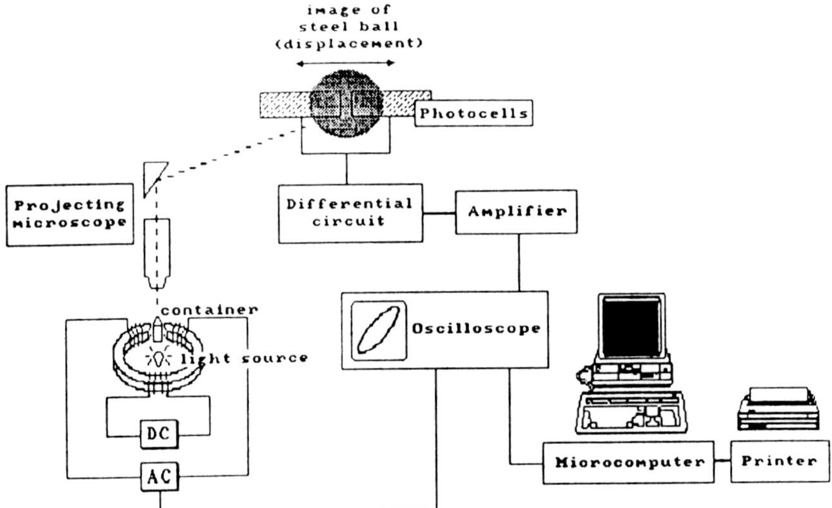

Figure 9 Schematic representation of the magnetic microrheometer. (From King, 1988; adapted by Silveira et al., 1992.)

tants, since the rheological probe lies completely within the mucus and "sees" only the bulk properties. As with all microrheological methods, one must be aware that mucus is inherently heterogeneous in its rheological properties, and testing of multiple aliquots is generally necessary. Recently, we have developed a computer-assisted, automated magnetic rheometer that improves the accuracy and speed of analysis (Silveira et al., 1992).

D. Filancemeter

Spinability (filance, *Spinnbarkeit*) is the thread-forming capacity of mucus under the influence of large amplitude elastic deformation. The Filancemeter measures spinability as thread formation in millimeters. This measurement is performed with a 10- to 20-μl mucus sample at a distraction velocity of 10 mm/s. An electric signal is conducted through the mucus sample. This signal is interrupted at the point where the stretched mucus thread is broken, permitting the reading of a spinability measurement (Zahm et al., 1986). Spinability has been correlated positively with mucociliary clearance on the frog palate (Puchelle, 1987a), but negatively with cough clearability using a simulated cough machine (King et al., 1989b). A major disadvantage with the measurement of spinability is that it does not correlate well with other more basic measures of viscoelasticity.

VI. Adhesivity

It is only in the last few years that the surface properties of mucus have been recognized as separate and distinct from bulk viscoelasticity. The surface properties of mucus are believed to be of critical importance for most aspects of mucus' function—its clearance by airflow and ciliary mechanisms, as well as its cytoprotective function. Adhesiveness is the ability of mucus to bond to a solid surface, and this can be measured as the force of separation between one or more solid surfaces and the adhesive material. Adhesiveness is dependent on mucus' surface tension, hydration, wettability, and contact (dwell) time.

Recent studies suggest that the sputum surface properties may be more important determinants of cough clearability than viscoelasticity (Agarwal et al., 1989; Zahm et al., 1989; King et al., 1989b, Girod et al., 1991). The absence of a strong relationship between sputum viscosity and cough clearability can be understood by the following analogy. If a peashooter is taken to represent the airway, and the blast of air that sends the pea to its target is a cough, a longer-distance shot (that is, increased "cough clearance") can be obtained using a whole pea, rather than pea soup—the equivalent to mucus that has been thinned by a mucolytic. Extending the analogy, the pea will go farther if it is first greased, reducing surface adhesion.

The hypothesis that cough clearability is directly related to the adherence of secretions to the underlying respiratory epithelium fits well with our present understanding of the basic defect in cystic fibrosis (CF) (Knowles et al., 1983). Ion transport hydrates the periciliary fluid layer to a greater extent than it could possibly affect the viscoelasticity of the mucus layer. Yet it is the periciliary fluid that separates the mucus from the epithelium, and we know that small alterations in hydration can lead to large changes in surface adhesion. Classic examples of this are a postage stamp or spilled fruit juice becoming tacky as the licked adhesive or juice dries. Puchelle's group in France has demonstrated the importance of a serous fluid layer in reducing adhesion tension of sputum, and that the presence of this type of serous layer is probably the strongest determinant of the cough clearability of mucus-simulant gels (Zahm et al., 1989). The results of our recent experiments using expectorated sputum (Rubin, 1992) reinforce this conclusion. In sputum from patients with CF we confirmed that, although there are minimal changes in CF sputum viscoelasticity, there is abnormally low cough clearability (Rubin et al., 1991a), and preliminary experiments suggest that treatment of expectorated CF sputum with surfactants can improve in vitro sputum cough clearability (Rubin, 1992).

Girod et al. (1992) have demonstrated that the phospholipid composition of CF sputum is different from that of sputum from patients with chronic bronchitis and bronchiectasis. In these studies, they showed that sputum phospholipid composition was related to the contact angle between the sputum sample and a negatively charged glass slide. As the contact angle is a measure of the wettability of the glass subsurface layer, it is one measurement of the properties of the surface of the sputum (Vaquez Girod, et al., 1988). Adhesion tension and interfacial tension (or surface tension, as it is called at the air–liquid interface) are the other critical surface properties of the sputum–glass interface. There is decreased phosphatidylcholine in CF secretions when compared with chronic bronchitis sputum. This compositional difference was associated with an increase in sputum surface tension (Gilljam et al., 1988). In vitro experiments have shown that the addition of surfactants to expectorated cystic fibrosis sputum reduces the sputum viscoelasticity (Motta et al., 1984) and that cystic fibrosis sputum phospholipid composition is related to sputum viscoelasticity (Galabert et al., 1987). Girod et al. (1991) recently demonstrated that certain forms of phospholipids are more capable of reducing mucus adhesion and improving cough clearability than others.

Lopez-Vidriero (1988) described the potential use of tack testing of sputum, but its use has been limited. Puchelle and co-workers (1987b) have used the platinum ring technique to measure the subsurface adhesion tension of sputum samples and mucus simulants. Our own group has developed a gravimetric distraction adhesiometer, which measures the force needed to pull a probe from the surface of a small sample of mucus while simultaneously measuring the contact angle (wettability) of the sample on a strip of Teflon tape (Rubin, 1992). For a reliable analysis of the adhesive properties of mucus, there must be a true separation of the solid surface from the mucus, otherwise one is measuring a combination of cohesiveness (bulk viscoelasticity) and adhesivity.

The measurement of interfacial properties is not a trivial matter, particularly because viscoelasticity can influence the relative degree of contact between the sputum and either the periciliary layer or the underlying epithelium. It is difficult to measure contact angle accurately on viscoelastic sputum, since it will not spontaneously assume the Laplacian profile necessary to accurately measure interfacial forces. We have approached this problem by taking each half of a sputum droplet resting on a Teflon surface, generating a mirror image of each half (using image-processing software and a personal computer), and then calculating a best-fit approximation of the Laplacian form most like each half of the original sputum droplet. Each half has a different contact angle and thus wets and adheres to the underlying surface slightly differently. Although the average of these two contact angles correlates fairly well with cough clearability, as measured in a simulated cough machine, we have found that both the measured contact angle of sputum and the difference in contact angle between each half of the droplet are also related to the bulk viscoelasticity of the specimen (unpublished data).

It is probable that surface-active phospholipids also play an important role in mucociliary clearance. A bronchial surfactant layer has recently been demonstrated between the mucus and periciliary fluid layers (Schürch et al., 1990). This bronchial surfactant may help the mucous layer to spread evenly across the periciliary layer surface and maintain the integrity of these layers. It probably also acts as a lubricant and so increases the efficiency of the mucociliary apparatus. Allegra and colleagues (1985) have put surfactant on the excised frog palate and showed that this markedly increases the mucociliary transport rate on this ciliated surface. We have recently demonstrated that the administration of exogenous surfactant to premature babies with neonatal respiratory distress syndrome dramatically improves the mucociliary clearability of their airway secretions (Rubin et al., 1992a). Finally, an artificial surfactant preparation instilled intrabronchially has recently been shown to enhance the in vivo rate of mucociliary clearance in anesthetized dogs (De Sanctis et al., 1992).

There are several lines of evidence supporting both the existence and importance of bronchial surfactant in the normal lung. Surfactant is probably cleared from the acinus into the airways, and there is evidence that the larger airways can secrete their own surfactant lipids (Widdicombe, 1987; Macklem et al., 1970; Lachmann, 1985). In biopsy and autopsy material, osmiophilic membranes containing surfactant have been demonstrated in airway mucus and, especially, along the border between sol and gel phases of bronchial mucus layers (Morgenroth and Bolz, 1985). It has been proposed that airway surfactant separates the sol and gel phases of the mucus (Morgenroth, 198b) and that the surfactant layer is responsible for the retention of some inhaled particles in the airway (Schürch et al., 1990).

VII. Rheology and Clearance of Mucus

There are two major mechanisms for clearing mucus from the airways: by ciliary action, the primary mechanism; and when this fails or is overloaded, by coughing or other forms of airflow interaction. Methods for studying mucociliary clearance range from in vitro direct observation (e.g., frog palate) to in vivo tracer methods (e.g., inhaled, radiolabeled particles). Cough or airflow clearance can be studied in both mechanical models, as well as in vivo, with the use of appropriate tracers.

The viscoelastic behavior of mucus is one of the primary determinants of mucociliary clearance rate. Giordano et al. (1978) studied the tracheal mucous velocity of dogs prepared with tracheal pouches and found a clear negative correlation between the in vivo tracheal clearance rate and the elasticity of the mucus secreted by the pouch. Results generally similar to this have been obtained in studies employing the frog palate as a model ciliated epithelium; that is, ciliary transport rate decreases with increasing rigidity or "thickness" of the mucus, whatever quantitative measure of this is used (King, 1989).

The *ratio* of viscosity to elasticity is also an important determinant of the transport rate. This relationship is illustrated in Figure 10a. The viscosity/

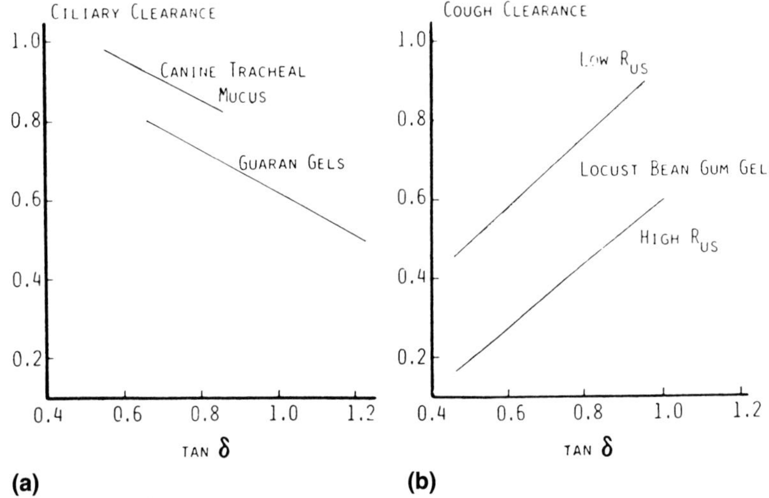

Figure 10 (a) Normalized ciliary clearance rate from frog palate studies; (b) cough clearance index determined with simulated cough machine. In each case, mechanical impedance **G*** was held constant. (From King, 1987.)

elasticity ratio (tan δ) represents the ratio of mechanical energy dissipated as friction per cycle versus that stored as kinetic energy. The result shown in Figure 10a thus implies that the decrease in mucous velocity with increasing tan δ is due to increased dissipation of ciliary energy by the mucus.

From the data in this and other studies, it appears that decreasing either the elasticity or the viscosity/elasticity ratio of mucus would be of benefit in enhancing the clearance of secretions. However, it has been demonstrated that as the mucus elasticity continues to decrease, the ciliary transport rate eventually passes through a maximum, and further decreases in mucous elasticity then result in a reduction in transport rate (Shih et al., 1977). Although this has not been observed with intact mucus from healthy animals, it has been seen in pathological human material (Puchelle et al., 1973b).

Cough clearance, represents the second line of airway defense, taking over in the case of mucous overload or when mucociliary clearance becomes inadequate. The phenomenology relating cough clearance with the rheology of mucus has been studied in vitro by means of a cough simulator (King et al. 1985b). The dependence of cough clearance on mucous viscosity, elasticity, and adhesivity is illustrated in Figure 11.

Not unreasonably, mucous viscosity (i.e., resistance to flow) is the major rheological variable affecting cough clearance. Elasticity enters the picture in terms of the recoil effect (i.e., a high degree of spinability or a low viscosity/

Viscosity

- Primary variable

- Newton's law

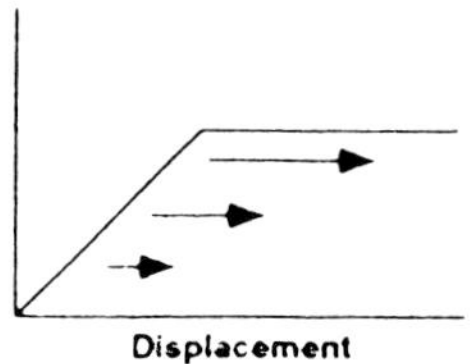

Spinability

- Large deformation elasticity,
  inhibiting deformation

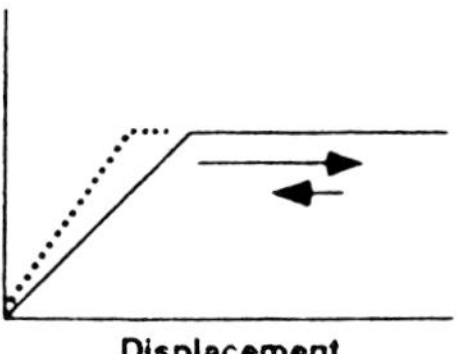

Adhesivity

- Surface tension, inhibiting
  wave formation, reducing
  air-mucus interaction

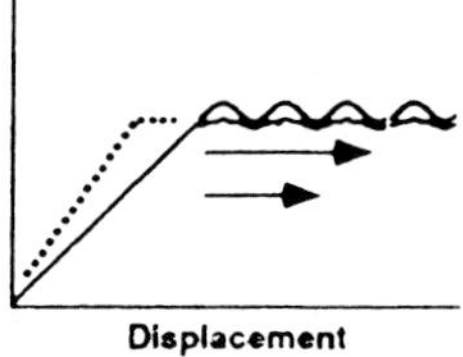

Figure 11 Schematic model of mucus clearance by airflow interaction, illustrating the effects of the three primary variables: viscosity, spinability, and surface tension. (From King et al., 1989b.)

elasticity ratio being inhibitive of cough clearance). Adhesivity or surface tension is inhibitive of cough clearance through the suppression of mucus–airflow interaction, which manifests itself as wave formation in the mucous layer during the cough (King et al., 1989b). In a recent study, Zahm et al. (1991) demonstrated that mucous thixotropy and shear-thinning were important in describing the movement of mucus in multiple, rapid coughs, and by extension high-frequency oscillation.

The existence of an optimal range of viscoelastic properties and because sometimes, both mucociliary and cough clearance should be optimized, would suggest that therapeutic measures designed to modify the rheology of secretions should consider the initial state of the mucus, and that monitoring the viscoelastic properties of mucus should be an essential part of any potential mucotropic therapy.

A. Ex Vivo Ciliary Transportability: Frog Palate Assay

The frog palate is a mucus-secreting ciliated epithelium. Leopard frogs (*Rana pipiens*) are prepared by pithing—bending the head forward and inserting an 18-gauge needle into the brain and the spinal cord. The jaw is disarticulated and the palate removed by cutting through from the junction of the posterior pharynx and esophagus out to the skin of the back. The excised palate is placed on a piece of gauze saturated with modified frog Ringer's prepared by mixing two parts of nonlactated Ringer's injection solution with one part sterile water. This gives a solution with an osmolarity of 206.5 mosm/L containing (mmol/L): NaCl, 98.3; KCl, 2.7; and $CaCl_2$, 1.5. The palate is placed in a dish and loosely covered with plastic wrap and allowed to rest in a refrigerator at 4–6°C for 12–18 h to deplete of mucus. The palate is then placed in a box with a glass top and fitted glass front. Humidity is maintained at 90–100% and temperature held constant. The palate is focused under a dissecting microscope so that a micrometer scale runs between the optic bulges to the opening of the esophagus (Fig. 12). The movement of a 2- to 5-μl aliquot of mucus is timed and three measurements of mucous transport rate are taken to minimize measurement variability. The average transport rate of a sample is normalized to the transport rate for collected endogenous frog mucus (King et al., 1974; Rubin et al., 1990b).

Alternatively, by using a standard preparation of mucus or collected frog mucus, one can measure the effect of drugs delivered differentially to the mucosal

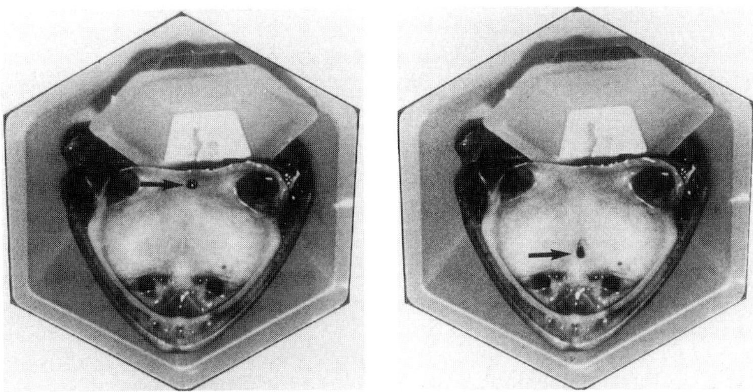

Figure 12 The mucus-depleted frog palate. (From Rubin et al., 1992b.)

side or air side of the frog palate. This technique has been widely used as a means of defining the inherent "transportability" of mucus, independent of systemic ciliary function.

B. In Vitro Cough Transportability: Simulated Cough Machine

A miniaturized simulated cough machine can be used to measure the airflow-dependent clearability and recoil of a mucous or sputum sample as small as 50 μl in volume. A model Plexiglas trachea, rectangular in cross section (dimensions 1.2 × 2 cm), is connected to an 8-L tank containing air pressurized to 8 psi (about 50 kPa), giving a flow rate of about 11 L/s (Fig. 13). A solenoid valve controls the release of this air through a flow-constrictive element used to mimic the airflow pattern of a natural cough maneuver. A sinusoidal obstruction (length 7.7 cm and height 8 mm) is used to decrease the airway diameter while minimizing the turbulence of the system. Peak linear air velocity is about 40 m/s in the unconstricted cough machine and 120 m/s with the 4-mm gap.

A sample of mucus, 40 μl in volume and 0.5 mm in depth, is placed in a thin line across the base of the Plexiglas trachea. Cough clearability can be measured both in the unobstructed cough machine, where the depth of the model trachea is 12 mm, and with an obstruction that narrows the depth of trachea to 4 mm at the point where the mucus is positioned. The bulk transport of the mucus is measured in millimeters after either a single cough maneuver or after multiple mechanical

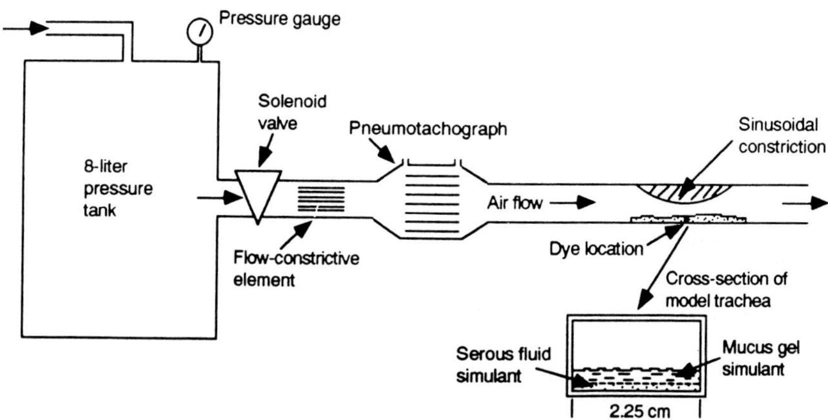

Figure 13   The miniaturized simulated cough machine. (From Agarwal et al., 1989.)

coughs (Agarwal et al., 1989; King et al., 1985b, 1989b). Different aliquots of the same sputum sample are used for three successive measurements, and the results are averaged. Measurement variability with different aliquots and in repeated measurements on the same sample is generally less than 10%.

C. Cough Versus Ciliary Clearance

Cilia beat at a frequency of 10–20 Hz and an amplitude of 5 μm, whereas the velocity (frequency times amplitude) in coughing is about 100 times greater. Also, at least in intact mucociliary systems, longer-range interactions between the mucous blanket at points of attachment should be considered (Macchione et al., 1992). Thus, low-shear rate or low-frequency viscoelasticity measurements are appropriate for relating to measurements of mucociliary clearance, whereas, high-shear rate, high-frequency measurements ought to be more predictive for cough clearance (King, 1987). A high tan δ (ratio of viscosity to elasticity) at high frequency suggests a viscous mucus that favors cough clearance (see Fig. 10). A low tan δ at low frequency characterizes an elastic mucus that favors ciliary clearance (see Fig. 10a). A high G^* (mechanical impedance or overall resistance to deformation) inhibits both forms of clearance.

VIII. Clinical Correlates of Mucous Clearance Defects

A. Primary Ciliary Dyskinesia (Immotile Cilia Syndrome)

We have studied the mucous properties from a patient with confirmed primary ciliary dyskinesia. The uninfected respiratory mucus obtained at the time of bronchoscopy had a high tan δ that would suggest poor ciliary clearability, but the viscoelasticity appeared to be optimal for cough clearance (unpublished data). It is tempting to speculate that the viscoelasticity was favorably altered for cough clearance in response to a signal from the epithelial cells that the cilia were dysfunctional.

B. Cystic Fibrosis

Numerous studies have demonstrated that sputum from patients with cystic fibrosis is not abnormally thick or viscous, but is rheologically comparable with sputum from patients with chronic bronchitis when corrected for the amount of purulence. Preliminary studies suggest that, although viscoelasticity might not differ from bronchitis sputum, sputum hydration is decreased in CF and cough clearability is decreased, probably owing to alterations in the surface properties of the mucus resulting from impaired chloride transport into the periciliary fluid layer.

C. Fucosidosis (Congenital Absence of α-L-Fucosidase)

Fewer than 100 patients with this rare, autosomal recessive defect have been described in the world literature. A prominent part of this disorder is recurrent sinus, ear, and pulmonary infections, but no evidence of systemic immune deficiency. Fucose and sialic acid are the preponderant terminal sugars of glycoprotein chains. We have studied one patient with infantile fucosidosis who had absence of cellular α-L-fucosidase activity as well as the characteristic elevation of sweat electrolytes and recurrent respiratory infections. This patient had an intact immune system as well as normally functioning cilia. Her respiratory mucus, obtained by bronchoscopy at the time of middle-ear surgery, was extremely watery (Rubin et al., 1991b). Our studies of mucous simulants on the frog palate and in the cough machine suggest that mucus this thin and watery can not be cleared well by either cough or ciliary mechanisms (King et al., 1974). The abnormal viscoelasticity could be explained by defective mucin cross-linking leading to poor formation of a cross-linked gel.

D. Allergy and Asthma

In sensitized experimental animals, the inhalation of *Ascaris suum* antigen in low dose releases a large volume of watery mucus. When sufficient antigen is inhaled to cause bronchoconstriction, a rigid, poorly cleared mucus is released. This biphasic response is similar to that seen with the administration of cholinergic drugs and can be blocked with anticholinergic medications (King et al., 1985a, Rubin et al., 1990c).

Sputum from patients with acute severe asthma has a high viscosity, and patients who die during an asthmatic attack have extensive mucous plugging of their airways. Active studies of mucus from well-controlled, asymptomatic asthmatic patients and from patients who have died from asthma are underway to determine when and how these changes occur and how they can best be prevented (Ramirez et al., 1991).

E. Neonatal Respiratory Distress Syndrome

Prematurely born babies fail to produce sufficient pulmonary surfactant to prevent alveolar collapse. In respiratory distress syndrome (RDS) there is also extensive plugging and collapse of conducting airways, which led us to speculate that surfactant deficiency might alter mucous viscoelasticity and clearability. We showed that babies with RDS have airway mucus that is extremely rigid—similar to that seen in patients with fatal asthma. Mucociliary clearability of this mucus on the frog palate is less than half of normal values. The early administration of surfactant aerosol to babies with RDS appears to correct these abnormalities (Rubin et al., 1992a).

F. Irritant Exposure, Smoking, and Lung Cancer

Acute exposure to irritants causes hypersecretion of a watery, easily cleared mucus that might be derived from preformed goblet cell secretions (King et al., 1989a). Similarly, asymptomatic smokers produce a watery mucus that is transported 30% faster than normal mucus on the frog palate (Rubin et al., 1992a). However, in vivo mucociliary clearance is not increased in the light smoker, probably because of ciliary damage.

Most chronic smokers produce a rigid, but elastic, mucus with more sialic acid and fewer fucose residues. This reduces ciliary clearability back to normal levels while further depressing cough clearance. It has been postulated that impaired mucous clearance in chronic smokers can lead to prolonged contact of irritants with the airway epithelium and so promote cellular metaplasia and cancer. However, some lifelong smokers seem to escape chronic obstructive pulmonary disease (COPD) and cancer. Preliminary evidence suggests that these smokers have mucus that retains viscoelasticity favorable for cough clearance. On the other hand, mucus from the few patients we have studied with primary adenocarcinoma who never actively smoked had viscoelasticity unfavorable for both cough and ciliary clearance (Zayas et al., 1990).

Although there are many reports of sputum analysis in patients with COPD, studies of mucus from smokers with the earliest pulmonary changes of COPD are lacking at this time.

IX. Therapy of Mucous Clearance Disorders

A. Physiotherapy and Postural Drainage

Chest physical therapy has been demonstrated to be most efficacious when it is accompanied by cough. Physiotherapy does not appear to alter mucociliary clearance, but may assist cough clearance by promoting the formation of easily expectorated mucous globules in the large airways, freeing adherent mucus from the epithelial surface, and by triggering cough receptors.

B. Medications

Cough suppressants have a limited role in the therapy of mucous clearance defects and the combination of a cough suppressant with an expectorant is illogical. Although expectorants can theoretically increase glandular secretions and so assist cough clearance, this has not been well studied. Expectorants do not alter ciliary beat frequency or mucociliary clearance favorably or unfavorably. It has not been conclusively demonstrated that expectorants have any true mucolytic properties. Although the mechanism of action of the expectorants is unclear, their use is supported by the demonstration of clinical efficacy. It may be that, by altering epithelial ion permeability, the expectorants loosen sputum that is adherent to the epithelial surface and, thereby, increase the effectiveness of coughing.

β-Agonists increase ciliary beat frequency and promote surfactant secretion. However, in vivo mucous clearance is surprisingly independent of ciliary beat frequency. Furthermore, it is unclear if β-agonists augment surfactant synthesis or secretion either in vivo or in damaged airways. Their role is limited in assisting sputum clearance, especially when there has been considerable ciliary damage. β-agonists may be ineffective mucokinetics in diseases, such as cystic fibrosis, in spite of their widespread clinical use. There is some evidence that the topical anticholinergic, ipratropium bromide, decreases the volume of airway secretions in patients with COPD, without altering the viscoelastic properties of mucus.

Few mucolytic agents have been demonstrated to be effective in assisting airway clearance. An ideal mucolytic medication should be well tolerated systemically and should thin abnormally viscous mucus and thicken mucus that is too watery for proper clearance. An alternative hypothesis is that the so-called mucolytics or mucus-hydrating agents alter the surface properties of secretions, without substantially modifying the bulk viscoelastic properties of these secretions— the peashooter analogy of airway clearance once again. It may be that surface-active agents will become the mucokinetic agents of the 1990s.

It is clear that techniques for the measurement of the physical and transport properties of mucus have been well standardized and must be employed when evaluating any new form of mucokinetic therapy. Not to do so would be as unthinkable as evaluating a new hypoglycemic agent without measuring the blood sugar of the subjects taking this medication, or to attempt to determine the efficacy of a novel antihypertensive by measuring the heart rate, but not the blood pressures, of test subjects.

References

Adams, G. K., Aharonson, E. F., Reasor, M. J., and Proctor, D. F. (1976). Collection of normal canine tracheobronchial secretions. *J. Appl. Physiol.* 40: 247–249.

Agarwal, M., King, M., Rubin, B. K., and Shukla, J. B. (1989). Mucus transport in a miniaturized simulated cough machine: Effect of constriction and serous layer simulant. *Biorheology* 26: 977–988.

Allegra L., Bossi, R., and Braga, P. C. (1985). Influence of surfactant on mucociliary transport. *Prog. Respir. Dis.* 19: 441–460.

App, E. M., and King, M. (1990). Tracheal mucus rheology and potential difference in two day old puppies. *Biorheology* 27: 515–526.

Barnett, B., and Dulfano, M. J. (1970). Sputum viscoelasticity I: New methodology. *Am. Rev. Respir. Dis.* 101: 773–776.

Bhaskar, K. R., O'Sullivan, D. D., Seltzer, J., et al. (1985). Density gradient study of bronchial mucus aspirates from healthy volunteers and from patients with tracheostomy. *Exp. Lung. Res.* 9: 289–308.

Boyd, E. M. (1972). *Respiratory Tract Fluid*. Springfield, IL, Charles C Thomas.

Braga, P. C. (1988). Sinusoidal oscillation method. In *Methods in Bronchial Mucology*. Edited by P. C. Braga and L. Allegra. New York, Raven Press, pp. 63–71.

Charman, J., and Reid, L. (1972). Sputum viscosity in chronic bronchitis, bronchiectasis, asthma and cystic fibrosis. *Biorheology* 9: 185–199.

Davis, S. S. (1973). Rheological examination of sputum and saliva and the effect of drugs. In *Rheology of Biological Systems*. Edited by H. L. Gabelnick and M. Litt. Springfield, IL, Charles C Thomas, pp. 158–194.

Davis, S. S., (1988). Mathematical description. In *Methods in Bronchial Mucology*. Edited by P. C. Braga and L. Allegra. New York, Raven Press, pp. 33–49.

Davis, S. S., and Dippy, J. E. (1969). The rheological properties of sputum. *Biorheology* 6: 11–21.

De Sanctis, G. T., Tomkiewicz, R., King, M., and Schürch, S. (1992). Improvement of in vivo tracheal mucus clearance following administration of artificial surfactant (Curosurf) in dogs. *Eur. Respir. J.* 5: 386s.

Eliezer, N. (1974). Viscoelastic properties of mucus. *Biorheology* 11: 61–68.

Galabert, C., Jacquot, J., Zahm, J. M., and Puchelle, E. (1987). Relationships between the lipid content and the rheological properties of airway secretions in cystic fibrosis. *Clin. Chim. Acta* 164: 139–149.

Gilljam, H., Andersson, O., Ellin, A., Robertson, B., and Strandvik, B. (1988). Composition and surface properties of the bronchial lipids in adult patients with cystic fibrosis. *Clin. Chim. Acta* 176: 29–38.

Giordano, A. M., Holsclaw, D., and Litt, M. (1978). Mucus rheology and mucociliary clearance: Normal physiological state. *Am. Rev. Respir. Dis.* 118: 245–254.

Girod, S., Galabert, C., Pierrot, D., Boissonade, M. M., Zahm, J. M., Baszkin, A., and Puchelle, E. (1991). Role of phospholipid lining on respiratory mucus clearance by cough. *J. Appl. Physiol.* 71: 2262–2266.

Girod, S., Galabert, C., Lecuire, A., Zahm, J. M., and Puchelle, E. (1992). Phospholipid composition and surface-active properties of tracheobronchial secretions from patients with cystic fibrosis and chronic obstructive pulmonary diseases. *Pediatr. Pulmonol.* 13: 22–27.

Hwang, S. H., Litt, M., and Forsman, W. C. (1969). Rheological properties of mucus. *Rheol. Acta* 8: 438–448.

Jeanneret-Grosjean, A., King, M., Michoud, M. C., Lioté, H., and Amyot, R. (1988). Sampling technique and rheology of human bronchial mucus. *Am. Rev. Respir. Dis.* 137: 707–710.

Keal, E., and Reid, L. (1970). Méthodes d'étude des modifications de la sécretion bronchique et de sa viscosité. *Poumon. Coeur.* 26: 52–58.

Kim, C. S. (1988). Capillary type viscometer. In *Methods in Bronchial Mucology*. Edited by P. C. Braga and L. Allegra. New York, Raven Press, pp. 93–103.

King, M. (1987). Role of mucus viscoelasticity in cough clearance. *Biorheology* 24: 589–597.

King, M. (1988). Magnetic microrheometer. In *Methods in Bronchial Mucology*. Edited by P. C. Braga and L. Allegra. New York, Raven Press, pp. 73–83.

King, M. (1989). Mucus, mucociliary clearance and coughing. In *Respiratory Function in Disease*, 3rd ed. Edited by D. V. Bates. Philadelphia, W. B. Saunders, Chap. 3.

King, M., and Macklem, P. T. (1977). Rheological properties of microliter quantities of normal mucus. *J. Appl. Physiol.* 42: 797–802.

King, M., Gilboa, A., Meyer, F. A., and Silberberg, A. (1974). On the transport of mucus and its rheologic simulants in ciliated systems. *Am. Rev. Respir. Dis.* 110: 740–745.

King, M., El-Azab, J., Phillips, D. M., and Angus, G. E. (1985a). Antigen challenge and canine tracheal mucus. *Int. Arch. Allergy Appl. Immunol.* 77: 337–342.

King, M., Brock, G., and Lundell, C. (1985b). Clearance of mucus by simulated cough. *J. Appl. Physiol.* 58: 1776–1782.

King, M., Wight, A., De Sanctis, G. T., et al. (1989a). Mucus hypersecretion and viscoelasticity changes in cigarette-smoking dogs. *Exp. Lung Res.* 15: 375–389.

King, M., Zahm, J. M., Pierrot, D., Vaquez-Girod, S., and Puchelle, E. (1989b). The role of mucus gel viscosity, spinability, and adhesive properties in clearance by simulated cough. *Biorheology* 26: 737–745.

Knowles, M. R., Stutts, M. J., Spock, A., Fisher, A. N., Gatzy, J. T., and Boucher, R. C. (1983). Abnormal ion permeation through cystic fibrosis respiratory epithelium. *Science* 221: 1067–1070.

Knowles, M. R., Church, N. L., Waltner, W. E., et al. (1990). A pilot study of aerosolized amiloride for the treatment of cystic fibrosis lung disease. *N. Engl. J. Med.* 332: 1189–1194.

Lachmann, B. (1985). Possible function of bronchial surfactant. *Eur. J. Respir. Dis.* 67(Suppl. 142): 49–60.

Leikauf, G. D., Ueki, I. F., and Nadel, J. A. (1984). Autonomic regulation of viscoelasticity of cat tracheal gland secretion. *J. Appl. Physiol.* 56: 426–430.

Lopez-Vidriero, M. T. (1988). Tack test technique. In *Methods in Bronchial Mucology.* Edited by P. C. Braga and L. Allegra. New York, Raven Press, pp. 141–150.

Lopez-Vidriero, M. T., Das, I., Smith, A. P., Picot, R., and Reid, L. (1977). Bronchial secretion from normal human airways after inhalation of prostaglandin $F_{2\alpha}$; acetylcholine, histamine, and citric acid. *Thorax* 32: 734–739.

Lutz, R. J., Litt, M., and Chakrin, L. W. (1973). Physical–chemical factors in mucus rheology. In *Rheology of Biological Systems.* Edited by H. L. Gabelnick and M. Litt. Springfield, IL, Charles C. Thomas, pp. 158–194.

Macchione, M., King, M., Lorenzi, G., Zin, W., Böhm, G. M., and Saldiva, P. H. N. (1992). Determinants of mucociliary transport in the nose of the rat. *J. Appl. Physiol.* (submitted).

Macklem, P. T., Proctor, D. F., and Hogg, J. C. (1970). The stability of peripheral airways. *Respir. Physiol.* 8: 191–203.

Majima, Y., Hirata, K., Takeuchi, K., Hattori, M., and Sakakura, Y. (1990). Effects of orally administered drugs on dynamic viscoelasticity of human nasal mucus. *Am. Rev. Respir. Dis.* 141: 79–83.

Marriott, C., and Richards, J. H. (1974). Studies on the variation in the viscosity of bronchial mucus and a technique for reducing such variation. *Biorheology* 11: 129–135.

Morgenroth, K. (1985). Morphology of the bronchial lining layer and its alteration in IRDS, ARDS, and COLD. *Eur. J. Respir. Dis.* 67(Suppl. 142): 7–18.

Morgenroth, K., and Bolz, J. (1985). Morphological features of the interaction between mucus and surfactant on the bronchial mucosa. *Respiration* 47: 225–231.

Motta, C., Touillon, A. M., Simon, G., and Dastugue, B. (1984). Active lipid: A potential fluididizer of cystic fibrosis mucus. In *Cystic Fibrosis: Horizons*. Edited by D. Lawson. Chichester, Wiley, p. 337.

Paul, A., Marelli, D., Shennib, H., et al. (1989). Mucociliary function in autotransplanted, allotransplanted, and sleeve resected lungs. *J. Thorac. Cardiovasc. Surg.* 98: 523–528.

Powell, R. L., Aharonson, E. F., Schwarz, W. H., Proctor, D. F., Adams, G. K., and Reasor, M. (1974). Rheological behavior of normal tracheobronchial mucus of canines. *J. Appl. Physiol.* 37: 447–451.

Puchelle, E., Benis, A. M., and Zahm, J. M. (1973a). Etude de la visco-élasticité de l'expectoration à l'aide d'un rhéometre rotatif. *Bull. Physiopathol. Respir.* 9: 113–126.

Puchelle, E., Zahm, J. M., and Havez, R. (1973b). Données biochimiques et rhéologiques dans l'expectoration. III Rélation des protéines et mucines bronchiques avec les propriétés rhéologiques. *Bull. Physiopathol. Respir.* 9: 237–256.

Puchelle, E., Tournier, J. M., Zahm, J. M., and Sadoul, P. (1984). Rheology of sputum collected by a simple technique limiting salivary contamination. *J. Lab. Clin. Med.* 103: 347–353.

Puchelle, E., Zahm, J. M., and Duvivier, C. (1987a). Spinability of bronchial mucus: Relationship with viscoelasticity and mucus transport properties. *Biorheology* 20: 239–249.

Puchelle, E., Zahm, J. M., Jacquot, J. Plotkowski, C., and Duvivier, C. (1987b). A simple technique for measuring adhesion tension properties of human bronchial secretions. *Eur. J. Respir. Dis.* 71(Suppl. 153): 281–282.

Ramirez, O., Rubin, B. K., Green, F., Zayas, J. G., and King, M. (1991). The properties of respiratory mucus from patients with stable asthma and fatal asthma. *Chest* 100: 47S.

Rubin, B. K. (1992). A superficial view of mucus and the cystic fibrosis defect. *Pediatr. Pulmonol.* 13: 4–5.

Rubin, B. K., Ramirez, O., Zayas, J. G., Finegan, B., and King, M. (1990a). Collection and analysis of respiratory mucus from individuals without lung disease. *Am. Rev. Respir. Dis.* 141: 1040–1043.

Rubin, B. K., Ramirez, O., and King, M. (1990b). The mucus depleted frog palate as a model for the study of mucociliary clearance. *J Appl. Physiol.* 69: 424–429.

Rubin, B. K., Ramirez, O., Zayas, J. G., App, E. M., and King, M. (1990c). Respiratory mucus from asymptomatic asthmatic humans and *Ascaris suum* antigen sensitized dogs has physical properties similar to cystic fibrosis sputum. *Am. Rev. Respir. Dis.* 141: A756.

Rubin, B. K., Ramirez, O., Gourishankar, S., Curtis, L., and King, M. (1991a). Cough clearability of human respiratory mucus. *Am. Rev. Respir. Dis.* 143: A707.

Rubin, B. K., MacLeod, P M., Sturgess, J. M., and King, M. (1991b). Recurrent respiratory infections in a child with fucosidosis: Is the mucus too thin for effective transport? *Pediatr. Pulmonol.* 10: 304–309.

Rubin, B. K., Ramirez, O., and King, M. (1992a). The role of mucus rheology and transport in neonatal respiratory distress syndrome and the effect of surfactant therapy. *Chest* 101: 1080–1085.

Rubin, B. K., Ramirez, O., Zayas, J. G., Finegan, B., and King, M. (1992b). Respiratory mucus from asymptomatic smokers is better hydrated and more easily cleared by mucociliary action. *Am. Rev. Respir. Dis.* 145: 545–547.

Schürch, S., Gehr, P., Im Hof, V., Geiser, M., and Green, F. (1990). Surfactant displaces particles toward the epithelium in airways and alveoli. *Respir. Physiol.* 80: 17–32.

Shih, C. K., Litt, M., Khan, M. A., and Wolf, D. P. (1977). Effect of nondialyzable solids concentration and viscoelasticity on ciliary transport of tracheal mucus. *Am. Rev. Respir. Dis.* 115: 989–995.

Shim, C. S., King, M., and Williams, M. H., Jr. (1987). Lack of effect of hydration on sputum production in chronic bronchitis. *Chest* 92: 679–682.

Silveira, P. S. P., Böhm, G. M., Wen, C. L., Guimarães, E. T., Parada, M. A. C., King, M., and Saldiva, P. H. N. (1993). Computer-assisted rheological evaluation of micro-samples of mucus. *Comput. Meth. Prog. Biomed.* (in press).

Sturgess, J., Palfrey, A. J., and Reid, L. (1970). The viscosity of bronchial secretion. *Clin. Sci.* 38: 145–156.

Vaquez Girod, S., Zahm, J. M., Dionisius, J. P., Pierrot, D., and Puchelle, E. (1988). Automatic measurement of the wetting properties of biological fluids. *Innov. Tech. Biol. Med.* 9: 402–412.

Widdicombe, J. G. (1987). Role of lipids in airway function. *Eur. J. Respir. Dis.* 71(Suppl. 153): 197–204.

Williams, I. P., Hall, R. L., Miller, R. J., and Richardson, P. S. (1982). Analyses of human tracheobronchial mucus from healthy subjects. *Eur. J. Respir. Dis.* 63: 510–515.

Zahm, J. M., Puchelle, E., Duvivier, C., and Didelon, J. (1986). Spinability of respiratory mucus. Validation of a new apparatus: The Filancemeter. *Bull. Eur. Physiopathol. Respir.* 22: 609–613.

Zahm, J. M., Pierrot, D., Vaquez-Girod, S., Duvivier, C., King, M., and Puchelle, E. (1989). The role of mucus sol phase in clearance by simulated cough. *Biorheology* 26: 747–752.

Zahm, J. M., King, M., Duvivier, C., Pierrot, D., Girod, S., and Puchelle, E. (1991). Role of simulated repetitive coughing in mucus clearance. *Eur. Respir. J.* 4: 311–315.

Zayas, J. G., Man, G. C. W., and King, M. (1990). Tracheal mucus rheology in patients undergoing diagnostic bronchoscopy: Interrelations with smoking and cancer. *Am. Rev. Respir. Dis.* 141: 1107–1113.

8

Gene Expression in Airway Mucus-Secreting Cells

CAROL BASBAUM

University of California
San Francisco, California

BERTHOLD H. JANY

Medizinische Poliklinik
Universität Würzburg
Würzburg, Germany

KAZUHIKO TAKEUCHI

Mie University School of Medicine
Tsu, Mie, Japan

TOHRU TSUDA

University of Occupational and
Environmental Health
Kitakyushu City, Japan

JEAN-MARIE TOURNIER

INSERM Unite 314
C.H.R.
Reims, France

I. Introduction

Three exocrine cell types contribute to the production of human airway mucus: epithelial goblet cells and submucosal gland serous and mucous cells. Goblet and mucous gland cells share a common structure and function. They contain electron-lucent secretory granules and synthesize mucin, a high relative molecular mass (M_r), heavily glycosylated protein that forms the bulk of the mucous polymer gel. Immunocytochemical studies have shown that mucin is present in mucous gland and goblet cells, but not serous gland cells (Perini et al., 1989; Jany et al., 1991b). The latter, in contrast, contain electron-dense secretory granules and synthesize the antibacterial proteins lysozyme (Bowers and Corrin, 1977) and lactoferrin (Bowes et al., 1981) as well as the low M_r proteinase inhibitor known as antileukoproteinase (also bronchial inhibitor) (De Water et al., 1986).

What is known about the development of serous and mucous cells? In light of the biochemical differences between them, it is interesting that they appear to arise from a single precursor cell. This cell originates in the airway surface epithelium (Bucher and Reid, 1961). During gland formation, this precursor cell undergoes proliferation, forms plaques, and migrates into the underlying connective tissue. The plaques are later "canalized" to form lumina. Cells examined during the early stages of this process contain abundant glycogen, but no secretory granules (Plopper et al., 1986), and appear to constitute a homogeneous population of precursor cells. Serous and mucous cells ultimately differentiate from these cells through mechanisms that are currently unknown. We are interested in identifying these mechanisms, not only because of their importance during early development, but also because of the likelihood that they play important roles during the hypertrophy and differentiation of glands seen in diseases such as asthma, chronic bronchitis, and cystic fibrosis.

Although the process of differentiation is unique for each cell type, certain general principles apply. One is that the commitment of a precursor cell to a specific phenotype involves the initiation of transcription of phenotype-specific genes (Blau, 1989). A second is that the regulation of transcription of such genes is under the control of extracellular stimuli, such as growth factors or extracellular matrix components (Maniatis et al., 1987).

With these principles in mind, we have undertaken two experimental strategies aimed at understanding the mechanisms by which precursor cells differentiate to mucous or serous cells. The first has been to isolate submucosal gland cells in culture (Finkbeiner et al., 1986), provide extracellular stimuli under controlled conditions, and then observe corresponding responses reflected by changes in cell phenotype. A second strategy has been to isolate cDNAs and genomic clones encoding serous and mucous cell-specific proteins with the goal of identifying the DNA regulatory regions (and ultimately transcription factors) that couple extracellular stimuli to the phenotype-specific response of selective gene transcription. Both strategies will be discussed.

II. The Properties of a Tracheal Gland Cell Can Be Altered by Varying the Extracellular Matrix Upon Which It Is Grown

We performed experiments in which we kept the growth medium of bovine tracheal gland (BTG) cells constant (serum-free medium modified slightly from Wu and Smith, 1982), and varied the nature of the substrate on which the cells were grown (Tournier et al., 1992). We found that the cells attached to collagen IV (Col IV), laminin (LN), and fibronectin (FN), in a concentration-dependent manner. Under phase microscopy, cells formed confluent monolayers on Col IV or LN, whereas on FN, they formed birefringent spheres. Metabolic-labeling experiments showed that [^{35}S]methionine-labeled protein bands at 68, 105, and 120 kd were prominent when cells were grown on Col IV or LN, but were lost or reduced when the cells were grown on FN. Collagen IV also enhanced the expression of proteins at 14, 16.5, 18, and 21.5 kd. Attachment to all substrates was inhibited by an antibody (antibody AIIB2, generously provided by Dr. C. Damsky) directed against the β_1-subunit of cell surface receptors, called integrins (Hynes, 1987). This antibody precipitated several integrin heterodimers from a BTG cell membrane extract, caused partial retraction of cells from all substrates, and strongly suppressed the expression of Col IV- and LN-dependent proteins (Tournier et al., 1992). Production of the 105-kd protein was completely inhibited by the antibody, even in the presence of the permissive Col IV or LM substrate. Control experiments indicated that the antibody's affects on protein synthesis did not require changes in cell shape. The results showed that gland cell protein production is regulated by integrin-mediated signals from the extracellular matrix (ECM). Since phenotype is a reflection of the specific proteins produced by a particular cell, the results suggest that the gland cell phenotype, itself, can be regulated by the ECM through integrins.

III. Collagenase Is Among the Gland Cell Proteins Regulated by the Extracellular Matrix

In the process of evaluating the effects of various substrates on gland cell differentiation, we noted that confluent BTG cell monolayers often contained "holes," possibly corresponding to focal degradation of the collagen substrate. Because of similar observations by other investigators (Niles, 1988), and that one of the aforementioned Col-IV-dependent proteins had an M_r of 68–72 kd (consistent with its possible identity as a collagenase), we examined BTG cells for their ability to secrete collagen-degrading enzymes. To detect these enzymes, we applied aliquots of BTG cell-conditioned medium to polyacrylamide gels impregnated with porcine skin gelatin. We detected progressively larger amounts of gelatin-degrading activity in conditioned medium left in contact with BTG cells for increasing lengths of time (Tournier and Basbaum, 1991). After purification, the activity from cultured BTG cells presented a single major band on reducing sodium dodecyl sulfate–polyacrylamide gel electrophoresis (SDS–PAGE) at 74 kd. After treatment of this enzyme with p-aminophenylmercuric acetate (APMA), we detected gelatinase activity at 68, 31, and 39 kd. To more precisely identify the enzyme, we performed Western blot assays using antibodies directed against matrix metalloproteinases 1 and 2 (MMP-1 and MMP-2). The BTG cell enzyme was recognized by the antibody directed against MMP-2 (a type IV collagenase also known as gelatinase), but not that directed against MMP-1. Consistent with identification of the enzyme as MMP-2, the immunoreactive band underwent a size reduction upon activation with APMA. This is due to the cleavage of the propeptide, exposing the Zn-binding site required for enzymatic activity. To determine the substrate specificity of this enzyme, we examined its ability to degrade both Col I and Col IV. The BTG cell gelatinase was able to degrade both types of collagen. Therefore, the enzyme is active against both the basal lamina (type IV) and interstitial connective tissue (type I) types of collagen. This unusual property has also recently been reported for a collagenase present in osteosarcoma cells (Overall and Sodek, 1991). Another interesting property of the enzyme lies in its susceptibility to regulation by extracellular signals. The 68-kd gelatinase decreased substantially if cultures were incubated with the AIIB2 antibody directed against the human β_1-integrin subunit (Tournier and Basbaum, 1991). Thus, as in fibroblasts (Werb et al., 1989), gelatinase synthesis in BTG cells is controlled by the composition of the ECM through integrins.

To examine the in vivo distribution of the enzyme, we raised a polyclonal antibody against collagenase purified from the BTG cells. This antibody recognized the 74-kd form of BTG cell gelatinase as well as ones at 68 and 39 kd observed only after APMA activation. By immunocytochemical techniques, we observed staining in tracheal submucosal glands and some epithelial basal cells of adult cows. By using an antibody recognizing the rat homologue of MMP-2, we stained tracheal sections from rats ranging in age from the day of birth to the adult. Although weak staining was present in epithelial cells at day 1, the staining was more pronounced in rats at the age of 5 days, when the enzyme was present discontinuously at the base of the tracheal epithelium. Some of the staining outlined convexities extending down into the connective tissue, suggesting the downgrowth of glands into the submucosa. Thus, collagenase is present not only in vitro, but also in vivo.

That collagenase expression is known to be modulated by cytokines and growth factors [interleukin-1_α and 1_β, tumor necrosis factor (TNF-β), basic fibroblast growth factor, interferon alpha, and transforming growth factor β] (Murphy et al., 1990) suggests that the control of collagenase synthesis by extracellular signals may be a component of the overall sequence of events leading to both gland morphogenesis and gland hypertrophy (Jones and Reid, 1973).

IV. The Search for Tracheal-Specific and Serous Cell-Specific Control Elements on the Lysozyme Gene

Immunocytochemical studies by previous investigators showed that lysozyme is present in serous, but not mucous, cells of the airway submucosal glands (Bowes and Corrin, 1977). In this sense, lysozyme represents a marker of the serous cell phenotype. For a precursor cell to differentiate into a serous cell, it will at some point have to initiate lysozyme transcription. We are interested in ultimately identifying the gene regulatory sequences, the transcription factors, and the extracellular signals regulating this event. To begin these studies, we have isolated lysozyme cDNAs and genomic clones.

To isolate lysozyme cDNAs, we screened a cow tracheal cDNA library with a cDNA probe encoding the "stomach 2" form of cow lysozyme (Irwin and

Wilson, 1989). We obtained three cDNAs, each encoding the entire lysozyme-coding region, 3′ untranslated regions (two with poly(A) tails), and 5′ untranslated regions of various sizes (Takeuchi et al., 1992). Within the coding region, the three clones showed approximately 90% homology. This, paired with the fact that the 3′ untranslated regions were dissimilar, indicated that each cDNA is related to a different gene. The cow trachea, therefore, expresses three lysozyme genes encoding similar, but nonidentical, proteins (the three genes correspond to cDNAs 5A, 1020 bp; 14D, 1258 bp; and 7A, 1060 bp). These genes encode mRNA transcripts of three different lengths, as determined by Northern blots of RNA extracted from tracheal tissue.

The 3′ untranslated region and lysozyme-coding region of clone 7A correspond exactly to that of the cDNA from stomach (stomach 2). Because of the tendency for untranslated regions of genes to diverge after duplication, the identity between the 3′ untranslated regions of the tracheal (7A) cDNA and the stomach 2 cDNA indicates that both are products of the same gene. In view of this, the substantial extension of the 5′ end of the tracheal 7A cDNA beyond that of the stomach 2 cDNA (determined by primer extension to be full length) denotes the occurrence of tracheal-specific RNA transcription or processing.

Primer extension data show that the transcription start site of the tracheal 7A cognate mRNA is approximately 220-bp upstream of that of the stomach 2 cognate mRNA. The presence of a TATA box in this region (approximately 30-bp upstream of the transcription start site of stomach 2) suggests that an alternative promoter drives expression of this gene in the trachea. This promoter presumably mediates tracheal-specific lysozyme transcription, although the specific cell type transcribing 7A is currently unknown.

Nondenaturing lysozyme overlay gel analysis of cow tracheal extracts revealed lysozyme proteins showing three distinct mobilities. Extracts from glands dissected free of connective tissue yielded a single band of intermediate mobility. Calculation of the isoelectric point of proteins encoded by each of our cDNAs suggested that clone 5A was most likely to encode the gland form of lysozyme. To obtain additional evidence for this, we purified lysozyme from gland tissue extract. The NH_2-terminal amino acid sequence of this lysozyme coincides exactly with that encoded by cDNA 5A. Most recently, we have shown by polymerase chain reaction (PCR) and Southern hybridization with a 5A-specific probe, that bovine tracheal gland (BTG) serous cells in culture transcribe 5A-specific mRNA. Two genomic clones (163 and 164), isolated by screening a cow genomic library with a 5A-specific probe, were digested with restriction enzymes and hybridized with probes corresponding to exons 1 and 2. The exon 1 probe hybridized strongly to a 12-kb fragment in clone 163. Additional analysis of this fragment revealed that it contains approximately 6 kb of sequence upstream of the transcription start site. Deletion analysis of this promoter-containing fragment of the *5A* lysozyme gene should identify regulatory elements controlling serous cell-specific transcription. These could potentially be incubated in vitro transcription assays together with nuclear extracts from cultured cells expressing high versus low levels of lysozyme to begin to identify nuclear transcription factors mediating serous cell-specific lysozyme transcription.

V. The Search for Regulatory Elements on the Mucin Gene: Relevance to Mucous Hypersecretion?

Immunocytochemical studies have shown that mucin is present in mucous, but not serous, cells of the airway submucosal glands (Perini et al., 1989). For a precursor cell to differentiate into a mucous cell, at some point, it will have to initiate mucin transcription. We are interested in ultimately identifying the gene regulatory regions, the transcription factors, and the extracellular signals regulating this event.

Our interest in mucin cDNAs is not limited to developmental issues, but also extends to the problem of overproduction of mucus in conditions such as asthma, chronic bronchitis, and cystic fibrosis. We wondered whether such overproduction might be at least partly mediated by up regulation of mucin gene transcription. To explore this possibility, we have induced overproduction of mucus in rats by infection or irritation, and compared mucin mRNA levels in the airways of these rats with those of specific pathogen-free controls (Jany et al., 1991a). One primary requirement for our studies was the availability of a mucin cDNA suitable for monitoring mucin mRNA in rat airways.

At the outset of our studies, three mucin cDNAs had been isolated. These were from a human mammary tumor (Gendler et al., 1987), pig submandibular gland (Timpte et al., 1988), and human intestine (Gum et al., 1989). On the basis of the similar amino acid compositions reported for mucins from the airways (Woodward et al., 1982; Feldhoff et al., 1979) and the intestine (Neutra and Forster, 1987), we used the human intestinal mucin cDNA SMUC-41 (Gum et al., 1989) generously provided by Drs. Y. Kim and J. Gum, to screen a human airway cDNA library. With SMUC-41 as probe, we isolated a human airway mucin cDNA, HAM-1, which was 96% homologous to SMUC-41 (Jany et al., 1991b). Gerard et al. (Gerard, 1990) isolated a similar cDNA from a human airway library by screening with a synthetic oligonucleotide designed from the SMUC-41 sequence. Southern blot analyses verified that SMUC-41 and the two cDNAs isolated from human airway libraries encoded mRNAs transcribed from a single gene, now referred to as *MUC-2*. In situ hybridization data obtained using HAM-1 as a probe revealed that the *MUC-2* gene is expressed at high levels in bronchial epithelial and intestinal goblet cells and at lower levels in bronchial gland cells in humans (Tsuda et al., 1991a). Our next step was to evaluate the ability of the human mucin probes to cross-hybridize with rat airway mRNA. Although our original intention was to use the human airway cDNA (HAM-1) to probe rat airways, we later found SMUC-41 itself to be more useful, based on its size.

In Southern blots, independent of hybridization conditions, SMUC-41 hybridized to a single approximately 8-kb major fragment in *Hinf* 1-digested and one major fragment at 6.5-kb in *Sau* 3A-digested human genomic DNA. DNA from dog, cow, and rat, digested with the same enzymes, yielded multiple bands. Pursuing studies in the rat, we performed Northern blots using RNA from the intestine, airways, and heart of specific pathogen-free (SPF) rats. As expected from the positive Southern blot results, rat RNA hybridized strongly with SMUC-41. In the SPF rats, intestinal RNA produced an intense, polydisperse signal (maximum size 13 kb) whereas that from the airways and heart was negative. The airway negativity is consistent with the fact that mucous cells are rare in SPF rats (Huang et al., 1989; Plopper et al., 1983).

The negative hybridization result in the airways of SPF rats was reversed in rats that lived in the animal colony for 1–3 weeks. Serum analysis revealed that some rats spontaneously became infected with Sendai virus, Corona virus or CAR bacillus. All rats with significant antibody titers for Sendai virus showed mucin hybridization signals. The SPF rats as well as those infected by other pathogens did not. Mucin hybridization signals obtained from airway RNA of Sendai virus-infected rats that were also exposed to SO_2 showed signals more intense than those from rats with infection alone (Jany et al., 1991a).

These data indicate that infection and irritation increase mucin mRNA steady state in rat airways. This does not seem to occur secondary to mucous cell mitosis because mucous cells (containing electron-lucent secretory granules) do not incorporate [³H]thymidine during the period of mucin mRNA induction (Royce and Basbaum, 1990). Furthermore, mucous cells have not been observed to incorporate [³H]thymidine during the period of rapid mucous cell increase following cigarette smoke exposure (Ayers and Jeffery, 1988). In the absence of mucous cell mitosis (as reflected by lack of DNA synthesis), it seems likely that the observed increases in mucin mRNA reflect new mucin gene transcription in previously existing cells, possibly an early event in mucous hypersecretion. Thus, the initiation of mucin gene transcription may figure importantly in a *trans-differentiation* event underlying hypersecretion as well as in a *differentiation* event underlying the early development of mucous cells. Since both process can be conveniently studied in a rat model, we have focused considerable effort on the isolation and characterization of rat airway mucin cDNA clones.

By screening a rat airway cDNA library with SMUC-41, we have isolated several positive clones. Clone RAM-7 encodes threonine/isoleucine repeats (Tsuda et al., 1991b). By screening the same library (constructed in λ ZAP 2) with an antibody directed against deglycosylated rat intestinal mucin (generously provided by Drs. Y Kim and J. Gum), we have isolated several cDNAs including RAM 35, which encodes threonine/arginine tandem repeats. Both cDNAs hybridize to airway RNA from Sendai virus-infected, SO$_2$-exposed rats, but not to that from SPF rats. We are now attempting to obtain additional cDNA sequence before screening a genomic library to isolate clones containing the mucin promoter.

Acknowledgments

We thank our collaborators who have contributed to this work: Drs. David Irwin, Beth Stewart, Eve Shinbrot, Marianne Gallup, Jim Gum, and Young Kim. This work was supported by NIH RO1HL43762 and NIH PPG HL24136.

References

Ayers, M. M., and Jeffery, P. K. (1988). Proliferation and differentiation in mammalian airway epithelium. *Eur. Respir. J.* 1: 58–80.

Blau, H. M. (1989). How fixed is the differentiated state? *Trends Genet.* 5(8): 268–272.

Bowes, D., and Corrin, B. (1977). Ultrastructural immunocytochemical localisation of lysozyme in human bronchial glands. *Thorax* 32: 163–170.

Bowes, D., Clark, A. E., and Corrin, B. (1981). Ultrastructural localisation of lactoferrin and glycoprotein in human bronchial glands. *Thorax* 36: 108–115.

Bucher, U., and Reid, L. (1961). Development of the mucus-secreting elements in human lung. *Thorax* 16: 219–225.

De Water, R., Willems, L. N. A., Van Muijen, G. N. P., Franken, C., Fransen, J. A. M., Dijkman, J. H., and Kramps, J. A. (1986). Ultrastructural localization of bronchial antileukoprotease in central and peripheral human airways by a gold-labeling technique using monoclonal antibodies. *Am. Rev. Respir. Dis.* 133: 882–890.

Feldhoff, P. A., Bhavanandan, V. P., and Davidson, E. A. (1979). Purification, properties, and analysis of human asthmatic bronchial mucin. *Biochemistry* 18: 2430–2436.

Finkbeiner, W. E., Nadel, J. A., and Basbaum, C. B. (1986). Establishment and characterization of a cell line derived from bovine tracheal glands. *In Vitro* 22: 561–567.

Gendler, S. J., Burchell, J. M., Dunig, T., Lamport, D., White, R., Parker, M., and Taylor-Papadimitriou, J. (1987). Cloning of partial cDNA encoding differentiation and tumor-associated mucin glycoproteins expressed by human mammary epithelium. *Proc. Natl. Acad. Sci. USA* 84: 6060–6064.

Gerard, C. (1990). The core polypeptide of cystic fibrosis tracheal mucin contains a tandem repeat structure. *J. Clin. Invest.* 86: 277–285.

Gum, J. R., Byrd, J. C., Hicks, J. W., Toribara, N. W., Lamport, D. T. A., and Kim, Y. S. (1989). Molecular cloning of human intestinal mucin cDNAs. *J. Biol. Chem.* 264: 6480–6487.

Huang, H. T., Haskell, A., and McDonald, D.M. (1989). Changes in epithelial secretory cells and potentiation of neurogenic inflammation in the trachea of rats with respiratory tract infections. *Anat. Embryol.* 180: 325–341.

Hynes, R. O. (1987). Integrins: A family of cell surface receptors.

Irwin, D. M., and Wilson, A. C. (1989). Multiple cDNA sequences and the evolution of bovine stomach lysozyme. *J. Biol. Chem.* 264: 11387–11393.

Jany, B., Gallup, M., Tsuda, T., and Basbaum, C. (1991a). Mucin gene expression in rat airways following infection and irritation. *Biochem. Biophys. Res. Commun.* 181: 1–8.

Jany, B., Gallup, M., Yan, P. S., Gum, J., Kim, Y., and Basbaum, C. (1991b). Human intestine and airways express the same mucin gene. *J. Clin. Invest.* 87: 77–82.

Jones, R., and Reid, L. (1973). Goblet cell glycoprotein and tracheal gland hypertrophy in rat airways: The effects of tobacco smoke with or without the anti-inflammatory agent phenylmethyloxadiazole. *Br. J. Exp. Pathol.* 54: 229–239.

Maniatis, T., Goodbourn, S., and Fischer, J. A. (1987). Regulation of inducible and tissue-specific gene expression. *Science* 236: 1237–1245.

Murphy, G., Hembry, R., Hughes, C., Fosang, A., and Hardingham, T. (1990). Role and regulation of metalloproteinases in connective tissue turnover. *Biochem. Soc. Trans.* 18: 812–815.

Neutra, M. R., and Forstner, J. F. (1987). *Gastrointestinal Mucus: Synthesis, Secretion, and Function.* New York, Raven Press.

Niles, R. K. K., Hyman, B., Christensen, T., Wasano, K., and Brody, J. (1988). Characterization of extended primary and secondary cultures of hamster tracheal epithelial cells. *In Vitro Cell Dev. Biol.* 24: 457–463.

Overall, C., and Sodek, J. (1991). Purification of rat osteosarcoma 72 kD gelatinase/type IV collagenase. Rat, but not human, 72 kD gelatinase degrades native collagen, 3/4 collagen fragments, and gelatin. *J. Cell Biol.* 115(Part 2): 139a.

Perini, J. M., Marianne, T., Lafitte, J. J., Lamblin, G., Roussel, P., and Mazzuca, M. (1989). Use of an antiserum against deglycosylated human mucins for cellular localization of their peptide precursors: Antigenic similarities between bronchial and intestinal mucins. *J. Histochem. Cytochem.* 37: 869–875.

Plopper, C. G., Mariassy, A. T., Wilson, D. W., Alley, J. L., Nishio, S. J., and Nettesheim, P. (1983). Comparison of nonciliated tracheal epithelial cells in six mammalian species: Ultrastructure and population densities. *Exp. Lung Res.* 5: 281–294.

Plopper, C. G., Weir, A. J., Nishio, S. J., Cranz, D. L., and St. George, J. A. (1986). Tracheal submucosal gland development in the rhesus monkey, *Macaca mulatta*: Ultrastructure and histochemistry. *Anat. Embryol.* 174: 167–178.

Royce, F. A., and Basbaum, C. B. (1990). Analysis of thymidine incorporation by airway epithelial cells in a rat model of chronic bronchitis. *Am. Rev. Respir. Dis.* 141: A107.

Takeuchi, K., Dohrman, A., Irwin, D., Gallup, M., Shinbrot, E., and Stewart, B. (1992). Multiple cDNA sequences and tissue localization of bovine tracheal lysozyme. *Am. Rev. Respir. Dis.* 145: A358.

Timpte, C. S., Eckhardt, A. E., Abernethy, J. L., and Hill, R. L. (1988). Porcine submaxillary gland apomucin contains tandemly repeated identical sequences of 81 residues. *J. Biol. Chem.* 263: 1081–1088.

Tournier, J.-M., and Basbaum, C. B. (1991). Production of a collagenase by bovine tracheal glands in culture. *Am. Rev. Respir. Dis.* 143: A403.

Tournier, J.-M., Goldstein, G. R., Hall, D. E., Damsky, C. H., and Basbaum, C. B. (1992). Extracellular matrix proteins regulate morphological and biochemical properties of tracheal gland serous cells through integrins. *Am. J. Respir. Cell Mol. Biol.* 6: 461–467.

Tsuda, T., Escudier, E., Cardone, M., Dohrman, A, Gum, J., Kim, Y., Jany, B., and Basbaum, C. (1991a). Localization of mucin mRNA in human bronchus and colon by in situ hybridization. [abstract] *J. Cell Biol.*

Tsuda, T., Jany, B., Gallup, M., and Basbaum, C. (1991b). Rat airway cDNA encoding mucin or mucin-like peptides. *Am. Rev. Respir. Dis.* 143: A141.

Werb, Z., Tremble, P. M., Behrendtsen, O., Crowley, E., and Damsky, C. H. (1989). Signal transduction through the fibronectin receptor induces collagenase and stromelysin gene expression. *J. Cell Biol.* 109: 877–889.

Woodward, H., Horsey, B., Bhavanandan, V. P., and Davidson, E. A. (1982). Isolation, purification, and properties of respiratory mucus glycoproteins. *Biochemistry* 21: 694–701.

Wu, R., and Smith, D. J. (1982). Continuous multiplication of rabbit tracheal epithelial cells in a defined, hormone-supplemented medium. *In Vitro* 18: 800–812.

9

Airway Submucosal Gland Secretion

SANAE SHIMURA and TAMOTSU TAKISHIMA

Tohoku University School of Medicine
Sendai, Japan

I. Introduction

Airway secretion of mucus has a principal role in mucociliary clearance and, thus, in the defense mechanisms against inhaled particles and pathogens as well as in the reflexes (bronchoconstriction and cough) and local immune responses. Secretory cells exist in both surface epithelium (goblet cells) and submucosal glands, which consist of serous and mucous cells. In healthy adult humans, the volume of submucosal gland cells exceeds that of the surface mucous cells (goblet cells) by a ratio of about 40:1 (Reid, 1960). Furthermore, a recent study has shown that the cystic fibrosis transmembrane conductance regulator (CFTR) expression is very low in the superficial epithelium and considerably higher in the submucosal glands (Collins, 1992), indicating that the submucosal glands probably make a greater contribution to the production of respiratory tract mucus in human lungs.

In the human respiratory tract, the submucosa consists of glands and cartilage, the two occurring together, with the gland mainly internal to the cartilage, lying between it and the epithelium, but also existing between the plates of cartilage. Glands are most numerous in the trachea, decreasing progressively distally, along with the cartilage. They are absent from airways smaller than 1 mm in diameter (i.e., bronchioles). The total volume and airway distribution of submucosal glands is species-related (Jeffery, 1983). In some species, such as the goose, rat, and rabbit, submucosal glands are scarce or absent and, therefore, goblet cells are presumably the primary source of mucus. In the rat, there is no cartilage in the intrapulmonary airway, and glands are concentrated centrally in the upper trachea. In the rabbit, gland-free cartilage extends into the small intrapulmonary bronchi. In cat, ferret, and pig trachea, submucosal glands are abundant, and in addition to human specimens, tracheas from these species are often used for the experimental study of submucosal gland secretion because of their basic anatomical similarity to human tracheobronchial trees (Goco et al., 1963; Jeffery, 1983).

Airway submucosal glands show tubuloacinar structures and consist of two functional units: the acinar portion that synthesizes, stores, and secretes granules and electrolytes; and the ductal portion that is speculated to have a role in electrolyte absorption (Meyrick et al., 1969, 1970). The ciliated portion of respiratory epithelium dips into the gland opening and leads to the first part of the duct, the ciliated duct, and then gives way in the collecting duct to an epithelium composed of tall, columnar, eosinophilic cells containing numerous large mito-chondria. These cell structures suggest that the collecting duct controls ionic and water concentration (Meyrick et al., 1969, 1970). In fact, there is an abundant supply of blood capillaries in the region of the collecting duct. However, no direct evidence supporting this speculation has yet been obtained because of lack of experimental tools suitable for this area.

From the collecting duct arise secretory tubules and acini that consist of three different morphological cell types: serous cells, mucous cells, and myoepi-thelial cells. Glycoproteins (mucins) are abundant in the mucous cells of sub-mucosal glands and the secretion or release of mucous glycoprotein has been investigated extensively. The major part of this chapter will deal with mucous glycoprotein secretion. Serous cells contain and secrete some antibacterial sub-stances: lysozyme, lactoferrin, immunoglobulins, and proteinase inhibitors of receptor-mediated responses. Furthermore, submucosal glands actively secrete electrolytes with fluid that is independent of mucin secretion, although it still remains unknown which acinar cells in the submucosal glands are responsible for the electrolyte secretion. Recent studies have given us some insights concerning its mechanism, and we will discuss some of these in this chapter. In addition, the myoepithelial cells, which surround acini and secretory tubules in airway sub-mucosal glands, and the contraction of these cells, which represents a short-term and initial secretory response, will also be discussed.

II. Experimental Preparations

Almost all the tools and methods available for functional research in other exocrine tissues have also been applied to the studies of airway submucosal gland secretion.

However, airway submucosal glands are unique in that they are embedded in the submucosal layers of airway walls, making it difficult to isolate these glands from surrounding tissues. Airway secretions are derived from both the surface epithelium and the submucosal glands of the tracheobronchial tree. It is also possible that the tissue surrounding submucosal glands affects secretion (Sasaki et al., 1990). Thus, investigations of airway submucosal gland secretion have been hindered by difficulties in adequately separating the physiological responses of submucosal gland cells from those of the surface epithelium and also in excluding the possible effects of surrounding tissues. To overcome these problems, various methods have been developed (Table 1).

A classic and conventional approach to such a problem is the histological study that includes morphometry and histochemistry of secretory granules. Another is to use markers specific to the secretions of submucosal glands: lysozyme, radiolabeled precursors, antibodies, and such. Recently, antibodies or other probes that specifically and sensitively measure secretion from airway submucosal glands have become available (Lin et al., 1989; Basbaum et al., 1986; Dwyer et al., 1992), and these will be described in detail in another section (see Sec. III). Another approach is to study a preparation of isolated tissue or cells enriched with specific cell types. Such a preparation enables one to study the function of a specific tissue or cell type without interference from other cellular, neural, connective tissue, or blood-borne factors.

Morphometry of granules in secretory cells of glands has been performed both in vitro and in vivo by stimulations with various secretagogues or exposure to tobacco smoke, air pollutants, or various proteinases (Basbaum et al., 1981; Gashi et al., 1986; Hayashi et al., 1979; Kollerstrom et al., 1977; Phipps et al., 1986; Tom-Moy et al., 1983). In interpreting such morphometric data related to secretory granules and products of submucosal glands, the following possibilities should be noted: First, the surrounding tissues and inflammatory cells affect the secretory responses. Second, the individual secretory granules will vary in their rates of production and secretion, and in their initial volumes; the alterations in the cell size are not precisely known. Lastly, morphometric analysis of secretory granules in response to various stimuli is suitable for the analysis of serous cells, but not for the analysis of mucous cells in submucosal glands. For example, Basbaum et al. (1981) and Gashi et al. (1986) have performed electron microscopic morphometric analysis of the alteration in secretory cell structure induced by adrenergic and cholinergic agonists and neuropeptides in incubated ferret tracheal segments. They have found that the volume of granules in the serous cells was significantly reduced by these agonists, suggesting the stimulation of secretion from serous cells, whereas they failed to see any significant alterations in the secretory granules of mucous cells in submucosal glands. This is because the granules in the mucous cells are large and fused.

The study of the control mechanism of submucosal gland secretion has been extensively examined by organ culture methods with tracheal or bronchial frag-

Table 1 Experimental Preparations for Study of Airway Submucosal Gland Secretion

Preparations	Secretory responses	Ref.
Morphometry of secretory granules	Degranulation in secretory cells	Tom-Moy et al., 1983; Phipps et al., 1986; Basbaum et al., 1981; Gashi et al., 1986
Airway explant organ culture	Mucous glycoprotein (mucin), glycoconjugate, and lysozyme secretion	Marom et al., 1981, 1984; Goswami et al., 1990; Baker et al., 1977; Cheng et al., 1981; Shelhamer et al., 1980
Isolated trachea in vivo	Whole (volume) secretion, mucous glycoprotein, glycoconjugate, and lysozyme secretion	Chakrin et al., 1972; Gallagher et al., 1975; Webber and Widdicombe, 1987
Micropipette method in vivo	Whole (volume, fluid?) secretion	Ueki et al., 1980; German et al., 1982
Hillock method (in vitro and in vivo)	Whole (volume, fluid?) secretion	Davis et al., 1976, 1980, 1982a,b, 1991; Schultz et al., 1985; Johnson et al., 1981, 1983, 1985; Haxihiu et al., 1991a,b,c
Isolated submucosal glands (in vitro)	Mucous glycoprotein secretion, ion transport, and glandular contraction	Ishihara et al., 1990, 1992; Sasaki et al., 1989a, 1986, 1990; Sasaki and Gallacher, 1990; Satoh et al., 1992; Shimura et al., 1986, 1987a,b, 1988, 1990a,b, 1991a,b, 1992a,b
Isolated gland cells (in vitro)	Mucous glycoprotein, glycoconjugate secretion, and ion transport	Madison et al., 1989; Dwyer et al., 1992; Finkbeiner et al., 1986; Sommerhoff et al., 1990; Yang et al., 1988b; Yamaya et al., 1991; Sommerhoff and Finkbeiner, 1990; Schuster et al., 1992; Paul et al., 1992

ments of the human, pig, dog, rat, and cat. Glycoconjugates and macromolecules secreted from tracheal and bronchial fragments (explants or whole trachea) contain both mucous glycoproteins and proteoglycans, the latter coming from the surrounding tissues as well as the secretory cells (superficial goblet cells and submucosal glands). Additionally, mucous glycoprotein (mucin) comes from both goblet cells and submucosal glands. The tracheal and bronchial airway explants employed in these experiments contain both submucosal glands and goblet cells. There appear to be many more submucosal gland cells than goblet cells, but we cannot differentiate the cellular origin of the biosynthetically labeled molecules. Some investigators, therefore, have used airway mucous membranes without cartilage for their experiments (Hartman et al., 1984; Hall, 1992). Culp et al. (1990) used cat tracheal explants in which the surface epithelium was removed by brushing, and Tandler et al. (1981) and Sherman et al. (1981) separated the surface epithelium by treatment with EDTA to exclude the superficial goblet cell secretion and possible effects of epithelium on submucosal gland secretion (Sasaki et al., 1989a). Some investigators (Borson et al., 1984; Corrales et al., 1984) have examined $^{35}SO_4$-labeled macromolecule release from airway tissues held between two half-chambers (an Ussing-like chamber). After incubation with $^{35}SO_4$ in the submucosal solution for 2–3 h, the tissue was stimulated and the effect was estimated as percentage increase from prior baseline value. The $^{35}SO_4$-macromolecule is believed to come from submucosal glands.

Some investigators have employed a whole trachea for studies of airway secretion in vivo. With use of a whole trachea, Chakrin et al. (1972) and Gallagher et al. (1975) describe a method for measuring the output of macromolecules and mucous proteins (especially the sulfated glycoproteins) from the trachea of anesthetized dog and cat. The animal breathed through the caudal of the cannulae, and the isolated tracheal segment was washed out with Krebs–Henseleit solution through the two cannules. The recurrent laryngeal nerves were left intact. Webber and Widdicombe (1987a) have developed an air-filled whole-trachea model of the ferret, suspended in a jacketed organ bath. The laryngeal end of the trachea, at the bottom of the bath, is fitted with a Perspex pump from which mucus can be extracted using a catheter. The caudal end is also cannulated and attached to a manometer that records intratracheal pressure, influenced by smooth-muscle tone. This preparation has the advantage of allowing simultaneous estimations of mucous secretion and smooth-muscle tone. As a marker of submucosal gland secretion, they measured ^{35}S-labeled mucin and lysozyme release into the trachea. This preparation of whole trachea has the advantage of providing in vivo secretory responses, although, in this experiment, they did not directly represent submucosal gland secretion.

Attempts to specifically measure the submucosal gland secretions, while avoiding those originating other than from submucosal glands, have been made by some investigators. Ueki et al. (1980) developed a method for studying fluid secretion from individual gland duct openings in vitro or in vivo using micropipettes. Micropipettes were used to collect timed samples from individual gland duct openings in exposed tracheal epithelium. Furthermore, Davis et al. (1976) and Quinton (1979) developed a method for the simultaneous visualization of secretions from many glands by coating the airway surface with powdered tantalum. Secreted mucus formed "hillocks" over each gland duct opening, the measurement of which provides an estimate of secretion rate in vitro and in vivo. With these techniques, the innervation of submucosal glands and the autonomical regulation of their secretion can be studied. These two methods, however, have a disadvantage in that we can know only the short-term response and not the relatively long-term responses, since, in the former method, it is difficult to continue a collection of secretion for more than a few minutes and, in the latter method, the number and size of the hillocks reach a plateau within 1 min after the stimulation (Davis et al., 1976; Davis and Nadel, 1980).

Recently, Shimura et al. (1986) have been successful in isolating single submucosal glands from trachea, which represent the functional unit of submucosal gland secretion (Fig. 1). Tracheas were removed from adult cats under anesthesia and fixed in Krebs–Ringer bicarbonate (KRB) solution. By applying a technique originally developed for the isolation of a single nephron (Burg et al., 1966), fresh, unstained submucosal glands were mechanically isolated from the membranous portion of the trachea using two pairs of sharpened tweezers and microscissors under a stereomicroscope (Shimura et al., 1986; Shimura, 1990). This isolated gland preparation allows the examination of submucosal gland secretion (mucin secretion, ion transport, and glandular contraction) in a well-defined condition by excluding the possible effects of surrounding tissues. Culp et al. (1983) have also developed a technique for isolating submucosal gland cells

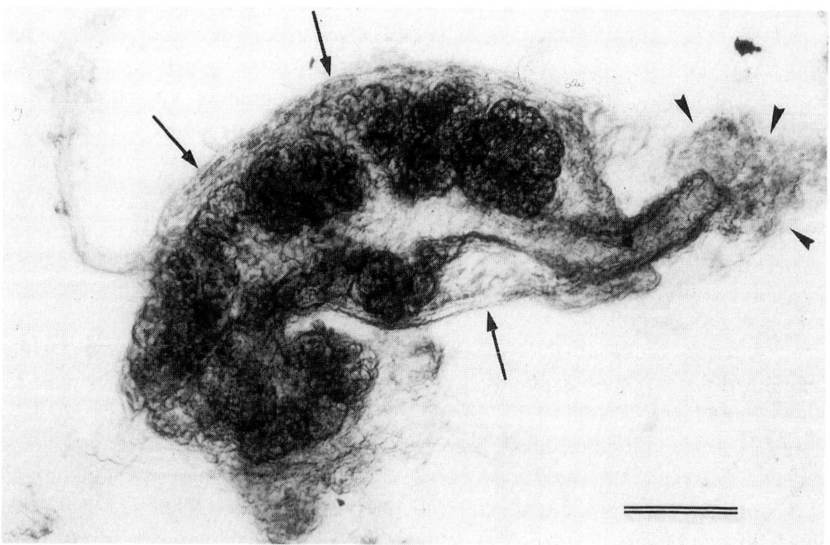

Figure 1 Single submucosal gland secreting mucus from the tip of a duct (arrowheads) in the fresh and unstained state, isolated from canine trachea. The gland has the appearance of a "bunch of grapes." Arrows indicate small vessels attached to the gland, which contain some blood cells (bar, 100 μm). (From Shimura et al., 1986)

from cat trachea. The excised trachea is stripped of surface epithelium, scraped free from underlying cartilage, minced into small pieces, and subjected to both enzymatic (collagenase and elastase) and mechanical treatment. Receptors assays and ion transports were examined with this cell preparation (Culp et al., 1986; Yang et al., 1988b), but it was difficult to examine mucin secretion from isolated gland cells (Culp et al., 1990). Unfortunately, they found the cell isolates to be extremely fragile and unable to withstand the extended incubation needed to permit a steady-state radiolabeling of glycoconjugates. Later, Dwyer et al. (1992) were successful in measuring mucous glycoprotein from submucosal gland cells isolated from swine trachea using monoclonal antibodies specific for lectins of the mucous glycoproteins. These gland cells prepared from tracheas contained both mucous and serous cells (Culp et al., 1983; Yang et al., 1988a). Finkbeiner et al. (1986) and Paul et al. (1988) have succeeded in isolating bovine tracheal gland serous cells that secrete hyaluronidase-sensitive glycoconjugates, but not mucous glycoproteins. This preparation is useful for the studies of serous cell secretion in airway submucosal glands (Sommerhoff and Finkbeiner, 1990; Sommerhoff et al., 1989, 1990). Finkbeiner et al. (1986) and Sommerhoff et al. (1990) established a gland cell line derived from bovine and human tracheal glands. By using this cell line, they have studied ion transport across glandular cells (Yamaya et al., 1991a,b).

III. Mucous Glycoprotein and Glycoconjugate Secretion

Secretory cells in airway submucosal glands consist of two morphologically different types of secretory cells: mucous and serous cells. Mucous cells are assumed to elaborate a viscous secretion that contains mucous glycoproteins (mucin) almost exclusively, whereas serous cells secrete a watery liquid that lacks mucin, but contains other glycoconjugates and proteins.

A. Mucous Glycoprotein (Mucin) Secretion

The presence of both neutral and acid glycoproteins has been histochemically demonstrated in the secretory cells (mainly mucous cells) of airway submucosal glands. The acid glycoproteins consist of sialated and sulfated mucin (Kollerstrom et al., 1977; Jones and Reid, 1973; Lamb and Reid, 1972; Sorvari, 1972; Spicer, 1965).

For the study of airway submucosal gland secretion, the amount of macromolecules and high relative molecular mass (M_r) glycoconjugates from culture medium and fluids secreted from airway explants and whole trachea in vitro and in vivo have been separated and measured. Dialysis (Coles and Reid, 1981; Coles et al., 1981), precipitation (Baker et al., 1977), and gel filtration (Cheng et al., 1981) methods have been used to determine the amount of macromolecules and glycoconjugates from airway explants and whole trachea in vitro and in vivo. For example, alcohol- (Marom et al., 1981; Shimura et al., 1987b) and trichloroacetic acid (TCA)-precipitable (Marom et al., 1984; Shimura et al., 1988) glycoconjugates in the airway secretions contain both mucous glycoprotein and glycoconjugates. The glycoconjugates come not only from submucosal glands, but also from the tissues surrounding the submucosal glands (cartilages, connective tissue) when airway explants and whole trachea are used for experiments. Generally, the high M_r glycoconjugates in the airways are separated into two types: hyaluronidase-resistant mucins (i.e., mucin or mucous glycoprotein) and hyaluronidase-susceptible glycosaminoglycans (Leigh et al., 1986a,b; Shimura et al., 1990).

Many radioactive precursors have now been used for in vitro and in vivo experiments of airway secretion: D-[U-^{14}C]glucose, D-[1-^{14}C]galactose, [^{14}C]threonine, Na$_2$[^{35}S]O$_4$ and [^{3}H]glucosamine. Incorporation of radioactive precursors in the secreted macromolecules or glycoconjugates is indicative of their active biosynthesis by the airway tissue. Earlier works (Lamb and Reid, 1970; Meyrick and Reid, 1975; Stahl and Ellis, 1973; Sturgess and Reid, 1972) on the metabolism of tracheal glycoproteins involved measurement of the incorporation of radioactive precursors into macromolecular products, but little information was obtained on the source and structure of these radioactive components. The trachea or bronchial explant (whole trachea), however, is a complex structure that consists of superficial ciliated epithelium, goblet cells, basement membrane, submucosal layer, various cells (fibroblasts, inflammatory cells), small vessels, and cartilage, in addition to submucosal glands. Nevertheless, the measurement of these macromolecules and glycoconjugates secreted from airway explants or whole trachea has been used for the studies of submucosal gland secretion by many investigators. This is based on the finding that superficial goblet cells are much fewer than the secretory cells of submucosal glands, especially in human airways (Reid, 1960), and that goblet cell secretion is not under any physiological pharmacological controls, nor under any neural control (Kim et al., 1989). Both Na$_2$[^{35}S]O$_4$ and [^{3}H]glucosamine are now frequently used for the study of airway mucous glycoconjugate and glycoprotein secretion. The [^{35}S]-labeled macromolecules represent mainly acid (sulfate) mucous glycoprotein, whereas the [^{3}H]glucosamine is incorporated into both acid and neutral mucous glycoproteins in human airway submucosal gland cells (Marom et al., 1981). Therefore, it is possible that different radiological precursors cause some variations in the reported levels of airway secretion in addition to those caused by species difference.

When airway explants or tissues are used to study airway secretory responses, we cannot know the number of submucosal glands in the samples. Therefore, a so-called secretory index is adopted for such experiments (Marom et al., 1981, 1982; Shimura et al., 1987b, 1988). After an incubation with radiolabeled precursors (usually 16 h or longer), the airway explants are allowed to incubate further for two successive periods (periods I and II). The *secretory index* is defined as the ratio of radioactivity collected in period II to that in period I. The effects of pharmacological agents are determined by comparing the secretory indices of the drug-treated samples with those of matched and control samples (Fig. 2). Thus, we can exclude the differences caused by the number of submucosal glands and those caused by environmental conditions.

Monoclonal antibodies are used for immunohistological characterization of secretory products from submucosal glands (Basbaum et al., 1984b; de Water et al., 1986; St. George et al. 1984, 1985). From use of a series of 12 monoclonal antibodies made against mucous and serous components of monkey trachea, St. George et al. (1985) have reported that the intracellular mucous products of tracheal secretory cells exhibit greater heterogeneity than is detectable by conventional histochemistry. Recently, some attempts to use monoclonal antibodies have been made to quantify mucous glycoprotein in the airway secretions (Basbaum et al., 1986; Lin et al., 1989; Dwyer et al., 1992). Lin et al. (1989) have used monoclonal antibodies, 17B1 and 17Q2, which are specific for large M_r mucous glycoproteins, to develop an enzyme-linked immunosorbent assay (ELISA) method to quantify the tracheal mucins of humans and rhesus monkeys. Dwyer et al. (1992) have developed an enzyme-linked lectin assay (ELLA) to measure mucous glycoproteins in their experiments. Lectins are plant and animal proteins of nonimmune origin and have the benefit of relative species-independence and of being relatively chemically defined molecules (Spiro, 1966). Therefore, they are useful as specific and sensitive probes for mucous glycoproteins These two ELISA and ELLA methods do not detect proteoglycans, but detect only mucous glycoproteins (Lin et al., 1989; Dwyer et al., 1992).

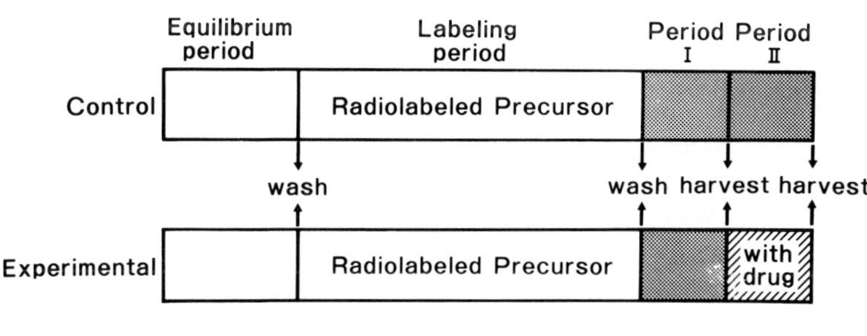

Figure 2   The secretory index is defined as the ratio of radioactivity (dpm) collected in period II to that in period I. The effects of pharmacological stimulation are determined by comparing the secretory indices of the drug-treated samples with those of matched and control samples.

B. Glycoconjugate and Lysozyme Secretion

Submucosal glands can secrete not only mucous glycoprotein (hylarulonidase-resistant glycoconjugates), but also hylarulonidase-sensitive glycoconjugates. Almost none of the conventional methods for measuring glycoconjugates can distinguish between these two types. Serous cells in airway submucosal glands are known to secrete hylarulonidase-sensitive glycoconjugates, because the glycoconjugates secreted from serous cells isolated from bovine trachea in response to various agonists were shown to be all hyaluronidase-sensitive (Leigh et al., 1986b; Paul et al., 1988, 1991). However, it has not yet been reported whether there are any differences between serous and mucous cell secretory responses in airway submucosal glands. Therefore, in most descriptions in this chapter, we do not distinguish between mucous glycoprotein and other hyaluronidase-sensitive glycoconjugate secretions. Lysozyme secretion is also thought to be a marker specific to submucosal gland secretion, and lysozyme release has been measured in the experiments concerned with airway submucosal gland secretion (Webber and Widdicombe, 1987a,b), especially when using airway explants and whole-trachea in vitro and in vivo conditions. This is based on the finding that lysozyme is localized in the granules of serous cells of airway submucosal glands in the airways, as described in the following.

Airway submucosal glands secrete not only mucous glycoprotein, but also other materials that are mainly secreted by serous cells and, moreover, have an antibacterial or defensive function in the airways. These include lysozyme, lactoferrin, carbonic anhydrase, IgA, proline-rich protein, and proteinase inhibitors.

Serous cells of the human respiratory tract evidence lysozyme and lactoferrin content at light microscopic level by immunocytochemical methods using rabbit antihuman lysozyme or lactoferrin (Bowes and Corrin, 1977; Mason and Taylor, 1975; Spicer et al., 1977). That ultrastructural, high-iron diamine (HID) staining localizes sulfated complex carbohydrate in the rim of many bizonal serous cell granules suggests that complex formation between the strongly cationic lysozyme and a sulfated glycoconjugate may occur in this region (Mason and Taylor, 1975). When the ultrastructural distribution of lactoferrin in human bronchial glands was studied by an immunoperoxidase method, the distribution of lactoferrin corresponded to that of lysozyme (Bowes and Corrin, 1977; Bowes et al., 1981). Another conspicuous component demonstrated immunocytochemically in human bronchial serous cell is carbonic anhydrase (Spicer et al., 1982). Tom-Moy et al. (1983) reported that electron microscopic and immunocytochemical analysis of incubated ferret tracheal segments showed a loss of serous granules and lysozyme immunoreactivity in response to cholinergic and α- and β-adrenergic drugs. Measurement of lysozyme assayed from the incubating medium indicated that these drugs stimulate lysozyme release. The biological significance of this glycosidase, lysozyme, which is widely encountered in epithelial cells, has not been precisely defined, but its presence is possibly related to an antimicrobial function. The presence of lactoferrin and carbonic anhydrase presumably is also related to an antimicrobial function in airway lumen.

Secretory IgA is the major immunoglobulin in bronchial secretions and other external body fluids in humans. Immunoglobulin A and the secretory component in human bronchial mucosa have been localized by immunohistological methods and immunoelectron microscopy (Goodman et al., 1981; Takemura et al., 1985). These morphological findings suggest that IgA dimers, synthesized in plasma cells, form complexes with the secretory component on the basolateral plasmalemma of epithelial cells in bronchial glands and are transported across the cells in endocytic vesicles to the gland lumen.

With use of antibodies to basic and acidic proline-rich protein (PRP) of salivary origin, Warner and Azen (1984) have detected PRP immunoreactivity in serous cells of human tracheobronchial glands by an immunoperoxidase technique. Immunoreactive PRP, detected by immunoblotting from sodium dodecyl sulfate (SDS) gels, was also found in culture media from tracheal explants. They hypothesized that PRP interacts with glycoproteins of mucus, as do other proteins, and may be necessary for maintaining the appropriate viscoelastic properties of respiratory secretions.

Bronchial secretion contains two proteinase inhibitors: the plasma-derived α_1-proteinase inhibitor and antileukoproteinase (ALP) (a bronchial mucous proteinase inhibitor), which is not present in the bloodstream. By immunoelectron microscopy, ALP was demonstrated in secretory granules of serous cells in human bronchial glands (Mooren et al., 1982). Moreover, de Water et al. (1986) examined the ultrastructural localization of ALP in human airways by using monoclonal ALP-specific antibodies and, in the serous cells of bronchial glands, ALP could be demonstrated in secretory granules.

IV. Fluid and Electrolyte Secretion

Submucosal glands in airway walls are the major source of airway mucous secretion which, to date, has been investigated mainly by measuring glycoconjugate or mucous glycoprotein (mucin) output from airways. There has been little knowledge of electrolyte and water secretion from airway submucosal glands, in spite of the fact that the fluid component (electrolyte and water) makes up 95% or more of airway secretions (Boat and Cheng, 1980) and, therefore, affects mucociliary transport in the airways.

Ion transport across airway wall preparations (or mucosa) has been examined by measuring potential difference (PD), short-circuit current (SCC), or ion fluxes using ^{22}Na and ^{36}Cl. However, the airway wall used in most of these studies contains not only surface epithelium, but also submucosal glands. By using airway wall preparations, it has been shown that Cl^- is secreted actively toward the airway lumen, and that the Cl^- secretion is stimulated by β-adrenergic agonists (Al-Bazzaz and Cheng, 1979). Studies, using monolayers cultured from surface epithelium (Widdicombe et al., 1985) and microelectrode techniques (Shorofsky et al., 1986), have demonstrated that surface epithelium can secrete Cl^-, especially when stimulated by β-agonists. In addition, acetylcholine and phenylephrine are reported not to alter either SCC or adenosine 3′,5′-cyclic monophosphate (cAMP) levels of surface epithelial cells scraped from canine trachea (Smith et al., 1982). In contrast, some investigators have found that acetylcholine increases SCC and stimulates electrolyte movement across the canine tracheal epithelium, which contains submucosal glands (Marin et al., 1976), but does not do so in rabbit tracheal epithelia, which contain few glands (Jarnigan et al., 1983). Furthermore, Phipps et al. (1986) have reported that chronic exposure of sheep to 0.5 ppm ozone increased net Cl^- secretion across tracheal mucosa and also increased the size of the submucosal gland in tracheal tissue.

More recent studies (Corrales et al., 1984; Leikauf et al., 1984; Sasaki et al., 1990, 1992; Yang et al., 1986b; Yamaya et al., 1991a,b) suggest that electrolyte and water secretion into airways comes from both epithelial cells and submucosal glands, and that they are subject to different mechanisms of regulation, although the precise mechanism of the fluid secretion from airway submucosal glands is still unknown. In general, it is believed that fluid movement is secondary to active ion transport (Curran and Solomon, 1957). This ion transport builds up local osmotic gradients across the epithelium that lead to water flow (Diamond and Bossert, 1967). If active ion transport is the source of the fluid in airway gland secretions, then the most likely candidate would be active Cl^- secretion, as in other exocrine cells (Frizzel et al., 1979). In contrast with this speculation, Corrales et al. (1984) have speculated that the phenylephrine-induced movement of Na^+ together with Cl^- across feline tracheal mucosa was the result of a passive process caused by mucin secretion from feline tracheal submucosal glands.

There have been recent studies supporting the idea of active ion transport with water movement in airway submucosal glands, as follows. Leikauf et al. (1984), using micropipette methods, examined the viscoelastic properties of secretions from feline tracheal submucosal glands. They found that cholinergic, α-adrenergic, and β-adrenergic agonists evoked ion-altered, less, and higher viscoelastic secretion, respectively. From these results, they speculated that both cholinergic and α-adrenergic agonists stimulated fluid secretion from submucosal glands and that β-agonist did not. Morphometric analysis using electron microscopy by Basbaum et al. (1981) has shown vacuole formation induced by a cholinergic agonist and by an α-adrenergic agonist in the acinar cells of feline tracheal submucosal glands, which supports this idea. This is compatible with the speculation that an active ion (water) secretion is stimulated by cholinergic and α-agonists (Sasaki et al., 1990).

Sasaki et al. (1990) examined ^{22}Na efflux as an indicator of electrolyte (or water) secretion from isolated feline tracheal submucosal glands. After incubation with ^{22}NaCl-containing KRB solution (pH 7.4) at 37°C, the ^{22}Na-loaded glands were transferred to a superfusion apparatus in which perfusate was continuously pumped to the glands at a constant flow rate and sampled at 18-s intervals for 10–15 min (Fig. 3). After 5 min of perfusion, a pharmacological or electrical field stimulation (FS) was given to the isolated glands. The instantaneous rate constant was calculated by measuring the radioactivity (cpm) of each effluent sample. The mean rate constant of the baseline ^{22}Na efflux was 0.21 min^{-1}, which fell significantly to 0.03 min^{-1} after treatment with ouabain. Both methacholine and phenylephrine significantly accelerated the ^{22}Na efflux to 3.6-fold and 1.8 times baseline efflux, respectively (Figs. 4 and 5). Field stimulation produced a significant increase in the rate constant, and the increase was abolished by pretreatment with ouabain or tetrodotoxin. Furthermore, atropine or phentolamine significantly suppressed the FS-evoked increase in the rate constant to 76 and 84%, respectively, of the maximal response evoked by FS alone. These results indicate that ^{22}Na efflux from feline tracheal submucosal glands, which is dependent on ouabain-sensitive NaK-ATPase activity in the secretory cells, is stimulated by both cholinergic and α-adrenergic agonists. Another possible pathway is that intracellular ^{22}Na is secreted together with mucous granules into the gland lumen as secreta (mucus) or that the secretion of osmotically active granule components into

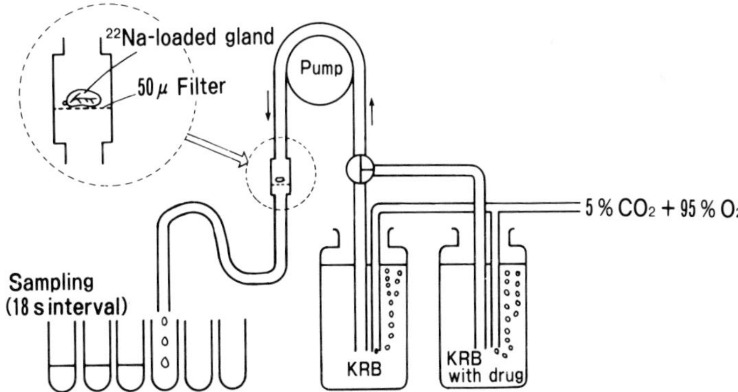

Figure 3 Schematic diagram of superfusion apparatus. The upper end of the sample chamber made of an acryl resin tube (6-mm ID and 30-mm length) is connected to perfusate reservoir through a peristaltic pump and the other end to a fraction collector. The ^{22}Na-loaded glands were placed on a 50-μm nylon mesh filter set in the sample chamber and superfused continuously at a flow rate of 2.5 ml/min. Drugs were applied to the glands by changing perfusate, which was gased with 5% CO$_2$–95% O$_2$ and warmed to 37°C. Sample chamber and most of the tubes were warmed in a 37°C water bath. KRB, Krebs–Ringer bicarbonate solution. (From Sasaki et al., 1990a)

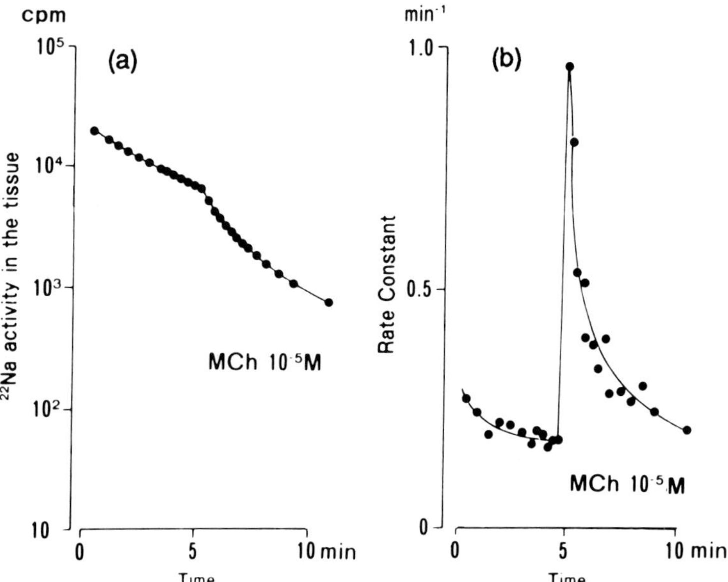

Figure 4 (a) Representative example of methacholine-evoked increase in ^{22}Na efflux from isolated feline glands; (b) A plot of instantaneous rate constant calculated from data in (a). (From Sasaki et al., 1990)

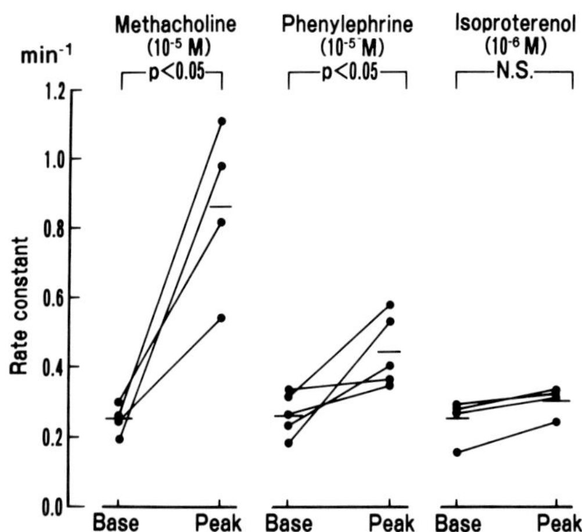

Figure 5 Changes in instantaneous rate constant after administration of three different agonists in isolated feline tracheal glands. "BaSE" represents mean rate constant during 3–5 min (usually seven points), whereas "Peak" indicates peak response after addition of the respective drugs. (From Sasaki et al., 1990)

the gland lumen draws water by simple osmosis, forming an NaCl gradient across the secretory epithelium, leading to secretion of Na^+ and Cl^+, as proposed by Corrales et al. (1984). In spite of previous reports that showed that mucous glycoprotein secretion from isolated feline submucosal glands is stimulated by β-adrenergic agonists (Sasaki et al., 1989a), isoproterenol produced no significant alteration in [22]Na release from isolated glands (see Fig. 5). This suggests that [22]Na efflux observed in their study does not result from mucous glycoprotein (granule) secretion.

A recent experiment using swine tracheal glandular cells by Yang et al. (1988b) has revealed that the intracellular Cl^- concentration fell rapidly with ouabain or furosemide, and that acetylcholine caused a decline in intracellular Cl^-. This decline in intracellular Cl^- was not accompanied by glycoprotein secretion, suggesting active ion transport through Cl^- channel activity, which is subject to regulation different from that in glycoprotein (granule) secretion in submucosal gland cells. They have speculated that chloride secretion from cells is stimulated by the activation of M_1 receptors, and that glycoprotein secretion is caused by the activation of $M_{2G}(M_3)$ receptors.

Yamaya et al. (1991a,b) isolated acini of human tracheobronchial submucosal glands by enzymatic digestion, then cultured and used confluent monolayers for bioelectric experiments with an Ussing chamber. The epithelial sheets showed high resistance, and mediators induced a significant increase in SCC. The potency sequence for stimulation of SCC by mediators was methacholine > bradykinin > isoproterenol = phenylephrine (Fig. 6). Amiloride decreased baseline SCC by 42%, but had little effect on the SCC response to mediators. However, a Cl^- channel blocker, diphenylamine-2-carboxylic acid, had no effect on baseline SCC, but markedly inhibited the SCC response to all mediators. These findings show that submucosal gland cells from human trachea can secrete Cl^- in response to cholinergic agonists and bradykinin.

To investigate the electrolyte secretion from airway submucosal glands, Sasaki et al. (1992) employed a standard patch–clamp technique on enzymatically digested acinar cells of isolated submucosal glands from human and feline trachea. Current responses were monitored in whole-cell voltage-clamp experiments. Acetylcholine (ACh) evoked bidirectional current responses; that is, an initial inward current at -80 mV (Cl^- current) followed by an outward current at 0 mV (K^+ current) (Fig. 7a). Lower concentrations (1–10 nM) of ACh evoked oscillations of both the currents, which are mimicked by the intracellular inositol triphosphate (IP_3). Removal of external Ca^{2+} with added EGTA did not alter the ACh-induced response, whereas a membrane-permeable Ca^{2+} chelator BAPTA-AM abolished the response completely, suggesting that the Ca^{2+} released from the internal store is responsible for both the currents. A large conductance (160 pS) K^+ channel was identified at the basolateral surface of the cells. To investigate the Ca^{2+}-mediated current response in detail, experiments were carried out in the

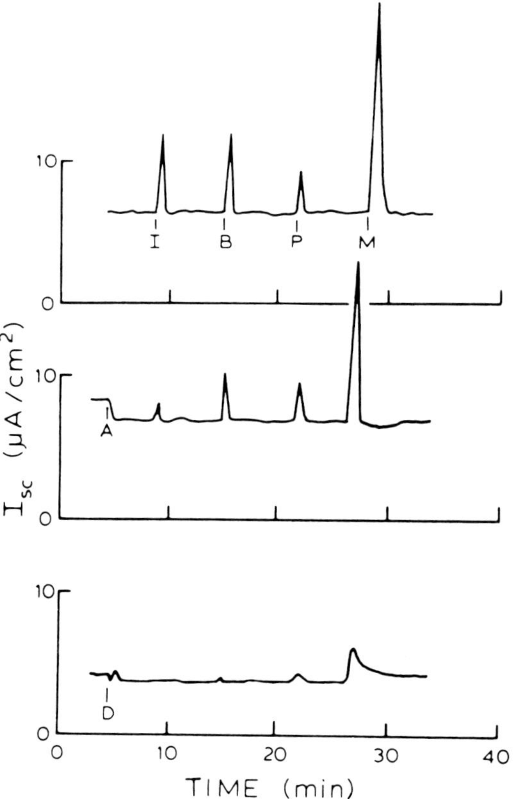

Figure 6 Effects of transport inhibitors on changes in short-circuit current (I_{sc}) in response to mediators. Top: responses in absence of inhibitor. Middle: effects of amiloride. Bottom: effects of diphenylamine-2-carboxylic acid (DPAC). Tissues from the same culture. A, 10^{-5} M amiloride; D, 10^{-3} M DPAC; I, 10^{-5} M isoproterenol; B, 10^{-6} M bradykinin; P, 10^{-5} M phenylephrine; M, 10^{-5} M methacholine. Mediators were added in same sequence and at approximately same times in all three traces. (From Yamaya et al., 1991a)

presence of either ionomycin (see Fig. 7) or caffeine. Ionomycin gradually increased both the currents; however, they were activated in reverse order, here, that is, the outward current was activated initially, followed by the inward current. On the other hand, caffeine evoked only a transient outward current. Moreover, analysis of intracellular Ca^{2+} concentration $[Ca^{2+}]_i$ images by Fura-2 showed the initial elevation at the apical portion when stimulated by ACh. These findings suggest that an IP_3-induced Ca^{2+}-release at the apical portion plays a crucial role in Cl^- secretion from airway submucosal gland cells.

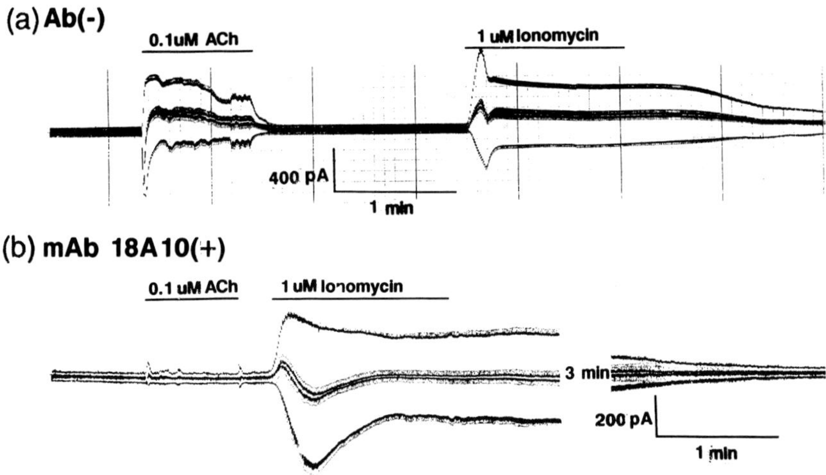

Figure 7 Effects of intracellular administration of IP_3 receptor antibodies (MAbs 18A10 and 10A6) on current responses in feline tracheal gland cells. (a) Control; (b) when one of the MAbs, 18A10 (200 μg/ml), was included in the intracellular solution, the response to acetylcholine (ACh) was abolished, whereas ionomycin evoked its normal response in the same cell. Another MAb, 10A6, did not affect the ACh response, suggesting that MAb 18A10 binds to an "active center" of the IP_3 receptors. (From Sasaki et al., 1992)

V. Glandular Contraction and Mucus Ejection

Myoepithelial cells surround acini and secretory tubules in airway submucosal glands. The myoepithelial cell is spindle-shaped, filled with masses of myofilaments, and lies on the basement membrane (Fig. 8). Dense bodies are seen in the filamentous part and small vesicles (caveolae) under the cell membrane (Shimura et al., 1986). These ultrastructural findings are similar to those from smooth-muscle cells, suggesting that myoepithelial cells are contractile. Myoepithelial cells in some exocrine glands are known to be contractile (Sato et al., 1979; Dreckhahn et al., 1977). However, this possibility has often been overlooked or ignored in studies of the secretion of airway submucosal glands, despite that the presence of the contraction may have a profound effect on the secretory response. Contractions in submucosal glands, attributed to the activity of myoepithelial cells, have been observed directly using isolated submucosal gland preparations. The glandular contraction results in the ejection of mucus that is secreted from secretory cells into secretory tubules and ducts, and exhibits an initial short response time (a few minutes) in submucosal gland secretion (Shimura et al., 1986).

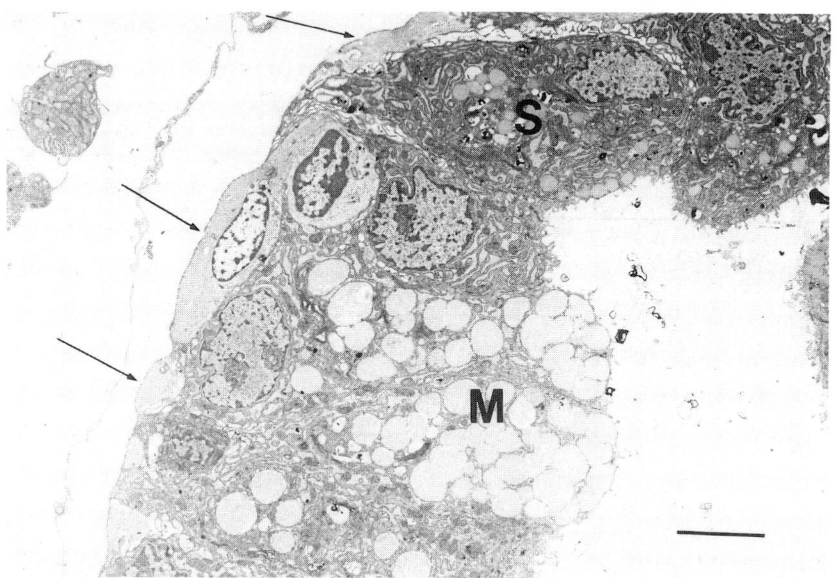

Figure 8 Electron micrograph of secretory tubule in an isolated gland from canine trachea. Myoepithelial cells (arrows) exist between membrane and secretory cells. S, serous cells; M, mucous cells (bar, 5 μm). (From Shimura et al., 1986)

For measuring the glandular contraction, isolated single glands were held by two sharp glass hooks in an experimental chamber in which warmed (37°C) KRB solution was circulated (Shimura et al., 1986). The upper hook was connected to a strain transducer for continuous recording of isometric tension. The isolated gland was stimulated with various drugs by superfusing the drug through a micropipette placed near the upper portion of the gland (Fig. 9).

Cholinergic muscarinic agonists (MCh and ACh) induced a significant contraction, which was blocked by atropine (Fig. 10). Furthermore, α-adrenergic agonist (phenylephrine) and substance P (SP) also induced contraction of isolated submucosal glands (Shimura et al., 1986, 1987b). However, β-adrenergic agonist (isoproterenol) failed to produced any significant contraction. Before the Shimura study (Shimura et al., 1987b), Coles et al. (1984) had reported the short time response to SP of ^{14}C-labeled mucous glycoprotein secretion from explants of canine tracheal mucosa in vitro. Because SP-evoked secretion is followed by a period (10–20 min after stimulation) of apparent secretion inhibition, they have speculated that SP acts to increase the rate of clearance of mucus from the ducts, probably by induced contraction of secretory tubules and ducts. The study by Shimura et al. (1987a) revealed that SP induces a dose-dependent contraction of

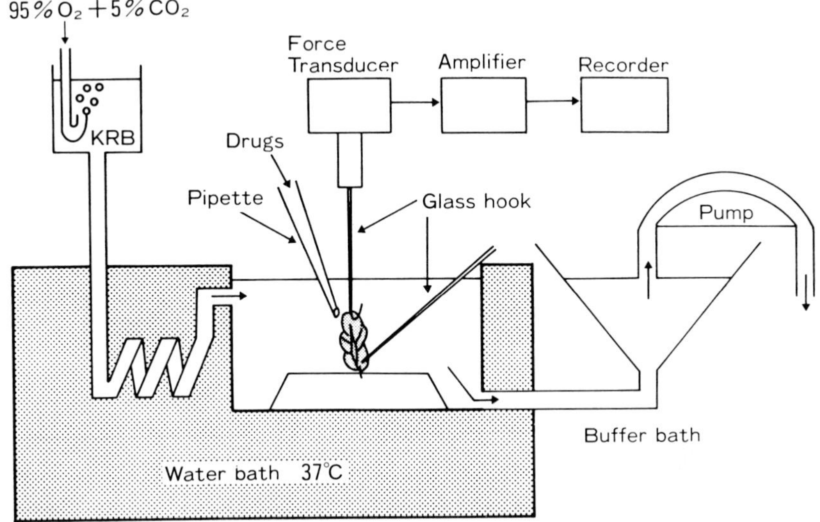

Figure 9 Block diagram of method for measuring tension induced by various drugs. Experimental chamber contains circulating (O_2-saturated Krebs–Ringer bicarbonate (KRB) and is connected to a buffer bath to prevent noise on drainage of medium. Samples are held in experimental chamber by two sharp glass hooks, one of which is connected to a force transducer. Samples were superfused with various drugs through a micropipette that is mounted on a micromanipulator and connected to a microsyringe containing agonist. (From Shimura et al., 1988)

isolated submucosal glands from feline trachea, confirming the speculation of Coles et al. (1984).

Bundles of unmyelinated axons are found between and in acini. Terminal axons (nerve endings) have been seen in the acinar portion, between secretory cells, between myoepithelial cells, and close to myoepithelial cells (Shimura et al., 1986). To stimulate intrinsic nerves, field electrical stimulation (FS) was applied to isolated glands from feline trachea. This stimulation induced a significant frequency-dependent contraction, which was abolished by atropine and slightly inhibited by phentolamine. These findings indicate that the contraction is mediated mainly by cholinergic nerves through muscarinic receptors and, in small part, by adrenergic nerves through α-receptors (Shimura et al., 1987a).

From these findings, Shimura et al. (1986, 1987a,b, 1992a) have postulated that the secretory response of submucosal glands consists of two actions: (1) secretion of mucus from secretory cells into tubules and ducts and (2) expulsion of mucus (mucin and fluid) into airway lumen through glandular contraction. The mucus-ejecting action through myoepithelial cell contraction represents the initial

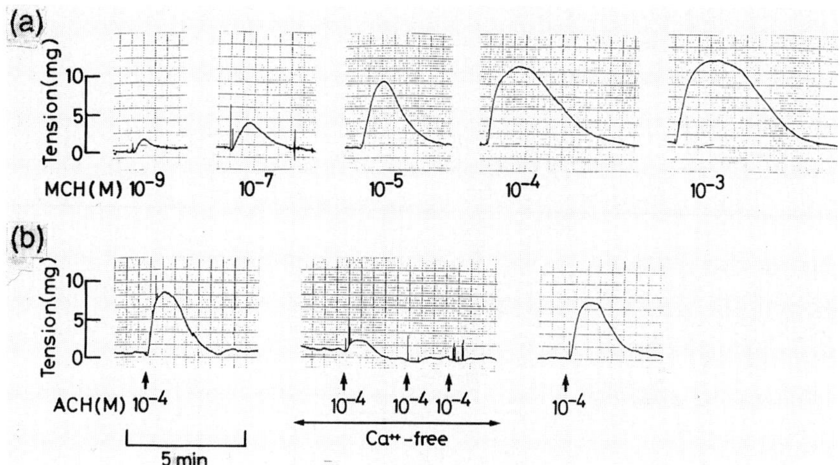

Figure 10 (a) An illustrative example of glandular contraction of dose–response relationships at 10^{-9} to 10^{-3} M methacholine (MCh) in a submucosal gland isolated from feline trachea. (b) An illustrative example of effect of a Ca^{2+}-free medium on the contraction induced by 10^{-5} M acetylcholine (ACh). In a Ca^{2+}-free medium, first application of ACh induced a tension 10% of that in Krebs–Ringer bicarbonate (a medium containing Ca^{2+}). A second or third application had no effect in this sample from canine trachea. (From Shimura et al., 1986)

short-term response that lacks a β-adrenergic contribution (Shimura et al., 1986, 1987a,b). The long-term response (up to a few hours) may be mediated by cholinergic, adrenergic, and noncholinergic, nonadrenergic nerves (Shimura et al., 1987a,b, 1992a). These two actions in submucosal gland secretion are under separate nervous control, and it is possible that not all neural stimuli are involved in either action (see Sec. IX).

Caffeine, which releases Ca^{2+} from sarcoplasmic reticulum (Lüttgan and Oetliker, 1968), induced myoepithelial contraction in isolated submucosal glands. Moreover, even in a Ca^{2+}-free solution, isolated glands contracted on the first application of cholinergic agonist, although the concentration was much smaller than that in a Ca^{2+}-containing solution (see Fig. 10b). These findings suggest that intracellular calcium ions stored in organelles as well as extracellularly play a major role in the contraction of myoepithelial cells (Shimura et al., 1986).

VI. Receptors

The presence of receptors in airway submucosal glands has been studied morphologically using autoradiography, with a receptor-binding assay of cell membranes, and functionally by the secretory response to agonist in the presence of each antagonist. In this section, we mainly discuss the presence of receptors that have been morphologically studied and also those examined by receptor-binding assay) (Table 2).

Localization of various receptors over airway submucosal glands has been examined by the autoradiographic method mainly at the light microscopic level using various ligands. In a study using autoradiographic techniques, muscarinic receptors were localized to both serous and mucous cells of ferret tracheal gland (Basbaum et al., 1984a). The muscarnic receptor distribution in ferret tracheal glands was determined using [^{3}H]propylbenzylcholine mustard ([^{3}H]PrBMC) binding and autoradiography. Specifically, atropine-sensitive [^{3}H]PrBMC binding was quantified autoradiographically in submucosal glands. Serous and mucous cells in the gland did not differ in receptor density. Binding sites on gland cells were associated with basolateral membranes. Barnes et al. (1983b) used the muscarinic antagonist [1-^{3}H]quinuclidinyl benzilate ([^{3}H]QHB) for the auto-radiographic localization of muscarinic receptors in lung and trachea. Culp and Martin (1986) used [^{3}H]QHB to functionally characterize glandular receptors. They found that muscarinic receptors on tracheal gland cells are of high affinity and density. The demonstration of muscarinic receptors on both serous and mucous cells confirms the capacity of both cell types to contribute to the secretory response on vagal or cholinomimetic stimulation.

Recently, muscarinic receptors of airways have been pharmacologically subclassified into three subtypes: M_1, M_2, and M_3 receptors (Barnes, 1989). Autoradiographic investigations of human lungs have demonstrated the coexistence of M_1 (36%) and M_3 (64%) receptors over human airway submucosal glands (Mak and Barnes, 1990). By receptor-binding assay of cell membranes, Yang et al. (1988a) have found the presence of both M_1 (27%) and M_3 (73%) receptors on isolated submucosal gland cells of swine trachea, and Ishihara et al. (1992) have reported mainly M_3 receptors in acinar cells of isolated submucosal glands from feline trachea.

Barnes et al. (1982, 1983a; Barnes and Basbaum, 1983) investigated the distribution of adrenergic receptors in ferret trachea using autoradiography. [^{3}H]Dihydroalprenolol, used to identify β-receptors, revealed a high density of specific-binding sites over surface epithelium and submucosal glands. Specific binding of [^{3}H]prazosin to lung section was used for autoradiography of the localization of α_1-receptors present in airway submucosal glands and epithelium. Comparison of adrenergic receptor densities in tracheal sections from the same animals showed a rank order for submucosal glands of α_1 greater than β. Within submucosal glands, α_1- and β-adrenergic receptors were differentially distributed, with α_1-receptors being significantly more numerous in serous than in mucous cells and β_1-receptors being significantly more numerous in mucous than in serous cells (Barnes and Basbaum, 1983; Barnes et al., 1983a). However, with cat gland cell membranes, Culp et al. (1990) have performed competition experi-

Table 2 Receptors of Secretory Cells in Airway Submucosal Glands
A. Receptors Visualized Autoradiographically

Receptors	Ligands	Antagonists	Localization		Species	Ref.
			Mucous cell	Serous cell		
Muscarinic	[^{3}H]PrBMC	(−)	++	++	Ferret	Basbaum et al., 1984a
	[^{3}H]QNB	(−)	++	++	Ferret	Barnes et al., 1983b
$M_1{:}M_3 = 36{:}64$	[^{3}H]QNB, [^{3}H]NMS	Pirenzepine	?	?	Human, guinea pig	Mak and Barnes, 1990
Adrenergic						
α_1 Receptor	[^{3}H]Prazosin	(−)	−/+	++	Ferret	Barnes et al., 1983a
	[^{3}H]Prazosin	(−)	−/+	++	Ferret	Barnes and Basbaum, 1983a
β-Receptor	[^{3}H]Dihydroalprenolol	(−)	++	−/+	Ferret	Barnes et al., 1982, 1983a
	[^{3}H]Iodocyanopindol	(−)	?	?	Ferret	Barnes and Basbaum, 1983
$\beta_1{:}\beta_2 = 1{:}9$	[^{125}I]Iodocyanopindol	ICI 118,551, Betaxolol	?	?	Human	Carstairs et al., 1985
Neuropeptides						
Substance P	[^{125}I]-Bolton–Hunter-labeled SP	(−)	+	?	Human, guinea pig	Carstairs and Barnes, 1986a
VIP	[^{125}I]-VIP	(−)	++	?	Human	Leys et al., 1986
	[^{125}I]-VIP	(−)	++	++	Human, guinea pig	Carstairs and Barnes, 1986b

Table 2 (Continued)

B. Receptors by Receptor Binding Assays of Cell Membranes

Receptor	Ligands	Antagonists	Species	Ref.
Muscarnic $M_1:M_2 = 27:73$	[³H]QNB, [³H]NMS	Pirenzepine	Swine	Yang et al., 1988a
$M_1 << M_3$	[³H]QNB	Pirenzepine, AF-DX116 4-DAMP	Cat	Ishihara et al., 1992
Adrenergic $\alpha_1:\alpha_2$	[³H]-Dihydroergocryptine	Prazosin, yomhibine	Cat	Culp et al., 1990

C. Other Receptors Proposed by Secretory Responses

Agonists or receptors	Antagonist	Species	Ref.
Histamine (H_2)	Cimetidine	Human	Shelhamer et al., 1980
Tachykinins (NK-1)		Dog	Coles et al., 1984
(substance P)	(DPro², DTrp⁷,⁹)SP	Cat	Shimura et al., 1987b
Leukotriene (LTD_4, LTC_4)	FPL-55712	Human	Marom et al., 1982
Thromboxane A_2	SQ-29548	Cat	Sasaki et al., 1989b
Purine (P_2) (ATP)	(−)	Cat	Shimura et al., 1992c
Bradykinin	(−)	Human	Yamaya et al., 1992a
Endothelin (ET-1)	(−)	Cat	Shimura et al., 1992b
Glucocorticosteroid	(−)	Human	Marom et al., 1984
		Cat	Lundgren et al., 1985
		Cat	Shimura et al., 1990
Protein kinase C (PMA)	H-7, shingosine	Cat	Rieves et al., 1991
		Cat	Shimura et al., 1991b
IP_3	Monoclonal antibodies (MAbs 18A10 and 10A6)	Cat, human	Sasaki et al., 1992

ments with α_1- and α_2-adrenergic selective antagonists (prazosin and yohimbine, respectively) which demonstrated high- and low-affinity sites for each antagonist, indicating the presence of both receptor subtypes. Carstairs et al. (1985) examined the localization of β-adrenoreceptors in human lungs by autoradiographic methods using [¹²⁵I]iodocyanopindolol (ICYO) to label β-receptors in tissue sections in competition with selective β-receptor antagonists ICI 118,551 (β_2-selective), and betaxolol (β_1-selective) to obtain the ratio of β_2 to β_1-receptors in the sections. In bronchial submucosal gland, the β_2/β_1-receptor ratio was 9:1, although the significance of the distribution of β-receptor subtypes remains to be determined.

Shimura et al. (1987b, 1988, 1991a) have shown that both exogenous substance P (SP) and vasoactive intestinal peptide (VIP) evoke [³H]-labeled mucous glycoprotein release from isolated submucosal gland; accordingly, gland cells are suggested to have their own receptors for SP or VIP. Few morphological findings concerning the neuropeptide receptors in airway submucosal glands have yet been obtained. Localizaton of specific receptors for SP and VIP in the submucosal glands of human and guinea pig airways has been demonstrated by autoradiography using ¹²⁵I-Bolton–Hunter-labeled SP([¹²⁵I]BH-SP) and ¹²⁵I-labeled VIP, respectively (Carstairs and Barnes, 1986a,b). Leys et al. (1986) have examined autoradiographic localization of VIP receptors in human lung using ¹²⁵I-labeled VIP and reported a lower density of VIP-binding sites over bronchial epithelium and submucosal gland than in pulmonary artery smooth-muscle and alveolar walls.

In addition, previous experiments of secretory responses have suggested the presence of histamine (H_2), leukotriene, bradykinin, endothelin-1, and purine (P_2) receptors on airway submucosal gland cells. These receptors will be described later in greater detail. Furthermore, from the findings of isolated glands from canine and feline trachea (Shimura et al., 1986, 1987a,b), myoepithelial cells in submucosal glands have been suggested to possess receptors for muscarinic cholinergic agonist, α-adrenergic agonist, and SP. However, no morphological investigations have yet demonstrated the presence of these receptors in myoepithelial cells of tracheobronchial glands.

VII. Cellular Mechanisms

Stimulation–secretion coupling in exocrine glands involves two different intracellular mechanisms: the adenylate cyclase adenosine 3′,5′-cyclic monophosphate (cAMP) system and the intracellular calcium ion ($[Ca^{2+}]_i$) messenger system (Case, 1973; Rasmussen and Barrett, 1984). Studies have also indicated that protein kinase A (PKA) and protein kinase C (PKC) also have important roles in the intracellular-signaling pathways in the coupling of these two intracellular mechanisms in exocrine glands (Gunther, 1981; McKinney and Rubin, 1988; Pandol and Schoeffield, 1986). In this section, we will address the significance of these second messengers in airway submucosal gland cells.

A. Second Messengers in Mucous Glycoprotein and Glycoconjugate Secretion

The function of airway submucosal glands is to secrete mucous glycoprotein or glycoconjugates. Some experiments (Lazarus et al., 1984, 1986; Sasaki et al., 1989a) have implicated cAMP as a second messenger in receptor-mediatd mucous glycoprotein secretion. For example, exogenous dibutyryl cAMP, which is permeant in secretory cells, stimulates glycoprotein secretion from feline tracheal submucosal glands (Sasaki et al., 1989a) and, by an immunocytochemical method, intracellular cAMP of secretory cells of ferret, feline, and canine tracheal glands has been shown by Lazarus et al. (1984, 1986) to increase in response to β-adrenergic agonist and vasoactive VIP, which are all known to stimulate mucous glycoprotein secretion through their receptors. Additionally, Paul et al. (1988, 1991) have shown that the release of chondroitin sulfate proteoglycans by cultured tracheal gland serous cells is subject to β-adrenergic regulation and that isoproterenol, a β-agonist, stimulated protein kinase A with an increase in $[cAMP]_i$.

There have been many reports concerning the role of $[Ca^{2+}]_i$ in mucous glycoprotein secretion from airway submucosal glands. Some experiments (Shimura et al., 1988) have shown that Ca^{2+} depletion of the medium produces a reduction of basal mucous glycoprotein secretion and abolishes methacholine (MCh)-evoked secretion from isolated feline tracheal glands. More directly, Ishihara et al. (1990) measured $[Ca^{2+}]_i$ of acinar cells in isolated feline tracheal submucosal glands in response to secretagogues using the Ca^{2+}-sensitive fluorescent dye Fura-2. The secretagogues included cholinergic, α- and β-adrenergic agonists, substance P, and VIP, which all induce mucous glycoprotein secretion from feline tracheal submucosal glands (Shimura et al., 1987b, 1988; Sasaki et al., 1989a). A cholinergic muscarinic agonist, methacholine (MCh) produced a significant increase in $[Ca^{2+}]_i$ of up to 9.8 times that of control in a dose-dependent fashion at concentrations of 10^{-8}–10^{-3} M. The $[Ca^{2+}]_i$ increase by MCh reached a peak within 30 s after stimulation and, thereafter, showed a sustained rise (Fig. 11a). In a Ca^{2+}-free solution, MCh produced only a smaller initial transient rise, without any sustained rise in $[Ca^{2+}]_i$ (see Fig. 11c). Later, to determine which muscarinic receptor subtypes regulate $[Ca^{2+}]_i$, Ishihara et al. (1992) examined the effects of atropine, pirenzepine (M_1 receptor antagonist), AF-DX116 (M_2 receptor antagonist) and 4-diphenylacetoxy-N-methylpiperidine (4-DAMP, M_3 receptor antagonist) on MCh-evoked $[Ca^{2+}]_i$ rise and compared these with mucous glycoprotein secretion from isolated feline submucosal glands. Half-maximal inhibitory concentrations (IC_{50}) of each antagonist against MCh-evoked $[Ca^{2+}]_i$ rise were compared. The 4-DAMP was 100-fold more potent than pirenzepine and was 1000-fold more potent than AF-DX116 in inhibiting the $[Ca^{2+}]_i$ rise induced by MCh. Furthermore, 4-DAMP produced an inhibitory curve similar to atropine (Fig. 12), a nonspecific muscarinic antagonist. These findings indicate muscarinic agonists stimulate $[Ca^{2+}]_i$ rise by activating M_3-muscarinic receptor subtypes in airway submucosal gland cells. An α-adrenergic agonist, phenylephrine produced a prolonged increase in $[Ca^{2+}]_i$ 240% greater than control, without any initial transient increase (see Fig. 11c), and this increase was abolished by an α_1-receptor antagonist, prazosin. This indicates that α-adrenergic stimulation by α_1-receptors induces $[Ca^{2+}]_i$ rise in feline tracheal submucosal glands (Sasaki et al., 1989a; Ishihara et al., 1990). The $[Ca^{2+}]_i$ rise

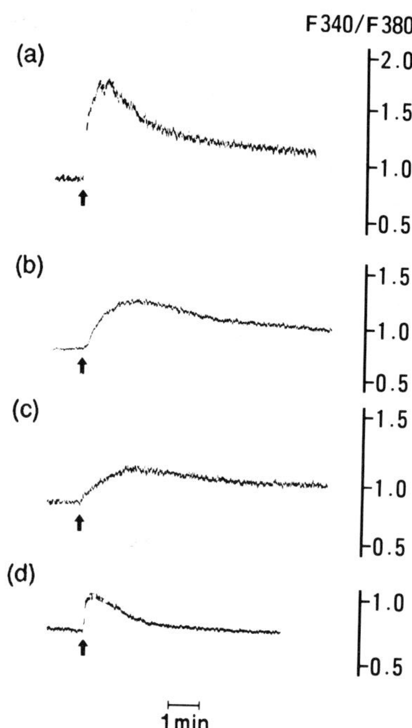

Figure 11 Time course of intracellular Ca^{2+} concentration expressed as ratio of fluorescence (F340/F380) in acinar cells of an isolated feline tracheal gland stimulated by secretagogues. (a), (b), and (c) Stimulated with 10^{-4} M methacholine (MCh), 10^{-5} M MCh, and 10^{-4} M phenylephrine, respectively, in Ca^{2+}-containing Krebs–Ringer bicarbonate solution. (d) Stimulated with 10^{-4} M MCh in a Ca^{2+}-free solution. (From Ishihara et al., 1990)

with phenylephrine was much smaller than that evoked by the cholinergic agonist, MCh, especially at higher concentrations. Substance P (up to 10^{-4} M) also evoked a prolonged increase in $[Ca^{2+}]_i$, 155% greater than control, which was abolished in a Ca^{2+}-free condition. The effect of SP on secretion of mucus is assumed to be dependent on $[Ca^{2+}]_i$ rise, mainly through Ca^{2+} influx. In some tissues, SP is known to accelerate both CA^{2+} release from intracellular stores and Ca^{2+} influx from extracellular fluid (Brown et al., 1985a; Putney, 1977). However, it remains to be determined whether SP stimulates Ca^{2+} release from the intracellular storage in airway submucosal gland cells as well as Ca^{2+} influx, since, in this study, the SP-induced $[Ca^{2+}]_i$ rise showed larger variations than those induced by MCh or phenylephrine. The large variation may be due to differences among samples in the amount of tissue peptidases, which rapidly inactivate SP (Borson et al., 1987). By contrast, both isoproterenol (up to 10^{-5} M) and VIP (up to 10^{-5} M) failed

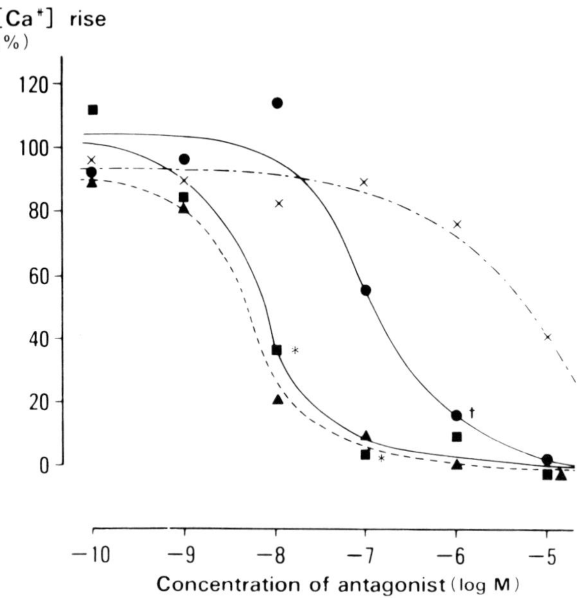

Figure 12 Inhibition curves of 10^{-5} M methacholine (MCh)-evoked intracellular calcium ion concentration ($[Ca^{2+}]_i$) rise for four muscarinic receptor antagonists in acinar cells of an isolated feline tracheal gland: pirenzepine (●); 11{[2-(diethylamino)methyl-1-piperidinyl]-acetyl}-5,11-dihydro-6*H*-pyrido(2,3-*b*) (1,4)-benzodiazepin-6-one (AF-DX116; X); 4-diphenylacetoxy-*N*-methylpiperidine methiodide (4-DAMP; ■), and atropine (▲). asterisk, $p < 0.05$, difference between 4-DAMP and pirenzepine. dagger, $p < 0.05$, difference between pirenzepine and AF-DX116. Results are means for 3–12 experiments. (From Ishihara et al., 1992)

to alter $[Ca^{2+}]_i$. These findings indicate that the mucous glycoprotein secretion evoked by muscarinic cholinergic, α-agonist, or SP may be mediated by intracellular Ca^{2+}, whereas that by β-agonists or VIP is not. In a Ca^{2+}-free solution, MCh produced an initial transient rise, which was 30% or less than that produced in a Ca^{2+}-containing solution, and lasted for 60 s with no prolonged sustained rise in $[Ca^{2+}]_i$ (see Fig. 11). Taken together, these data indicate that MCh produced $[Ca^{2+}]_i$ rise by both Ca^{2+} influx and Ca^{2+} release from intracellular storage. Furthermore, Ca^{2+} release from storage reflects the transient initial rise seen within 30 s after stimulation, and Ca^{2+} influx accounts for the sustained and prolonged rise in $[Ca^{2+}]_i$. The lower concentrations of MCh, phenylephrine, and SP, which all induce glycoprotein secretion from isolated glands (Sasaki et al., 1989a; Shimura et al., 1987b), did not produce the initial transient rise, but showed a sustained and prolonged rise only in $[Ca^{2+}]_i$. Therefore, it seems likely that Ca^{2+}

influx plays a more important role in mucous glycoprotein secretion than does the release of stored Ca^{2+}.

Recent studies indicate that phorbol esters stimulate a calcium-activated, phospholipid-dependent protein kinase (protein kinase C; PKC) by substituting 1,2-diacylglycerol (1,2-DAG), which is another hydroproduct of the phosphoinositides (Nishizuka, 1984). Phorbol esters have been reported to increase exocrine pancreatic secretion without increasing $[Ca^{2+}]_i$ (Gunther, 1981). Pandol and Schoeffield (1986) have reported that PKC has an inhibitory role in pancreatic stimulus–secretion coupling rather than a stimulus role. Models involving both changes in $[Ca^{2+}]_i$ and activation of PKC by 1,2-DAG have been proposed to account for the full biological response in a variety of tissues, including exocrine glands.

To determine the role of PKC in mucous glycoprotein secretion, Shimura et al. (1991b) examined the effects of a selective PKC stimulant, phorbol-12-myristate-13-acetate (PMA), or a PKC inhibitor, 1-(5-isoquinolinesulfonyl)-2-methylpiperazine (H-7), on both mucous glycoprotein secretion and $[Ca^{2+}]_i$ in feline tracheal submucosal glands. Use of PMA itself produced a significant increase in mucous glycoprotein secretion, whereas PMA failed to significantly alter the $[Ca^{2+}]_i$. Use of H-7 inhibited mucous glycoprotein secretion stimulated by MCh. These findings indicate that PKC has a direct stimulatory role in stimulus–secretion coupling of mucous glycoprotein secretion from airway submucosal glands. More recently, Rieves et al. (1991) examined the effect of the activation of the PKC family of cytosolic enzymes on the glycoconjugate release from feline airway explants. Chronic exposure to two known activators of PKC, PMA and mezerin (MEZ), resulted in profound increases in glycoconjugate release over a 7-day experimental period. Maximal glycoconjugate release was 90% above control. These data, combined with eicosanoid experiments, suggest that PKC activation induces prolonged, enhanced airway glycoconjugate production, and that a portion of this response is mediated by the alteration of arachidonic acid metabolism.

There is a recent report suggesting the presence of an interaction between the intracellular-signaling pathways in airway submucosal gland cells, as is true in other exocrine gland cells (McKinney and Rubin, 1988; Maruyama et al., 1985; Sato and Sato, 1981). Paul et al. (1991) examined the release of chondroitin sulfate proteoglycans, $[cAMP]_i$, PKA, and PKC activities in cultured bovine tracheal gland serous cells in response to isoproterenol, phenylephrine, PMA, and Ca^{2+} ionophor. Their findings indicate that the signaling pathways triggered by α- and β-adrenergic agonists converge at the level of adenylate cyclase in tracheal serous cells.

B. Second Messengers in Electrolyte or Fluid Secretion

Airway submucosal glands can secrete not only mucous glycoprotein, but also fluid or electrolytes with active ion transport. To investigate the cellular mechanism of electrolyte secretion, Sasaki et al. (1992) employed a patch–clamp technique on enzymatically digested acinar cells of isolated feline submucosal glands and examined the electrophysiological and $[Ca^{2+}]_i$ response to ACh. Also, the role of IP_3 and localization of IP_3 receptors were examined using monoclonal antibodies to IP_3 receptors. They found that the electrophysiological characteristics of the tracheal submucosal gland can be explained by the apical localization of the IP_3 receptors, which was confirmed immunohistochemically with monoclonal antibodies (Fig. 13). The IP_3 synthesis caused by the stimulation of ACh receptors at the plasma membrane leads to an initial apically localized increase of $[Ca^{2+}]_i$ which, in turn, activated the apical membrane Cl^- channels. The opening of the Cl^- channels results in Cl^- secretion (inward current) and simultaneous membrane depolarization. The following activation of K^+ channels at the basolateral membrane causes hyperpolarization, which is favorable both to maintain Cl^- secretion and to induce Ca^{2+} influx into the cytosol. In fact, imaging of

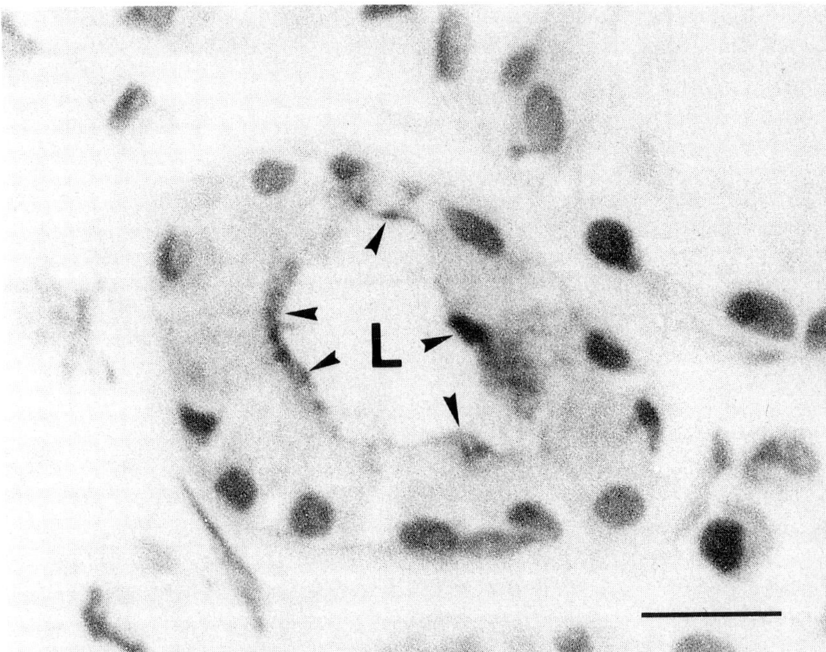

Figure 13 Immunohistological localization of IP_3 receptors in an acinar cell of human submucosal gland. Light microscopy: horseradish peroxidase (HRP)-label of MAb 18A10 (50 μg/ml) is localized at the apical pole of the human acinar cells (arrows). Some apical portions of acinar cells were HRP positive, but others were not. This may be due to the differences in cell types (serous and mucus) or in the physiological states of the cells (e.g., degranulation) (scale bar 30 μm). (From Sasaki et al., 1992)

$[Ca^{2+}]_i$ in Fura-2–loaded submucosal gland cells revealed that the ACh-induced rise of $[Ca^{2+}]_i$ began from the apical pole of the acinar cells. The Ca^{2+} responsible for the K^+-channel activation seems to be derived from the caffeine-sensitive (IP_3-insensitive) Ca^{2+} store because caffeine evoked only the outward K^+ current. These findings indicate that the binding of IP_3 to apically localized receptors plays a pivotal role in triggering a cascade of cellular events in electrolyte secretion, and that the Cl^- and K^+ channels are regulated separately by two distinct Ca^{2+} stores in airway glands (Fig. 14). Some investigators have found an initial rise in $[Ca^{2+}]_i$ at the apical pole of acinar cells after ACh stimulation in rodent exocrine pancreas and lacrimal glands (Kasai and Augustine, 1990; Toesu et al., 1992). Isoproterenol did not induce any significant currents from whole cells, suggesting that a β-agonist is not involved in the secretion of electrolytes.

There is a recent report (Shimura et al., 1991b) suggesting a stimulatory role of PKC in the electrolyte secretion from the airway submucosal glands. Shimura et al. (1991b) examined ^{22}Na efflux as an indicator of electrolyte secretion from isolated feline tracheal submucosal glands. Use of PMA produced a significant increase in ^{22}Na efflux (151% of baseline efflux at 10^{-5} M), and indomethacin did

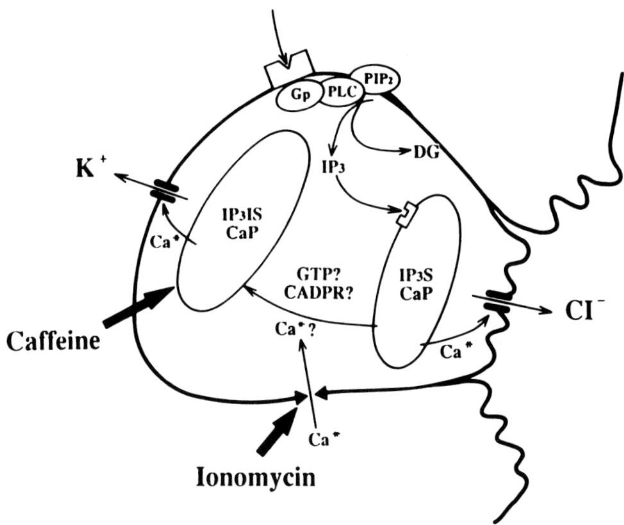

Figure 14 Intracellular mechanism proposed for the electrolyte secretion from airway submucosal glands. Acetylcholine receptor stimulation causes Ca^{2+} pool (IP_3SCap), in turn, activating the apical membrane Cl^- channels. The following activation of K^+ channels at the basolateral membrane by Ca^{2+} release from IP_3-insensitive Ca^{2+} pool (IP_3ISCaP) causes hyperpolarization, which is favorable both to maintain Cl^- secretion and to Ca^{2+} influx into the cytosol. (From Sasaki et al., 1992)

not alter the increase. Two PKC inhibitors, H-7 and shingosine, inhibited ^{22}Na efflux stimulated by PMA and partially inhibited that by MCh, thereby suggesting that PKC has a direct stimulatory role in the electrolyte secretion from airway submucosal glands.

C. Second Messengers in Glandular Contraction

The direct intracellular mechanisms of myoepithelial cell contraction have not yet been determined. However, an experiment of glandular contraction in a Ca^{2+}-free solution supports the idea that both intracellular Ca^{2+} release from storage and Ca^{2+} influx from extracellular solution play a role in the myoepithelial cell contraction (Shimura et al., 1986).

D. Microfilaments and Microtubules

Data obtained with various secretory cells show that microfilaments and microtubules play an obligatory role in the intracellular process (transport and degranulation) of protein or granule secretion of many exocrine glands (Brown et al., 1985b; Busson-Mabillot et al., 1982). Microtubules are 24-nm–diameter structural elements and microfilaments are 4- to 8-nm structures found in parallel arrays or lattice-like networks adjacent to the plasma membrane in airway submucosal glands (Fig. 15). Coles and Reid (1981) examined the effect of colchicine (an antimicrotubule agent) and cytochalasin B (an antimicrofilament agent) on glycoconjugate secretion from submucosal glands of human airways. They suggested that microtubules and microfilaments may be important in secretagogue-induced, but not in baseline, cellular glycoconjugate discharge, which implies that the mechanisms of the two processes differ substantially.

VIII. Cholinergic Regulation

It has been demonstrated morphologically that muscarinic receptors are present on airway gland cells (Barnes et al., 1983b) and are present in equal proportions on tracheal serous and mucous gland cells (Basbaum et al., 1984a). Acetycholinesterase molecules have also been histologically localized to gland cells (Wardell et al., 1970). Cholinergic muscarinic receptor stimulation is the most potent stimulant of tracheal secretion in vitro and in vivo in animals and human (Chakrin et al., 1973; Florey et al., 1932; Sturgess and Reid, 1972; Webber and Widdicombe, 1987a,b). By using a micropipette method, the secretions induced by cholinergic stimulation in feline tracheal submucosal glands were shown to be of the same viscosity as basal secretion (Leikauf et al., 1984), suggesting that muscarinic stimulation induces both glycoprotein and fluid secretions from airway submucosal glands. There have been many reports supporting this idea.

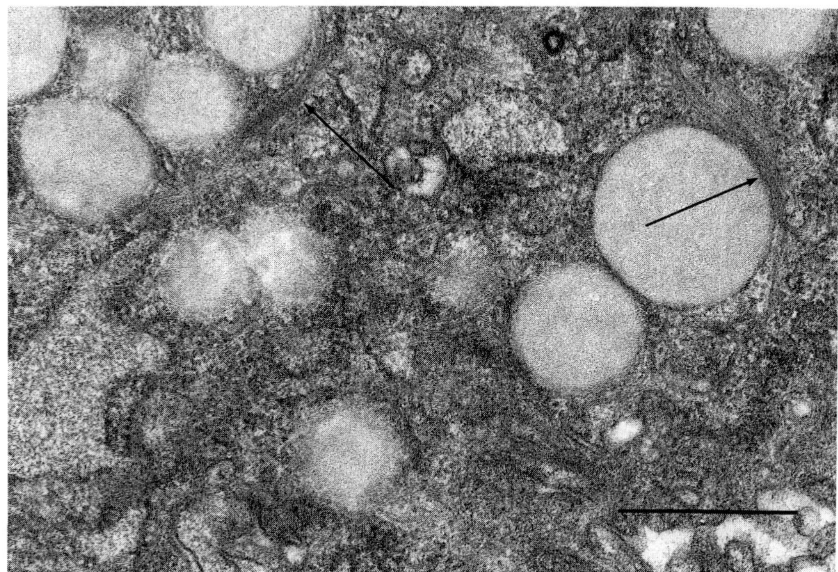

Figure 15   Electron microscopy of serous cell from an isolated gland of canine trachea. Microfilaments (arrows) are seen close to the granules in the cytoplasm (bar, 0.5 μm). (From Shimura, 1990)

Cholinergic muscarinic stimulation is reported to evoke mucous glycoprotein secretion from whole trachea in vivo (Webber and Widdicombe, 1987a), airway explants of animals and human (Yang et al., 1988a; Shelhamer et al., 1980), isolated submucosal glands (Sasaki et al., 1989a; Shimura et al., 1988; Ishihara et al., 1992), and isolated gland cells (Dwyer et al., 1992). There have been no controversies concerning the effect of cholinergic muscarinic stimulation. Because of the development of selective antagonists, muscarinic receptor subtypes have now been identified in several tissues (Eglan and Whiting, 1986), and as many as five different receptor subtypes have been cloned and identified (Bonner et al., 1987). Recently, muscarinic receptors of airways have been pharmacologically subclassified into three subtypes: M_1, M_2, and M_3 receptors (Barnes, 1989). Autoradiographic investigations of human lungs have demonstrated the coexistence of M_1 (36%) and M_3 (64%) receptors over airway submucosal glands (Mak and Barnes, 1990). Yang et al. (1988a, 1988b) have found the presence of both M_1 (27%) and M_3 (73%) receptors on isolated submucosal gland cells of swine trachea and speculated that mucous glycoprotein secretion is stimulated by activation of M_3 receptors. Meanwhile, Gater et al. (1989) have reported that the muscarinic receptor subtype mediating mucous secretion in cat trachea has an intermediate affinity for pirenzepine, suggesting the existence of an "intermediate" between M_1 and M_2 receptor subtypes.

Recently, Ishihara et al. (1992) examined the effects of M_1, M_2 and M_3 receptor antagonists on mucous glycoprotein secretion by cholinergic stimulation, using isolated feline tracheal submucosal glands. They demonstrated that 4-DAMP, an M_3 receptor antagonist, is 100-fold more potent than pirenzepine, a M_1 receptor antagonist, and is 1000-fold more potent than AF-DX116, a M_2 receptor antagonist, in inhibiting MCh-induced mucous glycoprotein secretion from isolated glands. Furthermore, 4-DAMP produced an inhibitory curve similar to atropine, a nonspecific muscarinic receptor antagonist (Fig. 16). These findings indicate that muscarinic agonists stimulate mucous glycoprotein secretion by activating M_3 muscarinic receptor subtypes in airway submucosal gland cells.

Fluid secretion from airway submucosal glands is stimulated by cholinergic muscarinic stimulation, as demonstrated by the following evidence: Yang et al. (1988b) showed that a rapid decline in intracellular ^{36}Cl was observed in response

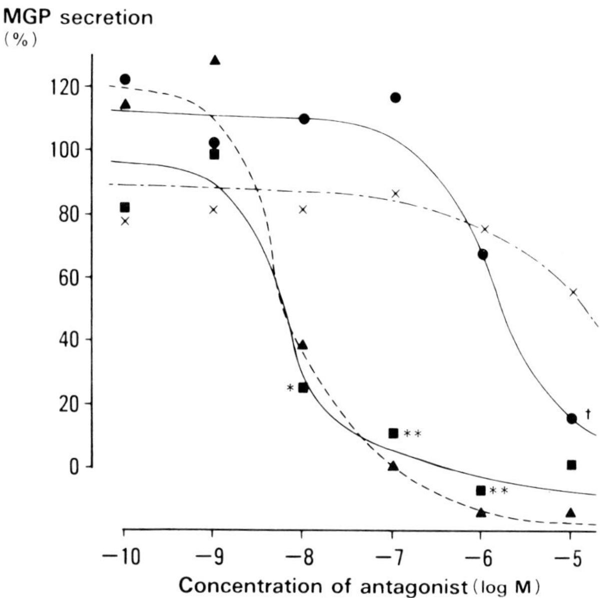

Figure 16 Inhibition curves of 10^{-5} M MCh-evoked, TCA-precipitable [^{3}H]glycoconjugate secretion for four muscarinic receptor antagonists in acinar cells of an isolated feline tracheal gland: pirenzepine, AF-DX116, 4-DAMP, and atropine. Symbols are the same as in Fig. 12: asterisk $p < 0.05$; double asterisk, $p < 0.01$, difference between 4-DAMP and pirenzepine; dagger, $p < 0.05$, difference between pirenzepine and AF-DX116. Results are means for 3–11 experiments. MGP, mucous glycoprotein. (From Ishihara et al., 1992)

to ACh in isolated swine trachea, which was inhibited by oubain. Sasaki et al. (1992) showed by a patch–clamp technique that, in response to ACh, both Cl^- and K^+ currents in a whole cell were evoked in enzymatically digested acinar cells of submucosal glands of human and feline trachea (see Fig. 7). Yamaya et al. (1991a) also showed that MCh is most potent in inducing short-circuit current across cultured human submucosal gland cells (see Fig. 6; see Sec. IV). Sasaki et al. (1990) showed that MCh is most potent in increasing ^{22}Na efflux, an indicator of electrolyte, from isolated feline tracheal submucosal glands (see Figs. 4 and 5). Ishihara et al. (1992) examined the effect of M_1 and M_3 receptor antagonists on the change in the rate constant of ^{22}Na efflux from isolated glands of feline trachea. The MCh-induced ^{22}Na efflux was significantly inhibited by both 4-DAMP and atropine, whereas it was not altered by pirenzepine (Fig. 17). This indicates that cholinergic stimulation induces electrolyte secretion as well as mucous glycoprotein secretion from airway submucosal glands by the activation of muscarinic M_3 receptors.

Cholinergic muscarinic stimulation is shown to induce glandular contraction (see Fig. 10), resulting in mucous ejection in the feline tracheal submucosal gland (Shimura et al., 1986; see Sec. V).

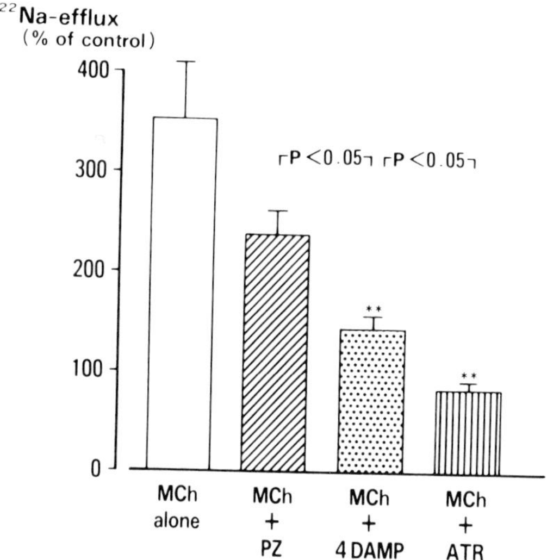

Figure 17 Methacholine (MCh $10^{-5}M$)-evoked ^{22}Na efflux from isolated glands in absence or presence of each antagonist [$10^{-7}M$ pirenzepine (PZ); $10^{-7}M$ 4-DAMP; or $10^{-7}M$ atropine (Atr)]. Results are expressed as percentage of baseline rate constant and means $\pm$ SE for three to five experiments: double asterisk $p < 0.05$, compared with MCh alone. (From Ishihara et al., 1992)

IX. Adrenergic Regulation

The adrenergic responses can be elicited by release of adrenergic neurotransmitters locally or by the release of circulating catecholamines from chromaffin cells.

A. α-Adrenergic Regulation

As seen from autoradiographic studies, the two major cell types of submucosal glands, serous and mucous cells, contain α-adrenergic receptor-binding sites (Barnes et al., 1983b). With isolated gland cells from cat trachea, Culp et al. (1990) have performed competition experiments with α_1 and α_2-adrenergic selective antagonists (prozosin and yohimbine, respectively) that demonstrated high- and low-affinity sites for each antagonist, indicating the presence of both receptor subtypes.

Airway submucosal glands have been demonstrated to secrete mucous glycoconjugates and glycoprotein in response to α-agonists in in vitro experiments of cat (Quinton, 1979; Phipps et al., 1980; Sasaki et al., 1989a), ferret (Tom-Moy et al, 1983) and human tissue (Shelhamer et al., 1980). Peatfield and Richardson (1982) showed that phenylephrine induced ^{35}S-labeled mucin secretion into cat trachea in vivo. Thus, the available evidence suggests mainly α_1-regulation in mucous glycoprotein and glycoconjugate secretion from airway submucosal glands. However, little or nothing is known of the possible role of α_2-receptors in the control of airway secretion.

Culp et al. (1990) reported that, in studies of glycoconjugate secretion by cat tracheal explants, α_1-receptor stimulation produced a significant response, whereas the α_2-adrenergic agonists (clonidine and UK-14,304) markedly inhibited β-adrenergic-stimulated secretion. α_2-Adrenergic receptors do not appear to play a significant role in directly stimulating glycoconjugate secretion. In other systems, α_2-adrenergic agonists have been demonstrated to attentuate cellular responses that are mediated by receptors associated with adenylate cyclase activation. The specific mechanisms of attenuation are unknown, but are, at least, associated with the inhibition of the membrane-bound adenylate cyclase enzyme complex (Gierschik and Jakobs, 1988).

From previous experiments with ferret trachea, both morphometric analysis (Basbaum et al., 1981) and studies of lysozyme secretion (a marker specific for serous cells) indicate that serous cells, but not mucous cells, are markedly stimulated to secrete in response to α-adrenergic stimulation (Tom-Moy et al., 1983). These results correlate with the greater density of α_1-adrenergic receptor sites found on serous cells than on mucous cells (Barnes and Basbaum, 1983).

There have been some reports indicating a role in fluid or electrolyte secretion from airway submucosal glands. Leikauf et al. (1984) examined the viscoelasticity of secretion from feline tracheal submucosal glands and found that phenylephrine evoked less viscoelastic and watery secretion. Sasaki et al. (1990) found that phenylephrine significantly accelerated ^{22}Na efflux (an indicator of electrolyte secretion) from isolated feline tracheal submucosal glands (see Fig. 5; see Sec. IV for details).

In addition, as described in Section V, α-agonist (phenylephrine) has a role in glandular contraction and mucous ejection that represents an initial and short-term secretory response.

B. β-Adrenergic Regulation

Experimental evidence acquired to date suggests that β-adrenergic agents modulate glycoprotein secretion in cat trachea (Liedtke et al., 1983; Sasaki et al., 1989a). Using cat tracheal fragments, Liedtke et al. (1983) found that β-adrenergic agonists increased the release of ^{35}So$_4$-radiolabeled mucin and mucosa–submucosal cAMP levels in a dose- and time-dependent manner. Isoproterenol routinely stimulated ^{35}SO$_4$-labeled chondroitin sulfate proteoglycan secretion in bovine tracheal serous cells (Finkebeiner et al., 1986; Madison et al., 1989; Paul et al., 1988).

β-Aderenergic receptors are seen over airway submucosal gland cells, and the ratio of β$_2$- to β$_1$-receptors is reported to be 9:1 in human bronchial glands (Carstairs et al., 1985). Peatfield and Richardson (1982b) reported that an β$_1$-receptor agonist, dobutamine, increased the output of ^{35}S-labeled mucin into cat trachea in vivo. Phipps et al. (1980) showed that the β$_2$-adrenergic agonist, terbutamine, increased release of ^{35}S-labeled glycoprotein from cat tracheal explants in vitro. Later, Sasaki et al. (1989a) have found that both β$_2$-adrenergic agonist, fenoterol and dbcAMP induced a prominent secretion of mucous glycoprotein from isolated submucosal glands of cat trachea, suggesting a principal role of β$_2$-adrenergic receptor stimulation in mucin secretion. Thus, the role of a subtype of β-adrenergic receptors in submucosal secretion remains to be elucidated.

β-Adrenergic stimulation has been variously reported to have no effect on human respiratory mucous glycoprotein secretion, or to stimulate mucous glycoprotein secretion (Kaliner et al., 1988). This may be due to differences in experimental design. For example, Shelhamer et al. (1980) have reported that the secretion macromolecules of explanted human tracheobronchial tissue are also responsive to adrenergic agonists, including β-adrenergic agonists.

In contrast with the findings that airway submucosal glands can secrete mucous glycoprotein, there has not yet been any direct evidence supporting the notion of an active ion transport with fluid movement in airway submucosal glands by β-adrenergic stimulation. Sasaki et al. (1990) reported that isoproterenol failed to significantly alter ^{22}Na efflux (an indicator of electrolyte secretion) from isolated feline submucosal glands (see Fig. 5). Later, they confirmed this by measuring K$^+$

and Cl$^-$ currents in a whole cell of feline tracheal submucosal gland by a patch–clamp method (1992). The absence of active ion transport supports the in vivo findings by Leikauf et al. (1984) that β-agonist induced higher viscoelastic secretion than the basal secretion, and that this was greater than that induced by cholinergic and α-agonists.

β-Adrenergic stimulation induces no significant glandular contraction or mucous ejection (Shimura et al., 1986).

X. Peptidergic Regulation

The neuropeptides include vasoactive intestinal peptide (VIP), peptide histidine isoleucine (PHI), peptide histidine methionine (PHM), substance P (SP), calcitonin gene-related peptide (CGRP), neurokinins A and B, neuropeptide Y, galanin, gastrin-releasing peptides, cholecytonin, and somatostatin (Lauweryns and Ranst, 1987; Lundberg et al., 1979; Polak and Bloom, 1982). Also, localization of the receptors for neuropeptides by autoradiography has been reported in lungs, showing a high density of binding over the submucosal glands of bronchi (Carstairs and Barnes, 1986a,b; Leys et al., 1986). Thus, neuropeptides are candidates for the transmitters of nonadrenergic and noncholinergic nerves (Dey et al., 1981) and have been implicated in the control of airway submucosal gland secretion. Among these neuropeptides the effects of SP, VIP, and bombesin on airway submucosal gland secretion have now been investigated (Baker et al., 1977; Borson et al., 1987; Coles and Reid, 1981; Coles et al., 1984; Gashi et al., 1986; Peatfield et al., 1983). These investigators used airway explants containing surface epithelium, submucosal tissues, and sometimes cartilage, in addition to submucosal glands. The potential effects of the surrounding tissues may include an epithelial inhibitory action on submucosal gland secretion (Sasaki et al., 1989a), tissue peptidases released during experiments (Borson et al., 1987; Keltz et al., 1980), and difficulty in the penetration of such high M_r peptides to the effector site of the submucosal gland. It is possible that differences in the environments of submucosal glands in different tissues may account for the observed variations in glandular secretory responses.

A. Tachykinins

Tachykinins in the airways include substance P and neurokinins (NK) A and B. There have been many reports that indicate SP-induced mucous glycoprotein and glycoconjugate secretion from airway submucosal glands, whereas neurokinins A and B are speculated to have less or no effect on the airway secretion by Baraniuk et al. (1991). Thus, airway submucosal gland secretion is thought to be mediated through the activation of NK 2 receptors.

Substance P is localized to nerves in the airways of several species, including humans (Lundberg et al., 1984), and autoradiographic studies have demonstrated SP receptors over submucosal glands in human airways using Boltan–Hunter [125I]SP (Carstairs and Barnes, 1986a). Baker et al. (1977) tested the effect of SP on the release of radiolabeled macromolecules from pieces of dog trachea in vitro and found a significant secretion in response to SP. Shimura et al. (1987b), using isolated feline tracheal glands, reported that SP produced a significant increase (74% above control at 10^{-7} M) in radiolabeled glycoconjugate release from isolated glands, whereas SP had no significant effect on glycoconjugate release from tracheal explants (Fig. 18), probably because of epithelial suppression (Sasaki et al., 1989a). Atropine abolished substance P-evoked glycoconjugate release in isolated glands. These findings indicate that SP stimulates radiolabeled glycoconjugate release in isolated submucosal gland, probably involving synthesis of mucus or cellular secretion, and that this action is also mediated by a peripheral cholinergic mechanism. There is some morphological evidence showing that the SP-induced increase in glycoconjugate release from

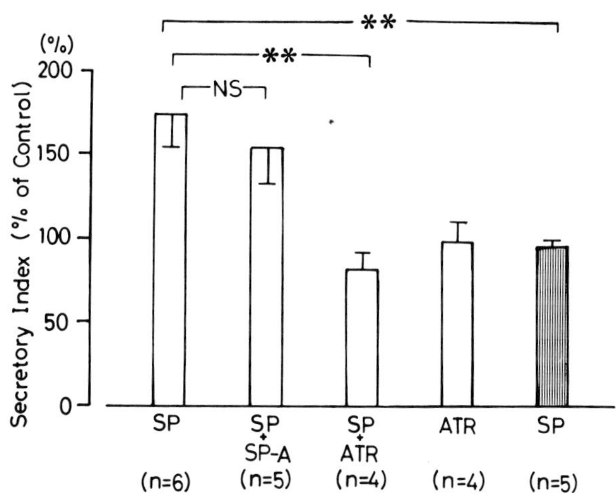

Figure 18   Labeled [3H]glycoconjugate release from isolated feline tracheal glands (open columns) and feline tracheal explants (shaded column). Substance P (SP, 10^{-7} M) induced significant increase in glycoconjugate release from isolated glands (174% of control). The SP antagonist (SP-A, 10^{-7} M), DPro[2], DTro[7.9])-SP, did not inhibit SP-induced glycoconjugate release, which did not differ significantly from SP-treated samples. Atropine (ATR, 10^{-6} M) abolished SP-induced release compared with SP-treated samples. In tracheal explants, however, SP failed to induce a significant increase in glycoconjugate release compared with control values. Single asterisk indicates $p < 0.05$; double asterisks indicate $p < 0.01$; NS, not significant. (From Shimura et al., 1987b)

isolated glands reflects the increase in cellular secretion or synthesis of mucus. From electron microscopy, Gashi et al. (1986) have reported that high doses of SP stimulate acinar cell degranulation in the ferret tracheal submucosal gland.

There have been some studies of the metabolism of SP in the airways. Borson et al. (1987) studied the roles of SP and endogenous peptidases in regulating mucous secretion from ferret trachea. They measured the SP-induced release of $^{35}SO_4$-labeled macromolecules after incubating segments of trachea in Ussing chambers in the presence and absence of selected inhibitors of proteolytic enzymes. The response to SP was concentration-dependent and reproducible. Both thiorphan and phosphoramidon potentiated SP-induced secretion, whereas other inhibitors of proteinases and peptidases had no effects. These results suggest that SP regulates mucous glycoconjugate secretion and that enkephalinase in the airways degrades SP in a physiologically significant fashion.

Coles et al. (1984) found that SP-evoked ^{14}C-labeled mucous glycoprotein release from dog tracheal explants was followed by a period of apparent inhibition and speculated that SP acted by contracting myoepithelial cells and mucous ejection into the medium. Shimura et al. (1987a) have confirmed this SP action using isolated submucosal glands of feline trachea as follows. Substance P (10^{-12}–10^{-4} M) produced dose-dependent increases in the contractile response, and maximal tension induced by SP was 70% of the response to MCh in the corresponding concentrations. The SP-induced contraction is blocked completely by atropine and augmented by neostigmine. Pretreatment with hemicholinium 3, an acetylcholine synthesis inhibitor, inhibited the contractile response to SP. Pretreatment with tetrodotoxin did not inhibit the contractile response to SP (Shimura et al., 1987b, 1991a). Capsaicin induced tension of a magnitude similar to that of SP. These findings indicate that SP induces glandular contraction, which is related to the mucous ejection in ducts and secretory tubules and that this action is mediated by a peripheral cholinergic mechanism.

B. Vasoactive Intestinal Peptide

Vasoactive intestinal peptide has also been implicated in the control of airway submucosal gland secretion. Coles et al. (1981) have reported that VIP causes inhibition of [^{14}C]glycoconjugate secretion by human bronchi, whereas Peatfield et al. (1983) and Gashi et al. (1986) have shown that VIP stimulates both ^{35}S-labeled macromolecule secretion and acinar degranulation in ferret tracheal submucosal glands. This discrepancy may be due to species differences. These investigators also used airway explants containing surface epithelium, submucosal tissues, and sometimes cartilage in addition to submucosal glands. These surrounding tissues possibly affect submucosal gland secretion. In fact, Shimura et al. (1988) found that VIP failed to produce a significant secretion from feline tracheal explants. In contrast, in isolated glands, VIP (10^{-10}–10^{-6} M) produced a dose-dependent increase in [³H]glycoconjugate release of as much as 300% of the control value (Shimura et al., 1988).

    An interaction of VIP receptors with muscarinic receptors in airway submucosal gland secretion has been proposed by Shimura et al. (1988, 1991a). At a low concentration that did not produce any significant increases over control values, VIP produced a 2.4- to 5-fold augmentation of the glycoconjugate release induced by 10^{-9}–10^{-7} M methacholine (Fig. 19; Shimura et al., 1988, 1991a). Atropine or VIP antiserum abolished the augmentation. Use of VIP did not pro-

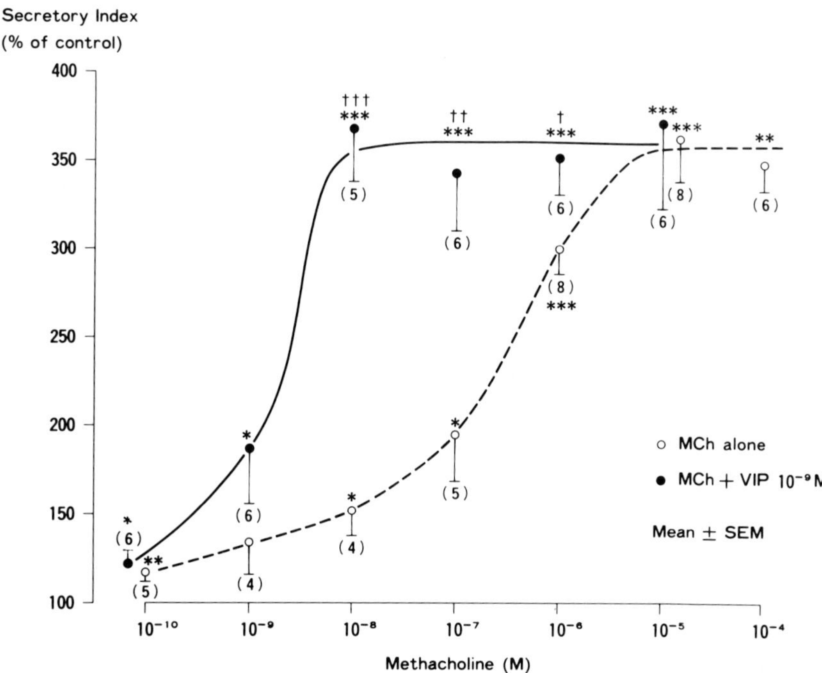

Figure 19 Dose–response curves to methacholine (MCh) only and MCh in addition to a low concentration of VIP (10^{-9} M) in [³H]-labeled glycoconjugate release from isolated feline tracheal glands. The VIP augmented MCh-evoked secretion by a 2.4- to 5.1-fold increment at concentrations of 10^{-9}–10^{-6} M MCh. NS, not significant: single asterisk indicates $p < 0.01$; triple asterisks indicate $p < 0.001$ compared with control values; single dagger indicates $p < 0.05$; double daggers indicate $p < 0.01$; three daggers indicate $p < 0.001$, differences between the response to MCh alone and that to MCh plus VIP. The number of experiments is shown in parentheses (bars represent SEM). Open circles, MCh alone; closed circles, MCh + VIP 10^{-9} M (mean ± SEM). (From Shimura et al., 1988)

duce any alteration in isoproterenol- nor in phenylephrine-evoked glycoconjugate secretion. These results indicate that VIP induces mucous glycoprotein release from secretory cells and also that it potentiates the secretion induced by cholinergic stimulation. From a calculation with the Hill coefficient, it is speculated that VIP enhances glycoconjugate secretion by switching muscarinic receptors to the high-affinity conformer from the low-affinity one in airway submucosal glands (Shimura et al., 1988), as was previously demonstrated in salivary gland (Lundberg et al., 1982). Because VIP is a transmitter that coexists with acetylcholine in the postganglionic neurons supplying exocrine glands (Johansson and Lundberg, 1981), this interaction of VIP receptors with mucarinic receptors is important for the understanding of submucosal gland secretion.

XI. Autonomic Innervation

Morphological examination has revealed the presence of nerve fibers over the submucosal glands and ganglia close to the glands in the airways (Bensch et al., 1965; Silva and Ross, 1974; Murlas et al., 1980; Baluk et al., 1985). Some differences relating to the functional autonomic innervation of airway submucosal gland secretion of macromolecules have been reported, even within the same species. Reflex-increased secretion in dog and cat tracheal submucosal glands in vivo has been reported to involve only a cholinergic efferent pathway (Davis et al., 1982a,b; German et al., 1982a,b; Schultz et al., 1985; Haxihiu et al., 1991a). Adrenergic mechanisms mediate the secretion of $^{35}SO_4$-labeled macromolecules from cat trachea, both in reflex to irritation of the upper airways and in vivo, when evoked by electrical stimulation of the satellite ganglion (Borson et al., 1980; Gallagher et al., 1975; Peatfield and Richardson, 1982; Phipps and Richardson, 1976). In addition, some investigators have found that nonadrenergic, noncholinergic neural mechanisms mediate the secretion of macromolecules from submucosal glands of ferret and cat trachea (Borson et al., 1984; Peatfield and Richardson, 1983). Different findings have been reported concerning autonomic innervation of airway submucosal gland secretion, even in the same species, depending on the methods in the experiments. Because, each preparation or method applied in the experiments has its own limitations, there are few preparations or methods by which we can obtain all three secretory responses (i.e., mucus ejection from glandular contraction, fluid (or electrolyte) secretion, and mucous glycoprotein secretion).

A. Neural Control of Glandular Contraction

With single, isolated submucosal glands from feline trachea, Shimura et al. (1986) have observed that mucous ejection is coincident with glandular contraction through the activity of myoepithelial cells, and that the glandular contraction is completed within 1 min. The glandular contraction is also mediated by cholinergic nerves through muscarinic receptors and, in small part, by adrenergic nerves through muscarinic receptors and, in small part, by adrenergic nerves through α-receptors (Shimura et al., 1987a). From these findings, the secretory response of submucosal glands is conjectured to consist of two actions: (1) discharge of mucus from secretory cells into tubules and ducts and (2) expulsion of mucus (mucin and fluid) into airway lumen through glandular contraction, which represents a rapid initial response. The previous experiments showing only cholinergic innervation all represented short-time (1 min or less) responses. For example, Davis et al. (1982a,b) and Schultz et al. (1985) have found a cholinergic pathway only in reflex-stimulated secretion from dog tracheal submucosal glands. These previous investigators all measured the hillock formation on tantalum-covered tracheal mucosa as an indicator of mucous secretion. German et al. (1982b), using a micropipette method, found that reflex submucosal gland secretion in cat trachea, evoked by gastric irritation, showed a peak within 1 min after stimulation and was only cholinergic, as indicated by its being blocked by atropine. Furthermore, reflex-increased secretion by hypoxemia or stimulation of bronchial or pulmonary C fibers in dog tracheal submucosal gland has been shown to involve only a cholinergic mechanism (Davis et al., 1980, 1982a,b; Schultz et al., 1985). Borson et al. (1980) have reported that fluid secretion from ferret tracheal submucosal glands is mediated by cholinergic and adrenergic nerves through α-receptors, but not β-receptors. These experiments described were all performed using a hillock formation on the tantalum-covered mucosa or a micropipette method, in which the response reached a plateau within 1 min, after which no response could be observed, even when nerve stimulation continued for up to 5 min (Borson et al., 1980; Davis et al., 1980, 1982a,b). However, when the responses to nerve stimulation for longer durations were observed by other methods, other innervations become apparent. The sympathetic nervous system, including the β-adrenergic mechanism, was involved in reflex secretion of radiolabeled sulfated glycoprotein in the cat trachea isolated in situ when there was irritation of the nose, pharynx, or larynx for 10 min or more (Phipps and Richardson, 1976). Gallagher et al. (1975) have also found β-adrenergic control in radiolabeled glycoprotein secretion from cat trachea in vivo using electrical stimulation for a duration of 15 min. Peatfield and Richardson (1982b, 1983) have reported β-adrenergic control and a noncholinergic, nonadrenergic mechanism in cat trachea in vivo, using an examination of radiolabeled glycoprotein that was released after electrical stimulation for 8 min. These findings, together with previous reports of airway submucosal gland secretion, seem to indicate that there are apparent differences in the functional innervation that are related to the differences in duration of observation or stimulation.

B. Neural Control of Mucous Glycoprotein and Glycoconjugate Secretion

To test the foregoing hypothesis, Shimura et al. (1992a) performed a study to determine whether functional innervation of submucosal gland secretion is dependent on the duration of neural stimulation, by examining radiolabeled mucous glycoprotein released from feline isolated tracheal submucosal glands when subjected to electrical field stimulation (FS) (Fig. 20). This stimulation produced an increase in the glycoconjugate release that was dependent on the duration of stimulation, reaching a maximum response of 215% of nonstimulated samples after 30 min of stimulation (Fig. 21). The FS-evoked secretion was abolished by tetrodotoxin, but was not altered by hexamethonium. Atropine alone abolished the response to FS, but for only 3 min or less. By contrast, a mixture of atropine, propranolol, and phentolamine blocked only part of the response to FS for 15 min or more. The mixture of three antagonists reduced the 30-min response to FS to 159% of control, which was significantly higher than control. Furthermore, atropine, propranolol, or phentolamine significantly reduced the 30-min response

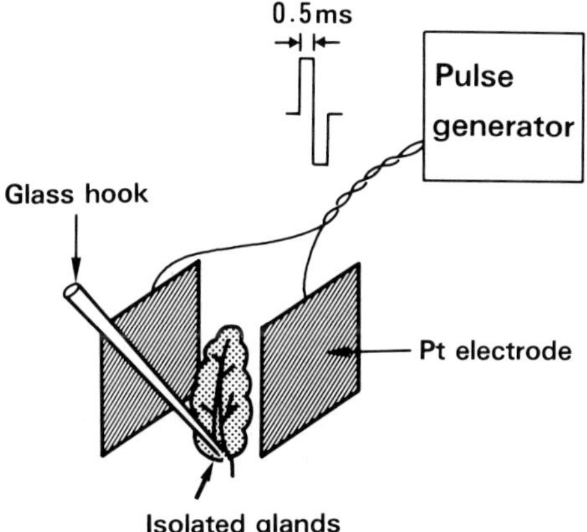

Figure 20 Block diagram of method used for measuring mucous glycoconjugate secretion induced by electrical field stimulation (FS). After 5-h incubation with [³H]glucosamine, isolated glands were held by glass hooks between two platinum electrodes in the experimental chamber containing 4 ml of medium 199 and placed in a controlled-atmosphere chamber and gased constantly with 5% CO_2, 55% N_2, and 40% O_2, at 37°C. Intrinsic nerves were stimulated with an electrical impulse, and radiolabeled glycoconjugates released to the medium were precipitated with trichloroacetic acid. Radioactivity (dpm) of glycoconjugates was divided by dry weight of sample and then compared with control samples. (From Shimura et al., 1992a)

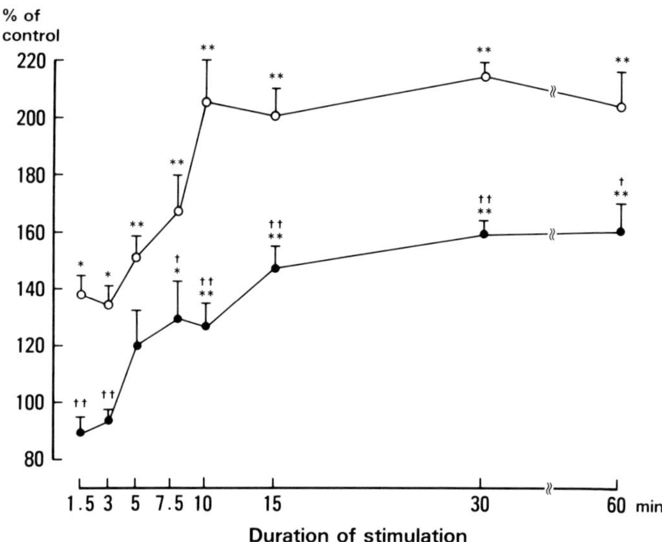

Figure 21 Stimulation duration-dependence in the secretory response to electrical field stimulation (FS) at 10 Hz, 10 V in [³H]glycoconjugate secretion from isolated feline tracheal glands, expressed as a percentage of control. Open circles, responses to FS without any antagonists; closed circles, those with a mixture of 10^{-6} M atropine, 10^{-5} M phentolamine, and 10^{-5} M propranolol, except those at 1.5- and 3-min stimulation, which were pretreated with 10^{-6} M atropine alone. When isolated glands were stimulated for 30 min or more, a mixture of three antagonists reduced response to 150% of control, which was a significantly higher response than that of controls. When stimulated for 60 min, the corresponding control gland was also incubated for 60 min. Bar, mean $\pm$ SE; number of experiments is four to seven; asterisk, $p < 0.05$; double asterisk, $p < 0.01$; compared with control; dagger, $p < 0.05$; double dagger, $p < 0.01$, compared with that without any antagonists. (From Shimura et al., 1992a)

to FS to 162, 193, and 195%, respectively, from 215% of the sample without blockers. These findings suggest that the functional innervation of mucous glycoprotein secretion from the airway submucosal gland is dependent on the duration of nerve stimulation. Taken together with a previous experiment on neural control of glandular contraction (Shimura et al., 1987a) and the reports by other investigators described earlier, it is deduced that short (a few minutes) nerve stimulation induces glandular contraction and ejection of mucous glycoprotein into the medium, which is mediated mainly by cholinergic nerves, whereas longer periods stimulate mucous glycoprotein secretion from secretory cells in submucosal glands, an action mediated by cholinergic, adrenergic, and noncholinergic, nonadrenergic (NANC) mechanisms. Generally, it takes 15 min or more to synthesize glycoproteins from the precursors in secretory cells (Castle, 1990).

Fung et al. (1992) used drugs that block neurotransmission at different sites in the autonomic nervous system to define the NANC nerve pathways regulating mucous glycoconjugate secretion into the trachea. In anesthetized cats, mucous glycoconjugates, radiolabeled biosynthetically with [^{35}S]sulfate and [^{3}H]glucose, were washed from a tracheal segment in situ, and dialyzed before scintillation counting and chemical assay by the periodic acid–Schiff (PAS) method. In the absence of autonomic blocking drugs, vagal stimulation significantly increased the output of radiolabeled and PAS-reactive glycoconjugates, and notable responses to vagal stimulation remained after combined muscarinic and adrenoceptor blockade with atropine, phentolamine, and propranolol. Subsequent treatment with the ganglion-blocking drug, hexamethonium, prevented most of the remaining response to vagal stimulation, significantly reducing the outputs of glycoconjugates. They concluded that the main NANC vagal pathway controls tracheal glycoconjugate secretions orthodromically through the mural ganglion cells in this species. Antidromic conduction along afferent nerves may also weakly stimulate secretion.

Opioid receptors modulate noncholinergic, nonadrenergic nerves in airway smooth-muscle contraction (Frossard and Barnes, 1987). There are some reports that suggest the presence of opioid receptor regulation of airway mucous secretion, probably from submucosal glands. Rogers and Barnes (1989) examined the releases of fucose and hexose from human bronchial explants, as markers of mucous secretion from submucosal glands, and found that capsaicin-induced mucous secretion was completely blocked by morphine, and this effect was reversed by naloxone.

C. Neural Control of Fluid and Electrolyte Secretion

There have been few experiments to determine whether fluid and electrolyte secretions, as well as mucous glycoprotein secretions, are also under autonomic nervous control. This is due to the lack of a suitable tool for the detection of the neural control of only electrolyte secretion, independent of that of mucous glycoprotein secretion in airway submucosal glands. Sasaki et al. (1990) examined the effect of FS on ^{22}Na efflux (an indicator of electrolyte secretion) from isolated feline submucosal glands (Fig. 22). They found that FS produced a significant frequency-dependent increase, which was partially inhibited by atropine or phentolamine (Fig. 23). These findings indicate that electrolyte secretion from airway submucosal glands is under autonomic nervous control and is mediated by both cholinergic and adrenergic nerves through α-receptors. Furthermore, a mixture of atropine, phentolamine, and propranolol abolished FS-evoked ^{22}Na efflux, indicating the absence of nonadrenergic, noncholinergic innervation to

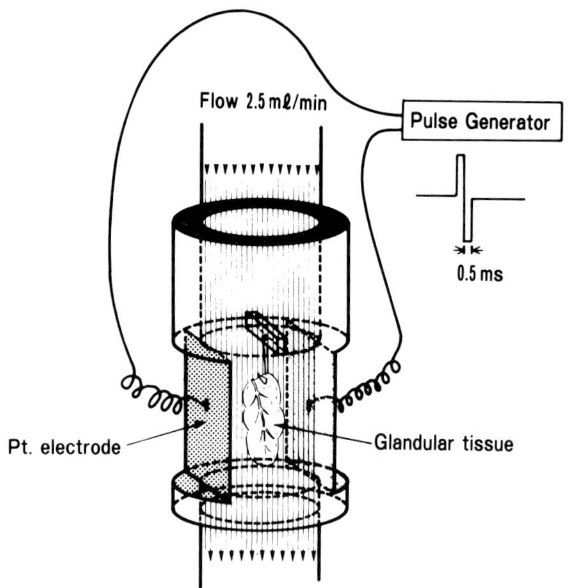

Figure 22 Schematic representation of the sample chamber used in the field stimulation experiments of ^{22}Na efflux from isolated glands. Platinum-plate electrodes (6 × 10 mm) are attached to windows at opposite sides of sample chamber. Glands are fixed by a glass hook which, in turn, was connected to a silicon rubber chip set inside the chamber. (From Sasaki et al., 1990)

electrolyte secretion from airway submucosal glands (see Fig. 23). This is clearly different from the neural control of mucous glycoprotein secretion in airway submucosal glands. Since autonomic innervation of airway epithelial cells has not yet been shown, the possible innervation of electrolyte (or water) secretion from airway submucosal glands may play a main role in airway electrolyte and fluid movement across the airway wall in response to neurological stimulation (i.e., neural reflexes).

D. Central Nervous System Control

There are recent studies indicating that airway gland secretion is under central nervous system control. Davis and Tseng (1991) investigated the effect of central and peripheral nerves on lysozyme secretion from tracheal submucosal glands in ferrets by injecting substance P intravenously and intracisternally in vivo. They found that intracisternal SP stimulated the central nervous system and activated secretomotor nerves of tracheal glands and that intravenous SP increased lysozyme secretion both directly, by activating tracheal glands, and indirectly, by

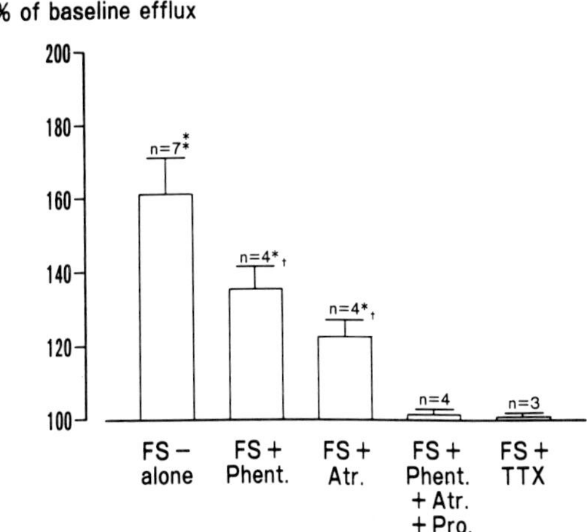

Figure 23   Electrical field stimulation (FS, 20 Hz, 20 V)-evoked ^{22}Na efflux from isolated feline glands and effects of antagonists on FS. Changes in instantaneous rate constant induced by application of FS are expressed as percentage increase of baseline rate constant. Phent, phentolamine (10^{-5} M); Atr, atropine (10^{-6} M); Pro, propranolol (10^{-6} M); TTX, tetrodotoxin (10^{-7} M), respectively. Significant differences from baseline efflux are indicated by asterisk, $p < 0.05$, and double asterisks $p < 0.01$, respectively, and those from FS-alone controls are dagger, $p < 0.05$. (From Sasaki et al., 1990)

activating secretomotor nerves through the central nervous system. More directly, Haxihiu et al. (1991b) studied the activation of nicotinergic receptors, located on the ventral surface of the medulla (VMS), and whether these may influence secretion from tracheal submucosal glands in anesthetized dog, by examining the changes in the number of hillocks of secretion appearing on submucosal glands. They concluded that the ventral medulla contains cells near its surface that influence and modulate the reflex response of tracheal submucosal gland secretion, probably by altering the level of general excitation within the central respiratory integrating circuits. By the same method, they also showed substance P, acting centrally, can increase tracheal submucosal gland secretion, mainly by cholinergic mechanisms, and that VMS is one of the sites of these actions (Haxihiu et al., 1991c).

In the neural control of airway smooth muscle, prejunctional inhibitory muscarinic receptors (autoreceptors) on cholinergic nerves are found in human and guinea pigs (Minette and Barnes, 1988). Dysfunctions of these autoreceptors (M_2 receptors) are known to exist in bronchial asthmatics (Ayala and Ahmed, 1989), thereby relating to their airway hyperresponsiveness. However, it has not yet been determined whether similar autoreceptors are also active in the neural control of airway submucosal gland secretion.

E. Augmentation by Chemical Mediators

Various chemical mediators, including serotonin, histamine, prostaglandins, and substance P augment airway smooth-muscle contraction by nerve stimulation through accelerated acetylcholine release from nerve terminals (Sheller et al., 1982; Walters et al., 1984). Among these agents, serotonin is known to be the most potent in augmentation of the response to nerve stimulation (Sheller et al., 1982). There have been some reports showing the presence of mechanisms in airway mucous secretion that are similar to those in smooth muscle.

One report (Shimura et al., 1987a) showed that serotonin potentiates glandular contraction by nerve stimulation in isolated feline tracheal submucosal glands. A short-time secretory response, measured by the hillock method, has also been reported to be augmented by serotonin in dog trachea (Popovac et al., 1979). More directly, Shimura et al. (1992a) examined the effect of serotonin on glycoprotein secretion from isolated submucosal glands, which was evoked by neural stimulation of different durations. Serotonin potentiated both glycoprotein secretion in response to FS for 3 min or less and that for 15 min or more. Since the former was mediated by cholinergic nerves alone, the potentiation was due to the interaction of these nerves. Cholinergic mechanisms are also probably responsible for the serotonin-induced potentiating response to FS because both atropine, a muscarinic receptor antagonist, and methysergide, a serotonin receptor antagonist, reduced the response to levels similar to those of the response to FS, both with and without atropine. The augmentation is due to the interaction of serotonin with the cholinergic action at the postganglionic nerve terminal, probably through accelerated acetylcholine release at the nerve terminal, since hexamethonium, an inhibitor of ganglionic transmission, had no effect. However, there have been other reports indicating that some chemical mediators act on ganglion neurons, accelating the transmission. For example, with use of a hillock method (Johnson et al., 1983a,b), it has been shown that leukotriene-C_4 (LCT_4) enhanced tracheal submucosal gland secretion over baseline values and that this enhancement could be blocked by hexamethonium. This indicates that leukotrienes have the ability to stimulate ganglionic motor neurons in the innervation of airway submucosal gland.

XII. Purigenic Regulation

There are two classes of purigenic receptors: P_2, those that recognize ATP, and P_1, those that recognize adenosine. ATP and other nucleotides produce an increase in IP_3 and an elevation of $[Ca^{2+}]_i$ in several cell types including exocrine cells (Sasaki and Gallacher, 1990, 1992; Soltoff et al., 1992). However, there have as yet been few experiments concerning purine receptors in airway submucosal glands.

To investigate the role of purine receptors in airway submucosal gland secretion, Shimura et al. (1992c) examined the effects of adenosine or ATP on both whole-cell current responses and on mucous glycoprotein secretion from isolated feline tracheal submucosal glands. A standard patch–clamp technique was employed on enzymatically digested acinar cells of isolated glands. Adenosine produced no significant current responses; ATP evoked bidirectional current responses in a dose-dependent fashion, an initial inward current (Cl^- current) followed by an outward current (K^+ current). Isoproterenol alone did not evoke any significant current responses, but did augment ATP-induced Cl^- and K^+ currents. Intracellular cAMP mimicked the augmentation by isoproterenol. Use of ATP evoked a significant dose-dependent mucous glycoprotein secretion, and isoproterenol enhanced ATP-induced secretion. These findings suggest that P_2 receptor stimulation induces both electrolyte and mucous glycoprotein secretion and that ATP-induced secretion is enhanced by β-receptor stimulation through an intracellular interaction in airway submucosal glands.

XIII. Chemical Mediators

The airways are exposed to a variety of mediators released locally in immediate hypersensitivity or inflammatory reactions. Mast cell degranulation, resulting from antigen interaction with cell-bound IgE, results in the release of the mediators of anaphylaxis, including histamine, as well as the production and release of prostaglandins, leukotrienes, other lipoxygenase pathway products, platelet-activating factor (PAF), and bradykinin. Inhalation of these chemical mediators (histamine, prostaglandin $F_{2\alpha}$) has been shown to stimulate sputum production in humans (Lopez-Vidriero et al., 1977).

A. Histamine

Shelhamer et al. (1980) examined the effects of histamine and several other chemical mediators on the release of [^{3}H]glucosamine-labeled glycoproteins in human airways in vitro. Exogenous histamine added to airway fragments increased mucous glycoprotein release, which was abolished by cimetidine, an H_2 receptor antagonist. Selective histamine H_2, but not H_1, agonists increased mucous glycoprotein release, suggesting the possibility that anaphylaxis of airways results in increased mucous glycoprotein release, partially through histamine H_2 receptor stimulation.

B. Prostaglandins

Arachidonic acid added to lung explants in vitro results in an increase in mucous glycoprotein secretion, an action presumably mediated by one of the metabolites of arachidonic acid (Marom et al., 1981). Products of the cyclooxygenase pathway of arachidonic acid metabolism include the prostaglandins (PGs), and arachidonic acid, PGA_2, PGD_2, and $PGF_{2\alpha}$ significantly increased [³H]glucosamine-labeled mucous glycoprotein release in human airway fragments, whereas PGE_2 significantly reduced the release (Marrom et al., 1981).

C. Leukotrienes and Other Lipoxygenase Products

Inhibition of the production of cyclooxygenase pathway products in vitro by the addition of nonsteroidal anti-inflammatory agents, however, results in a substantial increase in mucous glycoprotein secretion, implying that lipoxygenase pathway products of arachidonic acid metabolism may be important in the regulation of mucous glycoprotein production in human airways (Marom et al., 1981). Lipoxygenase products include the monohydroxy- and the hydroperoxyeicosatetraenoic acids as well as the leukotrienes. In fact, 5-, 8-, 11-, 12-, and 15-monohydroxy-eicosatetraenoic acids all stimulate mucous glycoprotein secretion when present in nanomolar concentrations (Shelhamer et al., 1980; Marom et al., 1982). Leukotriene C_4 and leukotriene D_4, when used in picomolar concentrations, are capable of stimulating mucous glycoprotein secretion from human airways in vitro (Marom et al., 1982). This effect is inhibited by the receptor antagonist of slow-reacting substances of anaphylaxis, FPL-55712 (Marom et al., 1981).

Peatfield et al. (1982) examined the effect of LTC_4 on the output of radiolabeled mucins from the trachea of the anesthetized cat and found that it stimulated mucin release. Johnson et al. (1985) have shown that 15-hydroxyeicosa-tetraenoic acid (15-HETE) but not 15-H(P) ETE or 5-HETE is a potent agonist for the secretion of glycoprotein-containing mucus into the in vivo canine trachea.

However, in in vitro experiments, LTC_4 failed to show any effect on mucin secretion (Peatfield et al., 1982). Sasaki et al. (1989a) also found no significant increase in response to LTC_4 and LTD_4 in glycoconjugate secretion in isolated feline tracheal glands. These findings suggest that leukotrienes have no direct action and mainly act on ganglionic neuron or postganglionic nerve terminals only under some conditions (Johnson et al., 1983a,b).

D. Platelet-Activating Factor

There have been several reports implicating platelet-activating factor (PAF) as an important mediator of inflammatory reactions since the original demonstration of PAF release by an IgE-dependent mechanism in rabbit (Benveniste et al., 1972). Platelet-activating factor induces airway mucous secretion in vitro in explants of rodent airways (Alder et al., 1987) and in vivo in ferret trachea (Hahn et al., 1986). With isolated glands from feline trachea, Sasaki et al. (1989b) examined the effect of PAF on radiolabeled glycoconjugate release and glandular contraction by measuring induced tension in the absence or presence of platelets. Use of PAF alone did not produce any significant glandular contraction, nor any significant change in glycoconjugate release from isolated glands. In the presence of purified platelets containing no plasma, PAF (up to 10^{-5} M) produced significant dose-dependent glycoconjugate secretion (Fig. 24), but no significant glandular contraction. The PAF-evoked glycoconjugate secretion was time-dependent, reaching a peak response of 277% of control 15–30 min after the exposure of isolated glands to 10^{-5} M PAF in the presence of platelets, and returning to 135% of controls at 2 h. Platelets alone did not produce any significant stimulation in glycoconjugate release. CV-3988, a known PAF antagonist, inhibited the secretory response to PAF (see Fig. 24). Methysergide, a known antagonist to receptors for 5-hydroxy-tryptamine, did not alter PAF-evoked glycoconjugate secretion from isolated submucosal glands. Epithiomethanothromboxane A_2, a stable thromboxane A_2 analogue, produced a significant dose-dependent increase in glycoconjugate

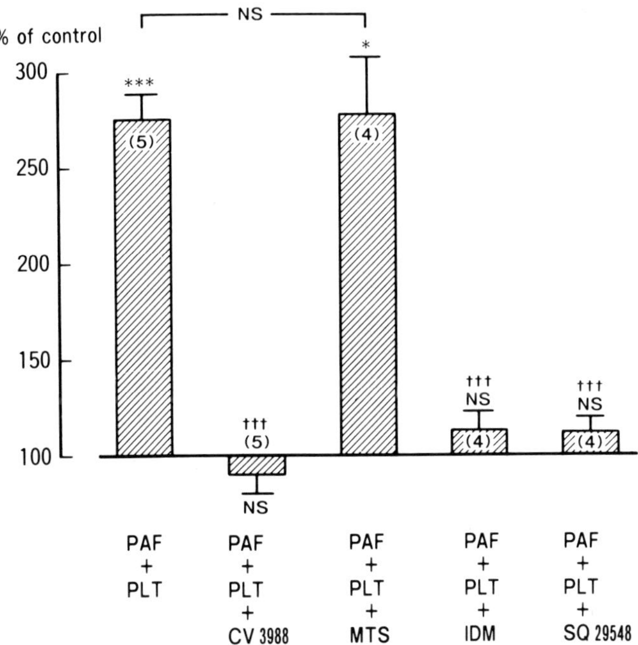

Figure 24 Effects of CV-3988 (10^{-5} M), methysergide (MTS, 10^{-5} M), indomethacin (IDM 10^{-5} M), and SQ-29548 (10^{-5} M) on glycoconjugate secretion induced by PAF (10^{-5} M) in presence of platelets. CV-3988, indomethacin, and SQ-29548, all significantly inhibited secretion induced by PAF, whereas methysergide did not inhibit secretion (number of experiments in parentheses). NS, not significant; asterisk, $p < 0.05$; triple asterisks, $p < 0.001$, compared with controls, and triple daggers, $p < 0.001$, compared with that induced by PAF (10^{-5} M) in presence of platelets. (From Sasaki et al., 1989b)

secretion. These findings indicate that PAF increases glycoconjugate release in the presence of platelets and that the increase is dependent on some aspect of platelet function, namely thromboxane generation.

E. Bradykinin

Bradykinin is released endogenously under various conditions and may play a role in the inflammatory process (Regoli and Varabe, 1980). Bradykinin may act on nervous pathways, secondarily affecting gland secretion. Thus, bradykinin reflexively stimulated fluid production from airway submucosal glands in vivo (Davis et al., 1982b), but had no significant effect on mucin release from airway explants (Sturgess and Reid, 1972). Yamaya et al. (1991a) reported that bradykinin induced an increase in short-circuit current (SCC) across a monolayer of cultured gland cells from human airways, indicating the active ion transport by bradykinin in airway submucosal glands. Basic polypeptides (kallidin and substance P) apparently stimulate macromolecule secretion in dogs, whereas hexadimethrine (a kallidin antagonist) decreases it (Baker et al., 1977).

XIV. Proteinases

Airway neutrophils are found in higher numbers in the airways and in the airway secretions of patients with chronic bronchitis and cystic fibrosis. Neutrophils are thought to play a major role in generating the pathological manifestations of airway inflammation, the features of which include increased and abnormal airway secretions. Neutrophils are a source of a variety of potentially important mediators of inflammation, including neutral proteinases. Prominent among these are the lysosomal proteinases cathepsin G and elastase, which are released from neutrophils during phagocytosis and cell death. Levels of catalytically active cathepsin G and elastase are negligible in normal airway secretions, but are greatly increased in purulent ones (Suter et al., 1986; Weitz et al., 1987). Neutrophils are infiltrate tissue lying beneath the airway mucosal surface in these conditions, where they may interact with subepithelial structures involved in secretion (i.e., submucosal glands).

To investigate the hypothesis that neutrophil proteinases stimulate airway gland secretion, Sommerhoff et al. (1990) studied the effect of human cathepsin G and elastase on secretion of [^{35}S]-labeled macromolecules from cultured bovine airway gland serous cells. Both proteinases stimulated secretion in a concentration-dependent fashion. Elastase was more potent than cathepsin G, causing a maximal secretory response of 1810% over baseline. The maximal response to cathepsin G was similar to the maximal response to elastase. These responses were tenfold larger than the responses to other agonists such as histamine. Proteinase-induced secretion was noncytotoxic and required catalytically active enzymes. The predominant sulfated macromolecule released by proteinases was chondroitin sulfate proteoglycan. Immunocytochemical staining demonstrated chondroitin sulfate in cytoplasmic granules and decreased granular staining after stimulation of cells with elastase. The neutrophil proteinases also degraded the proteoglycan released from serous cells. Cathepsin G and elastase in supernatant, obtained by degranulation of human peripheral neutrophils, also caused a secretory response. Thus, neutrophil proteinases stimulate airway gland serous cell secretion of chondroitin sulfate proteoglycan and degrade the secreted product. These findings suggest a potential role for neutrophil proteinases in the pathogenesis of increased and abnormal submucosal gland secretion in diseases associated with inflammation and neutrophil infiltration of the airways.

Later, Schuster et al. (1992) studied the effect of purified human neutrophil elastase on secretion of ^{35}S-labeled macromolecules from isolated tracheal tissues of ferrets, dogs, and humans. Human neutrophil elastase stimulated secretion in a concentration-dependent fashion, the secretory response being most pronounced in ferret tissues, with a maximal response of 1498% above baseline. In dog tissues, maximal secretory responses (509%) to human neutrophil elastase were much greater than to bethanechol (80%). Human tissues obtained several hours postmortem still responded to human neutrophil elastase significantly more strongly than to the combination of isoproterenol, phenylephrine, and bethanechol. Morphometric analysis of canine tracheal tissues showed degranulation of submucosal gland cells after exposure to human neutrophil elastase. A specific inhibitor of human neutrophil elastase (ICI 200,355) potently inhibited secretory responses in a concentration-dependent fashion. These findings suggest that human neutrophil elastase in airways of patients with cystic fibrosis and chronic bronchitis may cause hypersecretion and that treatment with ICI 200,355 may become a useful component of therapeutic intervention.

Mast cells are also recognized as important inflammatory cells and are implicated in various inflammatory lung diseases, including bronchial asthma. They are abundant in the airway mucosa, where they are in close contact with submucosal glands. Sommerhoff et al. (1989) and Nadel (1991) examined the effects of degranulation supernatant from mastocytoma cells and two mast cell proteinases (tryptase and chymase) on secretion of ^{35}S-labeled macromolecules from cultured bovine tracheal gland serous cells. They found a secretory response that was tenfold larger than those of other agonists, histamine, prostaglandins, and β-adrenergic agonists. None of the classic second messengers including [cAMP]$_i$ glycoconjugate, IP$_3$–Ca^{2+}, and PKC appears to be involved in chymase-induced secretion (Sommerhoff et al., 1989).

XV. Glucocorticoids

Although current pharmacological approaches to airway mucous hypersecretion are limited, glucocorticoid appears to be the most effective among the few useful drugs.

A. Mucous Glycoprotein Secretion

Several in vitro experiments using human and feline airway explants have suggested that glucocorticoids have an inhibitory effect on airway mucous glycoconjugate and glycoprotein secretion (Marom et al., 1984; Lundgren et al., 1985). Lundgren et al. (1985) reported that dexamethasone inhibits respiratory glycoconjugate secretion from feline airways in vitro by the induction of lipocortin (lipomodulin) synthesis. The precise mechanism by which glucocorticoids inhibit airway mucous secretion is still unknown. To study the direct effect of glucocorticoid on submucosal gland secretion, Shimura et al. (1990a) examined the effects of dexamethasone on the precursor uptake, biosynthesis, and release of mucous glycoprotein in isolated feline tracheal submucosal glands. Mucous glycoprotein release from isolated glands was estimated by measuring [^{3}H]glucosamine-labeled trichloroacetic acid (TCA)-precipitable glycoconjugates secreted into the medium. The released glycoconjugate per hour per dry weight of gland tissue was less than 7% of the total intracellular content. Treatment with 10^{-9}–10^{-5} M dexamethasone for 24–72 h significantly reduced basal glycoconjugate secretion to 22% of control (a 78% decrease) in a dose-dependent fashion, whereas the total intracellular [^{3}H]content was reduced to 70% of control (a 30% decrease) with no statistically significant differences from controls (Fig. 25). The ratio of released glycoconjugates to the total intracellular content decreased significantly to 30% of control (a 69% decrease) after the treatment with 10^{-10}–10^{-5} M dexamethasone. Dexamethasone also inhibited the glycoconjugate secretion stimulated by cholinergic muscarinic, dibutyryl cAMP, α- and β-adrenergic agonists (Fig. 26). Simultaneously, the ratio of released to total intracellular content also decreased significantly after dexamethasone treatment. These findings indicate that glucocorticoid directly inhibits both basal mucous glycoprotein secretion and stimulated secretion in airway submucosal glands, and that these inhibitions are due to a reduction in the release from secretory cells, but without significant alteration in synthesis or uptake of precursors, even at the low concentration at which the inhibitory effects are physiologically relevant.

B. Fluid or Electrolyte Secretion

To understand the effect of glucocorticoids on fluid movement across airway submucosal glands, Satoh et al. (1992) examined the effects of dexamethasone on ^{22}Na$^+$-efflux from isolated feline tracheal submucosal glands. Isolated glands were loaded with ^{22}Na and the rate constant of ^{22}Na$^+$-efflux was calculated by measuring the radioactivity of each effluent sample (Sasaki et al., 1990). After treatment with 10^{-9}–10^{-5} M dexamethasone for up to 6 h, isolated glands were stimulated with methacholine (MCh). Dexamethasone treatment did not significantly alter baseline values of the rate constant. However, dexamethasone treatment produced a dose-dependent attenuation of the MCh-evoked glandular rate constant (Fig. 27).

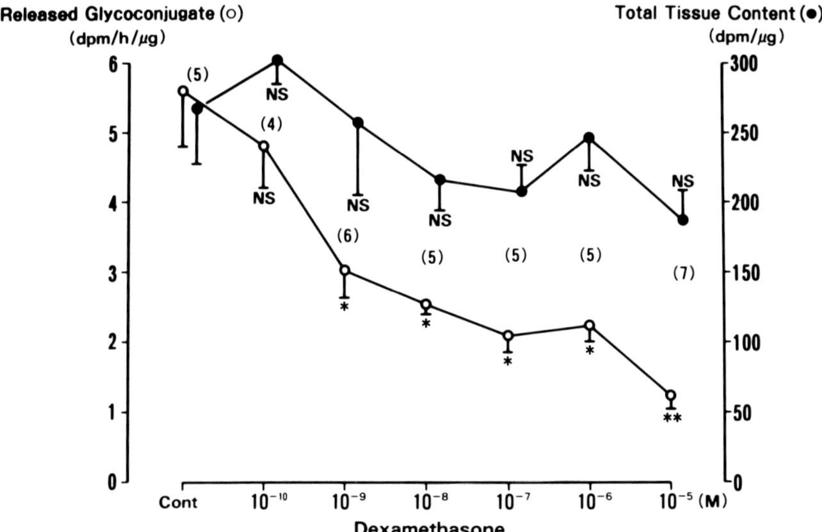

Figure 25 Radioactivity of glycoconjugates released to the medium ($\circ$, dpm h^{-1} μg^{-1} dry weight of sample) and that of gland tissue content ($\bullet$, dpm μg^{-1}) in isolated glands. Mucous glycoconjugate release was significantly reduced in a dose-dependent fashion up to 22% of control (a 78% decrease) after dexamethasone treatment, whereas gland tissue content did not change significantly after treatment. Mean $\pm$ SE; number of experiments in parentheses; cont, controls; NS, not significant; asterisk, $p < 0.05$ and double asterisk, $p < 0.01$ compared with controls. (From Shimura et al., 1990)

These findings suggest that glucocorticoid decreases the fluid secretion across the airway submucosal glands, especially when stimulated, as well as mucous glycoprotein secretion.

C.   Erythromycin

Empirical clinical experience and clinical study (Suez and Szefler, 1986) suggest that erythromycin is useful in decreasing mucous secretion in diseases associated with enhanced secretion, such as acute and chronic bronchitis and asthma. Goswami et al. (1990) have reported that erythromycin inhibits mucous glycoconjugate secretion from human airway explants and that other antibiotics, such as penicillin, ampicillin, tetracycline, and cephalosporin, do not have any effect on the secretion. However, it remains unknown whether erythromycin acts directly on submucosal gland secretion, although Marom and Goswami (1991) speculated that erythromycin has a steroid-sparing effect.

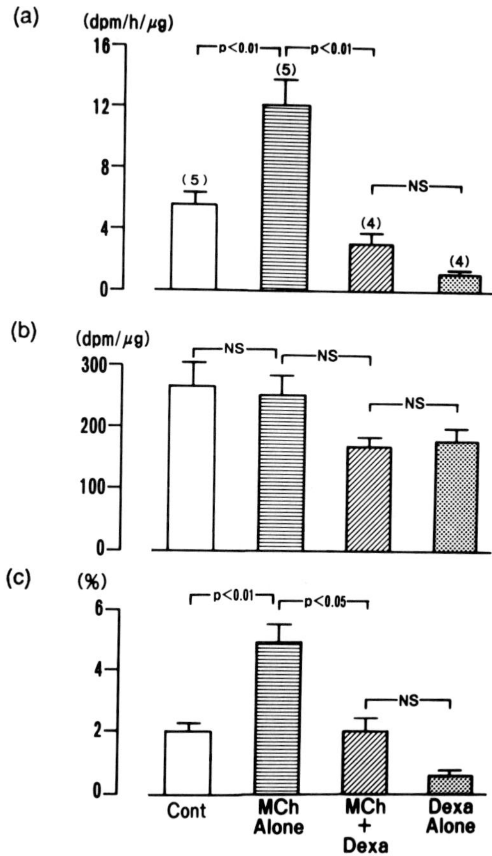

Figure 26 Effect of dexamethasone (Dexa, 10^{-5} M) treatment for 48 h on methacholine-evoked (MCh, 10^{-5} M) glycoconjugate secretion from isolated glands. (a) Glycoconjugates released to the medium (dpm $h^{-1}g^{-1}$), which was significantly reduced after Dexa treatment. (b) Radioactivity of total dissolved gland tissues, which did not significantly differ among 10^{-5} M MCh-evoked, MCh-evoked and 10^{-5} M Dexa-treated, or Dexa-treated isolated glands. (c) Ratio of released glycoconjugates to gland tissue content, which was also significantly reduced after Dexa treatment: cont, controls with no treatments. (From Shimura et al., 1990)

XVI. Epithelial Inhibition

Sasaki et al. (1989a) studied the influence of airway epithelium on mucous secretion by use of an isolated tracheal submucosal gland preparation. Mucous glycoconjugate release from submucosal glands of feline trachea was examined using [^{3}H]glucosamine as a mucous glycoprotein precursor. Isolated glands

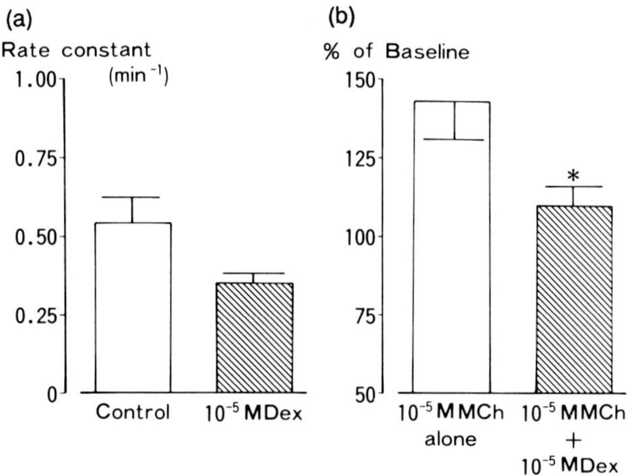

Figure 27 Effect of dexamethasone (Dex; 10^{-5} M) treatment for 6 h on ^{22}Na efflux from feline tracheal submucosal glands stimulated by 10^{-5} M methacholine (MCh). (a) Although not significant, dexamethasone reduced the baseline values of rate constants in ^{22}Na efflux. (b) When stimulated by MCh, Dex treatment produced a significant reduction in the rate constants. Mean $\pm$ SE of five experiments. (From Satoh et al., 1992)

showed significantly higher secretory responses to cholinergic, α- and β-adrenergic agonists, and dibutyryl cAMP (average 400% of control) than the tracheal explants, which contained epithelium and submucosal tissues in addition to submucosal glands. The addition of isolated epithelium depressed the secretory response of isolated glands to the same level as that of tracheal explants. Later, Masuda et al. (1990) confirmed this epithelial action using cultured epithelial cells from canine trachea. However, the supernatant from isolated epithelium failed to inhibit secretory responses to methacholine in isolated glands, suggesting that the epithelium-derived inhibitory factor to secretion may be short-lived. Leukotriene D_4 antagonist (FPL 55712), cyclooxygenase, or lipoxygenase inhibitors (indomethacin or BW 775C) caused no significant change in the inhibitory action of epithelium (Fig. 28), suggesting that the inhibition is not due to arachidonic acid metabolites. Although the precise action of this inhibitory factor on the stimulus–secretion coupling remains to be determined, we can speculate on a possible mechanism as follows: Because the factor has no effect on basal secretion, it seems unlikely that it alters synthesis or uptake of mucous precursor of the mucous glycoprotein in the secretory cells. Therefore, it is possible that the factor may inhibit secretagogue-evoked secretion by controlling the release of mucous glycoprotein. The secretory inhibitory action of the epithelium is of particular interest in the pathogenesis of hypersecretion associated with epithelial damage. Although a great deal remains to be elucidated about this potent epithelium-derived inhibi-

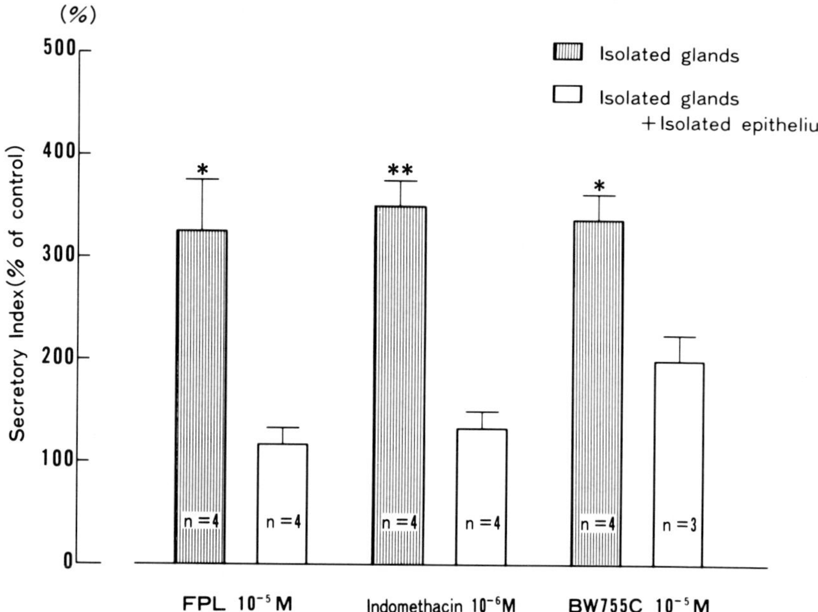

Figure 28 Effects of inhibitors (FPL 55712, BW 75c, or indomethacin) on methacholine (10^{-5} M)-induced secretion from isolated glands with (open columns) or without (closed columns) separated epithelium. Data (mean ± SE) are expressed as percentage of controls without added drugs. A significant difference between the two preparations was observed even in the presence of each inhibitor (*$p < 0.05$; **$p < 0.01$), showing that these three agents did not alter the inhibitory effect of secretion of isolated epithelium: n, number of experiments. (From Sasaki et al., 1989a)

tory factor of secretion, hypersecretion associated with epithelial dysfunction in various respiratory diseases may, in part, be due to a decreased ability of respiratory epithelial cells to generate the inhibitory signal.

XVII. Endothelin

Endothelin is a newly discovered polypeptide secreted from the vessel wall endothelium (Yanagisawa et al., 1988) that contracts airway smooth muscle (Lee et al., 1990; Turner et al., 1989). Nomura et al. (1989) have reported that an asthma patient showed bronchial-washing fluid with a raised endothelin immunoreactive level during status asthmaticus, suggesting that endothelin plays a part in bronchoconstriction in bronchial asthma. To determine the effect of endothelin on airway submucosal gland secretion, Shimura et al. (1992b) examined the effects of endothelin on both [^{3}H]glycoconjugate release and [Ca^{2+}]$_i$ in submucosal glands isolated from feline trachea. Endothelin-1 produced a significant dose-dependent increase in glycoconjugate release from the isolated glands, reaching a response of 161% of the control at 10^{-6} M (Fig. 29). Atropine, propranolol, phentolamine, or indomethacin produced no significant alterations in the endothelin-1-evoked glycoconjugate secretion from the isolated glands. In contrast, in tracheal explants that contained epithelium, endothelin-1 produced a significant dose-dependent reduction in the glycoconjugate secretion, reaching a response of 59% of the control at 10^{-6} M (Fig. 30). In the presence of cultured epithelial cells, endothelin-1 also produced a significant reduction in the glycoconjugate secretion from isolated glands. In isolated glands, endothelin-1 produced a sustained increase in the [Ca^{2+}]$_i$, which was abolished by the removal of Ca^{2+} from the medium or by the presence of cultured epithelial cells. Pretreatment with indomethacin failed to alter the epithelial inhibitory action evoked by endothelin-1 in both the glycoconju-

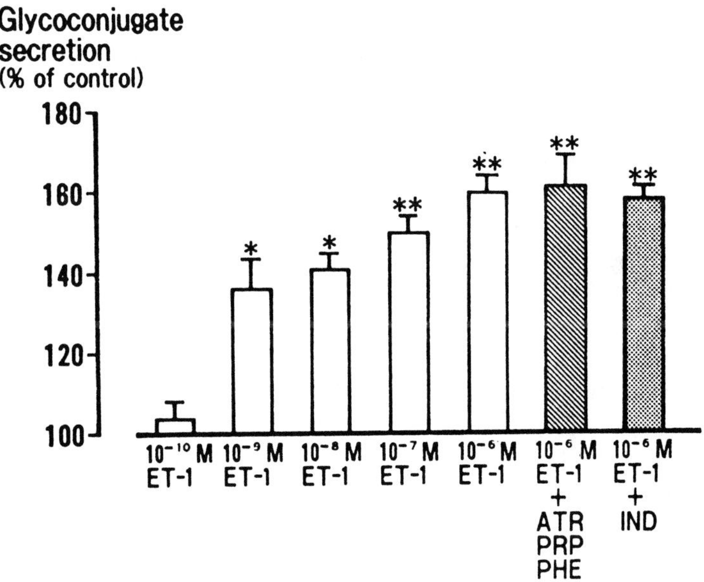

Figure 29 Endothelin-1 (ET-1)-induced glycoconjugate secretion from feline tracheal isolated glands. ET-1 produced a dose-dependent increase in glycoconjugate secretion, which was not altered by treatment with three antagonists or with indomethacin: ATR, 10^{-6} M atropine; PRP, 10^{-5} M propranolol; PHE, 10^{-5} M phentolamine, IND, 10^{-5} M indomethacin. Means ± SE of five to ten experiments. asterisk, $p < 0.05$; double asterisk, $p < 0.001$, compared with controls. (From Shimura et al., 1992b)

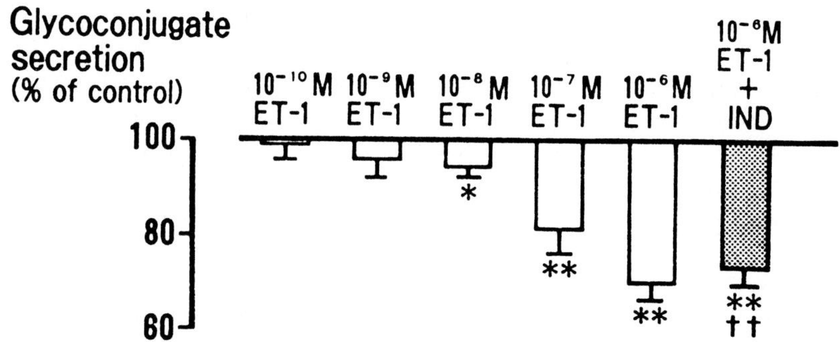

Figure 30   Effect of endothelin-1 (ET-1) on glycoconjugate secretion from feline isolated glands in presence of cultured epithelial cells. ET-1 produced a dose-dependent reduction in glycoconjugate secretion from isolated glands with culture epithelial cells, and reduction was not altered even after treatment with indomethacin. Means ± SE of four to eight experiments: double daggers, $p < 0.01$ compared with isolated glands alone stimulated by ET-1 (10^{-6} M). (From Shimura et al., 1992b)

gate secretion and the $[Ca^{2+}]_i$ in isolated glands. Endothelin-2 and endothelin-3 failed to produce significant alterations in the glycoconjugate secretion or $[Ca^{2+}]_i$. These findings indicate that endothelin-1 induces mucous glycoprotein secretion by a Ca^{2+} influx and that it possibly augments the epithelial action inhibitory to the mucous glycoprotein secretion from airway submucosal glands. Such an action of endothelin has also been observed in an in vivo experiment. Recently, Yurdakos and Webber (1991) have examined the effect of endothelin-1 on mucous and lyzozyme (a marker of submucosal gland secretion) secretion in whole ferret trachea. They found that endothelin-1 produced dose-dependent reductions in methacholine- and phenylephrine-induced mucous and lysozyme secretions.

XVIII. Future Investigations

Many physiological and functional aspects of airway submucosal gland secretion remain to be explored; the main areas are as follows:

1. Site-related physiological differences (tracheal vs bronchial or central vs peripheral) in submucosal gland secretion have not yet been found, despite some morphological differences.
2. Species differences have not yet been clearly defined.

3. The influences of surrounding tissue and cells, including cartilage, connective tissues, endothelium, epithelium, and migratory cells (lymphocytes, neutrophils, eosinophils, macrophages, basophils, and mast cells) remain to be elucidated.

4. Mechanical effects on the secretion: Mechanical strain causes surfactant secretion from alveolar type II cells (Wirtz and Dobbs, 1990) and also mucin from airway goblet cells (Kim and Brody, 1992). Similar effects have not been reported in spite of the fact that there are changes in airway caliber owing to respiration and smooth-muscle contraction, and also glandular contraction through the activation of myoepithelial cells.

5. Function of ductal cells: There have been no studies concerning the function of the ductal portion of airway submucosal glands because of the lack of a suitable experimental model.

6. Identification of each receptor on secretory cells by molecular biological techniques: This will provide an answer to whether each secretory response is receptor-operated.

7. Cellular mechanisms both in ion transport and in degranulation: What differences are there from other exocrine gland cells? Our present knowledge is mainly based on the findings from other exocrine glands.

8. Relationships of the three morphologically different acinar cells (mucous, serous, and myoepithelial cells) and the secretory responses (mucin, glycoconjugate, and fluid secretion).

9. Development of specific markers of airway submucosal gland secretion: This will enable us to estimate the functions not only in in vivo experimental conditions, but also clinically in the airways of diseased lungs.

10. Direct evidence for the role of airway submucosal glands in the defensive mechanisms of airways: Although lysozyme, lactoferrin, and IgA are known to be secreted from airway submucosal glands, there is little knowledge concerning the mechanisms of secretion and the significance of these substances.

Acknowledgments

We thank Ms. Kumiko Shibuya for typing and Mr. Brent Bell for reading the manuscript. This study was in part supported by scientific grants from the Ministry of Education, Science, and Culture of Japan (59570321, 60570342, 62570340, 21571422, and 04554249).

References

Al-Bazzaz, F. J., and Cheng, E. (1979). Effect of catecholamines on ion transport in dog tracheal epithelium. *J. Appl. Physiol.* 47: 397–403.

Alder, K. B., Schwartz, J. E., Anderson, W. H., and Welton, A. F. (1987). Platelet activating factor stimulates secretion of mucin by explants of rodent airways in organ culture. *Exp. Lung. Res.* 13: 25–43.

Ayala, L. E., and Ahmed, T. (1989). Is there loss of a protective muscarinic receptor mechanism in asthma? *Chest* 96: 1285–1291.

Baluk, P., Fujiwara, T., and Matsuda, S. (1985). The fine structure of the ganglia of the guinea-pig trachea. *Cell Tissue Res.* 239: 51–60.

Baker, A. P., Hillegass, L. M., Holden, D. A., and Smith, W. J. (1977). Effect of kallidin, substance P and other basic polypeptides on the production of respiratory macromolecules. *Am. Rev. Respir. Dis.* 115: 811–817.

Baraniuk, J. N., Lundgren, J. D., Okayama, M., Goff, J., Mullol, J., Merida, M., Shelhamer, J. H., and Kaliner, M. A. (1991). Substance P and neurokinin A in human nasal mucosa. *Am. J. Respir. Cell Mol. Biol.* 4: 228–236.

Barnes, P. J. (1989). Muscarinic receptor subtypes: Implications for lung disease. *Thorax* 44: 161–167.

Barnes, P. J., and Basbaum, C. B. (1983). Mapping of adrenergic receptors in the trachea by autoradiography. *Exp. Lung Res.* 5: 183–192.

Barnes, P. J., Basbaum, C. B., Nadel, J. A., and Roberts, J. M. (1982). Localization of β-adrenoreceptors in mammalian lung by light microscopic autoradiography. *Nature* 299: 444–447.

Barnes, P. J., Basbaum, C. B., Nadel, J. A., and Roberts, J. M. (1983a). Pulmonary α-adrenoceptors: Autoradiographic localization using [^{3}H]-prazosin. *Eur. J. Pharmacol.* 88: 57–62.

Barnes, P. J., Nadel, J. A., Roberts, J. M., and Basbaum, C. B. (1983b). Muscarinic receptors in lung and trachea: Autoradiographic localization using [^{3}H]quinuclidinyl benzilate. *Eur. J. Pharmacol.* 86: 103–106.

Basbaum, C. B., Ueki, I., Brezina, L., and Nadel, J. A. (1981). Tracheal submucosal gland serous cells stimulated in vitro with adrenergic and cholinergic agonists. A morphometric study. *Cell Tissue Res.* 220: 481–489.

Basbaum, C. B., Grillo, M. A., and Widdicombe, J. H. (1984a). Muscarinic receptors: Evidence for a nonuniform distribution in tracheal smooth muscle and exocrine glands. *J. Neurosci.* 4: 508–520.

Basbaum, C. B., Mann, J. K., Chow, A. W., and Finkbeiner, W. E. (1984b). Monoclonal antibodies as probes for unique antigens in secretory cells of mixed exocrine organs. *Proc. Natl. Acad. Sci. USA* 81: 4419–4423.

Basbaum, C. B., Chow, A., Macher, B. A., Finkebeiner, W. E., Veissiere, D., and Foresberg, L. S. (1986). Tracheal carbohydrate antigens identified by monoclonal antibodies. *Arch. Biochem. Biophys.* 249: 363–373.

Bensch, K. G., Gordon, G. B., and Miller, L. R. (1965). Studies on the bronchial counterpart of the Kulschitsky (argentaffin) cell and innervation of bronchial gland. *J. Ultrastruct. Res.* 12: 558–686.

Benveniste, J., Henson, P. M., and Cochrane, C. G. (1972). Leukocyte-dependent histamine release from rabbit platelets; role of IgE, basophils and platelet-activating factor. *J. Exp. Med.* 136: 1356–1377.

Boat, T. F., and Cheng, P. W. (1980). Biochemistry of airway secretion. *Fed. Proc.* 39: 3067–3074.

Bonner, T. I., Buckley, N. J., Young, A. C., and Brann, M. R. (1987). Identification of a family of muscarinic acetylcholine receptor genes. *Science* 236: 600–605.

Borson, D. B., Chinn, R. A., Davis, B., and Nadel, J. A. (1980). Adrenergic and cholinergic nerves mediate fluid secretion from tracheal glands of ferrets. *J. Appl. Physiol.* 49: 1027–1031.

Borson, D. B., Charlin, M., Gold, B. D., and Nadel, J. A. (1984). Neural regulation of $^{35}SO_4$-macromolecule secretion from tracheal glands of ferrets. *J. Appl. Physiol.* 57: 457–466.

Borson, D. B., Corrales, R., Varsano, S., Gold, M., Viro, N., Caughey, G., Ramachandran, J., and Nadel, J. A. (1987). Enkephalinase inhibitors potentiate substance-P induced secretion of $^{35}SO_4$-macromolecules from ferret trachea. *Exp. Lung Res.* 12: 21–36.

Bowes, D., and Corrin, B. (1977). Ultrastructural immunocytochemical localization of lysozyme in human bronchial glands. *Thorax* 32: 163–170.

Bowes, D., Clark, A. E., and Corrin, B. (1981). Ultrastructural localization of lactoferrin and glycoprotein in human bronchial gland. *Thorax* 36: 108–115.

Brown, J. H., Buxton, I. L., and Brunton, L. L. (1985a). The effects of substance P and related peptide on α-amylase release from rat parotid gland tissue. *Br. J. Pharmacol.* 73: 517–523.

Brown, L. A. S., Pasquale, S. M., and Longmore, W. J. (1985b). Role of microtubules in surfactant secretion. *J. Appl. Physiol.* 58: 1866–1873.

Burg, M., Grantham, M., Abramow, J., and Orloff, J. (1966). Preparation and study of fragments of single rabbit nephrons. *Am. J. Physiol.* 210: 1293–1298.

Busson-Mabillot, S., Chambaut-Gúerin, A.-M., Ovtracht, L., Muller, P., and Rossignol, B. (1982). Microtubules in portion secretion in rat lacrimal glands: Localization of short-term effects of colchicine on the secretory process. *J. Cell Biol.* 95: 105–117.

Carstairs, J. R., and Barnes, P. J. (1986a). Autoradiographic mapping of substance P receptors in lung. *Eur. J. Pharmacol.* 127: 295–296.

Carstairs, J. R., and Barnes, P. J. (1986b). Visualization of vasoactive intestinal peptide receptors in human and guinea pig lung. *J. Pharmacol. Exp. Ther.* 239: 249–255.

Carstairs, J. R., Nimmo, A. J., and Barnes, P. J. (1985). Autoradiographic visualization of beta-adrenoceptor subtypes in human lung. *Am. Rev. Respir. Dis.* 132: 541–547.

Case, R. M. (1973). Review. Cellular mechanisms controlling pancreatic exocrine secretion. *Acta Hepato-Gastroenterol.* 20: 435–444.

Castle, J. D. (1990). Sorting and secretory pathways in exocrine cells. *Am. J. Respir. Cell Mol. Biol.* 2: 119–126.

Chakrin, L. W., Baker, A. P., Spicer, S. S., Wardell, J. R., DeSanctis, N., Jr., and Dries, C. (1972). Synthesis and secretion of macromolecules by canine trachea. *Am. Rev. Respir. Dis.* 105: 368–381.

Chakrin, L. W., Baker, A. P., Christian, P., and Wardell, J. R. (1973). Effect of cholinergic stimulation on the release of macromolecules by canine trachea in vitro. *Am. Rev. Respir. Dis.* 108: 69–76.

Cheng, P.-W., Sherman, J. M., Boat, T. F., and Bruce, M. (1981). Quantification of radiolabeled mucus glycoproteins secreted by tracheal explants. *Anal. Biochem.* 117: 301–306.

Coles, S. J., and Reid, L. (1981). Inhibition of glycoconjugate secretion by colchicine and cytochalasin B. An in vitro study of human airway. *Cell Tissue Res.* 214: 107–118.

Coles, S. J., Said, S. I., and Reid, L. M. (1981). Inhibition by vasoactive intestinal peptide of glycoconjugate and lysozyme secretion by human airway in vitro. *Am. Rev. Respir. Dis.* 124: 531–537.

Coles, S. J., Neil, K. H., and Reid, L. N. (1984). Potent stimulation of glycoprotein secretion in canine trachea by substance P. *J. Appl. Physiol.* 7: 1323–1327.

Collins, F. S. (1992). Cystic fibrosis: Molecular biology and therapeutic implications. *Science.* 256: 774–779.

Corrales, R. J., Nadel, J. A., and Widdicombe, J H. (1984). Source of the fluid component of secretions from tracheal submucosal glands in cats. *J. Appl. Physiol.* 56: 1076–1082.

Culp, D. J., and Martin, M. G. (1986). Characterization of muscarinic cholinergic receptors in cat tracheal gland cells. *J. Appl. Physiol.* 61: 1375–1382.

Culp, D. J., Penny, D. P., and Martin, M. G. (1983). A technique for the isolation of submucosal gland cells from cat trachea. *J. Appl. Physiol.* 55: 1035–1041.

Culp, D. J., McBride, R. K., Graham, L. A., and Martin, M. G. (1990). α-Adrenergic regulation of secretion by tracheal glands. *Am. J. Physiol.* 259: L198–L205.

Curran, P. F., and Solomon, A. K. (1957). Ion and water fluxes in the ileum of rats. *J. Gen. Physiol.* 41: 143–168.

Davis, B., and Nadel, J. A. (1980). New methods to investigate the control of mucus secretion and ion transport in airways. *Environ. Health Perspect.* 35: 121–130.

Davis, B., and Tseng, H. C. (1991). Neural regulation of lyzosome secretion from tracheal submucosal glands of ferrets in vivo. *J. Appl. Physiol.* 71: 939–944.

Davis, B., Marin, M. G., Fisher, S., Graf, P., Widdicombe, J. G., and Nadel, J. A. (1976). A new method for study of canine mucous gland secretion in vivo: Cholinergic regulation. *Am. Rev. Respir. Dis.* 113: 257.

Davis, B., Chinn, R., Gold, J., Popovac, D., Widdicombe, J. G., and Nadel, J. A. (1982a). Hypoxemia reflexly increases secretion from tracheal submucosal glands in dogs. *J. Appl. Physiol.* 52: 1416–1419.

Davis, B., Roberts, A. M., Coleridge, H. M., and Coleridge, J. C. G. (1982b). Reflex tracheal gland secretion evoked by stimulation of bronchial C-fibers in dogs. *J. Appl. Physiol.* 53: 985–991.

de Water, R., Willens, L. N. A., Van Muijen, G. N. P., Franken, C., Fransen, J. A. M., Dijkman, J. H., and Kramps, J. A. (1986). Ultrastructural localization of bronchial antileukoprotease in central and peripheral human airways by a gold-labeling technique using monoclonal antibodies. *Am. Rev. Respir. Dis.* 133: 882–890.

Dey, R. D., Shannon, W. A., Jr., Said, S. I. (1981). Localization of VIP-immunoreactive nerves in airways and pulmonary vessels of dogs, cats, and human subjects. *Cell Tissue Res.* 220: 213–238.

Diamond, J. M., and Bossert, W. H. (1967). Standing-gradient osmotic flow. A mechanism for coupling of water and solute transport in epithelia. *J. Gen. Physiol.* 50: 2061–2083.

Dreckhahn, D., Gröschel-Stewart, U., and Unsicker, K. (1977). Immunofluorescence microscopic demonstration of myocin and actin in salivary glands and exocrine pancreas of the rat. *Cell Tissue Res.* 183: 273–279.

Dwyer, T. M., Szebeni, A., Diveki, K., and Farley, J. M. (1992). Transient cholinergic glycoconjugate secretion from swine tracheal submucosal gland cells. *Am. J. Physiol.* 262: L418–L426.

Eglan, R. M., and Whiting, R. L. (1986). Muscarinic receptor subtypes: A critique for the current classification and a proposal for a working nomenclature. *J. Auton. Pharmacol.* 5: 323–346.

Finkbeiner, W. R., Nadel, J. A., and Basbaum, C. B. (1986). Establishment and characterization of cell line derived from bovine tracheal glands. *In Vitro Cell. Dev. Biol.* 22: 561–567.

Florey, H., Carleton, H. M., and Wells, A. Q. (1932). Mucus secretion in the trachea. *Br. J. Exp. Pathol.* 13: 269–284.

Frizzel, R. A., Field, A. N., and Schultz, S. G. (1979). Sodium-coupled chloride transport by epithelial tissues. *Am. J. Physiol.* 236: F1–F8.

Frossard, N., and Barnes, P. J. (1987). μ-Opioid receptors modulate non-cholinergic constrictor nerves in guinea-pig airways. *Eur. J. Pharmacol.* 141: 519–522.

Fung, D. C. K., Allenby, M. I., and Richardson, P. S. (1992). NANC nerve pathways controlling mucus glycoconjugate secretion into feline trachea. *J. Appl. Physiol.* 73: 625–630.

Gallagher, J. T., Kent, P. W., Passatore, M., Phipps, R. J., and Richardson, P. S. (1975). The composition of tracheal mucus and the nervous control of its secretion in the cat. *Proc. R. Soc. Lond. B* 192: 49–76.

Gashi, A. A., Borson, D. B., Finkbeiner, W. E., Nadel, J. A., and Basbaum, C. B. (1986). Neuropeptides degranulate serous cells of ferret tracheal glands. *Am. J. Physiol.* 251: C223–C229.

Gater, P. R., Alabaster, V. A., and Piper, I. (1989). A study of the muscarinic receptor subtype mediating mucus secretion in the cat trachea in vitro. *Pulmonary Pharmacol.* 2: 87–92.

German, V. F., Ueki, I. F., and Nadel, J. A. (1982a). Micropipette measurement of airway submucosal gland secretion: Laryngeal reflex. *Am. Rev. Respir. Dis.* 122: 413–416.

German, V. F., Corrales, R., Ueki, I. F., and Nadel, J. A. (1982b). Reflex stimulation of tracheal mucus gland secretion by gastric irritation in cats. *J. Appl. Physiol.* 52: 1153–1155.

Gierschik, P., and Jakobs, K. H. (1988). Mechanisms for inhibition of adenylate cyclase by α-2 adrenergic receptors. In *The alpha-2 Adrenergic Receptors.* Edited by L. E. Limbird. Clifton, NJ, Humana Press, pp. 75–114.

Goco, R. V., Kress, M. B., and Brantigan, O. C. (1963). Comparison of mucus glands in the tracheobronchial tree of man and animal. *Ann. N.Y. Acad. Sci.* 106: 555–571.

Goodman, M. R., Link, D. W., Brown, W. R., and Nakane, P. K. (1981). Ultrastructural evidence of transport of secretory IGA across bronchial epithelium. *Am. Rev. Respir. Dis.* 123: 115–119.

Goswami, S. K., Kivity, S., and Marom, Z. (1990). Erythromycin inhibits respiratory glycoconjugate secretion from human airways in vitro. *Am. Rev. Respir. Dis.* 141: 72–78.

Gunther, G. R. (1981). Effect of 12-*O*-teradecanoyl-phorbol-13-acetate on Ca^{2+} efflux and protein discharge in pancreatic acini. *J. Biol. Chem.* 256: 12040–12045.

Hahn, H.-L., Purnama, I., Lang, M., and Sannuwald, U. (1986). Effects of platelet activating factor on tracheal mucus secretion, on airway mechanics and on circulating blood cells in live ferrets. *Eur. J. Respir. Dis.* 69(Suppl. 146): 277–284.

Hall, I. P. (1992). Agonist-induced inositol phosphate response in bovine airway submucosal glands. *Am. J. Physiol.* 262: L257–L262.

Hartmann, J. F., Hutchison, C. F., and Jewell, M. E. (1984). Pig bronchial mucous membrane: A model system for assessing respiratory mucus release in vitro. *Exp. Lung Res.* 6: 59–70.

Haxihiu, M. A., Cherniack, N. A., and Strohl, K. P. (1991a). Reflex responses of laryngeal and pharyngeal submucosal glands in dogs. *J. Appl. Physiol.* 71: 1669–1673.

Haxihiu, M. A., Van Lunteren, E., and Cherniack, N. S. (1991b). Influence of ventrolateral surface of medulla on tracheal gland secretion. *J. Appl. Physiol.* 71: 1663–1668.

Haxihiu, M. A., Van Lunteren, E., and Cherniack, N. S. (1991c). Central effects of tachykinin peptide on tracheal secretion. *Respir. Physiol.* 86: 405–414.

Hayashi, M., Sornberger, G. C., and Huber, G. L. (1979). Morphometric analyses of tracheal gland secretion and hypertrophy in male and female rats after experimental exposure to tobacco smoke. *Am. Rev. Respir. Dis.* 119: 67–73.

Ishihara, H., Shimura, S., Sato, M., Masuda, T., Ishide, N., Sasaki, H., Sasaki, T., and Takishima, T. (1990). Intracellular calcium concentration of acinar cells in feline tracheal submucosal glands. *Am. J. Physiol.* 259: L345–350.

Ishihara, H., Shimura, S., Satoh, M., Masuda, T., Nonaka, H., Kase, H., Sasaki, T., Sasaki, H., Takishima, T., and Tamura, K. (1992). Muscarinic receptor subtypes in feline tracheal submucosal gland secretion. *Am. J. Physiol.* 259: L345–350.

Jarnigan, F., Davis, J. D., Bromberg, P. A., Gatzy, J. A., and Boucher, R. C. (1983). Bioelectric properties and ion transport of excised rabbit trachea. *J. Appl. Physiol.* 55: 1884–1892.

Jeffery, P. K. (1983). Morphologic features of airway surface epithelial cells and glands. *Am. Rev. Respir. Dis.* 128: S14–S20.

Johansson, O., and Lundberg, L. M. (1981). Ultrastructural localization of VIP-like immunoreactivity in large dense-core vesicles of cholinergic type nerve terminals in cat exocrine glands. *Neuroscience* 6: 847–862.

Johnson, H. G., Chinn, R. A., Chow, A. W., Bach, M. K., and Nadel, J. A. (1983a). Leukotrience-C_4 enhances mucus production from submucosal glands in canine trachea in vivo. *Int. J. Immunopharmacol.* 5: 391–396.

Johnson, H. G., McNee, M., Johnson, M. A., and Miller, M. D. (1983b). Leukotriene C_4 and dimethylphenylpiperazinium-induced responses in canine airway tracheal muscle contraction and fluid secretion. *Int. Archs. Allergy Appl. Immunol.* 71: 214–218.

Johnson, H. G., McNee, M. L., and Sun, F. F. (1985). 15-Hydroxyeixosatetraenoic acid is a potent inflammatory mediator and agonist of canine tracheal mucus secretion. *Am. Rev. Respir. Dis.* 131: 917–922.

Jones, R., and Reid, L. (1973). The effect of pH on alcian blue of epithelial glycoproteins. II. Human bronchial submucosal glands. *Histochem. J.* 5: 19–27.

Kaliner, K. A., Shelhamer, J. H., Borson, D. V., Nadel, J. A., Patow, C. A., and Marom, Z.

(1988). Respiratory mucus. In *The Airways; Neural Control in Health and Disease*. Edited by A. Kaliner and P. T. Barnes. New York, Marcel Dekker.

Kasai, H., and Augustine, G. J. (1990). Cytosolic Ca^{2+} gradients triggering unidirectional fluid secretion from exocrine pancreas. *Nature* 348: 735–738.

Keltz, T. N., Straus, E., and Yalow, R. S. (1980). Degradation of vasoactive intestinal polypeptide by tissue homogenates. *Biochem. Biophys. Res. Commun.* 92: 669–672.

Kim, K. C., and Brody, J. S. (1992). Mechanical strain causes release of mucins from airway epithelial cells. *Am. Rev. Respir. Dis.* 145: A617.

Kim, K. C., Nassiri, J., and Brody, J. S. (1989). Mechanisms of airway goblet cell mucin release: Studies with cultured tracheal surface epithelial cells. *Am. J. Respir. Cell Mol. Biol.* 1: 137–143.

Kollerstrom, M., Lord, P. W., and Whimster, W. F. (1977). Distribution of acid mucus in the bronchial mucous glands. *Thorax* 32: 160–162.

Lamb, D., and Reid, L. (1970). Histochemical and autoradiographic investigation of the serous cells of the human bronchial glands. *J. Pathol.* 100: 127–138.

Lamb, D., and Reid, L. (1972). Quantitative distribution of various types of acid glycoprotein in mucous cells of human bronchi. *Histochem. J.* 4: 91–102.

Lauweryns, J. M., and Ranst, L. V. (1987). Calcitonin gene-related peptide immunoreactivity in rat lung: Light and electron microscopy. *Thorax* 42: 183–189.

Lazarus, S. C., Basbaum, C. B., and Gold, W. M. (1984). Prostaglandins and intracellular cyclic AMP in respiratory secretory cells. *Am. Rev. Respir. Dis.* 130: 262–266.

Lazarus, S. C., Basbaum, C. B., Barnes, P. J., and Gold, W. M. (1986). cAMP immunocytochemistry provides evidence for functional VIP receptors in trachea. *Am. J. Physiol.* 251: C115–C119.

Lee, H.-K., Leikauf, G. D., and Sperelaiks, N. (1990). Electromechanical effects of endothelin on ferret bronchial and tracheal smooth muscle. *J. Appl. Physiol.* 68: 417–420.

Leigh, M. W., Gambling, T. M., Carson, J. L., Collier, A. M., Wood, R. E., and Boat, F. (1986a). Postnatal development of tracheal surface epithelium and submucosal glands in the ferret. *Exp. Lung Res.* 10: 153–169.

Leigh, M. W., Cheng, P.-W., Carson, J. L., and Boat, T. F. (1986b). Developmental changes in glycoconjugate secretion by ferret trachea. *Am. Rev. Respir. Dis.* 134: 784–790.

Leikauf, G. D., Ueki, I. F., and Nadel, J. A. (1984). Autonomic regulation of viscoelasticity of cat tracheal gland secretions. *J. Appl. Physiol.* 56: 426–430.

Leys, K., Morice, A. H., Madonna, O., and Sever, P. S. (1986). Autoradiographic localization of VIP receptors in human lung. *FEBS Lett.* 199: 198–202.

Liedtke, C. M., Rudolph, S. A., and Boat, T. F. (1983). β-Adrenergic modulation of mucin secretion in cat trachea. *Am. J. Physiol.* 244: C391–C398.

Lin, H., Carlson, D. M., St. George, J. A., Plopper, C. G., and Wu, R. (1989). An ELISA method for the quantification of tracheal mucins from human and nonhuman primates. *Am. J. Respir. Cell Mol. Biol.* 1: 41–48.

Lopez-Vidriero, M. T., Das, I., Smith, A. P., Picot, R., and Reid, L. (1977). Bronchial secretion from normal airways after inhalation of prostaglandin $F_{2\alpha}$, acetylcholine, histamine, and citric acid. *Thorax* 32: 734–739

Lundberg, J. M., Hökfelt, T., Schultzgerg, M., Uvanas-Wallenstein, K., Köhler, C., and

Said, S. I. (1979). Occurrence of vasoactive intestinal peptide (VIP)-like immuno-reactivity in certain cholinergic neurons of the cat: Evidence from combined immunohistochemistry and acetylcholinersterase staining. *Neuroscience* 4: 1539–1559.

Lundberg, J. M., Hedlund, B., and Bartfai, T. (1982). Vasoactive intestinal polypeptide enhances muscarinic ligand binding in cat submandibular salivary gland. *Nature* 295: 147–149.

Lundberg, J. M., Hökfelt, T., Martling, C.-R., Saria, A., and Cuello, C. (1984). Substance P-immunoreactive sensory nerves in the lower respiratory tract of various mammals including man. *Cell Tissue Res.* 235: 251–261.

Lundgren, J. D. Hirata, F., Marom, Z., Logun, C., Steel, L., Kaliner, M., and Shelhamer, J. (1985). Dexamethasone inhibits respiratory glycoconjugate secretion from feline airways in vitro by the induction of lipocortion (lipomodulin) synthesis. *Am. Rev. Respir. Dis.* 137: 353–357.

Lüttgan, H. C., and Oetliker, H. (1968). The action of caffeine on the activation of the contractile mechanism in striated muscle fibers. *J. Physiol. (Lond.)* 194: 51–57.

McKinney, J. S., and Rubin, R. P. (1988). Enhancement of cyclic AMP modulated salivary amylase secretion by protein kinase C activators. *Biochem. Pharmacol.* 37: 4433–4438.

Madison, J. M., Basbaum, C. B., Brown, J. K., and Finkbeiner, W. E. (1989). Characterization of β-adrenergic receptors in cultured bovine tracheal glands. *Am. J. Physiol.* 256: C310–C314.

Mak, J. C. W., and Barnes, P. J. (1990). Autoradiographic visualization of muscarinic receptor subtypes in human and guinea pig lung. *Am. Rev. Respir. Dis.* 141: 1559–1568.

Marin, M. G., Davis, B., and Nadel, J. A. (1976). Effect of acetylcholine on Cl^- and Na^+ fluxes across dog tracheal epithelium in vitro. *Am. J. Physiol.* 231: 1546–1549.

Maron, Z. M., and Goswami, S. K. (1991). Respiratory mucus hypersecretion (bronchor-rhea): A case discussion—possible mechanisms and treatment. *J. Allergy Clin. Immunol.* 87: 1050–1055.

Marom, Z. M., Shelhamer, J. H., and Kaliner, M. (1981). Effects of arachidonic acid, monohyroxyeicosatetraenoic acid and prostaglandins on the release of mucus glyco-proteins from human airways in vitro. *J. Clin. Invest.* 67: 1695–1702.

Marom, Z., Shelhamer, J. H., Bach, M. K., Morton, D. R., and Kaliner, M. (1982). Slow-reacting substances, leukotriens C_4 and D_4 increase the release of mucus from human airways in vitro. *Am. Rev. Respir. Dis.* 126: 499–451.

Marom, Z., Shelhamer, J. H., Alling, D., and Kaliner, M. (1984). The effects of cortico-steroids on mucus glycoprotein secretion from human airways in vitro. *Am. Rev. Respir. Dis.* 129: 62–65.

Maruyama, N., Ruggles, B. T., Gapstur, S. M., Werness, J. L., and Dousa, T. P. (1985). Evidence for beta adrenoceptors in proximal tubules. Isoproterenol-sensitive adeny-late cyclase in pars of canine nephrone. *J. Clin. Invest.* 76: 474–481.

Mason, D. Y., and Taylor, C. R. (1975). The distribution of muramidase (lysozyme) in human tissue. *J. Clin. Pathol.* 28: 124–132.

Masuda, T., Shimura, S., Ishihara, H., Sato, M., Sasaki, T., Andoh, Y., Sasaki, H., and

Takishima, T. (1990). Cultured epithelial cells inhibit mucus glycoprotein secretion from isolated submucosal glands. *Am. Rev. Respir. Dis.* 141: A911.

Meyrick, B., and Reid, L. (1970). Ultrastructure of cells in the human bronchial submucosal glands. *J. Anat.* 107: 281–299.

Meyrick, B., and Reid, L. (1975). In vitro incorporation of [³H]-threonine and [³H]-glucose by the mucous and serous cells of the human bronchial submucosal glands. *J. Cell Biol.* 67: 320–344.

Meyrick, B., Sturges, J. M., and Reid, L. (1969). A reconstruction of the duct system and secretory tubules of the human bronchial submucosal gland. *Thorax* 24: 729–736.

Minette, P. A., and Barnes, P. J. (1988). Prejunctional inhibitory muscarinic receptors on cholinergic nerves in human and guinea pig airways. *J. Appl. Physiol.* 64: 2532–2537.

Mooren, H. W. D., Meyer, C. J. L. M., Kramps, J. A., Franken, C., and Dijkman, J. H. (1982). Ultrastructural localization of the low molecular weight protease inhibitor in human bronchial glands. *J. Histochem. Cytochem.* 30: 1130–1134.

Murlas, C., Nadel, J. A., and Basbaum, C. B. (1980). A morphometric analysis of the autonomic innervation of cat tracheal glands. *J. Auton, Nerv. Syst.* 2: 23–37.

Nadel, J. A. (1991). Role of mast cell and neutrophil proteases in airway secretion. *Am. Rev. Respir. Dis.* 144: S48–S51.

Nadel, J. A., Widdicombe, J. H., and Peatfield, A. C. (1985). Regulation of airway secretions, ion transport, and water movement. In *Handbook of Physiology*, Sec. 3, *The Respiratory System*. Vol. 1. Edited by A. P. Fishman, and A. B. Fisher. Washington, D. C., American Physiological Society, pp. 416–445.

Nishizuka, Y. (1984). The role of protein kinase C in cell surface signal transduction and tumor-promotion. *Nature* 308: 693–698.

Nomura, A., Uchida, Y., Kameyama, M., Saotome, M., Oki, K., and Hasegawa, S. (1989). Endothelin and bronchial asthma. *Lancet* 2: 747–748.

Pandol, S. T., and Schoeffield, M. S. (1986). 1, 2-Diacylglycerol, protein kinase C, and pancreatic enzyme secretion. *J. Biol. Chem.* 261: 4438–4444.

Paul, A., Picard, J., Mergey, M., Veisiére, D., Finkbeiner, W. E., and Basbaum, C. B. (1988). Glycoconjugates secreted by bovine tracheal serous cells in culture. *Arch. Biochem. Biophys.* 200: 75–84.

Paul, A., Mergey, M., Veissiére, D., Hermelin, B., Cherqui, G., Picard, J., and Basbaum, C. B. (1991). Regulation of secretion in cultured tracheal serous cells by protein kinases A and C. *Am. J. Physiol.* 261: L172–L177.

Peatfield, A. C., and Richardson, P. S. (1982). The control of mucin secretion into the lumen of the cat trachea by α- and β- adrenoceptors, and their relative involvement during sympathetic nerve stimulation. *Eur. J. Pharmacol.* 81: 617–626.

Peatfield, A. C., and Richardson, P. S. (1983). Evidence for non-cholinergic, non-adrenergic nervous control of mucus secretion into the cat trachea. *J. Physiol. (Lond.)* 342: 335–345.

Peatfield, A. C., Piper, P. J., and Richardson, P. S. (1982). The effect of leukotriene C_4 on mucin release into the cat trachea in vivo and in vitro. *Br. J. Pharmacol.* 77: 391–393.

Peatfield, A. C., Barnes, P. J., Bracher, C., Nadel, J. A., and Davis, B. (1983). Vasoactive intestinal peptide stimulates tracheal submucosal gland secretion in ferret. *Am. Rev. Respir. Dis.* 128: 89–93.

Phipps, R. J., and Richardson, P. S. (1976). The effects of irritation at various levels of the airway upon tracheal mucus secretion in the cat. *J. Physiol. (Lond.)* 261: 363–581.

Phipps, R. J., Nadel, J. A., and Davis, B. (1980). Effect of α-adrenergic stimulation on mucus secretion and on ion transport in cat trachea in vitro. *Am. Rev. Respir. Dis.* 121: 359–365.

Phipps, R. J., Denas, S. M., Sielczak, M. W., and Wanner, A. (1986). Effect of 0.5 ppm ozone on glycoprotein secretion, ion and water fluxes in sheep trachea. *J. Appl. Physiol.* 60: 918–927.

Polak, J. M., and Bloom, S. M. (1982). Regulatory peptides and neuron-specific enolase in the respiratory tract of man and other mammals. *Exp. Lung Res.* 3: 313–328.

Popovac, D., Chinn, R., Graf, P., Nadel, J. A., and Davis, B. (1979). Serotonin potentiates nervous stimulation of mucus gland secretion in canine trachea in vivo. *Physiologist* 22: 102.

Putney, J. W., Jr. (1977). Muscarinic, alpha-adrenergic and peptide receptors regulate the same calcium influx sites in the parotid gland. *J. Physiol. (Lond.)* 268: 139–149.

Putney, J. W., Jr. (1979). Stimulus-permeability coupling: Role of calcium in receptor regulation of membrane permeability. *Pharmacol. Rev.* 30: 209–245.

Quinton, P. M. (1979). Composition and control of secretions from tracheal bronchial submucosal glands. *Nature* 279: 551–552.

Rasmussen, H., and Barrett, P. Q. (1984). Calcium messenger system: An integrated view. *Physiol. Rev.* 64: 938–984.

Regoli, D., and Varabe, J. (1980). Pharmacology of bradykinin and related kinins. *Pharmacol. Rev.* 32: 1–46.

Reid, L. (1960). Measurement of the bronchial mucous gland layer: A diagnostic yardstick in chronic bronchitis. *Thorax* 15: 132–141.

Rieves, R. D., Lundgren, J. D., Logun, C., Wu, T., and Shelhamer, J. H. (1991). Effect of protein kinase C activating agents on respiratory glycoconjugate release from feline airways. *Am. J. Physiol.* 261: L415–L423.

Rogers, D. F., and Barnes, P. J. (1989). Opioid inhibition of neurally mediated mucus secretion in human bronchi. *Lancet* 1 (8644): 930–932.

Sasaki, T., and Gallacher, D. V. (1990). Extracellular ATP activates receptor-operated cation channels in mouse lacrimal acinar cells to promote calcium influx in the absence of phosphoinositide metabolism. *FEBS Lett.* 264: 130–134.

Sasaki, T., and Gallacher, D. V. (1992). The ATP-induced inward current in mouse lacrimal acinar cells is potentiated by isoprenaline and ATP. *J. Physiol. (Lond.)* 447: 103–118.

Sasaki, T., Shimura, S., Sasaki, H., and Takishima, T. (1989a). Effect of epithelium on mucus secretion from feline tracheal submucosal glands. *J. Appl. Physiol.* 66: 764–770.

Sasaki, T., Shimura, S., Ikeda, K., Sasaki, H., and Takishima, T. (1989b). Platelet-activating factor increases platelet-dependent glycoconjugate secretion from tracheal submucosal glands. *Am. J. Physiol.* 257: L373–L378.

Sasaki, T., Shimura, S., Ikeda, K., Sasaki, H., and Takishima, T. (1990). Sodium efflux from tracheal submucosal gland in feline trachea. *Am. J. Physiol.* 258: L112–L117.

Sasaki, T., Shimura, S., Wakui, M., Kakuta, Y., Satoh, M., Nagaki, M., Yamada, K., Nishiyama, A., and Takishima, T. (1992). Localization of IP_3-sensitive Ca^{2+}-release in Cl⁻ secretion from airway submucosal gland cells. *Am. Rev. Respir. Dis.* 145: A370.

Sato, K., and Sato, F. (1981). Role of calcium in cholinergic and adrenergic mechanisms of eccrine sweat secretion. *Am. J. Physiol.* 241: C113–C120.

Sato, K., Nishiyama, A., and Kobayashi, M. (1979). Mechanical properties and functions of the myoepithelium in the eccrine sweat gland. *Am. J. Physiol.* 237: C177–C184.

Satoh, M., Shimura, S., Ishihara, H., Yamada, K., Masuda, T., Sasaki, T., Sasaki, H., and Takishima, T. (1992). Effects of glucocorticoid on fluid secretion across airway mucosa. *Am. J. Physiol.* (in press).

Schultz, H. D., Roberts, A. M., Bratcher, C., Coleridge, M., Coleridge, C. G., and Davis, B. (1985). Pulmonary C-fibers reflexively increase secretion by tracheal submucosal glands in dogs. *J. Appl. Physiol.* 58: 907–910.

Schuster, A., Ueki, I., and Nadel, J. A. (1992). Neutrophil elastase stimulates tracheal submucosal gland secretion that is inhibited by ICI 200,355. *Am. J. Physiol.* 262: L86–L91.

Shelhamer, J. H., Marom, Z., and Kaliner, M. (1980). Immunologic and neuropharmacologic stimulation of mucous glycoprotein release from human airways in vitro. *J. Clin. Invest.* 66: 1400–1408.

Sheller, J. R., Holtzman, M. J., Skoogh, B.-H., and Nadel, J. A. (1982). Interaction of serotonin with vagal-ACh-induced bronchoconstriction in canine lungs. *J. Appl. Physiol.* 52: 964–966.

Sherman, J. M., Cheng, P.-W., Tandeler, B., and Boat, F. (1981). Mucous glycoproteins from cat tracheal goblet cells and mucous glands separated with EDTA. *Am. Rev. Respir. Dis.* 124: 476–479.

Shimura, S. (1990). Methods for the morphological study of tracheal and bronchial glands. In *Models of Lung Disease. Microscopy and Structural Methods*. Edited by J. Gil. New York, Marcel Dekker, pp. 309–358.

Shimura, S., Sasaki, T., Sasaki, H., and Takishima, T. (1986). Contractility of isolated single submucosal gland from trachea. *J. Appl. Physiol.* 60: 1237–1247.

Shimura, S., Sasaki, T., Okayama, H., Sasaki, T., and Takishima, T. (1987a). Neural control of contraction in isolated submucosal gland from feline trachea. *J. Appl. Physiol.* 62: 2404–2409.

Shimura, S., Sasaki, T., Okayama, H., Sasaki, H., and Takishima, T. (1987b). Effect of substance P on the mucus secretion of isolated submucosal gland from feline trachea. *J. Appl. Physiol.* 63: 646–653.

Shimura, S., Sasaki, T., Ikeda, K., Sasaki, H., and Takishima, T. (1988). Vasoactive intestinal peptide augments cholinergic-induced glycoconjugate secretion in tracheal submucosal glands. *J. Appl. Physiol.* 65: 2537–2544.

Shimura, S., Sasaki, T., Ikeda, K., Yamauchi, K., Sasaki, H., and Takishima, T. (1990). Direct inhibitory action of glucocorticoid on glycoconjugate secretion from airway submucosal glands. *Am. Rev. Respir. Dis.* 141: 1044–1049.

Shimura, S., Sasaki, T., Ikeda, K., Ishihara, H., Sato, M., Sasaki, H., and Takishima, T. (1991a). Neuropeptides and airway submucosal gland secretion. *Am. Rev. Respir. Dis.* 143: S25–S27.

Shimura, S., Ishihara, H., Nagaki, M., Satoh, M., Masuda, T., and Takishima, T. (1991b).

Role of protein kinase C in mucus glycoprotein secretion from feline tracheal submucosal glands. *Am. Rev. Respir. Dis.* 143: A705.

Shimura, S., Sasaki, T., Ishihara, H., Satoh, M., Sasaki, H., and Takishima, T. (1992a). Autonomic innervation of feline tracheal submucosal glands for mucus glycoprotein secretion. *Am. J. Physiol.* 262: L15–L20.

Shimura, S., Ishihara, H., Satoh, M., Masuda, T., Nagaki, M., Sasaki, H., and Takishima, T. (1992b). Endothelin regulation of mucus glycoprotein secretion from feline tracheal submucosal glands. *Am. J. Physiol.* 262: L208–L213.

Shimura, S., Sasaki, T., Yamada, K., Satoh, M., Nagaki, M., Sasaki, H., and Takishima, T. (1992c). Augmentation by isoproterenol in ATP-induced secretion from feline tracheal submucosal glands. *Am. Rev. Respir. Dis.* 145: A618.

Shorofsky, S. R., Field, M., and Fozzard, H. A. (1986). Changes in intracellular sodium with chloride secretion in dog tracheal epithelium. *Am. J. Physiol.* 250: C646–C650.

Silva, D. G., and Ross, G. (1974). Ultrastructural and fluorescence histochemical studies on the innervation of the tracheobronchial muscle of normal cats and cats treated with 6-hydroxydopamine. *J. Ultrastruct. Res.* 47: 310–328.

Smith, P. L., Welsh, M. J., Stoff, J. S., and Frizzel, R. A. (1982). Chloride secretion by canine tracheal epithelium: I. Role of intracellular cAMP levels. *J. Membr. Biol.* 70: 217–226.

Soltoff, S. P., McMillan, M. K., and Talamo, B. R. (1992). ATP activates cation-permeable pathway in rat acinar cells. *Am. J. Physiol.* 262: C934–C940.

Sommerhoff, C. P., and Finkbeiner, W. E. (1990). Human tracheobronchial gland cells in culture. *Am. J. Respir. Cell Mol. Biol.* 2: 41–50.

Sommerhoff, C. P., Caughey, C. H., Finkbeiner, W. E., Lazarus, S. C., Basbaum, C. B., and Nadel, J. A. (1989). Mast cell chymase: A potent secretagoues for airway gland serous cells. *J. Immunol.* 142: 2450–2456.

Sommerhoff, C. P., Nadel, J. A., Basbaum, C. B., and Caughey, G. H. (1990). Neutrophil elastase and cathepsin G stimulation from cultured bovine airway gland serous cells. *J. Clin. Invest.* 85: 682–689.

Sorvari, T. E. (1972). Histochemical observations on the role of ferric chloride in the high-iron diamine technique for localizing sulfated mucosubstances. *Histochem. J.* 4: 193–204.

Spicer, S. S. (1965). Diamine methods for differentiating mucosubstances histochemically. *J. Histochem. Cytochem.* 13: 211–234.

Spicer, S. S., Fraser, R., Virella, G., and Hall, B. J. (1977). Immunocytochemical localization of lysozymes in respiratory and other tissues. *Lab. Invest.* 36: 282–295.

Spicer, S. S., Hardin, J. H., and Setser, M. E. (1978). Ultrastructural visualization of sulphated complex carbohydrates in blood and epithelial cells with the high iron diamine procedure. *Histochem. J.* 10: 435–452.

Spicer, S. S., Sens, M. A., and Tashian, R. E. (1982). Immunocytochemical demonstration of carbonic anhydrase in human epithelial cells. *J. Histochem. Cytochem.* 30: 864–873.

Spiro, R. G. (1966). Analysis of sugars found in glycoproteins. *Methods. Enzymol.* 8: 3–26.

Stahl, G. H., and Ellis, D. B. (1973). Biosynthesis of respiratory-tract mucins. A comparison of canine epithelial goblet-cell and submucosal-gland secretions. *Biochem. J.* 136: 845–850.

St. George, J. A., Plopper, C. G., Etchison, J. R., and Dungworth, D. L. (1984). An immunocytochemical/histochemical approach to tracheobronchial mucus characterization in the rabbit. *Am. Rev. Respir. Dis.* 130: 124–127.

St. George, J. A., Cranz, D. L., Zicker, S. C., Etchison, J. R., Dungworth, D. L., and Plopper, C. G. (1985). An immunohistochemical characterization of rhesus monkey respiratory secretions using monoclonal antibodies. *Am. Rev. Respir. Dis.* 132: 556–563.

Sturgess, J., and Reid, L. (1972). An organ culture study of the effect of drugs on the secretory activity of the human bronchial submucosal gland. *Clin. Sci.* 43: 533–543.

Suez, D., and Szefler, S. (1986). Excessive accumulation of mucus in children with asthma: A potential role for erythromicin? A case discussion. *J. Allergy Clin. Immunol.* 77: 330–334.

Suter, S., Schaad, U. B., Tegner, H., Ohlsson, K., Desgrandchamps, D., and Waldvogel, F. A. (1986). Levels of free granulocyte elastase in bronchial secretions from patients with cystic fibrosis: Effect of antimicrobial treatment against *Pseudomonas aeruginosa*. *J. Infect. Dis.* 153: 902–909.

Takemura, T., and Eishi, Y. (1985). Distribution of secretory component and immunoglobulins in the developing lung. *Am. Rev. Respir. Dis.* 131: 125–130.

Tandler, B., Sherman, J., and Boat, T. F. (1981). EDTA-mediated separation of cat tracheal lining epithelium. *Am. Rev. Respir. Dis.* 124: 469–475.

Toesu, E. C., Lawire, A. M., Petersen, O. H., and Gallacher, D. V. (1992). Spatial and temporal distribution of agonist-evoked cytoplasmic Ca^{2+} signals in exocrine acinar cells: Analysis by digital image microscopy. *EMBO J.* 11: 1623–1629.

Tom-Moy, M., Basbaum, C. B., and Nadel, J. A. (1983). Localization and release of lysozyme from ferret trachea: Effects of adrenergic and cholinergic drugs. *Cell Tissue Res.* 228: 549–562.

Turner, N. C., Power, R. F., Polak, J. M., Bloom, S. R., and Dollery, C. T. (1989). Endothelin-induced contraction of tracheal smooth muscle and identification of specific endothelin binding sites in the trachea of rat. *Br. J. Pharmacol.* 98: 361–366.

Ueki, I., German, V. F., and Nadel, J. A. (1980). Micropipette measurement of airway submucosal gland secretion: Autonomic effects. *Am. Rev. Respir. Dis.* 121: 351–357.

Walters, E. H., O'Bryne, P. M., Fabbri, L. M., Graff, P. D., Holtzman, M. J., and Nadel, J. A. (1984). Control of neurotransmission by prostaglandins in canine trachealis smooth muscle. *J. Appl. Physiol.* 57: 129–134.

Wardell, J., Chakrin, L., and Payne, B. (1970). The canine tracheal pouch. A model for use in respiratory mucous research. *Am. Rev. Respir. Dis.* 101: 741–754.

Warner, T. F., and Azen, E. A. (1984). Proline-rich proteins are present in serous cells of submucosal glands. *Am. Rev. Respir. Dis.* 130: 115–118.

Webber, S. E., and Widdicombe, J. G. (1987a). The effect of vasoactive intestinal peptide on smooth muscle tone and mucus secretion from the ferret trachea. *Br. J. Pharmacol.* 91: 139–148.

Webber, S. E., and Widdicombe, J. G. (1987b). The actions of methacholine, phenylephrine, salbutamol and histamine on mucous secretion from in-vitro trachea. *Agents Actions* 22: 82–85.

Weitz, J. I., Crowley, K. A., Landman, S. L., Lipman, B. I., and Yu, J. (1987). Increased neutrophil elastase activity in cigarette smokers. *Ann. Intern. Med.* 107: 680–682.

Widdicombe, J. H., Colesman, D. L., Finkebeiner, W. E., and Tuet, I. K. (1985). Electrical properties of monolayers cultured from cells of human tracheal mucosa. *J. Appl. Physiol.* 58: 1729–1735.

Wirtz, H. R. W., and Dobbs, L. G. (1990). Calcium mobilization and exocytosis after one mechanical stretch of lung epithelial cells. *Science* 250: 1266–1269.

Yamaya, M., Finkbeiner, W. E., and Widdicombe, J. H. (1991a). Ion transport by cultures of human tracheobronchial submucosal glands. *Am. J. Physiol.* 261: L485–L490.

Yamaya, M., Finkbeiner, W. E., and Widdicombe, J. H. (1991b). Altered ion transport by tracheal glands in cystic fibrosis. *Am. J. Physiol.* 261: L491–L494.

Yanagisawa, M., Kurihara, H., Kimura, S., Tomobe, Y., Kobayashi, M., Mitsui, Y., Yazaki, Y., Goto, K., and Masaki, T. (1988). A novel potent vasoconstrictor peptide produced by vascular endothelial cells. *Nature* 332: 411–415.

Yang, C. M., Farley, J. M., and Dwyer, T. M. (1988a). Muscarinic stimulation of submucosal glands in swine trachea. *J. Appl. Physiol.* 64: 200–209.

Yang, C. M., Farley, J. M., and Dwyer, T. M. (1988b). Acetylcholine-stimulated chloride flux in tracheal submucosal gland cells. *J. Appl. Physiol.* 65: 1891–1894.

Yurdakos, E., and Webber, S. E. (1991). Endothelin-1 inhibits pre-stimulated tracheal submucosal gland secretion and epithelial albumin transport. *Br. J. Pharmacol.* 104: 1050–1056.

10

Ion and Fluid Transport by Airway Epithelium

JONATHAN H. WIDDICOMBE

University of California–San Francisco
San Francisco, California

I. Introduction

Fluid movement across epithelia is secondary to active transepithelial transport of solutes, which creates local concentration gradients across the epithelium and results in fluid movement by osmosis (Diamond, 1979). Such directional solute transport was first detected in airway epithelia by Melon (1968), and it is believed to play a critical role in mucociliary clearance by regulating the volume of the fluid layers that line the airway lumen.

Between the respiratory gases and the apical surface of airway epithelium is a film of fluid from 5 to 30 μm in depth. This fluid consists of a gel of mucus lying over the *periciliary sol layer*, a watery solution bathing the cilia (Lucas and Douglas, 1934; Yoneda, 1976). The mucous gel becomes thicker in bronchitis, asthma, and cystic fibrosis, but may be absent in healthy, uninflamed airways (Bhaskar et al., 1985). The presence of two layers is believed to be critical for effective *mucociliary clearance*, the process that keeps the airway surface clean. The cilia are able to beat in the low-viscosity sol layer, the depth of which is slightly less than the length of the cilia. Accordingly, on their forward propulsive strokes, the tips of the cilia contact the underside of the mucous blanket, driving it and any entrapped dirt to the mouth, where it is expectorated or swallowed.

Epithelial fluid transport, by altering the depth of the periciliary sol layer or the hydration of the mucous gel, could, thereby, markedly alter the efficiency of mucociliary clearance.

The major active ion transport processes of airway surface epithelia are active absorption of Na and active secretion of Cl (Table 1). Active secretion of chloride will make the airway lumen electrically negative, inducing net passive movement of Na toward the lumen, largely through the tight junctions. The resulting transfer of salt draws water into the lumen by osmosis. Similar arguments show that active absorption of Na should promote absorption of fluid from the luminal to serosal side of the epithelium.

Fluid movements have been measured across airway epithelia, and stimula-

Table 1   Major Active Transport Processes of Airway Epithelia

Only Cl secretion
    Fetal sheep trachea (Cotton et al., 1983)
    Fetal dog trachea (Gatzy et al., 1987)
    Newborn dog trachea (Gatzy et al., 1987)
Only Na absorption
    Pig nasal (Melon, 1968)
    Human nasal (Boucher et al., 1986)
    Human bronchus (Knowles et al., 1984)
    Dog bronchus (Boucher et al., 1981)
    Pig bronchus (Boucher et al., 1982)
    Human trachea (Yamaya et al., 1992)
    Sheep bronchus (Cotton et al., 1983)
    Sheep trachea (Cotton et al., 1983; Phipps et al., 1983)
    Monkey trachea (Boucher et al., 1982)
    Guinea pig trachea (Boucher et al., 1982)
Cl secretion and Na absorption
    Dog mainstem bronchus (Boucher et al., 1981)
    Rabbit trachea[a] (Melon, 1968)
    Ferret trachea[b] (Corrales et al., 1986)
    Cow trachea (Vulliemin et al., 1983)
    Cat trachea (Corrales et al., 1986)
    Dog trachea (Olver et al., 1975)

[a]Boucher and Gatzy (1983) reported that the rabbit trachea showed only Na absorption. However, their levels of I_{sc} were only about one-half those recorded by Melon (1968).
[b]Under resting conditions, the ferret trachea shows only Na absorption. However, Cl secretion can be induced by adrenergic agents and other mediators.

tion of Cl secretion has led to fluid secretion (Welsh et al., 1980), and stimulation of Na absorption has led to fluid absorption (Nathanson et al., 1983a). However, the most convincing evidence for a role of these ion transport processes in regulation of hydration and clearance of mucus comes from studies on cystic fibrosis. This genetic disease is characterized by an accumulation of mucous secretions in the airways, which has been linked to decreased airway Cl secretion (Widdicombe et al., 1985a), as well as increased absorption of Na (Boucher et al., 1986).

II. Methods

A. Cell Culture

In 1984, we demonstrated that primary cultures of dog tracheal epithelium showed qualitatively the same types of ion transport as the native epithelium (Coleman et al., 1984). Levels of transepithelial active ion transport of these cultures, however, were only one-tenth to one-fifth those of the original tissue. Improvements in culture techniques have now led to primary cultures of dog bronchus (Boucher and Larsen, 1988), dog trachea (Kondo et al., 1991; Van Scott et al., 1988), human nasal mucosa (Yankaskas et al., 1985), and human trachea (Yamaya et al., 1992), which show ion transport, both qualitatively and quantitatively, very similar to that of the original tissue. Such cultures have been very useful for a variety of ion transport studies (Widdicombe, 1990). In fact, patch–clamp studies have been performed only on cultured cells.

B. Ussing Chambers

For many epithelia, Ussing's short-circuit current technique (Ussing and Zerahn, 1951) represents the first approach to determining the types of active ion transport present. However, it can be applied only to relatively large sheets of epithelium, which show electrogenic transport processes (i.e., generate a transepithelial potential difference). Any transepithelial potential difference generated by the active transport process will cause net diffusional ion movements through shunt or leak pathways within the tissue. Thus, current will cycle within the tissue through the active and shunt pathways. If both sides of the tissue are connected by a wire of infinitely low resistance, the current normally flowing in the tissue shunt will be drawn off, and the transepithelial potential difference will be brought to zero, or short-circuited. In practice the external circuit is not a wire of infinitely low resistance, but rather, a circuit containing a variable current source. The current flowing through the external circuit is adjusted to maintain the transepithelial potential difference at zero. This current is known as the short-circuit current (I_{sc}). Provided that no forces exist to bring about net passive movement of ions (e.g., transepithelial gradients in ion concentration, osmotic or hydrostatic pressure), then the I_{sc} is generated by the tissue's metabolism, and it is equal to the sum of all the active transport processes operating across the tissue.

To determine what active processes are responsible for the I_{sc}, one can employ specific transport blockers and ion-substitution experiments. Alternatively, direct determination of the transport processes responsible for the I_{sc} can be made using radioactive tracers. For Na, both unidirectional fluxes (i.e., serosa-to-mucosa and mucosa-to-serosa) can be determined simultaneously with ^{24}Na and ^{22}Na. For other ions, the two unidirectional fluxes are measured on a pair of tissues that are closely matched in terms of their I_{sc} and electrical conductances. Unidirectional fluxes of several ions can be determined simultaneously taking advantage of differences in half-life and type of radiation between isotopes (Boucher et al., 1981).

C. Microelectrodes

Conventional microelectrodes can be used to determine the voltages across the apical and basolateral membranes, as well as the relative resistances of these membranes. Depending on whether the microelectrode inside an epithelial cell is referenced to the serosal or mucosal bath, it will record the apical or basolateral membrane potential (V_a, V_b). If the transepithelial potential difference (V_t) is also recorded, then the other membrane potential is easily derived from $V_t = V_a + V_b$.

When current pulses are passed across the epithelium, a certain amount of current passes between the cells (the paracellular route), whereas the remaining fraction of the current crosses the apical and basolateral membranes in series (transcellular pathway). Current flow through the cells causes change in V_a, V_b, and V_t. Because the same amount of current passes across both the apical and basolateral membrane resistances (R_a, R_b), one can readily derive the membrane resistance ratio (α) and the fractional apical membrane resistance (f_R) from:

$$f_R = \frac{\Delta V_a}{\Delta V_t} = \frac{R_a}{R_a + R_b},$$

and

$$\alpha = \frac{\Delta V_a}{\Delta V_b} = \frac{R_a}{R_b}.$$

Equivalent circuit analysis is an elegant way of analyzing microelectrode data, which treats the epithelium as an electrical circuit with a resistance and electromotive force (emf) at each membrane connected by a shunt or paracellular resistance (R_p). By assuming that only R_a, but not R_b or R_p, altered during the first 10 s of treatment with epinephrine, Welsh et al. (1983) were able to use changes in f_R and R_{te} (the transepithelial resistance) to determine R_p. By knowing R_p, they calculated R_a and R_b at different times after the addition of epinephrine. The membrane emfs (E_a and E_b) could also be calculated, because V_a and V_b are the sum of the membrane emf and the current drop across the membrane from flow of I_{sc} [e.g., $V_a = E_a - (I_{sc}R_a)$]. In this way, they calculated detailed time courses for E_a, E_b, R_a, and R_b during treatment with epinephrine. Equivalent circuit analysis has also been used, with somewhat different assumptions, to determine the membrane emfs and resistances of cultured nasal epithelium (Willumsen and Boucher, 1989a).

Finally, ion-selective microelectrodes have been used to determine intracellular activities of Na, K, and Cl in airway epithelia. In such experiments, electrically connected cells are penetrated by both a conventional microelectrode and an electrode containing a resin sensitive for the ion measured. The potential difference recorded by the ion-selective electrode (V_x) is given by:

$$V_X = V_a + S \ln\left(\frac{aX_c}{aX_m}\right),$$

where X is the ion being measured and aX_c and aX_m refer to its activities in the cell and mucosal solution. S is the calibration constant that gives the voltage change of the ion-selective electrode for a tenfold increase in aX. S is obtained by calibrating the electrode in solutions of known aX. For a perfectly selective electrode, S is given by RT/F, where R is the universal gas constant, T is the temperature in degrees Kelvin and F is Faraday's constant. At 37°C, RT/F is 26.7 mV. Knowing S, aX_m and V_a (from the conventional microelectrode), the reading from the ion-selective microelectrode (V_X) can be used to calculate aX_c.

D. Patch–Clamping

In patch-clamping, a small area of cell membrane (5–20 μm^2) is electrically isolated from the rest of the cell membrane by sucking it up into the tip of a fire-polished glass pipette (diameter = ~1.5 μm) (Sakmann and Neher, 1983). The resistance of the seal between the pipette and the membrane is in the order of gigohms (GΩ), ensuring that any clamp current from the pipette flows across the patch of membrane, and not through the narrow gap between the glass of the pipette and the cell membrane. Three types of patch are commonly used: the cell-attached patch, the cell-detached patch (in which the patch is mechanically excised from the cell), and the whole-cell patch, in which the membrane in the pipette tip is ruptured, and the remaining cell membrane, therefore, forms a sort of giant patch. Each technique has its own advantages and disadvantages (Hamill et al., 1981). In brief, receptor-mediated activation of channels can be studied in the cell-attached patch. In the cell-detached patch, macromolecular regulators of channel activity (e.g., protein kinases) can be added to the internal face of the patch membrane. Whereas both cell-attached and cell-detached patches are used to study the activity of single or small numbers of channels, the whole-cell patch is used to record currents from all the channels in the cell. Unwanted channels can be eliminated with blockers or by allowing nontransported ions to diffuse into the cell from the pipette.

The voltage across the patch is held at a particular value by passing clamp current across the membrane from the pipette to a reference electrode in the bathing medium. When channels in the patch open, the electrical resistance of the patch drops, and (by Ohm's law), more current is needed to maintain the selected holding potential. Opening and closing of channels is rapid, occurring within microseconds, and channel activity produces square waves in a typical patch–clamp current trace. The unit conductance of a particular channel is given by the product of the holding potential and the change in clamp current in going from open to closed.

Cultures of airway epithelial cells have been patch-clamped by many investigators. Comparatively dedifferentiated cultures are used, because the apical membrane specializations of native epithelium or more differentiated cultures prevent a tight seal between the pipette and the membrane. Also most patch–clamp studies have been performed on subconfluent cultures grown on a solid support. This poses some difficulties in comparing patch–clamp and Ussing chamber data, because the transport properties of such cells differ in some particulars from those of confluent cell sheets grown on permeant supports (Anderson and Welsh, 1991; McCann and Welsh, 1990).

E. Other Ion Transport Techniques

Langridge-Smith et al. (1983) developed an apical membrane preparation from bovine tracheal epithelium that has proved useful in several studies of ion and water transport (Elgavish et al., 1987; Fong et al., 1988; Landry et al., 1989; Valdivia et al., 1988; Worman et al., 1986). We have recently published a more rapid version of her procedure that has the advantage that contaminating basolateral membranes are eliminated by ouabain-affinity chromatography (Shen et al., 1991). There are no satisfactory preparations of basolateral membranes from airway epithelia.

The Cl-sensitive fluorescent probe, SPQ (Illsley and Verkman, 1987), has been used to study ion transport in intact airway cells (Chao et al., 1990), as well as apical membrane vesicles (Fong et al., 1988). Half-maximal quenching of this dye occurs with [Cl] of approximately 15 mM (Illsley and Verkman, 1987). Iodide and bromide are somewhat more effective quenchers than Cl. In most experiments, cells or vesicles are depleted of Cl (by incubation in a medium in which Cl is replaced by organic anions), and then Cl is readded. As Cl diffuses into the cell (or vesicle), the fluorescence is quenched, and the influx of Cl can be determined from the initial rate in decline of fluorescence. SPQ actually measures changes in the concentration of intracellular (or intravesicular) Cl and, therefore, is unsuitable for the measurement of transient changes in Cl influx, which may produce undetectable alterations in the rate of change of $[Cl]_i$.

Intracellular concentrations of ions can be measured by atomic absorption spectrophotometry (Widdicombe et al., 1981), or by determining equilibrium uptakes of radiotracers (Widdicombe et al., 1981). However, such measurements (especially of Na) are critically dependent on estimates of the extracellular space. Also, the concentrations so determined reflect bound and sequestered material as well as ion that is free in the cytoplasm. Consequently, concentrations determined by atomic absorption spectrophotometry are often considerably higher than activities determined with ion-selective microelectrodes.

F. Measurements of Transepithelial Fluid Movement

Three techniques have been used to measure fluid absorption across airway epithelia. In a modified Ussing chamber, the serosal half-chamber has been filled with fluid and connected to the exterior by a capillary tube. As the fluid moved across the epithelium, this was sensed by a photocell as movement of the meniscus along the tube (Durand et al., 1981). In a modification of the standing-drop technique, used in the kidney, physiological saline was introduced into a ferret trachea and sandwiched between mineral oil. Fluid movement was measured as the change in inulin concentration in the saline (Loughlin et al., 1982). Lastly, fluid transport has been measured with a capacitance probe (Fig. 1; Nathanson et al., 1983a; Welsh et al., 1980).

Fluid flow can also be estimated from net open-circuit ion fluxes. Under these circumstances (i.e., with no current flow in the external circuit, and the tissue at its spontaneous transepithelial potential difference), the sum of the transepithelial ion movements must be electrically neutral and, generally, take the form of NaCl secretion or NaCl absorption (Finkbeiner and Widdicombe, 1992). Assuming these ion movements reflect transport of isotonic fluid, then fluid movement can be estimated.

III. Results

A. Ion Transport by Surface Epithelium

Ussing Chambers

Melon (1968) was the first to apply Ussing's short-circuit current technique to airway epithelia. He demonstrated that the I_{sc} across nasal mucosae from pigs and other species could be accounted for entirely by active absorption of Na. Since then, a wide range of airway epithelial have been studied (Finkbeiner and Widdicombe, 1992). Many of these show only active absorption of Na; Cl secretion cannot be induced by mediators. In others, active secretion of Cl is the

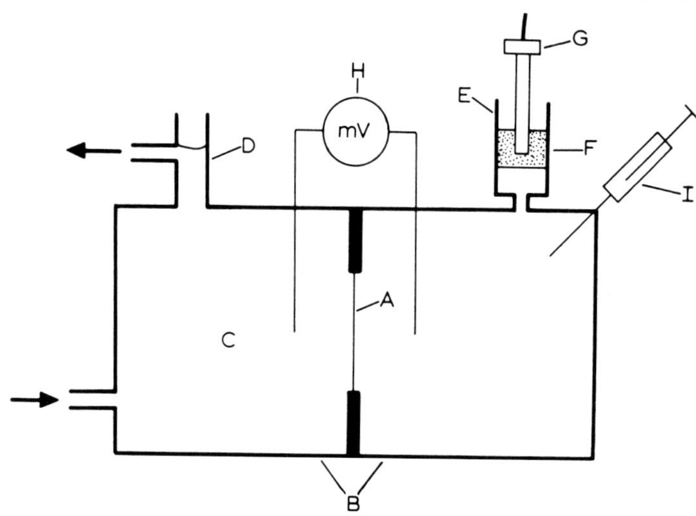

Figure 1 Apparatus for measurement of transepithelial fluid flow. A sheet of epithelium (A) is mounted between Lucite half-chambers (B). Warm, oxygenated physiological saline is circulated continuously across the mucosal face of the tissue (C). A tube (D) on the mucosal side allows one to apply a small hydrostatic pressure to press the tissue against a wire screen, thereby preventing bulging or flapping. The fluid on the serosal side of the tissue is introduced into a tube (E), and layered with paraffin oil (F). A capacitance probe (G) in the paraffin oil senses the distance between the probe tip and the meniscus of the serosal salt solution. Tissue viability is assessed from the transepithelial potential difference, which is measured with Ag/AgCl wires and a voltmeter (H). Calibration is performed by injecting fluid into the closed serosal chamber with a Hamilton syringe (I). Fluid movements across the tissue are registered as changes in the capacitance sensed by the probe.

major ion transport process. There is a tendency for larger airways to show Cl secretion, rather than Na absorption, and for a switch from Cl secretion to Na absorption during development. When adult airways show Cl secretion in the absence of added secretagogues, this is due to spontaneous release of prostaglandins, and it is abolished by indomethacin (Al-Bazzaz et al., 1981; Langridge-Smith et al., 1984). It may, therefore, reflect airway inflammation in the experimental animals used. In healthy, uninflamed adult airways, Na absorption may be the only major type of active ion transport present. Table 1 lists the predominant ion transport processes of airway epithelia.

Where it has been measured, most airway epithelia show a small amount of active K secretion (~ 0.1 $\mu Eq\,cm^{-2}h^{-1}$) (Finkbeiner and Widdicombe, 1992).

Calcium secretion ($\sim$1.5 nEq cm^{-2} h^{-1}) has been reported for the dog's tracheal epithelium (Jayaram and Al-Bazzaz, 1979).

Mechanism of Chloride Secretion

Directional transport of ions by epithelia requires the presence of different transport proteins in their apical and basolateral membranes. The apical membrane of airway epithelia contains Na and Cl channels, but has negligible K conductance. The basolateral membrane, however, is K-selective, containing cAMP- and Ca-activated K channels. Also restricted to the basolateral membrane are the Na,K-ATPase (Widdicombe et al., 1979a) and a Na,K–2Cl cotransporter (Fong et al., 1991).

Active secretion of Cl by tracheal epithelium is abolished by serosal ouabain (the inhibitor of Na,K-ATPase), and by removal of Na from the serosal bath (Widdicombe et al., 1979b). Addition of ouabain to, or removal of Na from, the mucosal medium, has no effect on active Cl secretion (Widdicombe et al., 1979b). These results suggest that Cl entry across the basolateral membrane is dependent on Na, and that Cl secretion requires an Na gradient across this membrane. Similar results on other Cl-secreting epithelia led to the model for Cl secretion illustrated in Figure 2 (Frizzell et al., 1979). In this model, entry of Cl across the

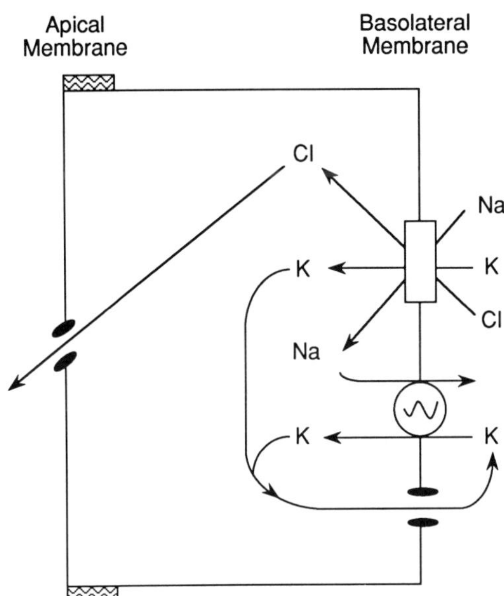

Figure 2   Model for active Cl secretion by airway epithelia. See text for details.

basolateral membrane is by cotransport with Na. The energy in the trans-membrane concentration gradient for Na allows Cl to be accumulated within the cells to a level greater than that predicted for passive distribution according to the apical membrane potential (V_a). Accordingly, there is net exit of Cl across this membrane, which is Cl-selective. The Na that enters by cotransport with Cl is removed from the cells by basolaterally located (Widdicombe et al., 1979a) Na,K-ATPase. The ATPase also pumps in K, which recycles across the K-selective basolateral membrane.

This model has been tested extensively for dog tracheal epithelium, and the following discussion refers to this tissue. However, all indications are that Cl secretion by other airway epithelia is very similar to that seen in dog trachea.

Intracellular ion activities and membrane potentials have been measured with microelectrodes (Table 2), and the driving forces for the movements of the various ions are in the appropriate directions. The sum of the transmembrane potential difference and the potential predicted by the Nernst equation for a particular ion gives the electrochemical driving force for that ion. The data for Cl in Table 2 yield a driving force for net exit across the apical membrane of 29 mV in resting, and 6 mV in stimulated, tissues (the reduction in driving force in stimulated tissues is due both to depolarization and to reduced aCl_i). For K, the electrochemical driving forces for net efflux across the basolateral membrane come to 19 mV (resting), and 13 mV (stimulated). Both electrical and chemical gradients favor Na entry, the driving forces across the apical membrane being 105 mV in resting and 77 mV in stimulated tissues.

Basolateral cotransport of Na and Cl is responsible for accumulation of Cl_i to levels greater than predicted for passive distribution according to V_a. Thus, in short-circuited tissues, Welsh (1983a) found aCl_i of 38 mM, considerably above the level of 14 mM predicted for passive equilibration. Removal of serosal Na,

Table 2 Membrane Potential and Ion Contents for Open-Circuited Dog Tracheal Epithelium

	Nonsecreting	Secreting	Ref.
V_a	−46	−34	Shorofsky et al., 1986
V_b	−64	−65	Shorofsky et al., 1986
aNa_i	11	21	Shorofsky et al., 1986
aCl_i	47	32	Shorofsky et al., 1984
aK_i	83	69	Smith and Frizzell, 1984

Membrane potentials are in mV; activities in mM. Nonsecreting tissues are those in which Cl secretion is essentially zero. Secreting tissues are those in which Cl secretion has been stimulated. For short-circuited tissues, $V_a = V_b = -60$ mV (Welsh, 1983a).

however, or inhibition of NaCl cotransport by loop diuretics, caused aCl_i to fall to levels not significantly different from those for passive distribution.

The apical membrane is conductive for Cl and Na; changes in the mucosal concentrations of these ions (but not of K) affect apical membrane potential. On the other hand, the basolateral membrane potential (V_b) is affected mainly by changes in serosal K concentration and not by changes in serosal Cl and Na (Welsh, 1983b; Welsh et al., 1982). Such ion substitution experiments, however, are complicated by current flow driven by diffusion potentials generated across the tight junctions. This current, flowing across the apical and basolateral cell membranes causes small changes in their potential differences. However, Welsh et al. (1983) showed by equivalent circuit analysis that E_b was equal to the equilibrium potential for K across this membrane (E_K), whereas E_a was equal to E_{Na} under resting conditions and E_{Cl} when stimulated with cAMP.

In an actively transporting epithelium, the turnover rates for the intracellular pools of transported ions are in the order of seconds or minutes (Schultz, 1981). Thus, when the rate of net Cl secretion increases, to avoid problems with intracellular tonicity and volume control, it is important that the turnover rates of all the transport proteins involved change in parallel (Schultz, 1981). In the trachea, studies by Welsh and Frizzell (Smith and Frizzell, 1984; Welsh et al., 1982), suggest the following sequence of events: An initial increase in apical membrane Cl conductance, G_{Cl}^a, causes V_a to depolarize. For a sustained increase in Cl secretion, the basolateral Na,K–2Cl cotransporter also turns over faster, bringing more Na into the cell, elevating $[Na]_i$, and stimulating the Na,K-ATPase, thereby increasing influx of K across the basolateral membrane. The G_K^{bl} now increases, serving two functions. First, by current flow in shunt pathways within the tissue, the increase in G_K^{bl} hyperpolarizes the apical membrane, thereby retaining the driving force for net Cl exit across this membrane. Second, the increased G_K^{bl} allows the increased amounts of K entering by the Na,K–2Cl cotransporter and the Na,K-ATPase to recycle across the basolateral membrane, thereby avoiding problems of volume control. In fact, the increases in turnover of the different transport proteins are so well matched that changes in intracellular ion contents on induction of Cl secretion are trivial (see Table 2).

Transport Proteins Involved in Chloride Secretion

The Na gradient across the basolateral membrane provides the energy for net Cl uptake across this membrane and for Cl secretion across the tissue as a whole. The Na,K-ATPase that generates this gradient has been localized exclusively to the basolateral membrane (Widdicombe et al., 1979a), where there are approximately 2400 pump units per square micron (Widdicombe et al., 1986). The properties of the Na,K-ATPase in trachea are much the same as for this enzyme in other tissues (Westenfelder et al., 1980).

Entry of Cl across the basolateral membrane is by NaCl or Na,K–2Cl cotransport. Loop diuretics, which inhibit Na-linked Cl transport (O'Grady et al., 1987), abolish Cl secretion when added to the basolateral side of dog tracheal epithelium (Welsh, 1983c; Widdicombe et al., 1983), but are about 100 times less effective when added to the mucosal side (Widdicombe et al., 1983). Two studies with isolated cells failed to demonstrate K dependence of this transport and found equal inhibition of Na and Cl influx by loop diuretics, suggesting that NaCl, rather than Na,K–2Cl cotransport, was the mechanism (Musch and Field, 1989; Widdicombe et al., 1983). However, isolated cells have lost the directionality of intact epithelium and may not retain all the components needed for vectorial Cl secretion. Thus, Welsh (1984), has shown in native epithelium that the ouabain-sensitive oxygen consumption associated with Cl secretion is twice that associated with Na absorption. This suggests that Cl secretion involves Na,K–2Cl, rather than NaCl cotransport. More direct evidence for involvement of K in NaCl cotransport has recently been obtained by us using cultured tracheal cells (Fong et al., 1991). We found negligible uptake of ^{86}Rb (a marker for K) across the apical membranes, but uptake of the same isotope across the basolateral membrane required Na and Cl and was inhibited by loop diuretics. Levels of loop diuretic-sensitive Rb uptake corresponded well with the I_{sc} of these cells. Liedtke (1989, 1990) has recently presented evidence for regulation of the Na,K–2Cl cotransporter by Ca. Thus, the loss of Cl from isolated human tracheal cells, and losses of both Na and Cl from rabbit tracheal cells were stimulated by α-adrenergic agents, and these stimulations were blocked by loop diuretics or preincubation with 1,2-bis(2-aminophenoxy)ethane-N,N,N′,N′-tetra acetic acid (BAPTA), a chelator of intracellular Ca. Furthermore, the Ca ionophore, ionomycin, stimulated effluxes by the same amount as α-adrenergic agents.

The Cl conductance of the apical membrane is in the form of channels (aqueous pores), which have been studied extensively by patch-clamping of primary tracheal cultures. Although several apical membrane Cl channels have been described (Shoemaker et al., 1986), attention in both dog and human tracheal cells (Frizzell et al., 1986; Welsh, 1986a,b), has focused on a channel that has a unit conductance of about 50 pS (at 0 mV, with 150 mM NaCl on both sides of a detached patch), and shows outward rectification (conductance doubles as the membrane potential, referenced to the cell's exterior, goes from -100 to $+100$ mV). At normal membrane potentials, in the unstimulated state, the probability of this channel being open (P_o) is negligible (0.001), but increases to about 0.15 on elevation of intracellular cAMP (Fong et al., 1988). At depolarizing (interior positive) potentials the P_o increases dramatically. Finally the halide-selectivity sequence for this channel is I(1.6) > Br(1.3) > Cl(1.0) > F(0.6) (Frizzell, 1987), which corresponds to Eisenmann's sequence I for a low-ionic–strength selectivity site (Wright and Diamond, 1977). The importance of this channel is that it is opened by cAMP in cell-attached patches and by the catalytic subunit of cAMP-dependent protein kinase in cell-detached patches (Li et al., 1988; Schoumacher et al., 1987) (cAMP is the major second messenger involved in physiological stimulation of Cl secretion). In cystic fibrosis (CF) epithelia, however, several authors have shown that protein kinase A fails to open this channel (Hwang et al., 1989; Li et al., 1988; Schoumacher et al., 1987). This led to the widespread belief that this channel represented the physiological defect in CF. Recently, however, the CF gene product, the cystic fibrosis transmembrane conductance regulator (CFTR), has been shown to be a 8-pS nonrectifying cAMP-regulated anion channel (Berger et al., 1991; Kartner et al., 1991; Tabcharani et al., 1991), closely resembling similar channels reported in apical membranes from pancreas (Gray et al., 1989), T_{84} cells (a human colonic carcinoma cell line) (Tabcharani et al., 1990), and dog tracheal cultures (Hagiwara et al., 1990). The role of the 50-pS outward rectifier in vectorial Cl transport, and its defective regulation by cAMP are now being questioned (Widdicombe and Wine, 1991). In fact, the rectifier closely resembles channels of nonepithelial cells that are involved in volume regulation (Solc and Wine, 1991).

Early patch–clamp experiments led to controversy over the effects of Ca on apical membrane Cl channels. Frizzell et al. (1986), for instance, with cultures of human tracheal cells, showed that the Ca ionophore, A23187, opened 50-pS outward rectifiers in cell-attached patches, and increasing the Ca on the inside of a cell-detached patch did likewise. However, Welsh and Liedtke (1986), who used the same cells and techniques, were unable to find any evidence for Ca-dependent regulation of this channel. More recently, measurements with microelectrodes and ^{125}I fluxes have provided evidence for Ca-dependent opening of Cl channels in cultures of human nasal and dog tracheal cells (Clancy et al., 1990a; Willumsen and Boucher, 1989b). This effect of Ca is probably not mediated by protein kinases, as kinase inhibitors or depletion of ATP did not alter the increased efflux of ^{125}I in response to A23187 (Clancy et al., 1990b). On the other hand, the same maneuvers markedly inhibited the increase in ^{125}I efflux induced by cAMP (Clancy et al., 1990b). Recently, Anderson and Welsh (1991) have provided clear evidence for separate Ca- and cAMP-activated Cl channels in the apical membrane of human tracheal epithelium. They permeabilized the basolateral membrane with nystatin and then imposed Cl concentrations gradients across the apical membrane. Addition of either Ca or cAMP led to Cl-generated currents that were additive and differed in their anion selectivity and sensitivity to blockers.

The basolateral K conductance is inhibited by Ba^{2+} (Smith and Frizzell, 1984; Welsh, 1983d). Basolateral K channels have been patch-clamped by Welsh and McCann (1985). They are Ca-activated with their P_o increasing dramatically between 10^{-7} and 10^{-6} M Ca_i. Other properties include inward rectification and a unit conductance of 20 pS (at 0 mV with 145 mM KCl on both sides). Later results showed that this channel was blocked by charybdotoxin, a scorpion venom (McCann et al., 1990). Indirect evidence also suggests the presence of cAMP-activated K channels in the basolateral membrane. Using confluent primary cultures of dog tracheal epithelium McCann and Welsh (1990) studied the effects of mediators on basolateral ^{86}Rb efflux (a marker for K channels). A23187 transiently stimulated Rb efflux and Cl secretion, and increases in both were prevented by charybdotoxin. They concluded that the Rb efflux was through a charybdotoxin-sensitive, low-conductance, inwardly rectifying, Ca^{2+}-activated channel (K_{CLIC}) previously discovered in subconfluent cell sheets grown on nonporous supports (McCann et al., 1990). In contrast with A23187, the I_{sc} response to isoproterenol shows two components (Hartmann et al., 1992; McCann and Welsh, 1990; Widdicombe et al., 1985b), with a large transient increase being followed by a sustained increase. The transient increase closely parallels changes in $[Ca^{2+}]_i$ (Hartmann et al., 1992; McCann and Welsh, 1990). Charybdotoxin blocked the transient increase, but not the sustained increase. In the presence of charybdotoxin, basolateral ^{86}Rb efflux still increased during the sustained increase in I_{sc} in response to isoproterenol. As Ca_i had returned to baseline values, and as K_{CLIC} channels close during the sustained increase, McCann and Welsh concluded that a second charybdotoxin-insensitive, cAMP-activated Cl channel had been opened by isoproterenol.

Second Messengers Regulating Chloride Secretion

Cyclic AMP stimulates Cl secretion across dog tracheal epithelium (Al-Bazzaz, 1981), and many mediators that stimulate Cl secretion also elevate intracellular cAMP (Smith et al., 1982; Lazarus et al., 1986; Table 3). Thus, a role for cAMP in regulation of airway Cl secretion has been recognized for some time. More recently, potential regulatory roles for Ca have been identified, and some secretagogues act preponderantly through cAMP and others through Ca. Treatment of dog tracheal epithelium with the phorbol ester 12-*O*-tetradecanoylphorbol-13-acetate (TPA) inhibits stimulation of Cl secretion by cAMP (Barthelson et al., 1987; Welsh, 1987a). Protein kinase C, therefore, may function as a negative-feedback control, reversing the stimulatory effects of Ca_i and protein kinase A.

Studies of the individual components of Cl secretion have shown that there are Ca-activated and cAMP-activated apical membrane Cl channels. Likewise Ca-activated basolateral K channels have been demonstrated directly by patch-clamping, and it is likely that cAMP-activated K channels also exist. Calcium activation of basolateral Na-dependent Cl transport has been demonstrated in isolated cells (Liedtke, 1989, 1990), in which β-adrenergic agents, which act through cAMP, were ineffective. However, this transporter loses its K-dependency on epithelial dispersion (Musch and Field, 1989; Widdicombe et al., 1983), and aspects of its regulation may also be altered. Thus, a regulation of this transporter by cAMP in intact epithelium remains possible. Na,K-ATPase is probably not modulated by second messengers, but responds directly to the increase in $[Na_i]$ produced by increased entry of Na by cotransport with Cl.

Table 3 Effects of Neurohumoral Agents on Chloride Secretion Across Dog Tracheal Epithelium

Agent	Side of action	PG release	cAMP increase	K_d (M)	Ref.
β-Adrenergic	S	No	Yes	100 nM	Al-Bazzaz and Cheng, 1979; Smith et al., 1982
PGE_2 and PGE_1	M or S	?	Yes	10 nM	Al-Bazzaz et al., 1981; Smith et al., 1982
$PGF_{2\alpha}$	M or S	?	No	100 nM	Al-Bazzaz et al., 1981; Smith et al., 1982
PGD_2, PGH_2	?	?	?	>100 nM	Eling et al., 1986
LTC_4, LTD_4	M or S	Yes	?	<10 nM	Leikauf et al., 1986
VIP	S	No	Yes	10 nM	Nathanson et al., 1983b
Adenosine	M	No	Yes	100 nM	Pratt et al., 1986
Bradykinin	M > S	Yes	?	1 nM (m) 100 nM (s)	Leikauf et al., 1985
Substance P	M	?	?	30 nM	Al-Bazzaz et al., 1985; Rangachari et al., 1987
Eosinophil MBP	M	?	?	2 μM	Jacoby et al., 1988
Neurokinin A, B	M > S	No	Yes	10 nM (m) 100 nM (s)	Tamaoki et al., 1988
Histamine	?	?	?	10 μM	Marin et al., 1977
Acetylcholine	?	?	?	<3 μM	Marin et al., 1976

PG, prostaglandin; LT, leukotriene; VIP, vasoactive intestinal peptide; MBP, major basic protein; M, mucosal; S, serosal.

Recently, cpt-cAMP has been shown to increase Ca_i in primary cultures of dog tracheal epithelium (McCann et al., 1989). This increase in Ca_i is not associated with an increase in inositol triphosphate (IP_3), the second messenger usually responsible for releasing Ca from intracellular stores (Berridge, 1987). Thus, a likely mechanism for receptor-mediated stimulation of Cl secretion is elevation of cAMP, leading to both opening of Cl channels and elevation of Ca_i. The Ca in turn increases both NaCl cotransport and basolateral G_K. Cyclic AMP, in addition, may activate a second population of K channels (McCann and Welsh, 1990). Isoproterenol increases intracellular diacylglycerol (DAG) (Anderson and Welsh, 1990), the natural stimulator of protein kinase C (Berridge, 1987). However, its lack of effect on the IP_3 levels suggests that the increase in DAG is not due to hydrolysis of phosphatidylinositol. Anderson and Welsh (1990) also found that the actions of isoproterenol were not associated with a change in phosphatidylcholine turnover. Therefore, the source of DAG generated by isoproterenol is unknown. However, stimulation of protein kinase C by the elevated DAG will exert a negative-feedback on the cAMP-dependent stimulation of Cl secretion. This regulatory scheme is illustrated in Figure 3a.

Much evidence also suggests that Ca can stimulate Cl secretion in the absence of charges in intracellular cAMP (Hartmann et al., 1992). Isoproterenol causes a large increase in I_{sc} followed by a smaller sustained increase. Other mediators, for example bradykinin in the presence of indomethacin, produce only a transient I_{sc} response. There is a close correspondence between the transient responses in I_{sc} and increases in Ca_i, suggesting that Ca is directly stimulating Cl secretion. Several other findings lend support to this hypothesis. First, there is a significant correlation between the maximal transient increase in I_{sc} and the maximal increase in Ca_i produced by different mediators. Second, preincubation of cells with the Ca-chelator, BAPTA, abolishes the transient responses of I_{sc} to isoproterenol and other mediators, but has no effect on the slower sustained response to isoproterenol, which is presumably due to cAMP. Third, mediators producing only transient increases in I_{sc} failed to elevate intracellular cAMP, even in cells pretreated with the phosphodiesterase inhibitor, 3-isobutyl-1-methyl-xanthine. Bradykinin does, however, increase both IP_3 and DAG in dog tracheal cells (Anderson and Welsh, 1990; McCann et al., 1989), presumably reflecting the cleavage of phophatidylinositol by phospholipase A. As with isoproterenol, stimulation of protein kinase C by DAG may act as a negative-feedback control.

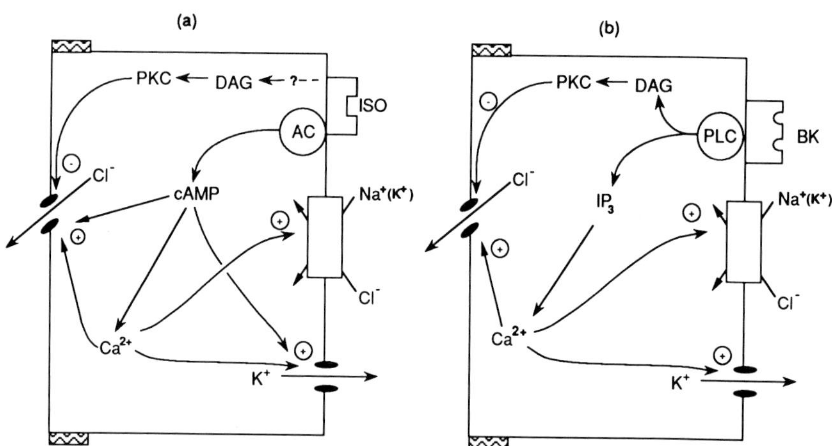

Figure 3 Regulation of Cl secretion by second messengers: (a) cAMP-dependent stimulation by isoproterenol; (b) Ca-dependent stimulation by bradykinin. Abbreviations: ISO, isoproterenol; AC, adenylate cyclase; DAG, diacylglycerol; cAMP, cyclic-AMP; PKC, protein kinase C; BK, bradykinin; PLC, phospholipase C; IP_3, inositol triphosphate. See text for further details.

This Ca-dependent, cAMP-independent regulation of Cl secretion is illustrated in Figure 3b.

The close correlation between I_{sc} and Ca_i suggests that Ca is directly activating one or more of the transport proteins involved in Cl secretion. An alternative possibility is that Ca causes prolonged opening of Cl or K channels, but fails to stimulate the Na,K–2Cl cotransporter. The K and Cl will run downhill across the basolateral and apical membranes, respectively, and the increase in I_{sc} will be matched by increased loss of Cl across the apical membrane and an equal flow of K across the basolateral membrane. The I_{sc} will then fall as Cl_i decreases, and eventually Cl loss across the apical membrane will come to equal Cl uptake across the basolateral, at which point I_{sc} will have returned to its original baseline value.

Neurohumoral Regulation of Chloride Secretion

Numerous mediators stimulate Cl secretion across dog tracheal epithelium (see Table 3). All those causing sustained increases in Cl secretion probably do so by elevating cAMP, either directly or, for bradykinin and the leukotrienes, secondarily to prostaglandin release. Several peptides (substance P, neurokinins A and B, bradykinin) cause transient increases in I_{sc} when applied mucosally. These transients may represent Ca-activated stimulation of K channels (accompanied by hyperpolarization and increased Cl loss through the apical membranes). The integral of current over time gives the charge lost during these transients in coulombs. The corresponding loss of KCl is less than the total KCl in these cells (Leikauf et al., 1985; Tamaoki et al., 1988), consistent with this interpretation.

The volume of airway secretions is sufficiently small (about 1 μl in a 1-cm length of airway of 2-mm radius), and the K_ds for many mediators are sufficiently low that very little mediator is needed in the respiratory tract fluid to reach a biologically active level. In fact, a single releasing cell (e.g., mucosal mast cell, APUD cell, or sensory nerve terminal) could release sufficient mediator on the mucosal side to stimulate Cl secretion along a 1-cm length of airway (Widdicombe, 1989).

Although studied in less detail, regulation of Cl secretion in other airway epithelia resembles that of dog trachea. Thus, in cow trachea, Cl secretion is stimulated by adrenergic agents and prostaglandins, and this stimulation is associated with increases in cAMP levels (Langridge-Smith et al., 1984). β-Adrenergic agents, prostaglandins, and bradykinin stimulate Cl secretion across cat trachea, and β-adrenergic agents, across ferret trachea (Corrales et al., 1986).

Sodium Ion Absorption

Active absorption of Na by airway epithelia follows the basic mechanism proposed 30 years ago by Koefoed-Johnsen and Ussing (1958) for frog skin (Fig. 4). Net

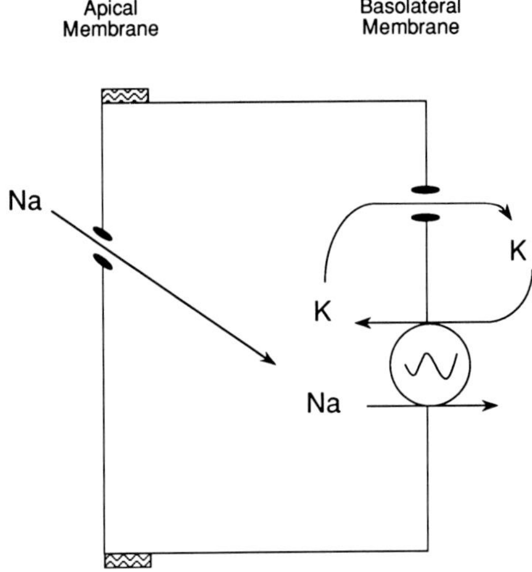

Figure 4 Model for active absorption of Na by airway epithelia. See text for details.

entry of Na occurs across the apical membrane down both chemical and electrical gradients (see Table 2). This Na is then extruded across the basolateral membrane by the Na,K-ATPase localized to this membrane. As with Cl secretion, the K pumped in by the Na,K-ATPase recycles across the K-selective basolateral membrane.

Amiloride, which blocks the apical membrane Na conductance of several nonairway epithelia (Benos, 1982), inhibits Na absorption across airway epithelia (Welsh, 1987b). However, at least in trachea, not all Na absorption is amiloride-sensitive (Widdicombe and Welsh, 1980). Cation-selective channels in airway epithelia are beginning to be identified by patch-clampers (Duszyk et al., 1989).

In dog tracheal epithelium, stimulation of Cl secretion is frequently associated with a small decline in active Na absorption (Al-Bazzaz et al., 1981; Widdicombe and Welsh, 1980). This presumably is due to the reduction in the driving force for Na entry because of both increased Na_i and apical membrane depolarization (see Table 2). However, there is no convincing evidence for neurohumoral regulation of Na absorption, independently of changes in Cl secretion. Al-Bazzaz (1986) has provided a list of the many negative findings. Cullen and Welsh (1987) bathed dog tracheal epithelium in Cl-free (gluconate) medium and identified the remaining I_{sc} as Na absorption. Elevation of intracellular cAMP increased this I_{sc}; depletion of cAMP in response to indomethacin inhibited it. However, the changes seen by these authors were small, and their sensitivity to pretreatment with amiloride was not rigorously tested. We found that cultures of dog tracheal epithelium, incubated in Cl- and HCO_3-free medium, and pretreated with amiloride, still showed increases in I_{sc} in response to isoproterenol (Widdicombe and Barthelson, 1988). The increases were unaffected by the loop diuretic, bumetanide. They were, however, abolished by the Cl channel inhibitor, diphenylamine-2-carboxylic acid (Wangemann et al., 1986), suggesting that they were due to Na movement through Cl channels, which are imperfectly selective for Cl over Na. The feasibility of Cl channels carrying some Na current is increased when one considers that the driving force for Na entry is some five to ten times greater than that for Cl exit (see Table 2).

B. Ion Transport by Gland Epithelium

Compared with the surface epithelium, little is known about ion transport by the epithelium of airway submucosal glands. Yang et al. (1988) showed that isolated swine gland cells actively accumulated Cl and that this process was inhibited by loop diuretics. These results suggest that fluid transport by gland acini is due to the same Na-dependent Cl secretion as present in the surface epithelium. Dwyer and Farley (1991) have presented indirect evidence, obtained with SPQ, that the Cl permeability of human gland cells from patients with cystic fibrosis is less than normal.

Confluent cell cultures of submucosal gland acinar cells from cow trachea were developed by Finkbeiner et al. (1986). More recently, Sommerhoff and Finkbeiner (1990) have shown that human gland acini, both non-CF and CF, can be grown to confluency. The cultures reacted immunocytochemically with antibodies to lysozyme and lactoferrin, known secretory products of gland cells (Bowes and Corrin, 1977, 1981), as well as with antibodies which stained gland but not surface epithelium of native tissue.

We have grown these human gland cells on porous supports and studied their transport processes with Ussing chambers (Yamaya et al., 1991a). Baseline R_{te} and I_{sc} were 600 $\Omega \cdot cm^2$ and 12 $\mu A\ cm^{-2}$. The I_{sc} was transiently increased by mediators in the potency sequence, methacholine > bradykinin > isoproterenol > phenylephrine. This sequence is of interest as methacholine has no effect on surface epithelium of human trachea or primary cultures of human trachea (Yamaya et al., 1992). Amiloride decreased baseline I_{sc} by 48 $\pm$ 8% (n = 5), but had little effect on the I_{sc} response to mediators. Diphenylamine-2-carboxylic acid, however, had no effect on baseline I_{sc}, but markedly inhibited the I_{sc} response to all mediators. These results suggest that the mediator-induced increases in I_{sc} are due to Cl secretion. Typical responses to mediators, and the effects of Na- and Cl-transport blockers are illustrated in Figure 5.

Cystic fibrosis submucosal gland cell cultures had R_{te} and baseline I_{sc} similar to those of non-CF. However, the I_{sc} responses to mediators of CF cultures were $\leq$5% those of non-CF cultures (Yamaya et al., 1991b) (Table 4). These results

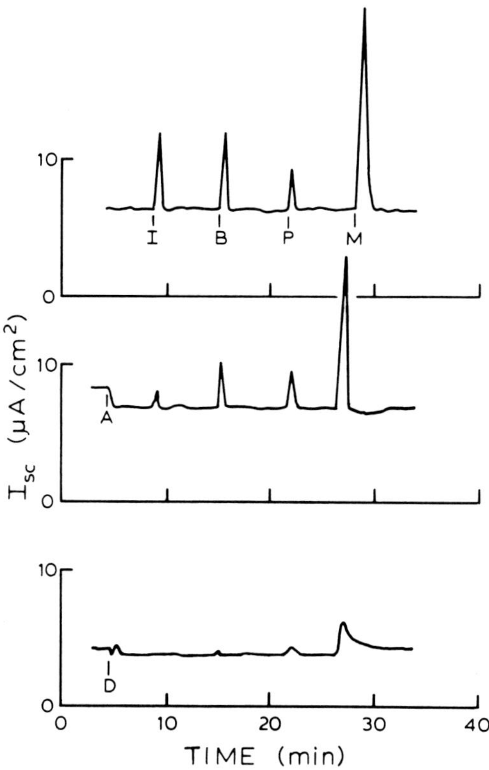

Figure 5 Effects of transport inhibitors on changes in I_{sc} of human airway gland cultures in response to mediators. Top: Responses in absence of inhibitor. Middle: Effects of amiloride. Bottom: Effects of DPAC. Tissues from the same culture. Key: A, 10^{-5} M amiloride; D, 10^{-3} M DPAC; I, 10^{-5} M isoproterenol; B, 10^{-6} M bradykinin; P, 10^{-5} M phenylephrine; M, 10^{-5} M methacholine. Mediators were added in the same sequence and at approximately the same times in all three traces. (From Yamaya et al., 1991a)

suggest that fluid secretion by submucosal airway glands is defective in cystic fibrosis. We speculate that this defect may play a role in the accumulation of mucous secretions, which is the major cause of mortality in this disease.

C. Fluid Transport

Transepithelial fluid transport occurs in response to local osmotic gradients set up by active solute transport. Dog tracheal epithelium possesses both a secretory and an absorptive ion-transport process. Thus, the net direction and volume of

Table 4 Electrical Properties of CF
and Non-CF Gland Cells

Property	Non-CF	CF
ΔI_{sc} (Iso)	1.9 ± 0.6	0.04 ± 0.04
ΔI_{sc} (MCh)	7.1 ± 1.7	0.2 ± 0.1
ΔI_{sc} (Bk)	5.0 ± 1.0	0.4 ± 0.1

Means $\pm$ SE, N = 5 from two tracheas for CF,
N = 14 from 12 tracheas for non-CF. Abbreviations: Iso, isoproterenol; MCh, methacholine;
Bk, bradykinin. All values for CF cells are
significantly different from those for non-CF
cells.

fluid flow across this epithelium may be regulated by altering the relative magnitudes of Cl secretion and Na absorption.

To test this hypothesis, Welsh et al. (1980) modified an apparatus described by Wiedner (1976) that measures transepithelial water movement by an electrical method. The net fluid movement across dog tracheal epithelium under resting conditions was not significantly different from zero. However, aminophylline (2×10^{-3} M), a drug that selectively stimulates active Cl secretion, always caused net fluid secretion. We also measured open-circuit Cl fluxes in paired tissues and found that there was no net movement of Cl under resting conditions, but that there was a significant net movement of Cl toward the lumen after administering aminophylline. The relative sizes of the net Cl flux and the fluid flow suggested that the secretion stimulated by aminophylline was approximately isosmotic with the bathing medium.

With the same apparatus, we showed that under certain conditions active Na absorption can also cause transepithelial fluid movement across dog tracheal epithelium (Nathanson et al., 1983a). Amphotericin B was used to stimulate Na absorption, and fluid flows were correlated with open-circuit ion fluxes. Under short-circuit conditions luminal amphotericin B (3×10^{-5} M) caused an inhibition of net Cl secretion and an increase in net Na absorption. Under resting open-circuit conditions, there was no significant net fluxes of Na or Cl. Amphotericin B, however, induced significant net movement of both Cl and Na toward the serosal side. In tissues from the same animals, there was no significant transepithelial fluid movement under resting conditions. Amphotericin B caused a net absorption of fluid. Ouabain abolished salt and fluid absorption.

Two other groups of workers directly measured fluid flow across airway epithelia. Durand et al. (1981) mounted bovine tracheal epithelium in a modified Ussing chamber and connected the closed serosal chamber to a horizontal glass tube. They measured volume flow by using a photocell to continuously record the movement of the meniscus along the tube. They found R_{te} of 200 $\Omega \cdot cm^2$ and V_t of 30 mV. No fluid flow was seen under baseline conditions or after histamine (10^{-4} M) was added. However, histamine doubled the hydraulic conductivity, as measured from fluid flows generated by adding sucrose to the bathing medium. Loughlin et al. (1982) introduced physiological saline into the lumen of a ferret trachea in vitro and sandwiched it between layers of mineral oil. They measured fluid movement as the change in inulin concentration in the saline. Under resting conditions, they found a significant net fluid absorption that carbamylcholine (10^{-6} M) converted to net secretion. Pretreatment with atropine prevented carbamyl-choline's effect on this tissue.

An alternative to directly measuring volume flows is to measure net open-circuit ion fluxes across paired tissues mounted in Ussing chambers. Net move-ments of both Na and Cl in the same direction presumably reflect fluid movement. Assuming isotonicity of the transported fluid, an estimate of the volume flow can be made. Boucher et al. (1988) report that epithelia from several airways show net absorption of both Na and Cl: adult sheep trachea and bronchi, monkey trachea, rabbit trachea, guinea pig trachea, human bronchi, and pig bronchi. In rabbit tracheal epithelium and dog bronchus, net Na and Cl absorption are equal at approximately 1.6 $\mu Eq\,cm^{-2}h^{-1}$ (Boucher et al., 1981; Jarnigan et al., 1983). Assuming these flows represent an isotonic NaCl solution, this then corresponds to a volume flow of about 10 $\mu l\,cm^{-2}h^{-1}$. Most other airway epithelia show net absorption or secretion of Na and Cl of about this magnitude (Finkbeiner and Widdicombe, 1992). In some cases the net absorption of Cl is less than net absorption of Na. This may reflect movement of $NaHCO_3$. Failure to detect net open-circuit movements of Na and Cl across airway epithelia may be due to the presence of both active Cl secretion and active Na absorption. Table 5 summarizes the forms of net open-circuit ion movements for airway epithelia. We have provided a detailed tabulation of the individual estimates of net open-circuit ion fluxes elsewhere (Finkbeiner and Widdicombe, 1992).

Semiquantitative estimates of submucosal gland secretion have been made by observing the upwellings of fluid from gland openings covered with a layer of tantalum dust (Borson et al., 1980; Davis et al., 1982). Quantitative estimates have been made with micropipette sampling from individual duct openings. Quinton (1979), for instance, covered the surface of cat trachea with mineral oil and then collected the droplets that formed at the duct openings. Although fluid output was essentially zero in the resting state (<1 nl min^{-1}), cholinergic and α-adrenergic agents induced fluid secretion of about 10 nl min^{-1}. The β-adrenergic agent isoproterenol was a less effective secretagogue. Figure 6 shows the results from one of these experiments. A very similar approach was taken by Ueki et al. (1980), who placed the fire-polished tips of microelectrodes directly over the duct openings of cat tracheal glands. Their results essentially confirmed those of

Table 5 Open-Circuit Ion Movements Across
Airway Epithelia

NaCl secretion
    Fetal sheep trachea (Cotton et al., 1983)
NaCl absorption
    Dog bronchus (Boucher et al., 1981)
    Sheep bronchus (Cotton et al., 1983)
    Pig bronchus (Boucher et al., 1982)
    Sheep trachea (Cotton et al., 1983)
    Rabbit trachea (Jarnigan et al., 1983)
    Monkey trachea (Boucher et al., 1982)
    Guinea pig trachea (Boucher et al., 1982)
Na absorption greater than Cl absorption
    Rabbit nasal (Melon, 1968)
    Rabbit trachea (Melon, 1968)
    Dog trachea (Boucher et al., 1981)
    Dog bronchus (mainstem) (Boucher et al., 1981)
    Human bronchus (Knowles et al., 1984)

Quinton, with the exception that they found a basal secretory rate of 9 nl min^{-1}. This, however, may have been in part an artifact created by the "slight negative pressure" needed to initiate flow into the pipette.

IV. Future Studies

The mechanisms of Na absorption and Cl secretion across airway epithelia have been well characterized. The driving forces for ion movements across basolateral and apical membranes have been determined, and there is general agreement on the basic types of carriers involved in the transport processes. Future research may concentrate on the intracellular regulation of transport and on the exact molecular nature of the transport proteins involved. Thus, the relative functional importance of Ca- and cAMP-dependent regulatory pathways remains to be fully determined, as does the identity of the transport proteins responding to these different second messengers. With the possible exception of the cystic fibrosis gene product (CFTR), which may be a cAMP-regulated apical membrane Cl channel, the molecular identity of virtually all the transport proteins is unknown. In particular, many Cl channels have been described for airway epithelia, and their manner of regulation and their roles (whether in Cl secretion or volume regulation) are uncertain. A similar plethora of Na channels may be developing (Chinet et al., 1990; Disser and Fromter, 1989; Duszyk et al., 1989).

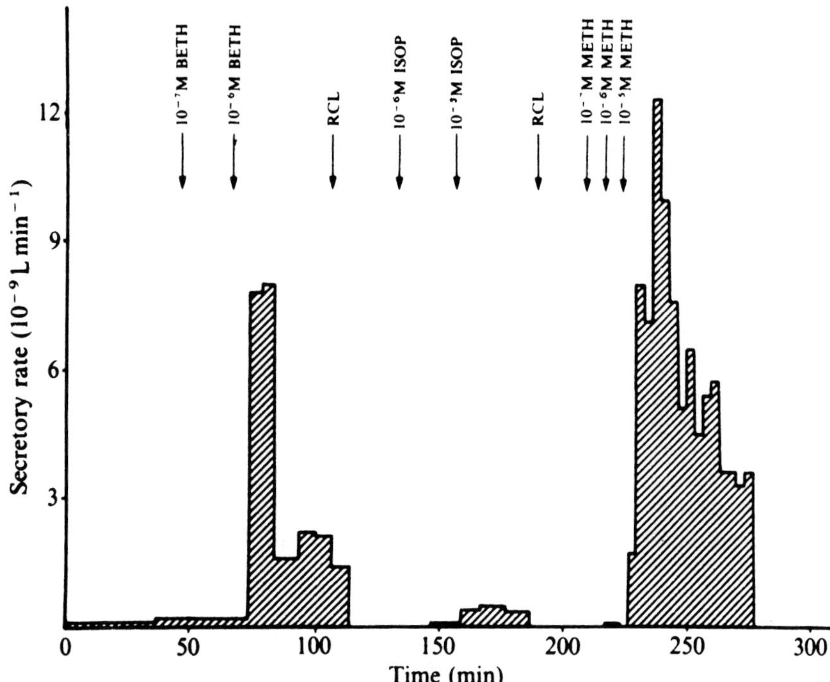

Figure 6 A typical secretory rate response (ordinate) of a single tracheal submucosal gland to increasing concentrations of bethanechol (BETH), isoproterenol (ISOP), and methoxamine (METH) in the bathing medium. At "RCL," bath was changed to Ringer's solution. Drugs were added at the arrows. (From Quinton, 1979)

Most disorders of mucociliary clearance (such as seen in asthma and cystic fibrosis) may result from abnormal fluid transport across airway epithelia. However, there have been very few measurements of fluid movement across these epithelia, and none in CF, even though much is known about defective ion transport in this disease. It is to be hoped that accurate measurements of transepithelial fluid movement and its responses to mediators will be forthcoming. Determination of the ion selectivity of the paracellular pathway of airway epithelia should also be made, as this could have profound effects on fluid movement. Finally, it is generally assumed that active transport processes regulate the depth of the periciliary sol layer. However, although this layer can be visualized in living material (Lucas and Douglas, 1934), its depth has never been measured. In fixed material, it is always exactly the same depth as the length of the cilia. Thus it seems possible that it is generated by means other than active fluid transport. One possibility is that ciliary motion has a thixotropic or liquifying action on cilia

(Negus, 1963). Another possibility is that its presence is due to forces of capillarity generated by the cilia (Widdicombe, 1988). It seems important to measure the depth of this layer in living material and determine how this changes in response to mediators. Perhaps microelectrodes could detect some subtle change in ion content (e.g., of $[Ca^{2+}]_i$) on passing from the gel to the sol. Microscopical measurements of the depth of the combined sol and gel mucous layers in living material have been initiated by Wanner and his colleges (Seybold et al., 1990).

References

Al-Bazzaz, F. J. (1981). Role of cyclic AMP in regulation of chloride secretion by canine tracheal mucosa. *Am. Rev. Respir. Dis.* 123: 295–298.

Al-Bazzaz, F. J. (1986). Regulation of salt and water transport across airway mucosa. *Clin. Chest Med.* 7: 259–272.

Al-Bazzaz, F. J., and Cheng, E. (1979). Effect of catecholamines on ion transport in dog tracheal epithelium. *J. Appl. Physiol.* 47: 397–403.

Al-Bazzaz, F. J., Kelsey, J., and Kaage, W. (1985). Substance P stimulation of chloride secretion by canine tracheal mucosa. *Am. Rev. Respir. Dis.* 131: 86–89.

Al-Bazzaz, F. J., Yadava, V. P., and Westenfelder, C. (1981). Modification of Na and Cl transport in canine tracheal mucosa by prostaglandins. *Am. J. Physiol.* 240: F101–F105.

Anderson, M. P., and Welsh, M. J. (1990). Isoproterenol, cAMP, and bradykinin stimulate diacylglycerol production in airway epithelium. *Am. J. Physiol.* 258: L294–L300.

Anderson, M. P., and Welsh, M. J. (1991). Calcium and cAMP activate different chloride channels in the apical membrane of normal and cystic fibrosis epithelia. *Proc. Natl. Acad. Sci. USA* 88: 6003–6007.

Barthelson, R. A., Jacoby, D. B., and Widdicombe, J. H. (1987). Regulation of chloride secretion in dog tracheal epithelium by protein kinase C. *Am. J. Physiol.* 253: C802–C808.

Benos, D. J. (1982). Amiloride: A molecular probe of sodium transport in tissues and cells. *Am. J. Physiol.* 242: C131–C145.

Berger, H. A., Anderson, M. P., Gregory, R. J., Thompson, S., Howard, P. W., Maurer, R. A., Mulligan, R., Smith, A. E., and Welsh, M. J. (1991). Identification and regulation of the cystic fibrosis transmembrane conductance regulator-generated chloride channel. *J. Clin. Invest.* 88: 1422–1431.

Berridge, M. J. (1987). Inositol trisphosphate and diacylglycerol: Two interacting second messengers. *Annu. Rev. Biochem.* 56: 159–193.

Bhaskar, K. R., O'Sullivan, D. D., Seltzer, J., Rossing, T. H., Drazen, J. M., and Reid, L. M. (1985). Density gradient study of bronchial mucus aspirates from healthy volunteers (smokers and nonsmokers) and from patients with tracheostomy. *Exp. Lung Res.* 9: 289–308.

Borson, D. B., Chin, R. A., Davis, B., and Nadel, J. A. (1980). Adrenergic and cholinergic nerves mediate fluid secretion from tracheal glands of ferrets. *J. Appl. Physiol.* 49: 1027–1031.

Boucher, R. C., and Gatzy, J. T. (1983). Characteristics of sodium transport by excised rabbit trachea. *J. Appl. Physiol.* 55: 1877–1883.

Boucher, R. C., and Larsen, E. H. (1988). Comparison of ion transport by cultured secretory and absorptive canine airway epithelia. *Am. J. Physiol.* 254: C535–C547.

Boucher, R. C., Narvarte, J., Cotton, C., Stutts, M. J., Knowles, M. R., Finn, A. L., and Gatzy, J. T. (1982). Sodium absorption in mammalian airways. In *Fluid and Electrolyte Abnormalities in Exocrine Glands in Cystic Fibrosis*. Edited by P. M. Quinton, J. R. Martinez, and V. Hopfer. San Francisco, San Francisco Press, pp. 271–287.

Boucher, R. C., Stutts, M. F., and Gatzy, J. T. (1981). Regional differences in bioelectric properties and ion flow in excised canine airways. *J. Appl. Physiol.* 51: 706–714.

Boucher, R. C., Stutts, M. F., Knowles, R. C., Cantley, L., and Gatzy, J. T. (1986). Na transport in cystic fibrosis respiratory epithelia. Abnormal basal rate and response to adenylate cyclase activation. *J. Clin. Invest.* 78: 1245–1252.

Boucher, R. C., Willumsen, N. J., Knowles, M. R., Yankaskas, J., and Gatzy, J. T. (1988). Na$^+$ and Cl$^-$ absorption in respiratory epithelia: the role of apical and basolateral membranes. In *Cellular and Molecular Basis of Cystic Fibrosis*. Edited by G. Mastella, and P. Quinton. San Francisco, San Francisco Press, pp. 107–114.

Bowes, D., and Corrin, B. (1977). Ultrastructural immunocytochemical localization of lysozyme in human bronchial glands. *Thorax* 32: 163–170.

Bowes, D., Clark, A. E., and Corrin, B. (1981). Ultrastructural localization of lactoferrin and glycoprotein in human bronchial glands. *Thorax* 36: 108–115.

Chao, A. C., Widdicombe, J. H., and Verkman, A. S. (1990). Chloride conductive and cotransport mechanisms in cultures of canine tracheal epithelial cells measured by an entrapped fluorescent indicator. *J. Membr. Biol.* 113: 193–202.

Chinet, T., Fullton, J., Yankaskas, J., Boucher, R. C., and Stutts, J. (1990). Characterization of sodium channels in the apical membrane of nasal epithelial cells. *Am. Rev. Respir. Dis.* 141: A164.

Clancy, J. P., McCann, J. D., Li, M., and Welsh, M. J. (1990a). Calcium-dependent regulation of airway epithelial chloride channels. *Am. J. Physiol.* 258: L25–L32.

Clancy, J. P., McCann, J. D., and Welsh, M. J. (1990b). Evidence that calcium-dependent activation of airway epithelia chloride channels is not dependent on phosphorylation. *Am. J. Physiol.* 259: L410–L414.

Coleman, D. L., Tuet, I. K., and Widdicombe, J. H. (1984). Electrical properties of dog tracheal epithelial cells grown in monolayer culture. *Am. J. Physiol.* 246: C355–C359.

Corrales, R. J., Coleman, D. L., Jacoby, D. B., Leikauf, G. D., Hahn, H. L., Nadel, J. A., and Widdicombe, J. H. (1986). Ion transport across cat and ferret tracheal epithelia. *J. Appl. Physiol.* 61: 1065–1070.

Cotton, C. U., Lawson, E. E., Boucher, R. C., and Gatzy, J. T. (1983). Bioelectric properties and ion transport of airways excised from adult and fetal sheep. *J. Appl. Physiol.* 55: 1542–1549.

Cullen, J. J., and Welsh, M. J. (1987). Regulation of sodium absorption by canine tracheal epithelium. *J. Clin. Invest.* 79: 73–79.

Davis, B., Chinn, R., Gold, J., Popovac, D., and Widdicombe, J. G. (1982). Hypoxemia reflexly increases secretion from tracheal submucosal glands in dogs. *J. Appl. Physiol.* 52: 1416–1419.

Diamond, J. M. (1979). Osmotic water flow in leaky epithelia. *J. Membr. Biol.* 51: 195–216.

Disser, J., and Fromter, E. (1989). Properties of Na^+ channels of the respiratory epithelium from CF and non-CF patients. *Pediatr. Pulmonol.* Suppl. 4: 115.

Durand, J., Durand-Arczynska, W., and Haab, P. (1981). Volume flow, hydraulic conductivity and electrical properties across bovine tracheal epithelium in vitro: effect of histamine. *Pflugers Arch.* 392: 40–45.

Duszyk, M., French, A. S., and Man, S. F. (1989). Cystic fibrosis affects chloride and sodium channels in human airway epithelia. *Can. J. Physiol. Pharmacol.* 67: 1362–1365.

Dwyer, T. M., and Farley, J. M. (1991). Intracellular chloride in submucosal gland cells. *Life Sci.* 48: 2119–2127.

Elgavish, A., DiBona, D. R., Norton, P., and Meezan, E. (1987). Sulfate transport in apical membrane vesicles isolated from tracheal epithelium. *Am. J. Physiol.* 253: C416–C425.

Eling, T. E., Danilowicz, R. M., Henke, D. C., Sivarajah, K., Yankaskas, J. R., and Boucher, R. C. (1986). Arachidonic acid metabolism by canine tracheal epithelial cells. Product formation and relationship to chloride secretion. *J. Biol. Chem.* 261: 12841–12849.

Finkbeiner, W. E., Nadel, J. A., and Basbaum, C. B. (1986). Establishment and characterization of a cell line derived from bovine tracheal glands. *In Vitro* 22: 561–567.

Finkbeiner, W. E., and Widdicombe, J. H. (1992). Control of nasal airway secretions, ion transport and water movement. In *Defence Capabilities of the Respiratory Tract.* Edited by R. Schlesinger. New York, Raven Press, pp. 633–657.

Fong, P., Chao, A. C., and Widdicombe, J. H. (1991). Potassium dependence of Na-Cl cotransport in dog tracheal epithelium. *Am. J. Physiol.* 261: L290–L295.

Fong, P., Illsley, N. P., Widdicombe, J. H., and Verkman, A. S. (1988). Chloride transport in apical membrane vesicles from bovine tracheal epithelium: characterization using a fluorescent indicator. *J. Membr. Biol.* 104: 233–239.

Frizzell, R. A. (1987). Cystic fibrosis: A disease of ion channels. *TINS* 10: 190–193.

Frizzell, R. A., Field, M., and Schultz, S. G. (1979). Sodium-coupled chloride transport by epithelial tissues. *Am. J. Physiol.* 236: F1–F8.

Frizzell, R. A., Rechkemmer, G., and Shoemaker, R. L. (1986). Altered regulation of airway epithelial cell chloride channels in cystic fibrosis. *Science* 233: 558–560.

Gatzy, J. T., Cotton, C. U., Boucher, R. C., Knowles, M. R., and Gowen, C. W. (1987). Development of epithelial ion transport in fetal and neonatal airways. In *Physiology of the Fetal and Neonatal Lung.* Edited by D. Walters, L. Strang, and F. Geubelle. Boston, MTP Press, pp. 77–89.

Gray, M. A., Harris, A., Coleman, L., Greenwell, J. R., and Argent, B. E. (1989). Two types of chloride channel on duct cells cultured from human fetal pancreas. *Am. J. Physiol.* 258: C240–C251.

Hagiwara, G., Muller, U. J., Krouse, M. E., Law, T. C., Ward, C. L., Widdicombe, J. H., and Wine, J. J. (1990). Quantitative single-channel studies of cultured canine airway epithelium. *Pediatr. Pulmonol.* Suppl. 4:28.

Hamill, O. P., Marty, A., Neher, E., Sakmann, B., and Sigworth, F. J. (1981). Improved patch–clamp techniques for high-resolution current recording from cells and cell-free membrane patches. *Pflugers Arch.* 319: 85–100.

Hartmann, T., Kondo, M., Mochizuki, H., Verkman, A. S., and Widdicombe, J. H. (1992). Calcium-dependent regulation of Cl secretion in tracheal epithelium. *Am. J. Physiol.* 262: L163–L168.

Hwang, T. C., Lu, L., Zeitlin, P. L., Gruenert, D. C., Huganir, R., and Guggino, W. B. (1989). Cl⁻ channels in CF: Lack of activation by protein kinase C and cAMP-dependent protein kinase. *Science* 244: 1351–1353.

Illsley, N. P., and Verkman, A. S. (1987). Membrane chloride transport measured using a chloride-sensitive fluorescent probe. *Biochemistry* 26: 1215–1219.

Jacoby, D. B., Ueki, I. F., Widdicombe, J. H., Loegering, D. A., and Gleich, G. J. (1988). Effect of human major basic protein on ion transport in dog tracheal epithelium. *Am. Rev. Respir. Dis.* 137: 13–16.

Jarnigan, F., Davis, J. D., Bromberg, P. A., Gatzy, J. T., and Boucher, R. C. (1983). Bioelectric properties and ion transport of excised rabbit trachea. *J. Appl. Physiol.* 55: 1884–1892.

Jayaram, T. H., and Al-Bazzaz, F. J. (1979). Calcium transport across canine tracheal mucosa. *Am. Rev. Respir. Dis.* 119: 319.

Kartner, N., Hanrahan, J. W., Jensen, T. J., Naismith, A. L., Sun, S., Ackerley, C. A., Reyes, E. F., Tsui, L.-C., Rommens, J. M., Bear, C. E., and Riordan, J. R. (1991). Expression of the cystic fibrosis gene in non-epithelial invertebrate cells produces a regulated anion conductance. *Cell* 64: 681–691.

Knowles, M. R., Murray, G. F., Shallal, J. A., Askin, F., Ranga, V., Gatzy, J. T., and Boucher, R. C. (1984). Bioelectric properties and ion flow across excised human bronchi. *J. Appl. Physiol.* 56: 868–877.

Koefoed-Johnsen, V., and Ussing, H. H. (1958). The nature of the frog skin potential. *Acta Physiol. Scand.* 42: 298–308.

Kondo, M., Finkbeiner, W. E., and Widdicombe, J. H. (1991). A simple technique for culture of highly differentiated cells from dog tracheal epithelium. *Am. J. Physiol.* 261: L106–L117.

Landry, D. W., Akabas, M. H., Redhead, C., Edelman, A., Cragoe, E. J., and Al-Awqati, Q. (1989). Purification and reconstitution of chloride channels from kidney and trachea. *Science* 244: 1469–1472.

Langridge-Smith, J. E., Field, M., and Dubinsky, W. P. (1983). Isolation of transporting plasma membrane vesicles from bovine tracheal epithelium. *Biochim. Biophys. Acta* 731: 318–328.

Langridge-Smith, J. E., Rao, M. C., and Field, M. (1984). Chloride and sodium transport across bovine tracheal epithelium: Effects of secretagogues and indomethacin. *Pflugers Arch.* 402: 42–47.

Lazarus, S. C., Basbaum, C. B., Barnes, P. J., and Gold, W. M. (1986). cAMP immunocytochemistry provides evidence for functional VIP receptors in trachea. *Am. J. Physiol.* 251: C115–C119.

Leikauf, G., Ueki, I. F., Nadel, J. A., and Widdicombe, J. H. (1985). Bradykinin stimulates chloride secretion and prostaglandin E₂ release by canine tracheal epithelium. *Am. J. Physiol.* 248: F48–F55.

Leikauf, G. D., Ueki, I. F., Widdicombe, J. H., and Nadel, J. A. (1986). Alteration of chloride secretion across canine tracheal epithelium by lipoxygenase products of arachidonic acid. *Am. J. Physiol.* 250: F47–F53.

Li, M., McCann, J. D., Liedtke, C. M., Nairn, A. C., Greengard, P., and Welsh, M. J. (1988). Cyclic AMP-dependent protein kinase opens chloride channels in normal but not cystic fibrosis airway epithelium. *Nature* 331: 358–360.

Liedtke, C. M. (1989). α-Adrenergic regulation of NaCl cotransport in human airway epithelium. *Am. J. Physiol.* 257: L125–L129.

Liedtke, C. M. (1990). Calcium and α-adrenergic regulation of Na-Cl(K) cotransport in rabbit tracheal epithelial cells. *Am. J. Physiol.* 259: L66–L72.

Loughlin, G. M., Gerencser, G. A., Crowder, M. A., Boyd, R. L., and Mangos, J. A. (1982). Fluid fluxes in the ferret trachea. *Experientia* 38: 1451–1452.

Lucas, A. M., and Douglas, L. C. (1934). Principles underlying ciliary activity in the respiratory tract II. A comparison of nasal clearance in man, monkey and other mammals. *Arch. Otolaryngol.* 20: 518–541.

Marin, M. G., Davis, B., and Nadel, J. A. (1976). Effect of acetylcholine on Cl^- and Na^+ fluxes across dog tracheal epithelium in vitro. *J. Appl. Physiol.* 231: 1546–1549.

Marin, M. G., Davis, B., and Nadel, J. A. (1977). Effect of histamine on electrical and ion transport properties of tracheal epithelium. *J. Appl. Physiol.* 42: 735–738.

McCann, J. D., Bhalla, R. C., and Welsh, M. J. (1989). Release of intracellular calcium by two different second messengers in airway epithelium. *Am. J. Physiol.* 257: L116–L124.

McCann, J. D., Matsuda, J., Garcia, M., Kaczorowski, G., and Welsh, M. J. (1990). Basolateral K^+ channels in airway epithelia. I. Regulation by Ca^{2+} and block by charybdotoxin. *Am. J. Physiol.* 258: L334–L342.

McCann, J. D., and Welsh, M. J. (1990). Basolateral K^+ channels in airway epithelia II. Role in Cl^- secretion and evidence for two types of K^+ channel. *Am. J. Physiol.* 258: L343–L348.

Melon, J. (1968). Activite secretoire de la muquese nasale. *Acta Otorhinolaryngol. Belg.* 22: 11–244.

Musch, M. W., and Field, M. (1989). K-dependent Na–Cl cotransport in bovine tracheal epithelial cells. *Am. J. Physiol.* 256: C658–C665.

Nathanson, I. T., Widdicombe, J. H., and Nadel, J. (1983a). Effect of amphotericin B on ion and fluid movement across dog tracheal epithelium. *J. Appl. Physiol.* 55: 1257–1261.

Nathanson, I. T., Widdicombe, J. H., and Barnes, P. J. (1983b). Effect of vasoactive intestinal peptide on ion transport across dog tracheal epithelium. *J. Appl. Physiol.* 55: 1844–1848.

Negus, V. E. (1963). Functions of mucus. *Acta Otolaryngol.* 56: 204–214.

O'Grady, S. M., Palfrey, H. C., and Field, M. (1987). Characteristics and functions of Na-K–Cl cotransport in epithelial tissues. *Am. J. Physiol.* 253: C177–C192.

Olver, R., Davis, B., Marin, M., and Nadel, J. A. (1975). Active transport of Na^+ and Cl^- across the canine epithelium in vitro. *Am. Rev. Respir. Dis.* 112: 811–815.

Phipps, R. J., Denas, S. M., and Wanner, A. (1983). Antigen stimulates glycoprotein secretion and alters ion fluxes in sheep trachea. *J. Appl. Physiol.* 55: 1593–1602.

Pratt, A. D., Clancy, G., and Welsh, M. J. (1986). Mucosal adenosine stimulates chloride secretion in canine tracheal epithelium. *Am. J. Physiol.* 251: C167–C174.

Quinton, P. M. (1979). Composition and control of secretions from tracheal bronchial submucosal glands. *Nature* 279: 551–552.

Rangachari, P. K., McWade, D., and Donoff, B. (1987). Luminal tachykinin receptors on canine tracheal epithelium: Functional subtyping. *Regul. Pept.* 18: 101–108.

Sakmann, B., and Neher, E. (1983). Geometric parameters of pipettes and membrane patches. In *Single-Channel Recording*. Edited by B. Sakmann, and E. Neher. New York, Plenum Press, pp. 37–51.

Schoumacher, R. A., Shoemaker, R. L., Halm, D. R., Tallant, E. A., Wallace, R. W., and Frizzell, R. A. (1987). Phosphorylation fails to activate chloride channels from cystic fibrosis airway cells. *Nature* 330: 752–754.

Schultz, S. G. (1981). Homocellular regulatory mechanisms in sodium-transporting epithelia: Avoidance of extinction by "flush through." *Am. J. Physiol.* 241: F579–F590.

Seybold, Z. V., Mariassy, A. T., Mariassy, D., and Kim, C. S. (1990). Mucociliary interaction in vitro: Effects of physiological and inflammatory stimuli. *J. Appl. Physiol.* 68: 1421–1426.

Shen, B.-Q., Yang, C.-M., and Widdicombe, J. H. (1991). A rapid procedure for obtaining tracheal apical membranes. *Am. J. Physiol.* 261: L102–L105.

Shoemaker, R. L., Frizzell, R. A., Dwyer, T. M., and Farley, J. M. (1986). Single chloride channel currents from canine tracheal epithelial cells. *Biochim. Biophys. Acta* 858: 235–242.

Shorofsky, S. R., Field, M., and Fozzard, H. A. (1984). Mechanism of Cl secretion in canine trachea: Changes in intracellular chloride activity with secretion. *J. Membr. Biol.* 81: 1–8.

Shorofsky, S. R., Field, M., and Fozzard, H. A. (1986). Changes in intracellular sodium with chloride secretion in dog tracheal epithelium. *Am. J. Physiol.* 250: C646–C650.

Smith, P. L., and Frizzell, R. A. (1984). Chloride secretion by canine tracheal epithelium: IV. Basolateral membrane K permeability parallels secretion rate. *J. Membr. Biol.* 77: 187–199.

Smith, P. L., Welsh, M. J., Stoff, J. S., and Frizzell, R. A. (1982). Chloride secretion by canine tracheal epithelium: I. Role of intracellular cAMP levels. *J. Membr. Biol.* 70: 215–226.

Solc, C. K., and Wine, J. J. (1991). Swelling-induced and depolarization-induced Cl⁻ channels in normal and cystic fibrosis epithelial cells. *Am. J. Physiol.* 261: C658–C674.

Sommerhoff, C. P., and Finkbeiner, W. E. (1990). Human tracheobronchial submucosal gland cells in culture. *Am. J. Respir. Cell Mol. Biol.* 2: 41–50.

Tabcharani, J. A., Chang, X.-B., Riordan, J. R., and Hanrahan, J. W. (1991). Phosphorylation-regulated Cl⁻ channel in CHO cells stably expressing the cystic fibrosis gene. *Nature* 352: 628–631.

Tabcharani, J. A., Low, W., Elie, D., and Hanrahan, J. W. (1990). Low-conductance chloride channel activated by cAMP in the epithelial cell line T_{84}. *FEBS Lett.* 270: 157–164.

Tamaoki, J., Ueki, I. F., Widdicombe, J. H., and Nadel, J. A. (1988). Stimulation of Cl secretion by neurokinin A and neurokinin B in canine tracheal epithelium. *Am. Rev. Respir. Dis.* 137: 899–902.

Ueki, I., German, V. F., and Nadel, J. (1980). Micropipette measurement of airway submucosal gland secretion: Autonomic effects. *Am. Rev. Respir. Dis.* 121: 351–357.

Ussing, H. H., and Zerahn, K. (1951). Active transport of sodium as the source of electric current in short-circuited isolated frog skin. *Acta Physiol. Scand.* 23: 110–127.

Valdivia, H. H., Dubinsky, W. P., and Coronado, R. (1988). Reconstitution and phosphorylation of chloride channels from airway epithelium membranes. *Science* 242: 1441–1444.

Van Scott, M. R., Lee, N. P., Yankaskas, J. R., and Boucher, R. C. (1988). Effect of hormones on growth and function of cultured canine tracheal epithelial cells. *Am. J. Physiol.* 255: C237–C245.

Vulliemin, P., Durand-Arczynska, W., and Durand, J. (1983). Electrical properties and electrolyte transport in bovine tracheal epithelium: Effects of ion substitutions, transport inhibitors and histamine. *Pflugers Arch.* 396: 54–59.

Wangemann, P., Wittner, M., Di Stefano, A., Englert, H. C., Lang, H. J., Schlatter, E., and Greger, R. (1986). Cl^--channel blockers in the thick ascending limb of the loop of Henle. Structure activity relationship. *Pflugers Arch.* 407: S128–S141.

Welsh, M. J. (1983a). Intracellular chloride activities in canine tracheal epithelium. Direct evidence for sodium-coupled chloride accumulation in chloride-secreting epithelium. *J. Clin. Invest.* 71: 1392–1401.

Welsh, M. J. (1983b). Evidence for a basolateral membrane potassium conductance in canine tracheal epithelium. *Am. J. Physiol.* 244: C377–C384.

Welsh, M. J. (1983c). Inhibition of chloride secretion by furosemide in canine tracheal epithelium. *J. Membr. Biol.* 71: 219–226.

Welsh, M. J. (1983d). Barium inhibition of basolateral membrane potassium conductance in tracheal epithelium. *Am. J. Physiol.* 244: F639–F645.

Welsh, M. J. (1984). Energetics of chloride secretion in canine tracheal epithelium: Comparison of the metabolic cost of chloride transport with the metabolic cost of sodium transport. *J. Clin. Invest.* 74: 262–268.

Welsh, M. J. (1986a). An apical-membrane chloride channel in human tracheal epithelium. *Science* 232: 1648–1650.

Welsh, M. J. (1986b). Single apical membrane anion channels in primary cultures of canine tracheal epithelium. *Pflugers Arch.* 407: S116–S122.

Welsh, M. J. (1987a). Effect of phorbol ester and calcium ionophore on chloride secretion in canine tracheal epithelium. *Am. J. Physiol.* 253: C828–C834.

Welsh, M. J. (1987b). Electrolyte transport by airway epithelia. *Physiol. Rev.* 67: 1143–1184.

Welsh, M. J., and McCann, J. D. (1985). Intracellular calcium regulates basolateral potassium channels in a chloride-secreting epithelium. *Proc. Natl. Acad. Sci. USA* 82: 8823–8826.

Welsh, M. J., and Liedtke, C. M. (1986). Chloride and potassium channels in cystic fibrosis airway epithelia. *Nature* 322: 467–470.

Welsh, M. J., Smith, P. L., and Frizzell, R. A. (1982). Chloride secretion by canine tracheal epithelium II. The cellular electrical potential profile. *J. Membr. Biol.* 70: 227–238.

Welsh, M. J., Smith, P. L., and Frizzell, R. A. (1983). Chloride secretion by canine tracheal epithelium: III. Membrane resistances and electromotive forces. *J. Membr. Biol.* 71: 209–218.

Welsh, M. J., Widdicombe, J. H., and Nadel, J. A. (1980). Fluid transport across the canine tracheal epithelium. *J. Appl. Physiol.* 49: 905–909.

Westenfelder, C., Earnest, W. R., and Al-Bazzaz, F. J. (1980). Characterization of Na-K-ATPase in dog tracheal epithelium: Enzymatic and ion transport measurements. *J. Appl. Physiol.* 48: 1008–1019.

Widdicombe, J. G. (1988). Force of capillarity tending to prevent drying of ciliary mucosa. In *The Airways*. Edited by M. A. Kaliner, and P. J. Barnes. New York, Marcel Dekker, p. 597.

Widdicombe, J. H. (1989). Airway diseases: Role of epithelium and inflammatory peptides. *Am. J. Physiol.* 257: L144–L146.

Widdicombe, J. H. (1990). Use of cultured airway epithelial cells in studies of ion transport. *Am. J. Physiol.* 258: L13–L18.

Widdicombe, J. H., and Welsh, M. J. (1980). Ion transport by dog tracheal epithelium. *Fed. Proc.* 39: 3062–3066.

Widdicombe, J. H., and Barthelson, R. A. (1988). Altered chloride transport across primary cultures of tracheal epithelium in cystic fibrosis. In *The Cellular and Molecular Basis of Cystic Fibrosis*. Edited by G. Mastella and P. Quinton. San Francisco, San Francisco Press, pp. 377–382.

Widdicombe, J. H., and Wine, J. J. (1991). The biochemical defect in cystic fibrosis. *Trends Biochem. Sci.* 16: 474–477.

Widdicombe, J. H., Basbaum, C. B., and Yee, J. Y. (1979a). Localization of Na pumps in the tracheal epithelium of the dog. *J. Cell Biol.* 82: 380–390.

Widdicombe, J. H., Ueki, I. F., Bruderman, I., and Nadel, J. A. (1979b). The effects of sodium substitution and ouabain on ion transport by dog tracheal epithelium. *Am. Rev. Respir. Dis.* 120: 385–392.

Widdicombe, J. H., Basbaum, C. B., and Highland, E. (1981). Ion contents and other properties of isolated cells from dog tracheal epithelium. *Am. J. Physiol.* 241: C184–C192.

Widdicombe, J. H., Nathanson, I. T., and Highland, E. (1983). Effects of "loop" diuretics on ion transport by dog tracheal epithelium. *Am. J. Physiol.* 245: C388–C396.

Widdicombe, J. H., Welsh, M. J., and Finkbeiner, W. E. (1985a). Cystic fibrosis decreases the apical membrane chloride permeability of monolayers cultured from cells of tracheal epithelium. *Proc. Natl. Acad. Sci. USA* 82: 6167–6171.

Widdicombe, J. H., Coleman, D. L., Finkbeiner, W. E., and Tuet, I. K. (1985b). Electrical properties of monolayers cultured from cells of human tracheal mucosa. *J. Appl. Physiol.* 58: 1729–1735.

Widdicombe, J. H., Basbaum, C. B., and Highland, E. (1986). Sodium-pump density of cells from dog tracheal mucosa. *Am. J. Physiol.* 248: C389–C398.

Wiedner, G. (1976). Method to detect volume flows in the nanoliter range. *Rev. Sci. Instrum.* 47: 775–776.

Willumsen, N. J., and Boucher, R. C. (1989a). Shunt resistance and ion permeabilities in normal and cystic fibrosis airway epithelia. *Am. J. Physiol.* 256: C1054–C1063.

Willumsen, N. J., and Boucher, R. C. (1989b). Activation of an apical Cl^- conductance by Ca^{2+} ionophores in cystic fibrosis airway epithelia. *Am. J. Physiol.* 256: C226–C233.

Worman, H. J., Brasitus, T. A., Dudeja, P. K., Fozzard, H. A., and Field, M. (1986). Relationship between lipid fluidity and water permeability of bovine tracheal epithelial cell apical membranes. *Biochemistry* 25: 1549–1555.

Wright, E. M., and Diamond, J. M. (1977). Anion selectivity in biological systems. *Physiol. Rev.* 57: 109–156.

Yamaya, M., Finkbeiner, W. E., and Widdicombe, J. H. (1991a). Ion transport by cultures of human tracheobronchial submucosal glands. *Am. J. Physiol.* 261: L485–L490.

Yamaya, M., Finkbeiner, W. E., and Widdicombe, J. H. (1991b). Altered ion transport by tracheal glands in cystic fibrosis. *Am. J. Physiol.* 261: L491–L494.

Yamaya, M., Finkbeiner, W. E., Chun, S. Y., and Widdicombe, J. H. (1992). Differentiated structure and function of cultures from human tracheal epithelium. *Am. J. Physiol.* 262: L713–L724.

Yang, C. M., Farley, J. M., and Dwyer, T. M. (1988). Acetylcholine-stimulated chloride flux in tracheal submucosal gland cells. *J. Appl. Physiol.* 65: 1891–1894.

Yankaskas, J. R., Cotton, C. U., Knowles, M. R., Gatzy, J. T., and Boucher, R. C. (1985). Culture of human nasal epithelial cells on collagen matrix supports. A comparison of bioelectric properties of normal and cystic fibrosis epithelia. *Am. Rev. Respir. Dis.* 132: 1281–1287.

Yoneda, K. (1976). Mucous blanket of rat bronchus: Ultrastructural study. *Am. Rev. Respir. Dis.* 114: 837–842.

11

Epithelial Goblet Cell Secretion

KWANG CHUL KIM

University of Maryland School of Pharmacy
Baltimore, Maryland

I. Introduction

The goblet cell is named because of its unique shape. It is characterized by the presence of secretory granules that are also unique in their appearance, as described in the earlier chapter. These granules are positively stained by periodic acid–Schiff (PAS), owing to the presence of carbohydrates, and are electron-lucent when conventionally osmicated for transmission electron microscopy (Jeffrey, 1978). It is believed that the substance responsible for this unique histocytochemical characteristic of goblet cells is mucous glycoprotein or mucin. However, these secretory granules have never been analyzed biochemically and likely contain not only mucins, but also non-mucin proteins (Christensen and Hayes, 1982; Water et al., 1986). These secretory granules are exocytosed through the apical cell membrane and then become part of airway luminal fluid. Since the amount of airway luminal fluid present under normal physiological conditions is small, lavage samples from pathological lungs have been used to study the biochemistry of airway secretions. However, the airway luminal contents from pathological samples are derived from various cell types and also contain various kinds of active proteinases. Therefore, it became necessary to develop a goblet cell culture system to study airway goblet cell secretions.

Epithelial cells from the trachea are easier to prepare for anatomical reasons than are epithelial cells from lower conducting airways. Wu and Smith (1982) were first able to grow tracheal epithelial (TE) cells from rabbits. Later, Lee et al. (1984) showed that the differentiated morphologic structure could be maintained if hamster TE cells were grown on a collagen gel matrix. With radiolabeling techniques, Kim et al. (1985) demonstrated that hamster TE cells grown on a thick collagen gel matrix produce mucin-like glycoproteins that are indistinguishable from in vivo airway mucins in carbohydrate structure. Thus, cultured TE cells have allowed us to study airway goblet cell secretions in vitro. For details of various TE cell cultures, see recent review articles (Van Scott et al., 1986; Wu, 1986). In this chapter, I will focus mainly on the cell biology of airway goblet cell mucin secretion.

II. Mucins Produced by Cultured Tracheal Epithelial Cells

Tracheal epithelial cells can be grown on either a plastic surface or a thick collagen gel. When confluent cultures of either type were metabolically labeled with [^{3}H]glucosamine, they both produced high relative molecular mass (M_r) glyco-conjugates, which were excluded from a Sepharose CL-4B column. However, the glycoconjugates produced by cells grown on plastic surface were completely digested by hyaluronidase, whereas those produced by cells grown on a thick collagen gel were only partially digested by hyaluronidase (Kim, 1985) (Fig. 1). Biochemical characterization of these hyaluronidase-resistant glycoconjugates showed that they were mucin-like glycoproteins (Kim et al., 1985), with the following structural characteristics: (1) multimillion dalton M_r glycoproteins; (2) O-linked glycoproteins (i.e., the glycosidic linkage between N-acetylgalactos-amine of the oligosaccharides and serine or threonine of the protein); (3) sugars consisting of N-acetylgalactosamine, N-acetylglucosamine, galactose, fucose, and sialic acids, but not mannose; (4) the presence of poly(N-acetyllactosamine) moiety (Rearick et al., 1984); (5) extreme heterogeneity in both size and charge, the latter being due to the presence of sulfate and sialic acids; (6) resistance to glycosaminoglycan-digesting enzymes; and (7) buoyant densities of about 1.5 g/ml, based on CsCl density gradient centrifugation (Adler et al., 1990b; Kim, 1991a).

The term *mucin-like glycoprotein*, has been interchangeably referred to as mucin or *high molecular weight mucin-like glycoprotein* in the literature, since there is not yet a clear structural definition of mucin. It is important to understand that the current structural information of mucins or mucin-like glycoproteins has been derived from a subpopulation of glycoproteins that has been *preselected* based on their high M_r. Since mucins are extremely heterogeneous in size, there

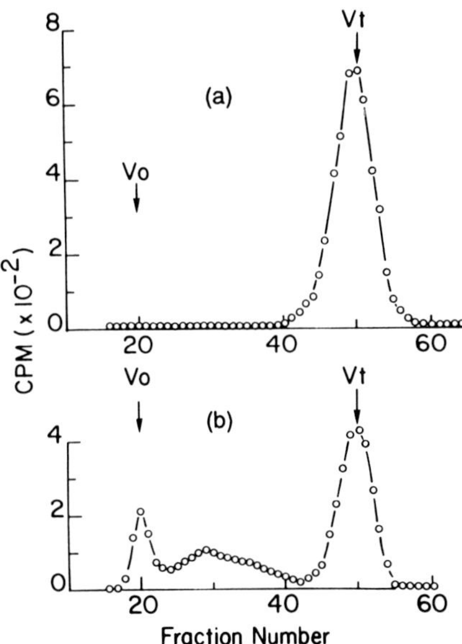

Figure 1   Gel filtration of high M_r glycoconjugates after hyaluronidase treatment. High M_r glycoconjugates released by confluent rabbit TE cells grown either (a) on a plastic surface or (b) on a thick collagen gel were treated with streptomyces hyaluronidase and subjected to Sepharose CL-4B column chromatography. V_0 and V_t represent void volume and total volume, respectively. Note that TE cells grown on a thick collagen gel produce hyaluronidase-resistant glycoconjugates. (Data from Kim, 1985)

may be mucins with "small" M_r. It seems that a clear structural definition of airway mucin awaits elucidation of its protein structure(s), which seems to depend heavily on the discovery of mucin genes. Until that time, mucin-like glycoprotein seems to be the most accurate term. Throughout this chapter, I will use the term *mucin* for both in vivo and in vitro mucins.

III.   Proteoglycans Produced by Cultured Tracheal Epithelial Cells

Both mucins and proteoglycans contain oligosaccharides attached to their core proteins. Since some proteoglycans are produced virtually by all cells grown in culture and since mucins may trap other macromolecules, presumably because of their viscoelastic property, it became necessary to check whether or not these high M_r mucin-like glycoproteins secreted from TE cells contain proteoglycans. A major structural difference between these glycoconjugates is that the protein backbone of proteoglycans is not only attached to oligosaccharides, as seen in mucins, but also to varying lengths of sugar chains called glycosaminoglycans (GAGs), consisting mainly of repeating disaccharide units that are sulfated to various degrees (Fig. 2). Therefore, individual proteoglycans can be separated using anion-exchange columns and identified using enzymes that can degrade the glycosaminoglycans. When confluent TE cells were metabolically double-labeled with Na^{35}SO$_4$ and [^{3}H]glucosamine, and the spent medium was subjected to DEAE-Sephacel anion-exchange column chromatography, followed by enzyme digestion, types of proteoglycans identified were hyaluronic acid, chondroitin sulfate proteoglycans (mainly 4-sulfated), and heparan sulfate proteoglycans (Kim et al., 1989). By using glycosaminoglycan-degrading enzymes, it was proved that the mucin preparation did not contain the foregoing proteoglycans (Kim et al., 1985, 1989). There still remains confusion concerning the possible contamination of type II keratan sulfate proteoglycan in the mucin preparation: this proteoglycan shares so many structural characteristics with mucins (Hascall, 1981) that a clear distinction between these two glycoconjugates is not yet possible. For details, see a recent review article (Kim, 1991b).

These proteoglycans are secreted by virtually all types of cultured cells, and their role in cellular function still seems unclear. In mast cells, some of these proteoglycans are found in secretory granules (Yurt et al., 1977; Stevens et al., 1985) and have been suggested to play a crucial role in minimizing autolysis by ionically binding basically charged carboxypeptidases (Everitt and Neurath, 1980)

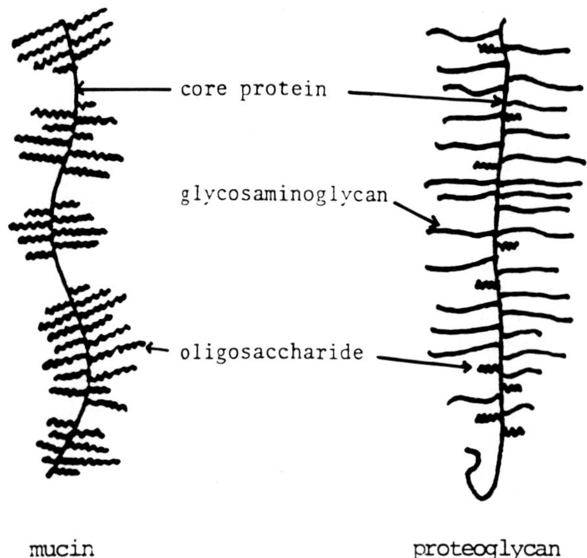

Figure 2   Schematic structures of mucins and proteoglycans.

and serine proteinases (Trong et al., 1987) inside the granules. The localization and function of these proteoglycans in the airway goblet cell is an interesting topic that remains to be explored.

IV. Localization of Mucin in Cultured Tracheal Epithelial Cells

Mucins contain terminal *N*-acetylgalactosamines that can bind to a lectin, *Helix pomatia* agglutinin (HPA). With use of gold-conjugated HPA lectin, Roth (1984) demonstrated that HPA binds to two major subcellular components of intestinal goblet cells, the Golgi and the secretory granule. The former binding is due to the presence of *N*-acetylgalactosamine as a linking sugar and the latter is due to the presence of terminal *N*-acetylgalactosamine in mature mucins inside the secretory granule. Mucin produced by cultured TE cells also contains *N*-acetylgalactosamine as both the linking and terminal sugars (Kim et al., 1985). With the same techniques used by Roth, Wasano et al. (1988) demonstrated that HPA can bind not only to the Golgi and the secretory granule, but also to the surface of TE secretory cells. No HPA binding was observed in ciliated cells either in vivo or in vitro. This cell surface HPA binding was not removed by extensive washing, suggesting the nature of tight binding. With sodium dodecyl sulfate–polyacrylamide gel electrophoresis (SDS–PAGE), followed by ^{125}I-HPA binding on the gel, it was shown that there were three HPA-binding glycoproteins in cultured TE cells (Wasano et al., 1988); a 120-kd glycoprotein, which is an integral glycoprotein and found throughout the culture period (i.e., both immature and mature cells), and 220-kd and high M_r glycoproteins, which are found in both soluble and membrane fractions, but only from confluent cultures (i.e., mature secretory cells). The term high M_r was chosen since they could not enter the 4–12% gradient gel. Purified mucin also bound to HPA and could not enter the same gradient gel. Thus, the high M_r HPA-binding glycoprotein band should contain mucins, whereas the 220-kd glycoprotein(s) likely represents immature mucins associated with the Golgi. We were particularly interested in the cell surface HPA-binding glycoproteins.

Both the cell surface HPA binding and mucin secretion increased concomitantly at confluence. However, there was no significant changes in the level of the 120-kd glycoprotein at confluence, suggesting that the cell surface HPA-binding glycoprotein at confluence may be mucin itself. About this time, we also found that human neutrophil elastase could release mucin from hamster TE cell cultures, apparently without granule exocytosis, and the same enzyme had an ability to degrade the released mucin (Kim et al., 1987). When human neutrophil elastase was added into confluent cultures, and both the degree of the cell surface HPA binding and the amount of the cellular HPA-binding glycoproteins were examined in the elastase-treated cultures, there was almost an equal degree of decrease in both the cell surface lectin binding and the density of the high M_r HPA band (Kim et al., 1987). From these data, it was clear that the high M_r HPA-binding glycoproteins released by human neutrophil elastase were mucins and were localized on the surface of secretory cells.

In summary, it appears that airway goblet cell mucins are localized in both secretory granules and on the surface of goblet cells.

V. Mucins are Associated with Lipids and Other Proteins

During the preparation of cellular mucin, some cellular mucin copurified as part of external membrane glycoproteins (Wasano et al., 1988), suggesting the hydrophobic nature of cellular mucins. Since some cellular mucins were hydrophobic and some were associated with the cell surface, we decided to see whether secreted mucins were also hydrophobic. By using metabolic radiolabeling with [³H]acetate, [³H]palmitate, or [³H]mevalonate, we were able to see that confluent TE cells synthesized and secreted a variety of lipids: neutral lipids, phospholipids, and glycolipids, and a significant portion of these lipids were associated with secreted mucin (Kim et al., 1989). Most of these lipids associated with mucin could be dissociated by treatment with detergents, such as 0.1% SDS and *N*-octylglucopyranoside, but about 3% of the lipids remained associated with mucin (Kim and Singh, 1990b). This trace amount of lipids could not be removed by CsCl density gradient centrifugation (unpublished data), strongly suggesting the presence of covalent binding between mucin and lipids. It was previously shown by Slomiany et al. (1983) that palmitic acid was covalently bound to intestinal mucins obtained from cystic fibrosis patients. However, the covalent binding of lipids is not generally believed to hold true for airway mucins (Carlstedt and Sheehan, 1984; Houdret et al., 1986). In any event, it was clear that mucins released by TE cells were extremely hydrophobic and associated with a variety of lipids.

In addition to lipids, these in vitro mucins were associated also with "small" glycoproteins and could be dissociated by heat denaturation and detergent treatment (Kim, 1991a), but not by 4 M guanidine HCl (Kim and Singh, 1990b). Several laboratories previously used 4–6 M guanidine HCl routinely as a "dissociative" agent during mucin preparation from pathological mucus samples. Neither the origin nor the biochemical nature of these small glycoproteins are now known. Nevertheless, both cellular and secreted mucins are extremely hydrophobic and associated with various macromolecules.

VI. Lipid Association with Mucin May Take Place Before Release

The association of mucins with lipids could take place after secretion, since mucins are hydrophobic. It is also possible that their association may have taken place before secretion, since cellular mucins are also hydrophobic, and some of them are even found associated with the cell surface, presumably with some membrane lipids. To examine these possibilities, confluent cells were metabolically labeled with radioactive lipid precursors, and lipids associated with both cellular and released mucin were analyzed quantitatively. The result showed that lipid profiles from both mucins were almost identical (Kim and Singh, 1990a), suggesting that the lipids were already associated with mucins before secretion and, accordingly, were released as an associated form. From these data, we have developed the following model of goblet cell mucin secretion.

VII. A Molecular Model of Goblet Cell Mucin Secretion

Airway goblet cell mucins seem to be secreted by two secretory pathways; a constitutive or nongranular pathway, and a regulated or granular pathway. Cultured TE cells secrete mucins continuously, most likely by a constitutive pathway (Wasano et al., 1988), and these mucins seem to be derived from a rapidly turning over mucin pool (Kim et al., 1987). A similar pathway of mucin secretion was also observed in intestinal goblet cells (Neutra et al., 1982). Given the hydrophobicity of mucins, we hypothesize the following model for goblet cell mucin secretion (Fig. 3):

1. Mucins are stored inside small vesicles or large secretory granules.
2. Secretory vesicles or granules contain not only mucins, but also other macromolecules such as small glycoproteins and lipids. These macromolecules are packaged in a rather polarized fashion: some hydrophobic moieties of mucins (i.e., portions of the protein backbone) are associated with the granule inner membrane through both the hydrophobic and covalent binding, whereas the hydrophilic portion of mucins including negatively charged groups (i.e., SO_4^{2-} and COO^- of sialic acids) are associated with other proteins and cations such as Ca^{2+} (Villalon et al., 1988), in such a way that they maximize the thermodynamic stability of the granules.
3. During exocytosis, these storage granules are fused with the plasma membrane. Some mucins are released along with lipids and proteins, whereas other mucins remain attached to the outer plasma membrane. These cell surface mucins can be released by proteinases, such as those released by neutrophils during airway inflammation, or possibly by some endogenous proteinases under normal physiological conditions.

Small secretory vesicles may be released through a constitutive pathway to supply a small amount of mucins constantly cleared from the airway lumen, whereas release of large secretory granules may take place only in response to abnormal physiological stimuli, such as inhalation of irritant gases or airway

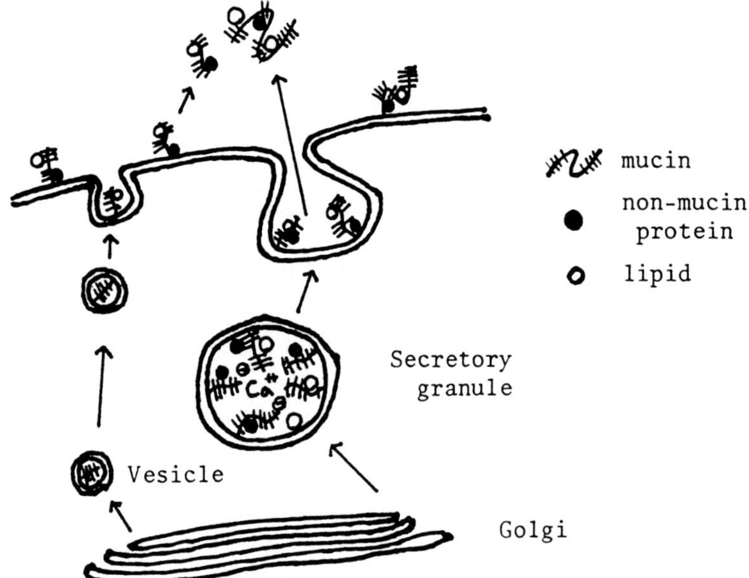

Figure 3   A proposed molecular model of goblet cell mucin secretion.

inflammation, to provide a rather large amount of mucins. It is also possible that mucins released constitutively may be different from mucins released by the granule exocytosis. However, validity of this model requires identification of a mechanism by which mucins are anchored to the plasma membrane.

VIII.   Regulation of Goblet Cell Mucin Release

Pharmacology of airway mucin secretion has been reviewed elsewhere (Widdicombe, 1978; Reid et al., 1983; Spicer and Martinez, 1984; Nadel, 1985; Marin, 1986; Adler, 1986; Kim, 1991b). However, our incomplete knowledge of airway mucin biochemistry has caused much confusion in studying the regulation of mucin secretion. In whole-animal models, the degree of secretion was monitored morphometrically by quantifying PAS-positive secretory granules. On the other hand, in in vitro culture systems, mucins were measured using biochemical assays. Since most of our current understanding of the regulation of airway goblet cell mucin secretion is based on these in vitro culture systems, I will discuss some potential problems related to use of in vitro systems for studying mucin secretion.

A. The Culture System

Most in vitro studies dealing with the regulation of airway mucin secretion have been carried out using tracheal organ or explant cultures that contain both surface epithelial goblet cells and submucosal glands. The coexistence of these two mucin sources in the same tissue makes it difficult to study regulation of individual mucin sources. Tracheas from rabbits and hamsters have been used in studying regulation of goblet cell mucin secretion because they contain few submucosal glands. However, organ cultures have other serious problems, such as instability of the culture system (Niles et al., 1986) and possible involvement of neighboring cells (e.g., smooth muscle) (Kim and Brody, 1987) and inflammatory cells, in regulation of mucin release. The recent availability of TE cell culture systems has made it possible to study the pharmacology of airway goblet cell mucin release at the cellular and biochemical levels (Kim and Brody, 1989).

B. Mucin Assays

Because of relatively low basal rates of mucin secretion from in vitro cultures, cultures are generally radiolabeled using metabolic precursors such as [^{3}H]- or [^{14}C]glucosamine, [^{3}H]- or [^{14}C]amino acids, and Na^{35}SO$_4$. The radiolabeled mucins released are then quantitated using one of the four assay systems as follows.

Precipitation with Trichloroacetic Acid–Phosphotungstic Acid or Ethanol

The precipitation method is based on the fact that macromolecules (radiolabeled glycoconjugates, here) can be precipitated by either trichloroacetic acid–phosphotungstic acid (TCA–PTA) or ethanol. It is quick and reproducible, and many samples can be handled in a short time. However, the method is extremely nonspecific and counts virtually all the glycoconjugates released, including mucins. The amount of mucins constitutes normally 20–50% of the total glyco-conjugates in the spent medium sample.

Gel Filtration

Gel filtration is based on an assumption that mucins are at least 1 million Da in size. Since each sample needs one separate column, which has to be completely washed before applying the next sample, this method is extremely slow and laborious. Multiple samples can be loaded into multiple columns at the same time and void volumes can be collected using a time-synchronized device, as described by Cheng et al. (1981). However, the variable performance among individual columns is a common problem; thus, constant monitoring of the column perfor-mance is required. The samples should be heat-denatured and run using an elution buffer containing detergents, owing to the hydrophobic nature of mucins (Kim, 1991a). One potential problem of this method would be that the small mucins (Kim et al., 1989) are not counted. Nevertheless, this is the most accurate method yet available, if used properly.

Helix Pomatia Agglutinin Lectin Binding

The lectin-binding method is based on the finding that purified mucins can bind to HPA. It is quick and reproducible, but seems to have a serious problem when one intends to use this method for measuring the amount of mucins in the sample. Since the lectin binds to terminal N-acetylgalactosamine of mucin molecules, the heterogeneity of oligosaccharide structure of mucins, for example, the variable number of N-acetylgalactosamines in each mucin molecule, will make it diffi-cult to determine the amount of mucin in the sample. We found that not all mucins produced by TE cells bind to an HPA affinity column (unpublished data).

Use of Antimucin Antibodies

The antimucin antibody method is based on the highly specific interaction of an antibody with its epitope in a mucin molecule. Virtually all the antibodies yet characterized seem to recognize the carbohydrate moiety of mucin molecules. Although this method is extremely sensitive and can handle a great number of samples with great reproducibility, it has exactly the same problems as the HPA method does. In addition, both the sample preparation and the assay condition should be carefully controlled, since the possible aggregation of these gigantic mucin molecules with other macromolecules may cause a significant steric hindrance to the antibody interactions.

In summary, none of the existing methods are perfect for various reasons. A better method can be developed only when the complete structure of mucins is elucidated. Meanwhile, the gel filtration method seems to be the most accurate from the biochemical point of view, if used accurately with properly radiolabeled samples. Following is a summary of studies of airway goblet cell mucin release employing various methods as described in the foregoing.

C.   Effects of Agents on Airway Goblet Cell Mucin Secretion

Irritant Gases

Chemical irritants are well known for their stimulatory effects on airway goblet cell mucus. Mucous granules of airway goblet cells were released by tobacco smoke in intact rat airways (Jones et al., 1973) and by sulfur dioxide inhalation in intact canine airways (Spicer et al., 1974). Ammonia vapor stimulated mucin release from intact cat tracheas (Gallagher et al., 1986). Inhaled irritant gases, such as sulfur dioxide, nitric oxide, or ammonia, will be dissolved in airway luminal fluid, changing the fluid pH to acidic or alkaline. In cultured hamster TE cells, a medium pH of either below 4 or above 9 caused mucin release as a result of plasma membrane damage (Kim et al., 1989).

Neuronal Control

Airway epithelium is free of autonomic innervation and, thus, it is not likely that neurotransmitters released from these nerve terminals have any direct influence on airway goblet cells. In the isolated cat tracheal epithelium, goblet cell mucin release was not stimulated by either adrenergic or cholinergic drugs (Sherman et al., 1981). Mucin release from cultured hamster TE cells was also resistant to these drugs (Kim, 1991b). However, in intact guinea pigs, vagal stimulation of the airway caused goblet cell granule exocytosis, indicating the presence of neural control of goblet cell mucous secretion (Tokuyama et al., 1990). In the same system, goblet cell granule exocytosis was also induced by either capsaicin or substance P, most likely through local axonal reflexes in which capsaicin causes release of neuropeptides from sensory nerves and the released neuropeptides induce mucous discharge (Kuo et al., 1990). The direct stimulatory effect of the neuropeptides has not yet been demonstrated in cultured cells. Neither histamine nor serotonin had any effect on mucin release from cultured hamster TE cells (Kim, 1991b).

Inflammatory Mediators

Prostaglandins (PG) E_2 and $F_{2\alpha}$, and leukotrienes-C_4 and D_4 did not influence mucin release in cultured hamster TE cells (Kim et al., 1989); however, in cultured guinea pig TE cells, mucin release was stimulated by prostaglandin $F_{2\alpha}$ (Adler et al., 1990c). In intact guinea pig airways, inhaled leukotriene-D_4 caused release of mucous granules from goblet cells (Hoffstein et al., 1990).

Platelet-activating factor (PAF) induced mucin release in rodent tracheal organ cultures as well as in human tracheal organ explants by two seemingly different mechanisms: (1) an increased intracellular leukotriene production by mucin-secreting cells, which seems responsible for their own mucin release in rodent tracheal organ explants (Adler et al., 1987); and (2) extracellular leuko-trienes released by other cells responsible for mucin release from mucin-secreting cells in human tracheal organ explants (Goswami et al., 1989). Platelet-activating factor also released mucin directly from cultured canine TE cells (Rieves, 1992) and guinea pig TE cells by stimulation of lipoxygenase metabolism of arachidonic acid to hydroxyeicosatetraenoic acids (HETEs) (Adler et al., 1992).

Proteinases

Proteinases released from bacteria associated with obstructive pulmonary diseases released mucins from cultured tracheal organ explants of rabbits (Klinger et al.,

1984) and from guinea pig tracheal explants (Adler et al., 1986), by proteolytic damage on the apical cell membrane or an apocrine mechanism (Klinger et al., 1984). Human neutrophil elastase released mucins from hamster tracheal organ explants (Niles et al., 1986) and also in cultured hamster TE cells (Kim et al., 1987) by proteolytic cleavage of mucins bound to the apical cell surface (Kim et al., 1987; Breuer et al., 1989). However, elastase from the porcine pancreas had no such effects (Kim et al., 1987).

Superoxide

Superoxide, which is produced by activated neutrophils during airway inflammation, released mucins from cultured guinea pig TE cells by increased $PGF_{2\alpha}$ production by the TE cells (Adler et al., 1990c). Neither hydrogen peroxide, a major product of superoxide, nor free radicals derived from hydrogen peroxide had any effect on mucin release in the same system. In response to superoxide, an increased phospholipase C activity was also observed in guinea pig TE cells (Adler et al., 1990a).

Nucleotides

Nucleotides are present in high concentrations inside cells (>5 mM ATP in the cytosol; Gordon, 1987), and may be present in high concentrations in inflamed airways owing to release from damaged cells. Some purine nucleotides have recently been shown to stimulate mucin release from cultured hamster TE cells by a P_2 purinoceptor-mediated mechanism (Kim and Lee, 1991; Kim et al., 1992). ATP, a prototype agonist of the P_2 purinoceptor released mucins through a mechanism involving an increased phosphatidylinositol turnover, which appears to be mediated, at least in part, by a pertussis toxin-sensitive mechanism (Kim et al., 1993). However, the detailed mechanism of P_2 purinoceptor-mediated mucin release remains to be elucidated.

Mechanical Strain

Hypoosmolarity increased mucin release, whereas hyperosmolarity decreased it in cultured hamster TE cells (Kim et al., 1989). On the other hand, contraction of the gel on which TE cells were cultured induced mucin release without causing cell damage (Kim and Brody, 1987). Since both the osmolarity change and the gel contraction can cause mechanical strain on secretory cells, the mechanical factor could be a cause of mucin release under the foregoing experimental conditions. We have recently demonstrated that a direct mechanical strain on culture TE cells could increase mucin release at least twofold, without cell membrane damage (unpublished data). This situation may exist in vivo: considering that airway epithelium is physically associated with underlying smooth muscles, contractility of airway smooth muscles can cause mechanical strain on goblet cells and, thereby, may stimulate mucin release. This might be an important regulator for physiological secretion of airway goblet cell mucins in vivo.

IX. Perspectives

Availability of airway epithelial cell culture systems has allowed us to begin to study airway epithelial secretions at the cellular and molecular levels. However, it is important to fully understand the culture system before using it as an in vitro model, since growth and differentiation of these mixed cells depend on the culture conditions, such as the matrix, the culture medium, and the polarity. Because of the limited amount of information, it may be premature to develop any molecular model of airway goblet cell mucin secretion at this moment. Nevertheless, there are some important questions that may be answered using one of these culture system, preferentially the air–liquid biphasic culture system. These include the following: (1) What is the mechanism by which mucins secrete constitutively? (2) What are the conditions and mechanisms for large granule secretion? (3) What substances are present in the secretory granules, and what are their roles? (4) What is the mechanism by which mucins are anchored on the cell surface? (5) Is the goblet cell membrane polarized in terms of its responsiveness to various secretion modulators?

Finally, it is worth emphasizing that, despite the advantages the cell culture system can provide in terms of stability and relative homogeneity of the cell population, it has possible limitations, especially when one uses the cell culture as a model for studying certain functions in vivo. This seems to be especially important in studying the regulation of airway goblet cell mucin secretion.

Acknowledgments

I thank Dr. Kenneth Adler at North Carolina State University Veterinary Medicine and Dr. Jeffrey Berman at Boston University Pulmonary Center for their comments and suggestions throughout the manuscript. Preparation of this chapter was supported by a grant from NIH, HL-47125.

References

Adler, K. B. (1986). Mucin secretion by explants of respiratory tissue in vitro. In *In Vitro Models of Respiratory Epithelium*. Edited by L. J. Schiff. Boca Raton, CRC Press, pp. 27–50.
Adler, K. M., Hendley, D. D., and Davis, G. S. (1986). Bacteria associated with obstructive

pulmonary disease elaborate extracellular products that stimulate mucin secretion by explants of guinea pig airways. *Am. J. Pathol.* 125: 501–514.

Adler, K. B., Schwarz, J. E., Anderson, W. H., and Welton, A. F. (1987). Platelet activating factor stimulates secretion of mucin by explants of rodent airways in organ culture. *Exp. Lung Res.* 13: 25–43.

Adler, K. B., Akley, N. J., and Lee, J. (1990a). Oxygen metabolites stimulate inositol turnover in guinea pig airway epithelial cells in organotypic culture. *Am. Rev. Respir. Dis.* 141: A107.

Adler, K. B., Cheng, P. W., and Kim, K. C. (1990b). Characterization of guinea pig tracheal epithelial cells maintained in biphasic organotypic culture: Cellular composition and biochemical analysis of released glycoconjugates. *Am. J. Respir. Cell Mol. Biol.* 2: 145–154.

Adler, K. B., Holden-Stauffer, W. J., and Repine, J. D. (1990c). Oxygen metabolites stimulate release of high molecular-weight glycoconjugates by cell and organ cultures of rodent respiratory epithelium via an arachidonic acid-dependent mechanism. *J. Clin. Invest.* 85: 75–85.

Adler, K. B., Akley, N. J., and Glasgow, W. C. (1992). Platelet-activating-factor provokes release of mucin-like glycoproteins from guinea pig respiratory epithelial cells via a lipoxygenase-dependent mechanism. *Am. J. Respir. Cell Mol. Biol.* 6: 550–556.

Breuer, R., Christensen, T. G., Niles, R. M., Stone, P. J., and Snider, G. L. (1989). Human neutrophil elastase causes glycoconjugate release from the epithelial cell surface of hamster trachea in organ culture. *Am. Rev. Respir. Dis.* 139: 79–782.

Carlstedt, I., and Sheehan, J. K. (1984). Is the macromolecular architecture of cervical, respiratory and gastric mucins the same? *Biochem. Soc. Trans.* 12: 615–617.

Cheng, P. W., Sherman, J. M., Boat, T. F., and Bruce, M. (1981). Quantitation of radiolabeled mucous glycoproteins secreted by tracheal explants. *Anal. Biochem.* 117: 301–306.

Everitt, M. T., and Neurath, H. (1980). Rat peritoneal mast cell carboxypeptidase: Localization, purification, and enzymatic properties. *FEBS Lett.* 110: 292–296.

Christensen, T. G., and Hayes, J. A. (1982). Endoperoxidase in the conducting airways of hamsters: Morphological evidence of synthesis and secretion. *Am. Rev. Respir. Dis.* 125: 341–346.

Gallagher, J. T., Hall, R. L., Phipps, R. J., Jeffrey, P. K., Kent, P. W., and Richardson, P. S. (1986). Mucus-glycoproteins (mucins) of the cat trachea: Characterization and control of secretion. *Biochim. Biophys. Acta* 886: 243–254.

Gordon, J. L. (1986). Extracellular ATP: Effects, sources and fate. *Biochem. J.* 233: 309–319.

Goswami, S. K., Lhashi, M., Stathas, P., and Marom, Z. M. (1989). Platelet-activating factor stimulates secretion of respiratory glycoconjugate from human airways in culture. *J. Allergy Clin. Immunol.* 84: 726–734.

Hascall, V. C. (1981). Proteoglycans: Structure and function. In *Biology of Carbohydrates*, Vol. 1. Edited by C. Ginsburg. New York, John Wiley & Sons, pp. 1–50.

Hoffstein, S. T., Malo, P. E., Bugelski, P., Wheeldon, E. B. (1990). Leukotriene D4 induces mucus secretion from goblet cells in the guinea pig respiratory epithelium. *Exp. Lung Res.* 16: 711–725.

Houdret, N., Perini, J. M., Galabert, C., Scharfman, A., Humbert, P., Lamblin, G., and Roussel, P. (1986). The high lipid content of respiratory mucins in cystic fibrosis is related to infection. *Biochim. Biophys. Acta* 880: 54–61.

Jeffrey, P. K. (1978). Structure and function of mucus-secreting cells of cats and goose airway epithelium. In *Respiratory Mucus*. (A Ciba Foundation Symposium). Amsterdam, Elsevier/Excerpta Medica/North-Holland, pp. 5–20.

Jones, R., Boldue, P., and Reid, L. (1973). Goblet cell glycoprotein and tracheal gland hypertrophy in rat airway: the effect of tobacco smoke with or without the anti-inflammatory agent, phenylmethyloxidiazole. *Br. J. Exp. Pathol.* 54: 229–239.

Kim, K. C. (1985). Possible requirement of collagen gel substratum for production of mucin-like glycoproteins by primary rabbit tracheal epithelial cells in culture. *In Vitro* 21: 617–621.

Kim, K. C., Rearick, J. I., Nettesheim, P., and Jetten, A. M. (1985). Biochemical characterization of mucous glycoproteins synthesized and secreted by hamster tracheal epithelial cells in primary culture. *J. Biol. Chem.* 260: 4021–4027.

Kim, K. C., and Brody, J. S. (1987). Gel contraction causes mucin release in primary hamster tracheal epithelial cells growing on a collagen gel. *J. Cell Biol.* 105: 158a.

Kim, K. C., Wasano, K., Niles, R. M., Schuster, J. E., Stone, P. J., and Brody, J. S. (1987). Human neutrophil elastase releases cell surface mucins from primary cultures of hamster tracheal epithelial cells. *Proc. Natl. Acad. Sci. USA* 84: 9304–9308.

Kim, K. C., and Brody, J. S. (1989). Use of primary cell culture to study regulation of airway surface epithelial mucus secretion. In *Mucus and Related Topics*. Edited by E. N. Chantler, and N. A. Ratcliffe. Cambridge, Company of Biologists Limited, pp. 231–239.

Kim, K. C., Opaskar-Hincman, H., and Bhaskar, K. R. (1989). Secretions from primary hamster tracheal surface epithelial cells in culture: Mucin-like glycoproteins, proteoglycans, and lipids. *Exp. Lung Res.* 15: 299–314.

Kim, K. C., and Singh, B. N. (1990a). Association of lipids with mucins may take place prior to secretion: Studies with primary tracheal epithelial cells in culture. *Biorheology* 27: 491–501.

Kim, K. C., and Singh, B. N. (1990b). Hydrophobicity of mucin-like glycoproteins secreted by cultured tracheal epithelial cells: Association with lipids. *Exp. Lung Res.* 16: 279–292.

Kim, K. C. (1991a). Mucin-like glycoproteins secreted from cultured hamster tracheal surface epithelial cells: Their hydrophobic nature and amino acid composition. *Exp. Lung Res.* 17: 65–76.

Kim, K. C. (1991b). Biochemistry and pharmacology of mucin-like glycoproteins produced by cultured airway epithelial cells. *Exp. Lung Res.* 17: 533–545.

Kim, K. C., and Lee, B. C. (1991). P_2 purinoceptor regulation of mucin release by airway goblet cells in primary culture. *Br. J. Pharmacol.* 103: 1053–1056.

Kim, K. C., Wilson, A. K., and Lee, B. C. (1992). Nucleotides and mucin release from cultured airway epithelial cells. *Chest* 101: 68S–69S.

Kim, K. C., Zheng, Q. X., and Van Seuningen, I. (1993). Involvement of a signal transduction mechanism in ATP-induced mucin release from cultured airway goblet cells. *Am. J. Resp. Cell Mol. Biol.* 8: 121–125.

Klinger, J. D., Tandler, B., Liedke, C. M., and Boat, T. F. (1984). Proteases of *Pseudomonas aeruginosa* evoke mucin release by tracheal epithelium. *J. Clin. Invest.* 74: 1669–1678.

Kuo, H.-P., Rohde, J. A. L., Tokuyama, K., Barnes, P. J., and Rogers, D. F. (1990). Capsaicin and sensory neuropeptide stimulation of goblet cell secretion in guinea-pig trachea. *J. Physiol.* 431: 629–641.

Lee, T. C., Wu, R., Brody, A. R., Barrett, J. C., and Nettesheim, P. (1984). Growth and differentiation of hamster tracheal epithelial cells in culture. *Exp. Lung Res.* 6: 27–45.

Marin, M. G. (1986). Pharmacology of airway secretion. *Pharmacol. Rev.* 38: 273–289.

Nadel, J. A. (1985). Regulation of airway secretions. *Chest* 87(Suppl.): 111S–113S.

Neutra, M. R., O'Malley, L. J., and Specian, R. D. (1982). Regulation of intestinal goblet cell secretion. II. A survey of potential secretagogues. *Am. J. Physiol.* 242: G380–G387.

Niles, R. M., Christensen, T. G., Breuer, R., Stone, P. J., and Snider, G. L. (1986). Serine proteases stimulate mucous glycoprotein release from hamster tracheal ring organ culture. *J. Lab. Clin. Med.* 108: 489–497.

Rearick, J. I., Kim, K. C., Nettesheim, P., and Jetten, A. M. (1984). Hamster mucin secreted in vitro contains poly-*N*-acetyllactosamine oligosaccharides. *Fed. Proc.* 43: 1969.

Reid, L., Bhaskar, K., and Coles, S. (1983). Control and modulation of airway epithelial cells and their secretion. *Exp. Lung Res.* 4: 157–170.

Rieves, R. D., Goff, J., Wu, T., Larivee, P., Logun, C., and Shelhamer, J. H. (1992). Airway epithelial cell mucin release: Immunologic quantitation and response to platelet-activating factor. *Am. J. Respir. Cell Mol. Biol.* 6: 158–167.

Roth, J. (1984). Cytochemical localization of terminal *N*-acetyl-D-galactosamine residues in cellular compartments of intestinal goblet cells: Implications for the topology of *O*-glycosylation. *J. Cell Biol.* 98: 399–406.

Sherman, J. M., Cheng, P. W., Tandler, B., and Boat, T. F. (1981). Mucous glycoproteins from cat tracheal goblet cells and mucous glands separated with EDTA. *Am. Rev. Respir. Dis.* 124: 476–479.

Slomiany, A., Witas, H., Aono, M., and Slomiany, B. L. (1983). Covalently linked fatty acids in gastric mucus glycoprotein of cystic fibrosis patients. *J. Biol. Chem.* 258: 8535–8538.

Spicer, S. S., and Martinez, J. R. (1984). Mucin biosynthesis and secretion in the respiratory tract. *Environ. Health Perspect.* 55: 193–204.

Spicer, S. S., Chakrin, L. W., and Wardell, J. R., Jr. (1974). Effect of chronic sulfur dioxide inhalation on the carbohydrate histochemistry and histology of the canine respiratory tract. *Am. Rev. Respir. Dis.* 110: 13–24.

Stevens, R. L., Otsu, K., and Austen, K. F. (1985). Purification and analysis of the core protein of the protease-resistant intracellular chondroitin sulfate E proteoglycan from the interleukin 3-dependent mouse mast cell. *J. Biol. Chem.* 260: 14194–14200.

Tokuyama, K., Kuo, H. P., Rohde, J. A., Barnes, P. J., and Rogers, D. F. (1990). Neural control of goblet cell secretion in guinea pig airways. *Am. J. Physiol.* 259: L108–L115.

Trong, H. L., Neurath, H., and Woodbury, R. G. (1987). Substrate specificity of the chymotrypsin-like protease in secretory granules isolated from rat mast cells. *Proc. Natl. Acad. Sci. USA* 84: 364–367.

Van Scott, M. R., Yankaskas, J. R., and Boucher, R. C. (1986). Culture of airway epithelial cells: Research techniques. *Exp. Lung Res.* 11: 75–94.

Villalon, M., Basbaum, C. B., Johnson, D. E., and Verdugo, P. (1988). X-ray microanalysis of secretory granules from respiratory goblet cells. *FASEB J.* 2: A958.

Wasano, K., Kim, K. C., Niles, R. M., and Brody, J. S. (1988). Membrane differentiation markers of airway epithelial secretory cells. *J. Histochem. Cytochem.* 36: 167–178.

Water, R. de, Willems, L. N. A., van Muijen, G. N. P., Franken, C., Fransen, J. A. M., Dijkman, J. H., and Kramps, J. A. (1986). Ultrastructural localization of bronchial antileukoprotease in central and peripheral human airways by a gold-labeling technique using monoclonal antibodies. *Am. Rev. Respir. Dis.* 133: 882–890.

Widdicombe, J. G. (1978). Control of secretion of tracheobronchial mucus. *Br. Med. Bull.* 34: 57–61.

Wu, R. (1986). In vitro differentiation of airway epithelial cells. In *In Vitro Models of Respiratory Epithelium*. Edited by L. L. Schiff. Boca Raton, CRC Press, pp. 1–26.

Wu, R., and Smith, D. (1982). Continuous multiplication of rabbit tracheal epithelial cells in a defined, hormone-supplemented medium. *In Vitro* 18: 800–812.

Wu, R., Nolan, E., Turner, C. (1985). Expression of tracheal differentiated function in serum-free hormone-supplemented medium. *J. Cell. Physiol.* 125: 167–181.

Yurt, R. W., Leid, R. W., Jr., Austen, K. F., and Silbert, J. E. (1977). Native heparin from rat peritoneal mast cells. *J. Biol. Chem.* 252: 518–521.

12

Airway Mucosal Exudation of Plasma

CARL G. A. PERSSON

University Hospital of Lund
Lund, Sweden

I. Introduction

During the era of Hippocrates, Aeretus, and Galen, the belief became established that a cerebral catarrh produced the airway symptoms of asthma and rhinitis: "Cerebral secretions seeped down into the nasal cavity and further to the bronchi." Curiously enough, this view of hypersecretion was to last until the end of the 17th century. It was replaced by an interesting speculation suggesting that the evil airway fluid came directly from the blood, a notion well compatible with the contemporary use of blood-letting therapies. For some time now, it has been realized that significant amounts of plasma proteins can enter the airway lumen and be found in samples of sputum and "mucous" plugs. However, "leak" of the large proteins into the airway lumen is generally considered a sign of a severely injured mucosa. For this or other reasons (Persson, 1992a) it has not been as accepted to carry out research on exudation mechanisms as it has been to examine mucosal secretion.

My group had a special reason for studying airway luminal entry of plasma exudates. We had observed that a wide variety of exudative agents, applied on the tracheobronchial mucosa, produced plasma extravasation, but did not induce any clear-cut edema, not even at high doses (Persson et al., 1986; Erjefält, 1991).

During the last 8 years we have been able to show that inflammatory stimuli evoke an airway mucosal response whereby a largely nonsieved plasma exudate enters the lumen (Persson and Erjefält, 1986; Erjefält and Persson, 1989, 1991a; Alkner et al., 1991). This is a finely regulated process that is subject to physiological and pharmacological control. These recent observations demonstrating that mucosal exudation of plasma may not cause or be associated with any mucosal damage (Persson et al., 1987; Luts et al., 1990) are in contrast with previously held notions.

One increasingly important way of learning facts about asthma and rhinitis is to explore the pharmacology of those drugs that significantly affect the symptoms and the progression of these diseases (Persson, 1989a). Also the pharmacological approach suggests that secreted products may not be the only important mucosal outputs in asthma and rhinitis. The major drugs in inflammatory airway diseases, the glucocorticoids, may not have dramatic effects on airway secretions, particularly in vivo (Maron et al., 1984; Persson, 1988a; Shimura et al., 1990). In contrast, they effectively inhibit the mucosal exudation of plasma (Persson, 1988a; Svensson et al., 1991; Van der Graff et al., 1991). The latter action should be expected because the exudative response appears to be a specific and quantitative sign of ongoing airway inflammation (Persson, 1991a).

This chapter briefly discusses the physiology and pathophysiology of airway mucosal exudation of plasma and attempts to relate this process both to the normal airway defense system (Persson et al., 1991a) and to the pathogenesis of airway diseases (Persson, 1986). The pharmacology of airway plasma exudation will be mentioned, because it may help clarify the distinction between secretion and exudation. Since mucosal exudation mechanisms have not yet been studied or conceptualized in many laboratories, an autobiographical bias has been difficult to avoid.

II. Definition

Mucosal or airway exudation is used in this text to describe inflammatory stimulus-induced bulk flow of plasma, plasma-derived mediators, and attracted fluid across the airway microvascular and mucosal barriers into the airway lumen.

The mucosal exudate may have attracted substantial amounts of fluid on its way to the mucosal surface. However, in contrast with the "transudation" of protein-poor fluid, the mucosal exudate is nonsieved and contains also the large plasma proteins.

Airway exudation of unfiltered plasma proteins reflects dramatic increases in the microvascular and mucosal permeabilities. However, the airway absorption ability remains unaltered during and after the plasma exudation process.

The mechanisms involved and the largely nonsieved nature of the plasma exudate distinguish mucosal exudation from secretory processes and cell traffics in the airway.

III. The Asymmetry of the Airway Mucosal Barrier

A. The Outward Exudative Flux of Solutes

The mucosal exudation of plasma has been characterized in in vivo studies involving particularly guinea-pig tracheobronchial airways and human nasal airways. Inflammatory stimuli, ranging from single histamine-type mediators to allergens and occupational factors, variably produce prompt, biphasic and, by repeated exposures, sustained mucosal exudation of plasma (Erjefält and Persson, 1989; Persson et al., 1991b; Svensson et al., 1990). The luminal entry usually involves little sieving (Persson and Erjefält, 1986; Erjefält and Persson, 1989; Alkner et al., 1991). Plasma molecules of different sizes and different charges thus appear together on the mucosal surface in much the same proportion as in the circulation. Since the exudative mucosal permeability during a brief period "freely" allows the passage of macromolecules with relative molecular masses (M_r) of several hundred kilodaltons, the passage across the airway endothelial and epithelial barriers must be through paracellular routes. The mucosal exudation of plasma is also a specific outward flux of molecules, because the mucosal absorption ability may not be affected by it (Persson et al., 1991a; Erjefält and Persson, 1991b; Gustafsson and Persson, 1991; Greiff et al., 1991a,b).

B. Misconceptions Based on the View of Bidirectional Mucosal "Permeability"

The normal rates of airway absorption of tracer molecules, such as ^{99m}Tc-DTPA (M_r 500 Da), ^{131}I-albumin (M_r 69,000 Da) and FITC-dextran (M_r 70,000 Da), vary greatly, depending on the size of the molecules. It seems likely that paracellular routes are responsible for the inward mucosal passage of these polar and a hydrophilic molecules. Since both the outward, exudative route and the inward, absorptive route would be paracellular, it might be expected that an increased exudation should be associated with increased absorption across the mucosa. The prevailing view in discussions of mucosal permeability changes in airway disease has also been that any increase in "permeability" is bidirectional (see Persson et al., 1991a). The abundant presence of plasma proteins in airway surface material of asthmatic subjects has even been taken as good evidence in support of the notion that abnormally increased absorption of inhaled material characterizes this disease. However, this appears to be a misconception.

C. Plasma Exudation Without Increased Airway Absorption

Work in tracheobronchial and nasal airways has demonstrated that neither during the airway mucosal exudation process nor in the immediate postexudation phase have the rates of absorption of the aforementioned polar tracers been significantly affected (Erjefält and Persson, 1991b; Gustafsson and Persson, 1991; Greiff et al., 1991a,b). The lack of interaction between exudation and absorption mechanisms suggests the possibility that different paracellular routes are used for the absorption and exudation processes, respectively. This is not an unlikely event, because the vast stretches of interepithelial linings (1 cm² of mucosa may have about 50 m of apical epithelial cell circumference) would hypothetically provide an abundance of paracellular pathways. The actual mucosal routes for absorption or the exudation have not been characterized in great detail. It has been speculated that the tightness of the epithelial lining cells may be compromised more easily at corners where three cells meet or between epithelial cells and goblet cells, particularly if the latter type of cell has discharged its contents. Still more speculations exist.

If the epithelium had been disrupted or even shed as a result of plasma exudation, one would expect that the absorptive perviousness should be increased. The lack of an increased mucosal absorptive ability thus suggests that the plasma exudation response has not caused any damage to the epithelial lining. This conclusion is supported by light, fluorescence, and electron microscopy examinations of the airway mucosa in which marked mucosal exudation of plasma has occurred. Beneath large sheets of plasma exudates the structure of the epithelial lining is normally tight (Luts et al., 1990).

IV. Mucosal Exudation Mechanisms

How can the plasma exudate traverse the normal airway mucosa? Which noninjurious mechanism can move a nonsieved "soup" of peptides–proteins, including very large plasma molecules, across the mucosa into the airway lumen, also without compromising the normal barrier function of the epithelial lining? Several observations have provided clues for the formulation of a *hydrostatic pressure* hypothesis for the mucosal crossing of plasma exudates (Persson, 1989b).

A. Extravasation of Plasma May Increase the Subepithelial Hydrostatic Pressure

The extravasation of plasma is known to be secondary to inflammatory mediator-induced separation of endothelial cells in the microvascular wall. This occurs specifically in postcapillary venules, which are abundant just beneath the airway epithelium. The concentration gradient of vasoactive mediators after a topically induced mucosal inflammation would favor the formation of venular holes on the luminal side. Nonsieved plasma is moved through the interendothelial holes by an intravascular to interstitial hydrostatic pressure difference amounting to about 20 cm H_2O. The microvascular basement membrane evidently offers little resistance to the passage of extravasated plasma, and the direction of the spreading of tissue plasma may be preferably toward the epithelium. Outside the microvessels, the plasma protein systems would be activated to produce many more molecules and attract much more fluid than that of its original composition in the circulation. Hence, although it has not been directly measured, a slightly increased hydrostatic pressure in the subepithelium is a likely immediate consequence of mucosal stimulus-induced extravasation of plasma.

B. Only a Small Increase in Pressure Would Be Needed

Our in vivo observations have provided further prerequisites that may be helpful in the search for the mechanism of mucosal crossing of plasma exudates. First, mucosal edema has not been detectable after application of exudative stimuli on the airway surface. Second, the luminal entry of plasma exudates has occurred promptly, being measurable in the lumen within 2 min after mucosal provocation. Third, threshold exudative effects have frequently been detected even better in the luminal samples than in the tissue samples. These three pieces of information suggest that the extravasated plasma is not allowed to accumulate and produce edema, nor would large increases in subepithelial hydrostatic pressure be induced.

C. The First Demonstration of Pressure-Induced Movement of Macromolecules Into the Airway Lumen

The idea has now been tested in vitro that small increases in hydrostatic pressure beneath the mucosa might be sufficient to move macromolecular solutes into the airway lumen. As demonstrated in isolated tracheal tubes, increases in the submucosal pressure of only 5 cm H_2O produced significant luminal entry of macromolecular solutes (Persson et al., 1990; Gustafsson and Persson, 1991). This in vitro process was noninjurious, reversible, repeatable, and strictly unidirectional (the absorption ability did not increase), in good accord with our previous in vivo observations. Furthermore, inflammatory mediators that induce mucosal exudation of plasma in vivo did not interfere with the hydrostatic pressure-induced luminal entry of macromolecules in vitro (Gustafsson and Persson, 1991). The latter observation suggests that the exudative mediators themselves may not produce any destabilizing effect on the epithelial junctions.

Taken together, the experimental data support the notion that the plasma exudate itself, soon after its extravasation, is responsible for the creation of pathways for its luminal entry. This idea fits nicely with the finding that all types of mucosal provocation that have produced extravasation of plasma into the airway tissue have also resulted in plasma exudate entering the lumen.

D. The Importance of a Lateral Pressure Effect

The structural asymmetry of the epithelial cells, with the tight connections being present toward the apical pole area, whereas there is a more loose juxtaposition toward the base, is well known and would allow the spreading of extravasated plasma up along the sides of the epithelial cells. Hence, not only a subepithelial pressure but also a lateral hydrostatic pressure influence on the epithelial cells may be important to bring about pathways for the luminal entry of plasma exudates. This is supported by observations in vivo. When the airway intraluminal pressure is elevated 5–10 cm H_2O above baseline in vivo, the inflammatory stimulus-induced mucosal exudation of plasma is reduced, but it is not completely prevented (Miller-Larsson, Brattsand, and Persson, unpublished observations). Inferentially, a pressure increase acting laterally and tending to separate the epithelial cells along their entire sides may be decisive in the process of creating paracellular pathways.

V. Mucosal Exudation of Plasma in Normal Airway Defense

A. A Novel Notion

The data that have been discussed in the foregoing ought to be interpreted also in a teleological way. It does seem purposeful to me that the increased microvascular permeability should not lead to primarily a tissue edema in the challenged airway. Rather, the purpose should be that the extravasated plasma, with its powerful protein systems, is swiftly moved to the airway mucosal surface where the load of provocating factors has been deposited. It would, indeed, serve the airway defense system best if as much as possible of threatening microbes, allergens, and other offensive materials in the airways could be already neutralized on the mucosal surface. The complement, kinin, coagulation, fibrinolysis, and other systems, as well as plasma enzymes, immunoglobulins, and such, should enter the airway lumen in bulk, and the entry should occur without compromising the normal barrier function of the mucosa.

According to the views of current textbooks, the foregoing reasoning is merely wishful thinking. However, data have now accumulated to support the new concept that airway plasma exudation, as outlined here, has a major role in the first-line defense of the airway mucosa (Persson et al., 1991a; Persson, 1991a). Plasma exudates may thus operate on the surface of an intact airway mucosa together with other established mechanisms, including airway secretions and mucociliary transport activities.

B. A Graded and Brief Burst of Exudate

Mucosal exudation of plasma is a graded response. The larger the dose of provocative agent that is applied on the mucosal surface, the larger the amount of plasma that is promptly exuded. A limited mucosal stimulus, such as a small dose of histamine-type mediators, will cause a brief localized burst of plasma exudate into the airway lumen. The duration of the exudation is somewhat prolonged with increasing doses. Only if the stimulus becomes stronger or novel inflammatory agents are deposited on the mucosal surface, will the mucosal exudation response last longer than the few minutes that constitute the usual duration of an isolated initial response. The mechanism behind the normally brief duration of the exudation response is a strong tendency for the separated venular endothelial cells to resume contact. The extravasation process is, thereby, closed, despite continuous presence of the initiating stimulus (Svensjö and Joyner, 1984; Greiff et al., 1990). Again, it seems purposeful to allow the first burst of plasma exudate some time to produce its defensive actions in the airways. More plasma exudate is needed and poured out only if the provocation is not dealt with or becomes worse.

C. Noninjurious and Injurious Stimuli

Inflammatory stimuli that release or mimic the effect of endogenous mediators and autacoids have been demonstrated to induce the mucosal exudation of plasma response, without causing any damage to the mucosa itself and without increasing its absorptive perviousness (Erjefält and Persson, 1991b; Gustafsson and Persson, 1991; Greiff et al., 1991a,b). By repeated stimulation of mediator release, for example, by allergen inhalations, the mucosal exudation process may occur for months and perhaps chronically without causing damage.

Plasma exudation is also induced by stimuli that are toxic and injurious. Frank damage to the mucosa will result in large and prolonged exudative responses. The application of membrane-toxic agents, such as ethanol, a detergent, or H_2O_2, will thus evoke large exudative responses (Greiff et al., 1991a; Erjefält, I., et al., unpublished work). These foreign membrane-active chemicals will not only produce mucosal exudation of plasma, but will directly disrupt the epithelial lining so that also the mucosal absorptive ability is greatly increased. In these latter cases, plasma exudation may have the additional defense capacity of sealing the injured sites by providing fibrinogen and fibronectin, which would form fibrin–fibrinonectin gels. Such a gel provides a matrix for cell adhesion and migration; it may also promote angiogenesis and reepithelialization (Crouch, 1990).

VI. Mucosal Exudation of Plasma Reflects Ongoing Airway Inflammation

A. The Classic Signs of Inflammation Are of Little Use

Basically all inflammatory mechanisms would serve a defensive purpose; however, the opposite may not be true. Rather, most airway defensive reactions appear as nonspecific end-organ effects that may occur as normal baseline variations, or may be induced by simple irritants that merely evoke neural activity and neurogenic actions. Increased blood flow, increased pooling of blood, increased secretion, altered mucociliary efficacy, cough, and sneezes, all may belong to this nonspecific category. These airway responses can be secondary to an inflammatory process, but they can equally well be induced by noninflammatory provocations. The classic signs rubor, dolor, calor, tumor, and functio laesa, may likewise be of little help when it comes to determining whether or not airway inflammation is present. Indeed, dolor, calor, and funtio laesa may not apply. Pain and heat thus are not characteristic of allergic airways, and many of the end-organ functions in airway inflammation, including secretion, are hyper-, rather than hypofunctional (Klementsson et al., 1991; Persson, 1992b). Finally, the problem with tumor is to know what is behind it. Is the swelling due to edema or is it intravascular pooling of blood? Is it due to bronchoconstriction, cell accumulation, tissue growth, or other factors?

B. Can the Presence of Inflammatory Cells and Their Biology Be Equated With Airway Inflammation?

It is widely accepted that studies of certain cells in the airways, particularly when complemented with cell and molecular biology analyses of the status and capacity of these cells, can tell beyond any doubt whether or not inflammation is present. However, the presence of antigen-presenting cells and activated lymphocyte populations, as well as the presence of a range of inflammatory cells and their products, may demonstrate only a high degree of immunocompetence and a high potential for inflammation (Persson, 1992b). The cellular capacity in the airways can, alternatively, be a sign of successful defensive operations, with little involvement of the airway tissue itself. Cell accumulation may further reflect airways in a phase of successful repair. Hence, the cell biology may reveal what is potentially fueling an airway inflammation, but may not provide the crucial information on whether a significant inflammatory process is going on (Persson, 1992b).

C. Mucosal Exudation as an Inflammatory End-Organ Response

It is implied by the foregoing discussion that specific indexes of end-organ involvement would be needed to decide about airway inflammation. In this context, mucosal exudation of plasma is an interesting response. Plasma extravasation (and the subsequent mucosal exudation of plasma) is not an exaggeration of the normal baseline exchange of fluid and solutes between the capillary circulation and the mucosa. It is a specific response of postcapillary venules (Grega et al., 1988), and inflammatory factors or mediators are required to induce it. Particularly in human airways, irritant-induced neurogenic actions do not include a plasma exudative response (Greiff et al., 1991c; Persson, 1991b). (Neurogenic airway exudation–inflammation appears to be a rat and guinea-pig phenomenon; Persson, 1991b). Whereas plasma exudation is specific to inflammation, it is a general response in the sense that it does not distinguish which particular cellular or noncellular mechanism is driving the inflammatory process.

Plasma exudation is a graded response. The more pronounced the inflammation the greater the airway exudative response (Erjefält and Persson, 1989; Greiff et al., 1990). Decisively important for human studies is the observation that exudative indexes in luminal airway samples promptly and quantitatively reflect the process in the underlying mucosa–submucosa (Persson and Erjefält, 1986; Erjefält and Persson, 1989). The luminal entry of plasma seems little hindered, even in airways with a normal epithelial lining having uncompromised barrier functions. Hence, the relevance of luminal samples would be equally good in mild inflammation, with no tissue damage, as in severe conditions in which the epithelial lining may have been disrupted.

D. Which Exudative Indexes Should Be Analyzed?

Many proteins are fairly specific to plasma and can be used. However, the most common plasma protein, albumin, is not always a good index. It is a small protein that normally enters the airway lumen by diffusion and by secretory mechanisms. Albumin can thus accumulate in the airways to produce large and variable baseline values. In the nasal airways, this problem may be overcome by repeated lavages that produce low and stable baseline values of mucosal albumin. Unfortunately, this technique cannot be employed in the lower airways. Hence, bronchoalveolar lavage fluid levels of albumin may not always tell whether or not exudation has occurred. Larger proteins, such as fibrinogen and α_2-macroglobulin, which are scarcely present in normal airway surface liquids, seem to be more specific exudative indexes than albumin (Persson, 1991a; Salomonsson et al., 1992). The nonsieved nature of mucosal plasma exudates underlines the usefulness of the large proteins.

Selected exudative indices may give more detailed information. If particular roles of mucosal exudation are being investigated, the analyses have to be directed accordingly. For example, exuded enzymes, immunoglobulins, and other factors, are of interest as such, but may not be particularly useful as a general measure of the mucosal exudation response. By measuring kinins, complement fragments, and other plasma-derived peptides, knowledge is gained about the degree of activation of the exuded protein systems.

VII. The Role of Mucosal Exudation of Plasma in Airway Diseases

A. Airway Edema in Asthma and Rhinitis, Does It Exist?

Plasma exudation naturally has a reputation for causing airway edema; however, actual edema has not been well demonstrated in airway tissue challenged with exudative mediators or allergen. Wet/dry weight ratios have not been increased (Persson et al., 1986; Erjefält, 1991), and quantitative histological methods to prove that edema exists do not seem to be available (Persson, 1988b; Laitinen et al., 1992). Indeed, it was our inability to induce edema in the airway mucosa that prompted Dr. Erjefält and myself to study escape routes for the extravasated plasma, particularly its luminal entry (Persson and Erjefält, 1986). We also observed that lymphatic transport of extravasated molecules was not, or was only marginally, increased in challenged airways (Erjefält et al., 1992). This latter observation agreed with a lack of edema formation and supported our conclusion that luminal entry was a rapid and efficient elimination of the plasma exudates.

Also in asthma and rhinitis, the evidence for true airway edema is poor (Persson, 1988b; Laitinen et al., 1992). Quantitative histological procedures are now lacking, and the impression of mucosal swelling that one obtains from looking at nasal and bronchial surfaces is only suggestive of edema. The edema look may rather or equally well stem from bronchoconstriction and intravascular pooling of blood. The possibility that edema formation may not be an obligatory consequence of plasma exudation in asthma and rhinitis is supported by findings of largely nonsieved plasma on the bronchial and nasal surface soon after topical allergen challenges (Alkner et al., 1991; Salomonsson et al., 1992). Hence, mucosal exudation of plasma does not reflect the presence of a large and saturated mucosal edema. Rather, it should be viewed as a mechanism that prevents edema formation in upper and lower airways.

B. Increased Absorption Permeability in Asthma and Rhinitis, Is It a Myth?

Plasma exudation has been associated with at least four physical abnormalities in the airways. Three of these may not be as well founded as the fourth. Besides the reputed edema, the plasma exudate has been thought to cause epithelial shedding, and if shedding has not occurred, mucosal exudation of plasma "surely must be associated with an increased perviousness for absorption." As discussed in the foregoing in some detail, airway plasma exudation may cause neither of these abnormalities; and neither of these abnormalities may always characterize asthma and rhinitis. Although epithelial shedding in asthma has been widely reported and even assumed a de facto status, the documentation of this effect in preterminal stages of the disease is in doubt because of possible artifacts induced by the techniques employed for obtaining bronchial biopsies (Laitinen et al., 1992). As with the edema and the epithelial shedding, an increased mucosal absorption has not been well demonstrated in asthma and rhinitis. On the contrary, a decreased absorption ability has been found in studies of the human allergic airway (Persson et al., 1991a; Greiff et al., 1992).

C. "Hypersecretion" May Not Be Secretion

The fourth physical pathology is hypersecretion. Mucous plugs are known to contain large amounts of plasma proteins, and elevated plasma protein levels have been found in both nasal and bronchial discharges and also in nasal and bronchial lavage liquids in rhinitis and asthma (reviewed by Persson, 1988b; Persson et al., 1991a). Detailed analyses of the relative proportion of exudative and secretory products have not been carried out. Mucosal exudation of plasma thus contributes to the luminal material that may cause symptoms and worsening of inflammatory airway diseases. The appearance of too much and too viscous material in the airway lumen, including the formation of so-called mucous plugs in asthma, should perhaps be renamed as hyperexudations–hypersecretions and plasma–mucous plugs, respectively.

What is the actual volume of either secretions or plasma exudates? There is little likelihood that the plasma exudate entering the airway lumen has retained the original volume that it previously occupied in the circulation. Although the exudation is a nonsieved, bulk flow of solutes the measurement of albumin, fibrinogen, α_2-macroglobulin, or other tracer levels in airway surface liquids cannot tell how large a volume has entered the airway lumen along with these macromolecules. After extravasation, the protein systems will be activated and, as a consequence, plasma-derived molecules will multiply. By osmotic forces, this process will attract more fluid to the exudate both in and on the mucosa. On the other hand, the exudate may be subject to some drying action both by water-absorbing extracellular matrix molecules and, in the airway lumen, by the incoming air.

Interactions between mucosal plasma exudates and mucosal secretions can take place at different levels. The plasma proteins and mucins may form complexes that have a high viscosity. The plasma proteins may also stimulate glandular secretion. An interesting observation, made by Aitken and Verdugo (1989), is that plasma proteins (albumin) potently prevent the normal hydration of secreted mucins.

D. Plasma-Derived Extracellular Matrix Macromolecules

Fibronectin, fibrinogen, and clotting factors of the plasma exudate may produce fibrin–fibronectin gels. This not only would be a physical change, but would also involve potentially significant pathophysiology. Inflammatory fibrin degradation products may be released and fibrin-fibronectin may provide a matrix and adhesion for macrophage, fibroblast, and other cell migration (Dvorak et al., 1986; Brown, 1989). Fibrin–fibronectin in the subepithelium can provide a matrix for angiogenesis and fibroplasia. On the luminal surface, at sites where the mucosa is damaged, it may provide a matrix for migration of connective tissue cells and reepithelialization (Crouch, 1990). Conceivably, this latter process may also reduce the free airway lumen. Plasma-derived fibrin–fibronectin matrix formation may characterize severely injured airways, as well as allergic airways.

E. Plasma-Derived Active Agents

The plasma exudate provides a wide range of inflammatory enzymes and peptide mediators. Besides fibrinolysis peptides, bradykinins, complement fragments, and coagulation peptides, many as yet unidentified peptides may be produced. The formation of several of these mediators may be an obligatory consequence of the plasma exudation process. For example, bradykinins seem always to be produced independently of how the plasma exudation has been brought about, whether by acute histamine doses or by prolonged seasonal allergen exposure (Svensson et al., 1989, 1990).

The importance of the plasma-derived molecules in fueling pathophysiological processes is not clear from their mere presence in the airways. As with factors released from inflammatory cells, the plasma-derived proinflammatory mediators and enzymes may be coproduced with agents that are anti-inflammatory. Hence, the sum of the activities is more important than the presence and actions of single factors. The final assessment of the contribution of any plasma-derived agent will have to await the advent of specific antagonizing compounds. The role of bradykinins in airway disease is now being evaluated by employment of increasingly potent antagonists of bradykinin or inhibitors of tissue kallikrein, the enzyme responsible for bradykinin formation.

VIII. Pharmacological Regulation of Mucosal Exudation of Plasma

Microvascular endothelial cells harbor surface receptors for common inflammatory mediators. Thus, histamine, bradykinin, leukotriene D_4, and presumably many other exudative agents, have direct effects on the microvascular wall. Interestingly, this possibility was predicted by Cohnheim, who made a series of fundamental observations on inflammation and plasma exudation processes over 100 years ago.

A. Airway Blood Flow Changes May Be of Little Consequence

In addition to increasing vascular permeability, the inflammatory mediators may exert vasodilation and increase local blood flow. In the airways the abundant subepithelial microvessels are richly perfused with blood already under baseline conditions. Hence, the vasodilating effect that hypothetically could contribute to the exudation by increasing the supply of plasma, may not be particularly important in the regulation of airways plasma exudation. This view is supported by the observation that a potent vasoconstrictor, that may have halved the blood flow, was without effect on histamine-induced exudation in human nasal airways (Svensson et al., 1992a). Interestingly, a major secretory stimulant and a vasodilator, carbachol (or methacholine), does not produce any mucosal exudation of plasma, even when given in very large doses (Erjefält and Persson, 1989, 1991b).

The direct effect on the microvascular wall that dramatically increases the permeability appears to be the important vascular mechanism regulating plasma extravasation and, hence (see foregoing), the mucosal exudation of plasma into the airways.

B. Luminal Entry of White Cells Is Distinct from Mucosal Exudation of Plasma

There is a clear distinction between the inflammatory movement of plasma and the traffic of white cells. Cellular diapedesis and migration into the airway lumen are not regulated by the plasma exudation mechanisms. Thus, histamine-type mediators can produce massive exudation of plasma without inducing any cell traffic. On the other hand, the white cells may traverse the vascular–mucosal barriers by mechanisms that maintain the protein-tight seal of these barriers. Inferentially, pharmacological inhibition of white cell traffic into the airway lumen may not of itself reduce the mucosal exudation of plasma. Inhibition of cell priming and activation is a different matter (see following).

C. Pharmacological Antagonists and Other Vascular Antipermeability Drugs

The direct vascular permeability effect of mediators is antagonized by the proper receptor antagonist. This effect is exerted with the usual pharmacological specificity, meaning, for example, that antihistamines cannot inhibit the effects of bradykinins and leukotrienes. Animal work has also demonstrated a direct drug effect on vascular endothelium, which is a more general inhibitory effect than that exerted by pharmacological antagonists. The β-receptor agonists belong to this category. Stimulation of endothelial β_2-receptors will thus reduce the plasma exudation effect of a wide variety of mediators. In guinea pig tracheobronchial airways, β_2-agonists, such as terbutaline, reduce exudation despite that they increase blood flow (Persson et al., 1986; Erjefält and Persson, 1991a). Another β_2-agonist, formoterol, has both potent and long-lasting antiexudative effects in the guinea pig airways (Erjefält and Persson, 1991a). β-Blockers antagonize the antiexudative effect of terbutaline, formoterol, and other β-agonists. The antiexudative effect of β_2-agonists contrast their prosecretory actions as shown in animal and in vitro studies (Webber and Widdicombe, 1989). Hence, the distinction between exudation and secretion is evident both in terms of which agents are inducing and which drugs are antagonizing these mucosal responses.

Also other types of antiasthma or antirhinitis drugs—xanthines, glucocorticoids, and cromoglycates—may exert general vascular antipermeability actions and variably reduce mediator-induced plasma exudation in guinea pig airways (Erjefält and Persson, 1991a). However, all these types of drugs as well as the β_2-agonists appear to produce only weak antiexudative effects in the airways. If the dose of the provocating exudative mediator is increased, perhaps only doubled, the entire antiexudative action of these vascular antipermeability drugs may be lost (Erjefält and Persson, 1991a). This relative lack of efficacy can be interpreted as a safeguard mechanism, because when required in airway defense, a mucosal exudation response can always be induced, despite the presence of these drugs.

D. Anti-Inflammatory Drug Effects, Rather Than Direct Effects, on Vascular Permeability Inhibit Plasma Exudation in Asthma and Rhinitis

Clinical experimental data are now emerging suggesting that direct vascular antipermeability action of topical glucocorticoids, such as budesonide, may not be produced in human airways, even if the exudative stimulus is kept at low threshold levels (Svensson et al., 1992b). However, in active rhinitis, asthma, and bronchitis, the institution of glucocorticoid treatment very effectively inhibits the mucosal exudation of plasma (Svensson et al., 1991; Persson, 1988a, 1989b; Persson and Pipkorn, 1990; Van der Graaf et al., 1990). This effect may best be interpreted as a general anti-inflammatory effect, rather than a specific vascular antipermeability action. An abundance of potentially important anti-inflammatory effects of glucocorticoids have now been demonstrated at the cellular level. Thus, glucocorticoid drugs will reduce the immunocompetence and inhibit the accumulation and activation of several proinflammatory cells in the airway mucosa. When the mucosal exudation of plasma is inhibited by budesonide in airway diseases, it may be concluded that a critical mechanism that is fueling the airway inflammation has been effectively inhibited. Any contribution of a direct vascular antipermeability action to drug-induced antiexudative effects in airway diseases now remains speculative.

Acknowledgments

I thank Mrs. M. Broman for excellent secretarial assistance. This study was supported by the Swedish Medical Research Council (Project No. 8308) and Astra Draco, Lund, Sweden.

References

Aitken, M. L., and Verdugo, P. (1989). Donnan mechanism of mucin release and conditioning in goblet cells: The role of polyions. In *Mucus and Related Topics*. Edited by E. N. Chantler. New York, Plenum Press, pp. 1–8.

Alkner, U., Svensson, C., Andersson, M., Pipkorn, U., and Persson, C. G. A. (1991). Fibrinogen and albumin on the surface of allergen- and histamine-exposed human nasal mucosa. *J. Allergy Clin. Immunol.* 87: 217.

Brown, L. F., Dvorak, A. M., and Dvorak, A. M. (1989). Leaky vessels, fibrin deposition, and fibrosis: A sequence of events common to solid tumors and to many other types of disease. *Am. Rev. Respir. Dis.* 140: 1104–1107.

Crouch, E. (1990). Pathobiology of pulmonary fibrosis. *Am. J. Physiol.* 259: L159–L184.

Dvorak, H. F., Galli, S. J., and Dvorak, A. M. (1986). Cellular and vascular manifestations of cell-mediated immunity. *Hum. Pathol.* 17: 122–137.

Erjefält, I. (1991). Plasma exudation in tracheobronchial airways. Thesis, Lund, pp. 1–57.

Erjefält, I., and Persson, C. G. A. (1991a). Pharmacological control of plasma exudation in guinea-pig lower airways. *Am. Rev. Respir. Dis.* 143: 1008–1014.

Erjefält, I., and Persson, C. G. A. (1989). Inflammatory passage of plasma macromolecules into airway tissue and lumen. *Pulmonary Pharmacol.* 2: 93–102.

Erjefält, I., and Persson, C. G. A. (1991b). Allergen, bradykinin, and capsaicin increase outward but not inward macromolecular permeability of guinea-pig tracheobronchial mucosa. *Clin. Exp. Allergy* 21: 217–224.

Erjefält, I., Luts, A., and Persson, C. G. A. (1993). The appearance of airway absorption and exudation tracers in guinea-pig tracheobronchial lymph nodes. *J. Appl. Physiol.* 74: 817–824.

Grega, G. J., Persson, C. G. A., and Svensjö, E. (1988). Endothelial cell reactions to inflammatory mediators assessed in vivo by fluid and solute flux analysis. In *Endothelial Cells*. Edited by U. S. Ryan. Boca Raton, CRC Press, pp. 103–122.

Greiff, L., Pipkorn, U., Alkner, U., and Persson, C. G. A. (1990). The "nasal pool-device" applies controlled concentrations of solutes on human nasal airway mucosa and samples its surface exudations/secretions. *Clin. Exp. Allergy* 20: 253–259.

Greiff, L., Erjefält, I., Wollmer, P., Pipkorn, U., and Persson, C. G. A. (1991a). Different patterns of inflammatory effects on airway barriers: Plasma exudation with and without increased absorption of small or large luminal solutes. *Thorax* 46: 700–705.

Greiff, L., Pipkorn, U., Alkner, U., and Persson, C. G. A. (1991b). Unchanged absorption of ^{51}Cr-EDTA during histamine-induced plasma exudation. *Thorax* 146: 630–632.

Greiff, L., Erjefält, I., Wollmer, P., Andersson, M., Pipkorn, U., Alkner, U., and Persson, C. G. A. (1991c). Nicotine evokes neurogenic mucosal exudation of plasma into guinea-pig but not into human airways. Thesis, Lund, pp. 109–123.

Greiff, L., Wollmer, P., Svensson, C., Andersson, M., and Persson, C. G. A. (1993). Airway mucosal absorption of ^{51}Cr-EDTA is reduced in seasonal allergic rhinitis. *Thorax* (in press).

Gustafsson, B., and Persson, C. G. A. (1991). Asymmetrical effects of increase in hydrostatic pressure on macromolecular movement across the airway mucosa. *Clin. Exp. Allergy* 21: 121–126.

Klementsson, H., Svensson, C., Andersson, M., Venge, P., Pipkorn, U., and Persson, C. G. A. (1991). Eosinophils, secretory responsiveness and glucocorticoid-induced effects on the nasal mucosa during a weak pollen season. *Clin. Exp. Allergy* 21: 705–710.

Laitinen, L. A., Laitinen, A., and Persson, C. G. A. (1993). Role of epithelium. In *Bronchial Asthma*, 3rd ed. Edited by E. B. Weiss, and M. Segal. Boston, Little, Brown & Co., 296–308.

Luts, A., Sundler, F., Erjefält, I., and Persson, C. G. A. (1990). The airway epithelial lining is intact promptly after the mucosal crossing of a large amount of plasma exudate. *Arch. Allergy Appl. Immunol.* 91: 385–389.

Maron, Z. V. I., Shelhamer, J., Alling, D., and Kaliner, M. (1984). The effect of corticosteroids on mucous glucoprotein secretion from human airways in vitro. *Am. Rev. Respir. Dis.* 129: 62–65.

Persson, C. G. A. (1986). Role of plasma exudation in asthma. *Lancet* 2: 1126–1129.

Persson, C. G. A. (1988a). Plasma exudation and asthma. *Lung* 166: 1–23.

Persson, C. G. A. (1989a). On the medical history of asthma and rhinitis. In *Rhinitis and Asthma. Similarities and Differences*. Edited by N. Mygind, U. Pipkorn, and R. Dahl. Copenhagen, Munksgaard, pp. 9–20.

Persson, C. G. A. (1989b). Permeability changes in obstructive airway diseases. In *Bronchitis IV*. Edited by H. J. Sluiter, and R. Van Der Lende. Assen, Van Gorcum, pp. 236–248.

Persson, C. G. A. (1991a). Mucosal exudation mechanisms. *Allergy Clin. Immunol. News* 3: 142–149.

Persson, C. G. A. (1991b). Mucosal exudation in respiratory defence: Neural or non-neural control? *Arch. Allergy Appl. Immunol.* 104: 222–226.

Persson, C. G. A. (1992a). Plasma exudation from tracheobronchial microvessels in health and disease. In *The Bronchial Circulation*. Edited by J. Butler. New York, Marcel Dekker, pp. 443–473.

Persson, C. G. A. (1992b). What is airway inflammation? *Clin. Exp. Allergy* (in press).

Persson, C. G. A., and Erjefält, I. (1986). Inflammatory passage of plasma macromolecules from vascular compartment into the tracheal lumen. *Acta Physiol. Scand.* 126: 615–616.

Persson, C. G. A., and Pipkorn, U. (1990). Glucocorticoids. In *1939–1989—Fifty Years Progress in Allergy*. Edited by B. Waksman. *Allergy* 90: 264–277.

Persson, C. G. A., Erjefält, I., and Andersson, P. (1986). Leakage of macromolecules from guinea pig tracheobronchial microcirculation. Effects of allergen, leukotrienes, tachykinins, and antiasthma drugs. *Acta Physiol. Scand.* 127: 95–106.

Persson, C. G. A., Erjefält, I., and Sundler, F. (1987). Airway microvascular and epithelial leakage of plasma induced by PAF-acether and capsaicin. *Am. Rev. Respir. Dis.* 135: A401.

Persson, C. G. A., Erjefält, I., Gustafsson, B., and Luts, A. (1990). Subepithelial hydrostatic pressure may regulate plasma exudation across the mucosa. *Int. Arch. Allergy Appl. Immunol.* 92: 148–153.

Persson, C. G. A., Erjefält, I., Alkner, U., Baumgarten, C., Greiff, L., Gustafsson, B., Luts, A., Pipkorn, U., Svensson, C., and Wollmer, P. (1991a). Plasma exudation/transudation as a first line mucosal defence. *Clin. Exp. Allergy* 21: 17–24.

Persson, C. G. A., Gustafsson, B., Luts, A., Sundler, F., and Erjefält, I. (1991b). Toluene diisocyanate produces an increase in airway tone that outlasts the inflammatory exudate phase. *Clin. Exp. Allergy* 21: 715–724.

Salomonsson, P., Grönneberg, R., Gilljam, H., Andersson, O., Billing, B., Enander, I., Alkner, U., and Persson, C. G. A. (1992). Immediate exudation of plasma macro-molecules at endobronchial allergen challenge in subjects with allergic asthma. *Am. Rev. Respir. Dis.* 146: 1535–1542.

Shimura, S., Sasaki, T., Ikeda, K., Yamauchi, K., Sasaki, H., and Takishima, T. (1990). Direct inhibitory action of glucocorticoid on glucoconjugate secretion from airway submucosal glands. *Am. Rev. Respir. Dis.* 141: 1044–1049.

Svensjö, E., and Joyner, W. L. (1984). The effects of intermittent and continuous stimulation of microvessels in the cheek pouch of hamsters with histamine and bradykinin on the development of venular leakage sites. *Microcirc. Endothelium Lymphatics* 1: 381–396.

Svensson, C., Baumgarten, C. R., Pipkorn, U., Alkner, U., and Persson, C. G. A. (1989). Reversibility and reproducibility of histamine-induced plasma leakage in the human nasal airways. *Thorax* 44: 13–18.

Svensson, C., Andersson, M., Persson, C. G. A., Alkner, U., Venge, P., and Pipkorn, U. (1990). Albumin, bradykinins, and eosinophil cationic protein on the nasal mucosal surface in hay fever patients during natural allergen exposure. *J. Allergy Clin. Immunol.* 85: 828–833.

Svensson, C., Klementsson, H., Alkner, U., Pipkorn, U., and Persson, C. G. A. (1991). A topical glucocorticoid reduces the levels of fibrinogen and bradykinins on the allergic mucosa during natural pollen exposure. *J. Allergy Clin. Immunol.* 87: 147.

Svensson, C., Alkner, U., Baumgarten, C. R., Pipkorn, U., and Persson, C. G. A. (1992a). Topical α-adrenoceptor stimulation may not reduce histamine-induced plasma exudation in human nasal airways. *Clin. Exp. Allergy* 22: 411–416.

Svensson, C., Greiff, L., Andersson, M., Alkner, U., and Persson, C. G. A. (1992b). Topical steroids may not inhibit microvascular permeability in human airways. *Clin. Exp. Allergy* (in press).

Van der Graaf, E. A., Out, T. A., Roos, C. M., and Jansen, H. (1991). Respiratory membrane permeability and bronchial hyperreactivity in patients with stable asthma. *Am. Rev. Respir. Dis.* 143: 362–368.

Webber, S. E., and Widdicombe, J. G. (1989). The transport of albumin across the ferret in vitro whole trachea. *J. Physiol.* 408: 457–472.

13

Airway Inflammation and Mucous Hypersecretion

PIERRE LARIVÉE

Centre Hospitalier Universitaire de
  Sherbrooke
Sherbrooke, Quebec, Canada

RAFEL DWAINE RIEVES

University of Mississippi School of
  Medicine
Jackson, Mississippi

STEWART J. LEVINE
and JAMES H. SHELHAMER

National Institutes of Health
Bethesda, Maryland

I. Introduction

In healthy individuals, the volume of tracheobronchial secretions (mucus) elaborated per day is approximately 10–100 ml. Mucus is a complex mixture of water (95%), proteins and glycoproteins (3%), lipids (1%), and salts (1%). These secretions, along with the ciliary transport, provide a protective barrier against airborne physicochemical insults and invading microorganisms. However, alterations in the quality or quantity of airway mucus, as encountered in many respiratory tract disorders, can result in impaired mucociliary clearance. A variety of events may lead to excessive production of respiratory secretions. The quantity of airway mucus can increase by hypersecretion of mucous glycoproteins and other macromolecules from mucus-secreting cells, an increase in the total number of mucus-secreting cells, an increase in transepithelial chloride secretion, leakage of plasma products into the airway space, or any combination thereof. This chapter will primarily address the mechanisms underlying the hypersecretion of mucous glycoproteins. Mucous glycoproteins or mucins (MGP) are important constituents of airway mucus and are responsible for its viscoelastic properties. Mucous glycoprotein is a large, acidic macromolecule composed of a protein core (20–30%) to which are attached oligosaccharide side chains (70–80%). Mucous glycoproteins are produced by the goblet cells of the surface epithelium and the submucosal gland mucous cells. Since, under normal circumstances, the submucosal glands (comprising mucous and serous cells) far outnumber the goblet cells (40:1), it is estimated that the former constitute the principal source of MGP.

This chapter reviews the current concepts concerning the pathogenesis of mucous hypersecretion in inflammatory airway disorders. Over the past decade, numerous studies have provided important insights concerning the modulation of respiratory MGP secretion by neuronal influences, inflammatory mediators, bacterial products, and physicochemical factors. Specifically, progress has been made in understanding the pathogenesis of mucous hypersecretion associated with airway inflammatory diseases such as asthma, chronic bronchitis, cystic fibrosis, bronchiectasis, and acute infection. Hypersecretion of mucus contributes to the morbidity of these airway diseases by predisposing patients to respiratory infections and by contributing to airflow obstruction and patients' discomfort. Furthermore, results of a long-term mortality survey conducted over 22 years in a population of 1061 men (Annesi and Kauffmann, 1986), revealed a significant association between chronic production of mucus and an increased risk of mortality (relative risk = 1.35). This relationship is an important public health concern because of the high prevalence rates of respiratory mucous hypersecretion.

Inflammation has been increasingly recognized to be an important etiological factor in the pathogenesis of many airway diseases. Consequently, basic research efforts have been directed toward obtaining a better understanding of the various components of the inflammatory response. These components include the inflammatory effector cells, the mediators of inflammation, and the dynamic interactions between these and the target cells of the airways. This chapter will discuss the general characteristics of the inflammatory response in the airway, the methods used to assay mucous secretion, and the response of airway secretory cells to various components of airway inflammation. The discussion of airway secretory cell responses will include an overview of the neuronal control of mucous secretion, with special attention to the concept of neurogenic inflammation; a summary of the modulation of MGP release by inflammatory cells, mediators, and bacterial products; and an analysis of the contribution of inflammation to the development of secretory cell hyperplasia. The final section provides a proposed sequence of events culminating in mucous hypersecretion in airway inflammatory diseases.

II.   Airway Inflammation: An Overview

A.   General Characteristics of the Inflammatory Response

Inflammation arises in vascularized tissue in response to noxious stimuli. The goal of the inflammatory response is to orchestrate a complex series of events that ultimately lead to healing and repair of the damaged tissue. Although inflammation and repair have useful functions, deleterious sequelae may also occur. Airway inflammation can be elicited by several stimuli, such as tobacco smoke, allergens, infectious agents, and air pollutants. Both the host response and the type of injurious agent determine the magnitude of inflammation.

The acute inflammatory response, usually of a relatively short duration (hours to days), exhibits similar features, regardless of the nature of the inciting agent. These features include vasodilation with increased blood flow, microvascular leakage, and the subsequent generation of a local exudate composed of plasma proteins and leukocytes (mainly neutrophils). A myriad of chemical compounds mediating the acute inflammatory response have been identified. Acute bacterial bronchitis is a common example of acute inflammation involving the airways.

The chronic inflammatory response is more heterogeneous and of longer duration (weeks to years) than acute inflammation. It can occur not only in response to persistent inflammatory stimuli, but can also arise after repeated episodes of acute inflammation or supervene more insidiously as a first-line response. Chronic bronchitis is a good example of chronic inflammation. The characteristics of chronic inflammation include infiltration by chronic inflammatory cells (mainly mononuclear cells) and proliferation of connective tissue and small blood vessels. The nature of the cellular infiltrate may vary according to the specific causative factor or disease process. For example, typical eosinophilic infiltration of the airways in asthma is sometimes referred to as chronic eosinophilic bronchitis (Barnes, 1989). Exposure of airways to an injurious agent can stimulate airway resident cells (i.e., mast cells, epithelial cells, macrophages) to release products with chemoattractant properties for leukocytes. Examples of these chemotactic factors include arachidonate-derived products, such as leukotriene B_4 (LTB_4) and 15-hydroxyeicosatetraenoic acid (15-HETE); platelet-activating factor (PAF), and various cytokines, such as interleukin-5 (IL-5; Plaut et al., 1989) and interleukin-8 (IL-8; Nakamura et al., 1991). It is conceivable that the nature of the injurious agent may determine both the specific profile of chemotactic factors produced and the subsequent type of cellular infiltrates. Other cardinal features of airway inflammation specifically related to mucous membranes include (1) mucous hypersecretion and (2) desquamation or shedding of epithelial cells, with subsequent remodeling of the epithelial cell population (Florey, 1962).

The mediators of the inflammatory response may originate from airway resident cells, recruited inflammatory cells (i.e., neutrophils, eosinophils, and mononuclear cells), sensory nerves, and plasma. The mediators of inflammation have diverse actions on airway target cells (smooth muscle, epithelial cells including mucus-secreting cells, or bronchial vessels) and other inflammatory cells. This will lead to the expression, at least in part, of the pathophysiological features of inflammatory airway diseases. As detailed later, several mediators of the inflammatory response have the ability to enhance airway mucous secretion. Thus, it should be stressed that mucous hypersecretion, which characterizes airway diseases, such as asthma, chronic bronchitis, and cystic fibrosis, constitutes an integral component of the inflammatory response.

B. Morphological Changes and Cellular Infiltrates of Airway Inflammatory Diseases

Airway inflammation is a key event in asthma. Uncontrolled chronic inflammation presumably represents a basic abnormality of asthmatic airways (Barnes, 1989; O'Byrne, 1990; Kay, 1991; Djukanovic et al., 1990). Pathological findings of airways obtained from cases of fatal asthma show substantial evidence of inflammatory changes (Dunnill, 1960). The airways are characterized by extensive bronchial lumen plugging with mucus, inflammatory exudates, and cellular debris. Other findings include bronchial vascular congestion, submucosal edema, bronchial smooth-muscle enlargement, subepithelial collagen deposition, and an intense bronchial wall inflammatory cell infiltration with a preponderance of eosinophils. The surface epithelium is disrupted, and hyperplasia or metaplasia of the mucus-producing cells and enlarged submucosal glands are present. More recently, bronchial biopsies and lavages have documented the presence of an inflammatory process, even in mild asthmatics (Azzawi et al., 1990; Beasley et al., 1989; Wardlaw et al., 1988).

Because the early recognition that mast cells and their bronchoactive degranulation products play a pivotal role in the early asthmatic response, much of the asthma literature has addressed the role of inflammation in the late asthmatic response and in bronchial hyperresponsiveness. Literature focusing on the role of infiltrating inflammatory cells, such as eosinophils, macrophages, neutrophils, and lymphocytes, in the pathogenesis of asthma is extensive and continues to accumulate. A prominent feature of asthma is eosinophilic infiltration of the airways. Studies have shown that the quantity of eosinophils in bronchoalveolar lavage correlates with the degree of bronchial hyperresponsiveness or asthma severity (Durham and Kay, 1985; Lam et al., 1987; Wardlaw et al., 1988). Once activated, eosinophils release granule-derived basic proteins that are toxic to the airway epithelium. Membrane phospholipid-derived mediators (platelet-activating factors, eicosanoids) are also released and may contribute to the asthmatic process (Frigas and Gleisch, 1986). Macrophages, through their low-affinity IgE receptors (Godard et al., 1982; Joseph et al., 1983; Metzger et al., 1987), and T lymphocytes (Hamid et al., 1991) are also thought to play a pathogenic role. Uncertainties exist about the role of neutrophils in asthma (Hutson et al., 1990). Attention has also been focused on neurogenic inflammation as a component of the inflammatory events occurring in asthmatic airways (Barnes, 1986).

Some of the pathological abnormalities seen in asthmatic airways are also present in airways from cystic fibrosis or chronic bronchitis patients. These shared features include hyperplasia and hypertrophy of the mucus-secreting cells, bronchial smooth-muscle enlargement (to a lesser degree than in asthma), and various degrees of squamous and goblet cell metaplasia (Bedrossian et al., 1976; Mullen et al., 1985). In chronic bronchitis, the airway wall is infiltrated principally by mononuclear cells (Mullen et al., 1985), whereas cytological examinations of sputum (Chodosh, 1979) and bronchial lavage suggest the presence of an intraluminal airway neutrophilia (Thompson et al., 1989). Interestingly, a study of 45 patients undergoing lung surgery (Mullen et al., 1985) showed that chronic bronchitis, as clinically defined in 1965 by the British Medical Research Council, was closely associated with inflammation of the cartilaginous airways (>2 mm in diameter). However, continued sputum production did not significantly correlate with either hypertrophy of mucous glands or the Reid index. Consequently, the authors suggested that mucosal inflammation, rather than mucus-secreting cell hypertrophy, is mainly responsible for the excessive production of mucus seen in chronic bronchitics. The pathological and pathophysiological effects of cigarette smoking on small airways (<2 mm in diameter) have also been studied (Niewoehner et al., 1974; Cosio et al., 1978, 1980). This so-called small or peripheral airways disease anatomically corresponds to mural inflammation, fibrosis, goblet cell metaplasia, mucous plugging, and distortion of bronchioles.

The inflammatory response in cystic fibrosis involves all sizes of conducting airways. Abnormalities include mucopurulent plugging of the airway lumen, severe inflammation of the bronchial wall, and bronchiectasis. The cellular infiltrate is characterized by the presence of both acute and chronic inflammatory cells. The increased number of neutrophils and their various products, such as phospholipid-derived mediators, proteolytic enzymes, and toxic oxygen metabolites, are likely to participate in the disease process.

To what extent the presence of these inflammatory cells in the airways contribute to the process of mucous hypersecretion is a question that has been evaluated in the past decade. It is the main objective of this chapter to summarize the findings of this research area.

III. Methods Used to Assay Mucous Secretion

A variety of approaches have been used to study respiratory secretions (Table 1). Collection of secretions produced in vivo has the advantage for the study of a living intact organism, but may be complicated by the uncertainty of the cellular origin of specific secretory components and by the uncertainty of the effect of the collection system on the characteristics of secretions studied (i.e., reflex-mediated effects). The study of organ cultures in vitro involves the study of denervated tissue that

Table 1 Approaches Used to Study Airway Mucus

Method	Applicability	Measurable parameters	Refs.
Collection of tracheobronchial mucus	In vivo	A,B,C,D	Puchelle et al., 1984
Spontaneous or protected expectoration			Chase et al., 1985
Bronchoscopic aspiration			Rahmoune et al., 1991
Whole trachea preparation	In vitro	A,B,C,D	Robinson et al., 1983
Tantalum dust hillocks methods	In vitro; In vivo	A	Davis and Nadel, 1980
Micropipetting of submucosal glands	In vitro; In vivo	A,C,D	Ueki et al., 1980 Leikauf et al., 1984
Culture of airway tissue			
Organ cultures	In vitro	B,C	Shelhamer et al., 1980 Adler et al., 1987
Isolated submucosal glands	In vitro	B,C	Shimura et al., 1986, 1988a,b
Primary cultures of			
Surface tracheal epithelial cells	In vitro	B,C	Wu, 1986, 1990 Kim and Brody, 1989 Rieves et al., 1992a
Submucosal gland cells	In vitro	B,C	Culp et al., 1983 Tournier et al., 1990
Cell lines	In vitro	B,C	Finkbeiner et al., 1986 Goswami et al., 1990

Parameters: A, secretion flow rate; B, measurement of macromolecules using either radiolabeling or immunological (ELISA) methods; measurement of cell-specific secretory proteins (e.g., lysozyme, lactoferrin); C, biochemical analyses (e.g., pH, osmolality, ion concentrations, proteins); D, rheological properties (e.g., viscoelasticity, adhesiveness, spinability).

has in it a variety of cell types that may interact in an inflammatory process. The study of cell cultures of specific secretory cells has the advantage of a greater simplicity, but may be devoid of the potential for relevant cell–cell interactions, as might occur in tissue or in the living organism.

The composition of respiratory tract secretions is altered in many airway inflammatory diseases, with resultant typical rheological and biochemical patterns (Dulfano et al., 1971; Sahu and Lynn, 1978; Chase et al., 1985; Rahmoune et al., 1991). Collection of tracheobronchial secretions, in vivo, by spontaneous expectoration, protected expectoration (Puchelle et al., 1984), or bronchoscopic techniques, has allowed investigators to analyze the rheological and biochemical characteristics of human mucus in both healthy and diseased states. The two latter methods offer the advantage of greatly diminishing salivary contamination; thereby, providing a high-quality specimen for rheological studies. The in vivo hillocks method was introduced by Davis and his colleagues (Davis et al., 1976) to study the role of neuronal influences and reflexes on tracheal mucous gland secretion. It consists of a semiquantitative estimation of submucosal gland secretion by visualizing the emergence of mucus from secretory ducts, with the consequent formation of hillocks on the airway surface previously sprayed with powdered tantalum. An elegant micropipette method (Ueki et al., 1980) has also been employed for in vivo analysis of mucous secretion. By using this technique, both the secretion flow rate and physicochemical properties of mucus can be studied from single submucosal glands. Both the hillocks technique and the micropipette method can be adapted for in vitro studies, thereby excluding the influence of neural reflexes and circulating mediators in the secretion process. An alternative in vitro method of assaying mucous secretion, principally applied to the ferret, uses the whole trachea mounted in an organ bath (Robinson et al., 1983; Webber and Widdicombe, 1987).

Studies on regulation of mucous secretion have been facilitated by the improvement of cell culture methods. Available strategies consist of cultures of tracheobronchial segments (airway organ culture), primary cultures of cells from submucosal glands and surface tracheobronchial epithelium, and cultures of cell lines. Although it is beyond the scope of this chapter to provide a detailed description of these individual cell culture methods, this subject has been extensively reviewed in several recent references (Wu et al., 1990; Van Scott et al., 1986, 1991). *Organ culture* is best defined as the maintenance of intact airway segments in vitro. It refers to a heterogeneous cell population that includes mucus-secreting cells of the surface epithelium and submucosal glands, along with a variety of nonepithelial cell types. Although organ culture offers the advantage of a prolonged preservation of morphology, the heterogeneous cell population precludes the establishment of a direct causal relation between the studied factor and specific mucus-secreting cells. A distinction is sometimes made between the terms *organ* and *explant* culture (Van Scott et al., 1986). Tracheal explants represent the culture of airway segments that additionally allows the epithelial cells to grow onto a supporting matrix from the original airway section. Monolayer cultures of cells from tracheal surface epithelium have been successfully used by several groups to further elucidate the specific mechanisms involved in mucous secretion. Experimental animal (Lee et al., 1984; Wu, 1986; Kim and Brody, 1989; Rieves et al., 1992a) and human (Wu et al., 1990) tracheobronchial surface epithelial cells are usually obtained by enzymatic dissociation of freshly excised airway tissues or autopsy material. Several investigators have found that the use of both serum-free, hormone-supplemented medium containing vitamin A, and a thick collagen gel substratum are required to maintain the mucous secretory phenotype in vitro by the tracheal surface epithelial cells (Kim, 1985; Rearick et al., 1987; Wu et al., 1990). In addition, some reports have described techniques concerning the isolation and culture of cells from submucosal glands (Culp et al., 1983; Finkbeiner et al., 1986; Tournier et al., 1990). In particular, a line of bovine tracheal gland serous cells has been developed by Finkbeiner and co-workers (1986), thereby providing investigators with a valuable tool to study the regulation of serous cell secretion. No airway epithelial cell line expressing a mucous secretory cell phenotype has yet been identified. However, a line of human endometrial adenocarcinoma cells (Ishikawa cells) that secretes a mucinlike glycoprotein has been used by some investigators to study the modulation of mucin secretion (Goswami et al., 1990; Amin et al., 1991; Sperber et al., 1991).

With use of these cell culture strategies, several studies have analyzed the secretion of respiratory glycoconjugates (RGC). The use of radioactive precursors, such as [^{3}H]glucosamine, [^{14}C]threonine, or [^{35}S]sulfate, for the quantitation of RGC secretion relies on the principle that cultured cells will incorporate radio-labeled precursors from nutrient medium into newly synthesized and secreted macromolecules. Quantification of secreted RGC is then carried out by scintillation counting of the culture medium after dialysis or precipitation with trichloro-acetic acid or ethanol. However, the radiolabeled respiratory glycoconjugates represent not only mucous glycoproteins, but are also composed of various proteoglycans, such as hyaluronic acid, heparan sulfate, keratan sulfate, and chondroitin sulfate. To more specifically quantitate MGP secretion, size-exclusion chromatography (Cheng et al., 1981; Klinger et al., 1984) or treatment with proteoglycan-degrading enzymes (Adler et al., 1987) have been used in conjunction with the radiolabeling method. Therefore, mucous glycoprotein (MGP) specifically refers to the high relative molecular mass (M_r), hyaluronidase-resistant, mucinlike glycoproteins, whereas RGC includes several glycoconjugates. The measurement of radiolabeled macromolecules has also been used in secretion studies performed with airway segments mounted in a Ussing chamber (Borson et al., 1984) and with in vivo animal studies (Gallagher et al., 1975). Autoradiographic studies, using [^{35}S]sulfate as precursor, have also been useful in the study of various secretagogues on ferret tracheal segments (Gashi et al., 1987).

Although the measurement of certain marker molecules, such as lysozyme or lactoferrin, may provide a method to assay serous cells secretory activity, the lack of a sensitive and specific method to identify cell-specific glycoconjugate products has resulted in the use of monoclonal antibodies in studies of airway mucous glycoproteins (Basbaum et al., 1984, 1986; Finkbeiner and Basbaum, 1988; Koshino et al., 1990). Of great interest is that some of the developed monoclonal antibodies appear to be specific for high M_r mucinlike glycoproteins. Use of these monoclonal antibodies in an enzyme-linked immunosorbent assay (ELISA) system provides a fairly sensitive and specific method for the quantitation of MGP secretion from human airway tissues (Lin et al., 1989; Logun et al.,

1991). With the ELISA technique, concentrations of MGP of as little as 1.5 ng/ml can be measured (Logun et al., 1991). Some of the monoclonal antibodies directed against MGP have shown various degrees of cross-reactivity among species. For example, immunofluorescent studies of one such antibody (the 7F10, a murine antibody initially raised against human MGP), have demonstrated cross-reactivity with feline tracheal surface mucous cells (Rieves et al., 1992). Consequently, the use of this monoclonal antibody in an ELISA provides a useful approach to study mucous secretion from human or animal (feline) airway tissues.

IV. Neural Control of Mucous Secretion

Because of its complexity, the neural control of mucous secretion in health and diseased states is still not well understood. The diverse neural influences involved in the regulation of mucous secretion are briefly summarized here. In particular, attention is directed to the concept of neurogenic inflammation and its relation to airway mucous secretion.

A. Cholinergic, Adrenergic, and Nonadrenergic– Noncholinergic Influences

The autonomic nervous system regulates mucous secretion from submucosal glands. Motor innervation supplying the submucosal glands includes adrenergic, cholinergic, and nonadrenergic–noncholinergic (NANC) influences (Barnes, 1986). In contrast, the goblet cells of the surface epithelium receive no autonomic motor nerve fibers. The use of neuropharmacological agonists to stimulate the secretion of macromolecules from goblet cells has been traditionally unsuccessful. Although it was generally believed that mucous secretion from goblet cells is not under neural control, increasing evidence suggests that goblet cell secretion may be influenced by NANC neural influences (McDonald, 1988; Tokuyama et al., 1990; Kuo et al., 1990).

Electrical stimulation of the vagus nerve in animals (Davis et al., 1976; Borson et al., 1984) or pharmacological stimulation of human airways in vitro with cholinergic agonists (Sturgess and Reid, 1972; Boat et al., 1975; Shelhamer et al., 1980) causes profound mucous secretion from submucosal glands. This effect is mediated by muscarinic receptors. Muscarinic receptors are present on submucosal glands and subtypes of these receptors have been identified by autoradiographic studies (Mak and Barnes, 1990). The finding of two muscarinic receptor subtypes located on human submucosal glands, M_1 and M_3 in the proportions of 36 and 64%, respectively, prompted a study of the role of these subtypes on cholinergic stimulation of mucous secretion. Following cholinergic stimulation (methacholine at 0.1 mM) of human airways in vitro, MGP release can be completely inhibited by antagonists of the M_3 muscarinic receptor subtype

(100% inhibition with 4-diphenylacetoxy-*N*-methylpiperidine-methiodide at 0.1 and 0.01 mM) and partially inhibited by an M_1 receptor antagonist (74% inhibition with pirenzipine at 0.1 mM). However, the M_2 muscarinic receptor antagonist gallamine did not exert an inhibitory effect on methacholine-induced secretion (Johnson et al., 1990). Thus, both M_1 and M_3 receptor subtypes may mediate the secretion of mucus elicited by cholinergic stimulation.

The sympathetic nervous system is also involved in the regulation of mucous secretion. Phenylephrine, a pure α-adrenergic agonist, increases RGC secretion from human airways in vitro (Shelhamer et al., 1980; Phipps et al., 1982). In animal species, β-agonists also enhance airway mucous secretion in vitro (Lietdke et al., 1983). However, their effect on mucous secretion in human studies has been variable. For example, following β-agonist stimulation in vitro, Phipps et al. (1982) found the release of RGC from human bronchi to be augmented, whereas it was unchanged in other reports (Boat and Kleinerman, 1975; Shelhamer et al., 1980).

Data from animal experiments suggest that selective stimulation of muscarinic, α-adrenergic, or β-adrenergic receptors produces secretions with different physicochemical characteristics (Ueki and Nadel, 1981; Leikauf et al., 1984). This phenomenon has been explained, in part, by the heterogeneous distribution of the α- and β-adrenergic receptors on mucous and serous cells of the submucosal glands (Barnes and Basbaum, 1983). β-Agonists appear to preferentially stimulate submucosal gland mucous cells with resultant increases in both MGP secretion and mucous viscosity. In contrast, α-adrenergic agonists seem to preferentially stimulate serous cells, thereby increasing secretion of fluid and lysozyme, which diminishes the viscosity of mucus. Stimulation of muscarinic receptors, which are distributed equally on mucous and serous cells, results in a marked increase in both fluid and MGP secretion, with an unaltered viscosity. It should be mentioned that this concept is derived from animal studies, and caution should be taken in extrapolating to human physiology.

Over the past few years, much information has become available concerning the role of the NANC system in the control of mucous secretion. In 1983, Peatfield and Richardson made the observation that the release of mucus following vagal nerve stimulation in cats in vivo could not be totally inhibited by atropine. The administration of phentolamine and propranolol, in addition to atropine, also failed to reduce the vagal-mediated mucous secretion. From segments of ferret trachea mounted in a Ussing chamber, Borson and associates (1984) demonstrated that a combination of the same three antagonists was insufficient to totally suppress the secretion of $^{35}SO_4$ macromolecules in response to electrical field stimulation. Consequently, it was postulated that a NANC pathway may also control the secretion of mucus from submucosal glands. Originally, the presence of distinct NANC nerves supplying the airways was suspected. Now, there is convincing evidence that the NANC or peptidergic system consists of several neuropeptides that exert their effect after being released from classic autonomic nerves. Cotransmission of these neuropeptides has been described with adrenergic, cholinergic, and sensory nerves. Table 2 lists neuropeptides that have been identified in the lower respiratory tract that may influence airway mucous secretion.

B. Reflex-Mediated Mucous Secretion: Transspinal Reflexes and Intra-airway Antidromic Reflexes

Airways are richly supplied by afferent sensory nerves. Up to 80% of vagal afferent nerves consist of nonmyelinated sensory nerve endings (also called capsaicin-sensitive sensory nerve or C fiber) that have been identified throughout the tracheobronchial tree, including the epithelial cell layer. One important feature of the cholinergic system is its role in the mediation of reflex hypersecretion that arises following stimulation of sensory nerve receptors (Widdicombe, 1988). A variety of sensory nerve stimuli have induced submucosal gland mucous secretion by transspinal vagal reflexes, primarily involving a cholinergic efferent pathway. Such cholinergic reflex mechanisms have been proposed to mediate the secretion of airway mucus that occurs in various situations such as laryngeal irritation, hypoxemia, mechanical or chemical stimulation of airway sensory nerve receptors, and gastric distension (Kaliner et al., 1988).

In addition, animal studies have shown that mucous secretion from submucosal glands, and possibly from goblet cells, may also be mediated by intra-airway axon reflexes elicited following stimulation of C fiber endings. Lundberg and Saria (1982) elegantly demonstrated that vagal stimulation of atropine-treated rats results in an increase in vascular permeability in the respiratory tract, presumably by vagal sensory axon stimulation. Furthermore, they discovered that once sensory C fibers are depleted of their neuropeptides by pretreatment with capsaicin (the pungent agent of hot peppers), respiratory tract inflammation induced by cigarette smoke, and mechanical or chemical irritants is prevented (Lundberg and Saria, 1983). In addition to the vapor-phase component of tobacco smoke, similar activation of C fiber endings can be produced by capsaicin, hydrochloric acid, histamine, or bradykinin (Lundberg et al., 1988). Thus, these stimuli can induce inflammation through an intra-airway axon reflex mechanism that involves antidromic conduction down afferent nerve collaterals, with subsequent release of bioactive neuropeptides.

Neuropeptides that have been identified in airway sensory nerves include substance P, neurokinin A (NKA), neuropeptide K, and calcitonin gene-related peptide (CGRP). Gastrin-releasing factor may also be contained in the sensory nerves (Panula et al., 1983; Holtzer, 1988). Substance P, a potent mucous secretagogue, is thought to be the neuropeptide that primarily accounts for axon reflex-induced mucous secretion. The local release of these neuropeptides in the airways

Table 2 Effects of Neuropeptides on Mucous Secretion

| Peptide | Nerve localization | Mucous secretion | Receptor location | | Refs. |
			Submucosal glands	Surface epithelium	
Substance P	Sensory nerve	Increase	Present (NK-1)	Present (NK-1)	Carstairs and Barnes, 1986a; Lundgren et al., 1989; Baraniuk et al., 1991
Neurokinin A	Sensory nerve	Increase	Absent[a]	Absent[a]	
Gastrin-releasing peptide	Sensory nerve Neuroendocrine cells	Increase	Present	Present	Baraniuk et al., 1990b, 1992
Calcitonin gene-related peptide	Sensory nerve	No effect	Absent	Absent	Mak and Barnes, 1988; Baraniuk et al., 1990a
Vasoactive intestinal peptide	Parasympathetic	Variable	Present	Present	Carstairs and Barnes 1986b; Lazarus et al., 1986; Baraniuk et al., 1990d
Other peptides					
Dynorphin A	?	Increase			
Endothelin-1		Increase	Present	Present	Mullol et al., 1991; Wu, T., personal communication

[a]Substance P is more potent than NKA for inducing airway mucous secretion, suggesting that NK-1 receptors (SP receptors) are involved. The effect of NKA on mucous secretion in vitro could reflect the action of NKA on NK-1 receptors, rather than an action on NKA-specific receptors (NK-2 receptors).

causes smooth-muscle contraction and mucous hypersecretion as well as pro-inflammatory effects such as vasodilation, increased vascular permeability, and possibly modulation of immune and inflammatory cell functions. The term *Neurogenic inflammation* describes this inflammatory phenomenon. Figure 1 represents a speculative schema illustrating the events involved in axon reflex-mediated mucous secretion.

C. Neurogenic Inflammation in Airway Diseases

It has also been proposed that neurogenic inflammation may be involved in the pathogenesis of asthma (Barnes, 1986). For example, airway epithelial damage and desquamation are prominent pathological abnormalities in asthmatic airways. Signs of epithelial damage are also encountered in other conditions, such as upper respiratory tract infections (Jacoby et al., 1988), cystic fibrosis (Bedrossian et al.,

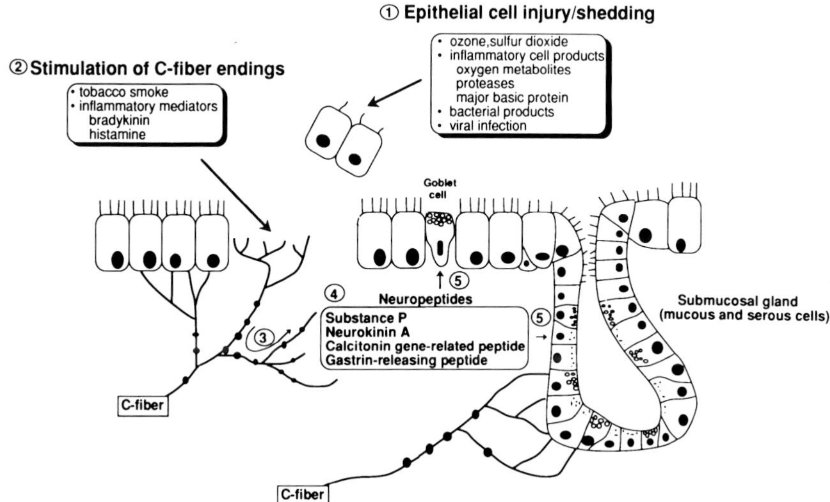

Figure 1 Speculative schema of axonal reflex-induced mucous secretion. (1) Injury and shedding of the surface epithelial cells following exposure to cytotoxic agents. (2) The exposed C fiber endings can be easily activated by inflammatory mediators. (3) Stimulation of the C fiber endings leading to axon reflex with antidromic conduction down collateral sensory endings. (4) Release of proinflammatory sensory neuropeptides in the airways. (5) Among the sensory neuropeptides released, substance P, neurokinin A, and gastrin-releasing peptide may stimulate mucous secretion from both submucosal glands and surface epithelial goblet cells. Furthermore, a decrease in neutral endopeptidase (tachykinin-degrading enzyme) activity may occur in the presence of surface epithelium shedding, thereby potentiating the effects of tachykinins on mucus-secreting cells.

1976), chronic bronchitis, and sulfur dioxide and ozone exposure (Murlas and Roum, 1985). The epithelial damage seen in these airway conditions may, in part, be attributed to the presence of toxic products released from infiltrating inflammatory cells. Examples include eosinophil granule-derived proteins (Frigas and Gleich, 1986), toxic oxygen metabolites, and various proteinases (Amitami et al., 1991). In turn, the shedding of the surface epithelium may expose large numbers of C fiber endings. Consequently, the exposed C fiber endings can be easily activated by noxious stimuli to create axon reflexes, with local liberation of proinflammatory peptides. Again, it should be emphasized that allergic (histamine) and inflammatory (bradykinin) reaction products are capable of activating C fiber endings. Thus, this illustrates that airway inflammation can predispose to C fiber activation which, in turn, can contribute to mucous hypersecretion and amplification of the inflammatory reaction.

D. Modulation of Neurogenic Inflammation by Neutral Endopeptidase

The tachykinins, substance P, and neurokinin A, released by an axon reflex mechanism, are subject to degradation by the enzyme neutral endopeptidase, or enkephalinase (EC 3.4.24.11). The presence of this enzyme has been reported in airway epithelium, submucosal glands, sensory nerves, and smooth muscles (Nadel and Borson, 1991). Because this enzyme can inactivate tachykinins, it has been suggested that neutral endopeptidase may modulate the neurogenic inflammation. For example, Nadel and associates postulated that a decrease in airway neutral endopeptidase activity can result in an exaggerated tissue response to neurogenic inflammation. Such a reduction in neutral endopeptidase activity has been reported during respiratory tract infection (Jacoby et al., 1988) and after exposure to cigarette smoke (Dusser et al., 1989), ozone (Murlas et al., 1990), and toluene diisocyanates (Sheppard et al., 1988). Also, decreased neutral endopeptidase activity may also occur following mechanical removal of the airway epithelium in vitro (Sekizawa et al., 1987), suggesting that a similar reduction in enzyme activity may be found in airway diseases associated with shedding of the superficial epithelium.

The case for a modulating role of neutral endopeptidases in neurogenic inflammation has been strengthened by several in vitro and in vivo studies that demonstrated that neutral endopeptidase inhibitors (thiorphan, phosphoramidon) can potentiate tachykinin-mediated effects, including mucous hypersecretion (Borson et al., 1987; Rogers et al., 1989). Furthermore, neutral endopeptidase appears to be capable of modulating the effects of other peptides that may be involved in inflammatory reactions and mucous secretion. For example, endothelin-1, a 21-amino acid peptide possessing potent vasoconstrictive and broncho-constrictive properties, has been recently reported to increase mucous secretion from human nasal mucosa (Mullol et al., 1991) and human bronchi (Johnson et al., 1991). Phosphoramidon, when added simultaneously with endothelin-1 to human organ cultures, markedly potentiates the effect of endothelin-1 on MGP secretion (Johnson, C., personal communication). Since the airway epithelium is an important source of neutral endopeptidase, it represents another potential way for it to participate in the modulation of airway inflammatory reactions.

E. Neuropeptides and Mucous Secretion

Among all the sensory neuropeptides that are released by axon reflexes, the effect of substance P on airway mucous secretion is the best characterized. Substance P and neurokinins A and B are the mammalian members of a family of peptides designated tachykinins. The observation that substance P acts as a potent mucous secretagogue has been reported in studies involving several species including canines (Coles et al., 1984b), ferrets (Borson et al., 1987; Gashi et al., 1986), felines (Shimura et al., 1987; Lundgren et al., 1989), and humans (Rogers et al., 1989). With use of a feline tracheal isolated submucosal gland preparation, Shimura and associates (1987) demonstrated that substance P may exert its secretagogue activity by two mechanisms. First, substance P can cause glandular duct contraction through stimulation of myoepithelial cells, thereby expelling the previously accumulated mucus into the airway lumen. Second, substance P can also stimulate submucosal gland cells to release RGC. Studies from feline (Lundgren et al., 1989) and human airway organ cultures (Rogers et al., 1989) showed that substance P is more potent secretagogue than neurokinin A or B, thereby suggesting the presence of a NK-1 tachykinin receptor subtype on submucosal glands. Autoradiographic studies of human bronchi have further confirmed the presence of a NK-1 receptor on submucosal glands (Carstairs and Barnes, 1986a). Additionally, substance P has also been reported to induce goblet cell discharge from guinea pig tracheas in vivo (Barnes et al., 1990). Coincubation of substance P with selective neutral endopeptidase inhibitors (phosphoramidon, thiorphan) clearly potentiates the substance P-induced secretion (Borson et al., 1987).

Calcitonin gene-related peptide is another bioactive peptide localized in C fibers and released by an axon reflex mechanism. It is a potent vasodilator of bronchial vessels (Salonen et al., 1988; McCormack et al., 1989). Baraniuk and colleagues (1990a) have reported that calcitonin gene-related peptide failed to increase the release of RGC when added exogenously to human nasal mucosal organ cultures. Thus, little evidence exists for a direct role of this peptide in the control of mucous secretion.

Vasoactive intestinal peptide (VIP), a 28-amino acid peptide, is colocalized and released with acetylcholine from cholinergic nerves. This peptide is known for its capacity to relax airway smooth muscle (Palmer et al., 1986). More recently, attention has focused on the diverse anti-inflammatory properties of VIP, which include inhibition of inflammatory cell functions, antagonism of the effects of inflammatory mediators, and attenuation of inflammation-induced injury (Said, 1991). The effect of VIP on airway mucous secretion remains controversial. Both inhibitory and stimulatory effects on mucous secretion have been reported. This discrepancy can be explained, in part, by differences in the systems and species employed to assess airway secretion. Vasoactive intestinal peptide increased mucous secretion in vitro from ferret (Peatfield et al., 1983) and dog (Coles et al., 1984a) tracheas. Shimura and colleagues also found that VIP increased mucous secretion from feline tracheal isolated submucosal glands (Shimura et al., 1988a), but not from tracheal explants of the same species. In the same study, VIP potentiated mucous secretion induced by cholinergic stimulation. Conversely, in human airway organ cultures, VIP has caused a dose-dependent inhibition of both baseline and methacholine-induced release of RGC and lysozyme (Coles et al., 1981). Interestingly, VIP did not inhibit baseline or methacholine-induced RGC release in bronchi obtained from chronic bronchitics. The authors suggested that the absence of VIP inhibition of RGC release may represent a functional abnormality that contributes to mucous hypersecretion in these patients.

With a line of human epithelial cells secreting a mucinlike glycoprotein (Ishikawa cells derived from endometrial adenocarcinoma), Amin and associates (1991) have recently demonstrated that both basal and methacholine-induced MGP secretion could be blocked by VIP. The inhibitory effect of VIP on MGP secretion was accompanied by an increase in membrane adenylate cyclase activity and cytosolic cyclic adenosine $3',5'$-monophosphate (cAMP) formation. Similar results were found with isoproterenol and forskolin, suggesting that MGP secretion is inhibited by increases in cytosolic cAMP. No definite conclusion can yet be drawn for the role of VIP on mucous secretion from human airways. However, current theory suggests that VIP might have an inhibitory effect on mucous secretion and that either a depletion or a functional defect of VIP in the airways may contribute to mucous hypersecretion.

Gastrin-releasing peptide, the mammalian counterpart to bombesin (an amphibian peptide), stimulates the release of RGC from feline (Lundgren et al., 1990a) and human nasal (Baraniuk et al., 1990b) organ cultures. Binding sites for gastrin-releasing peptide have been identified on submucosal glands and surface epithelium of human tracheal (Baraniuk et al., 1992) and nasal mucosa (Baraniuk et al., 1990b). Gastrin-releasing peptide has been found located in pulmonary neuroendocrine cells, in pulmonary macrophages, and colocalized with substance P in some neurons (Baraniuk, 1991). Thus, gastrin-releasing peptide represents another peptide of the NANC system that may modulate airway mucous secretion.

The effect of endorphins on airway mucous secretion has also been evaluated. Lundgren and colleagues (1987) demonstrated that dynorphin A, when exogenously added to feline organ cultures in micromolar concentration, increased the release of RGC. Naloxone in equimolar concentration totally inhibited the dynorphin-induced secretion, suggesting a κ–receptor-mediated response. However, Rogers and Barnes (1989) reported that activation of the subtype μ endorphin receptor caused an inhibition of NANC-mediated stimulation of fucose (used as a MGP marker) release from human bronchi. The precise role and relevance of endorphins in the regulation of mucous secretion remains to be clarified.

Adenosine 5′-triphosphate (ATP) was originally considered to be the neurotransmitter of the NANC nervous system (Burnstock, 1972). Subsequently, numerous studies have identified and proposed a large list of peptides that could mediate NANC transmission. There has been increasing interest in the signaling roles of extracellular purines and their importance in cell communication. The diverse modulatory effects of purine nucleotides (ATP) and nucleosides (adenosine) on cellular functions are mediated by specific purinoceptors that have been localized on several cell types. Purinoceptors have been classified into two major categories, P_1- and P_2-purinoceptors. The effects of ATP are mediated by P_2-purinoceptors, whereas those of its hydrolysis product, adenosine, are mediated through P_1-purinoceptors. Additionally, P_1-purinoceptors have been further subclassified as P_1A_1 and P_1A_2 on the basis of their selectivities for various adenine analogues and of their effects on cAMP level. Similarly, on the basis of relative pharmacological potencies of structural ATP analogues and selective antagonism, P_2-purinoceptors have been subclassified as P_{2x} and P_{2y} (Burnstock and Kennedy, 1985).

Adenosine causes bronchoconstriction in asthmatic patients (Cushley et al., 1984) and potentiates mediator release from activated human lung mast cells (Peachell et al., 1988). By radioligand techniques, Joad (1990) demonstrated the presence of an adenosine receptor, probably of the A_2 subtype, on membrane preparations from human peripheral lung. The potential role of purines in the regulation of mucous secretion was first suggested by Johnson and McNee (1985). By employing the tracheal hillock method to assess mucous secretion from canine trachea, they found that adenosine stimulated the secretion of mucus. Furthermore, *N*-ethylcarboxyadenosine (NECA) enhanced the secretion of mucus, suggesting that this effect was mediated by a P_1A_2-type purinoceptor. Recently, Kim and Lee (1991) examined the effect of purines on MGP secretion from primary cultures of hamster tracheal epithelial cells. In this system, adenosine failed to stimulate the secretion of MGP. However, ATP clearly stimulated the release of mucin, presumably by a P_2–receptor-mediated mechanism. Conceivably, cells from submucosal glands and surface epithelium may express different purinoceptors. Additional studies are required to characterize the effect of purines on mucous secretion from human airways.

V.   Inflammatory Modulation of Mucous Secretion

The excessive production of mucus that is an important component of airway inflammation may also be mediated by nonreflex mechanisms. This section elaborates on the ability of cellular and soluble endogenous mediators of inflammation, as well as bacterial products, to directly stimulate mucous secretion. In addition, data concerning a possible role of airway inflammation in the pathogenesis of secretory cell hyperplasia will be examined.

A.   Cell-Derived Mediators

A variety of mediators released from resident cells and recruited inflammatory cells are known to cause mucous hypersecretion (Table 3). In particular, platelet-activating factor (PAF) and eicosanoids deserve a special attention because they

Table 3   Inflammatory Cell Products that May Cause
Mucous Hypersecretion

Mast cells
Histamine
Eicosanoids[a]
Platelet-activating factor
Chymase
Prostaglandin-generating factor of anaphylaxis (PGF-A)
Neutrophils
Elastase
Cathepsin G
Eicosanoids[a]
Platelet-activating factor
115-kd protein
Oxygen species
Eosinophils
Eosinophilic cationic protein (ECP)
Eicosanoids[a]
Platelet-activating factor
Oxygen species
Macrophages
Eicosanoids[a]
Platelet-activating factor
Macrophage mucous secretagogue (MMS)
Oxygen species

[a]See text for specific cellular eicosanoid profile.

are lipid mediators produced by many of the cellular components of the inflammatory response.

Eicosanoids

Eicosanoids are oxygenated, 20-carbon fatty acids derived from arachidonic acid (5,8,11,14-eicosatetraenoic acid) metabolism. The bulk of arachidonic acid (AA) in mammalian cells is esterified in the cell membrane phospholipids (Irvine, 1982). The hydrolysis of AA through phospholipase A_2 activation results in the liberation of free AA from the membrane phospholipids (Fig. 2). Oxidative metabolism of free AA through the cyclooxygenase pathway leads to the forma-

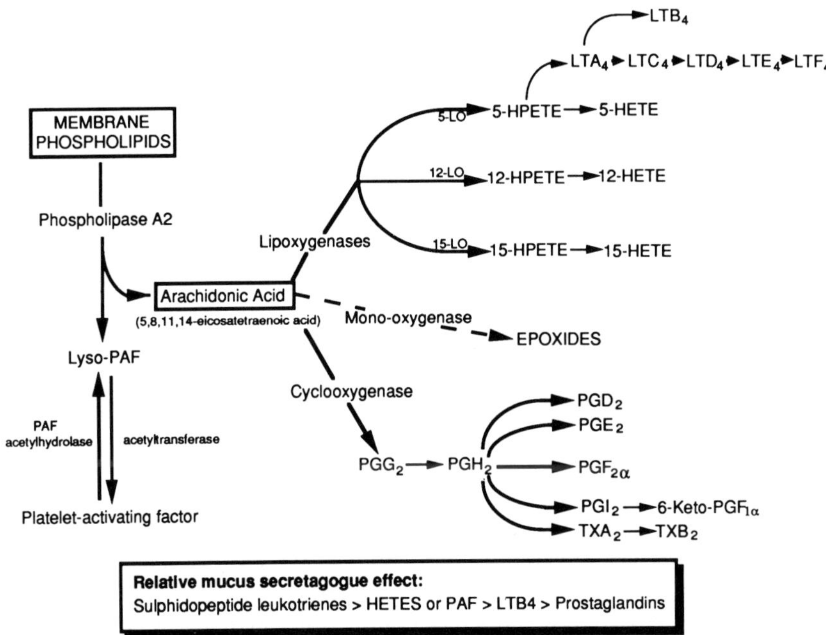

Figure 2 Arachidonic acid metabolism and PAF biosynthesis. Both arachidonic acid and the precursor of PAF, lyso-PAF, are formed by the action of phospholipase A_2 on membrane phospholipids. Acetylation of lyso-PAF forms PAF. Oxidation of arachidonic acid can be effected through the cyclooxygenase or the lipoxygenase pathway. The major end products of these pathways are shown. A third pathway, the cytochrome P-450 monooxygenase, may also be present in the airways. Also shown is the relative potency of PAF and diverse arachidonate-derived metabolites on mucous secretion. The relative mucous secretagogue effect is estimated from animal and human studies using organ and primary cell cultures. See text for details.

tion of prostaglandins (PGs) and thromboxanes (TXs). Arachidonic acid oxidation through the lipoxygenase pathway results in the production of leukotrienes (LTs) and unstable hydroxyperoxyeicosatetraenoic acids (HPETEs) that are transformed to hydroxyeicosatetraenoic acids (HETEs). The lipoxygenase pathway consists of a variety of distinct enzymes, including the 5-, 12-, and 15-lipoxygenases. The sulfidopeptide leukotrienes (LTC_4, LTD_4, and LTE_4), formerly called slow-reacting substance of anaphylaxis (SRS-A), and LTB_4 are generated by the action of the 5-lipoxygenase enzyme. A third pathway of arachidonate acid oxygenation is the cytochrome P-450 monooxygenase enzyme system. Metabolism of AA in this system may result in the production of epoxides. By immunocytochemical techniques, the presence of cytochrome P-450–dependent monooxygenase has been documented in the nonciliated bronchiolar epithelial cells (Clara cells) of the small airways in certain animal species (Boyd, 1977; Serabjit-Singh et al., 1979).

Each type of airway inflammatory cell generates a distinct profile of eicosanoids after stimulation (Henderson, 1991). For example, human lung mast cells release preponderantly PGD_2 and LTC_4 (MacGlashan et al., 1982; Schleimer et al., 1986), whereas neutrophils produce primarily LTB_4 (Henderson and Klebanoff, 1983). Eosinophil activation leads mainly to the production of the sulfidopeptide leukotriene LTC_4 (Weller et al., 1983). Alveolar macrophages produce 5-lipoxygenase pathway products (LTB_4, LTC_4; Fels et al., 1982; Goldyne et al., 1984) and cyclooxygenase products (TXA_2, PGE_2; Laviolette et al., 1981; Godard et al., 1982). Human airway epithelial cells also exhibit a distinct pattern of arachidonate-derived products that exhibits interspecies variability. In human airway epithelial cells, AA is predominantly metabolized by the 15-lipoxygenase and cyclooxygenase pathway products (Holtzman, 1991; Sigal et al., 1991). In contrast, release of LTB_4 (Holtzman et al., 1983; Bigby et al., 1985) and LTC_4 (Eling et al., 1986) has been documented from tracheal epithelial cells of certain animal species.

Some of the eicosanoids, when added exogenously to human airways organ culture, enhance RGC secretion (Marom et al., 1981, 1982, 1983). The estimated rank order of potency of eicosanoids on RGC secretion, according to previous studies, is sulfidopeptide leukotrienes > HETES > LTB_4 > prostaglandins. From a series of experiments performed on human bronchi in vitro, picomolar concentrations of sulfidopeptide leukotrienes, nanomolar concentrations of HETES, and micromolar concentrations of prostaglandins, have been the lowest dose to effectively increase RGC release (Lundgren and Shelhamer, 1990). The sulfidopeptide leukotriene-induced secretion can be blocked in vitro, as well as in vivo, with a sulfidopeptide leukotriene receptor antagonist, FPL 55712 (Marom et al., 1982; Peatfield et al., 1982b; Johnson et al., 1983). In contrast with the powerful secretory effect of other eicosanoids, PGE_2 inhibited RGC release from human airways (Marom et al., 1981).

Eicosanoids have also been reported to increase mucous secretion in primary surface tracheal epithelial cells. For example, $PGF_{2\alpha}$ has been reported to induce mucinlike glycoproteins release from primary cultures of guinea pig tracheal epithelial cells (Adler et al., 1990). In the same in vitro model, a combination of 5-, 12-, and 15-HETE provoked MGP secretion, only when all three were added simultaneously (Glasgow et al., 1991). In contrast, Kim and associates reported that physiological concentrations of prostaglandins (PGE_2 and $PGF_{2\alpha}$) and leukotrienes (LTC_4 and LTD_4) did not increase release of mucus from primary cultures of hamster tracheal epithelial cells (Kim et al., 1989). In monolayer cultures of bovine tracheal serous cells, PGE_1, PGE_2, PGA_1, and PGD_2 have been reported to increase the release of ^{35}S-labeled macromolecules (mainly chondroitin sulfate proteoglycans) (Sommerhoff et al., 1989). Thus, we can reasonably postulate that eicosanoids released from recruited inflammatory cells and airway resident cells can contribute to mucous hypersecretion, as encountered in diverse airway inflammatory diseases or immediate hypersensitivity reactions.

In addition, intracellular eicosanoid metabolism also seems to regulate mucous secretion in normal states. In vitro, normal human airways spontaneously elaborate various prostaglandins and HETEs. Arachidonic acid added to airway organ cultures induces a dose-related increase in RGC release, but only after a latent period, suggesting that arachidonate-derived metabolites are responsible for the enhanced secretion (Marom et al., 1981). The inhibitory action of various glucocorticoids on RGC secretion has been examined in isolated feline sub-mucosal glands (Shimura et al., 1988b) and in human (Marom et al., 1984a), ferret (Cheng et al., 1986), and feline (Lundgren et al., 1988a) tracheal organ cultures. For example, dexamethasone inhibited the baseline secretion of RGC from human (Marom et al., 1984a) and feline (Lundgren et al., 1988a) airways, with a peak effect observed at 18–24 h (human) and at 24–60 h (feline) after initiation of treatment. In addition, dexamethasone induced the synthesis of lipocortin in the feline model. Thus, one effect of dexamethasone may be to reduce RGC secretion by inducing lipocortin synthesis which, in turn, inhibits the action of phospho-lipase A_2 on AA cleavage from cell membrane phospholipids. Blockade of the cyclooxygenase pathway using nonsteroidal anti-inflammatory drugs (NSAID), such as acetylsalicylic acid (ASA) or indomethacin, has been reported to increase RGC release from human airways (Marom et al., 1981). This effect may be due to either a decrease in PGE_2, an inhibitor of mucous glycoprotein secretion, or a shift of AA metabolism toward the production of lipoxygenase pathway metabolites, which are capable of increasing MGP secretion in nanomolar concentrations. Furthermore, exposure of airways to nordihydroguaiaretic acid (NDGA) or eicosatetraynoic acid (ETYA), both combined cyclooxygenase and lipoxygenase inhibitors, inhibits the baseline release of RGC. The concept that eicosanoids are important modulators of mucous glycoprotein secretion is further supported by the observation that a variety of mucous secretagogues may exert their effect by altering airway eicosanoid metabolism. Examples include platelet-activating factor (Rieves et al., 1992a; Glasgow et al., 1991), oxygen metabolites (Adler et al., 1990), bradykinin (Baraniuk et al., 1990c), protein kinase C activators (Rieves et al., 1991), and prostaglandin-generating factor of anaphylaxis (Marom et al., 1984c).

Platelet-Activating Factor

Platelet-activating factor (1-*O*-alkyl-2-acetyl-*sn*-glyceryl-3-phosphocholine) is a phospholipid mediator that possesses potent proinflammatory properties relevant to many biological systems (Snyder, 1987). It has been proposed that PAF is an important mediator of airway inflammation, and several studies have focused on its role in the pathophysiology of asthma and bronchial hyperreactivity (Cuss et al., 1986; Barnes et al., 1988; Smith, 1991). In fact, several reports have demonstrated that PAF can induce mucous hypersecretion and, thereby, contribute to the airway obstruction found in asthma (Adler et al., 1987; Sasaki et al., 1989; Goswami et al., 1989; Lundgren et al., 1990b; Rieves et al., 1992a).

The cellular origin of PAF is multiple. It is neither stored nor preformed, but, similar to eicosanoids, is synthesized on cellular activation. A wide variety of inflammatory and noninflammatory airway cells can produce PAF when stimulated. Although PAF can be synthesized by endothelial and epithelial cells, most of the extracellular PAF is thought to originate from inflammatory cells, such as eosinophils, neutrophils, macrophages, and mast cells. It is formed by the action of phospholipase A_2 on a cell membrane phospholipid (1-alkyl-2-acylglycero-phosphocholine). This action results in the synthesis of the biologically inactive PAF precursor, lyso-PAF, which is then converted to PAF by a specific acetyl-transferase enzyme.

Many groups have attempted to elucidate the precise mechanisms underlying PAF-evoked mucous secretion. Some of these studies have been performed in human (Goswami et al., 1989; Lundgren et al., 1990b), feline (Lundgren et al., 1990b), and rodent (Adler et al., 1987) organ cultures. From these organ culture studies and in vivo studies (Hahn et al., 1986; Lang et al., 1987), one can hypothesize that PAF may indirectly enhance secretion by a stimulatory effect on other resident or migratory cells of the airways. In turn, these stimulated cells may release other potential secretagogues. In a model using isolated feline submucosal glands, Sasaki and associates (1989) found that PAF increased the release of glycoconjugates only in the presence of platelets. Furthermore, this action was dependent on thromboxane generation by platelets. However, PAF has been reported to directly induce the release of MGP when tested on a monolayer culture of tracheal epithelial cells from cats (Rieves et al., 1992) and guinea pigs (Adler et al., 1992). It is unlikely that this action reflects a nonspecific lipophilic interaction of PAF with cell membranes, since lyso-PAF, the nonactive PAF analogue, failed to enhance the release of MGP from these primary cultures. In addition, both studies demonstrated that PAF-induced secretion can be blocked by various PAF receptor antagonists, such as Ro 19-3704, WEB 2086, and CV-3988, suggesting a receptor-mediated mechanism.

When PAF interacts with its receptor, a complex series of biochemical events are initiated through diverse signal transduction pathways. Some of the intracellular responses triggered by PAF include protein kinase C activation, phosphoinositide and arachidonic acid metabolite production, and elevation of intracellular free-calcium concentration. There are at least three lines of evidence suggesting that PAF-induced secretion is dependent on the generation of arachidonic acid metabolites, especially lipoxygenase products, by the airway epithelium: (1) PAF is capable of inducing the release of a variety of eicosanoids from airway explants and tracheal epithelial cell cultures (Adler et al., 1987; Goswami et al., 1989; Wu et al., 1991; Glasgow et al., 1991). (2) Coincubation of PAF with *p*-bromophenacyl bromide (BPB), an inhibitor of arachidonic acid release, results in a complete inhibition of PAF-stimulated secretion in cultured feline tracheal epithelial cells (Rieves et al., 1992). Dexamethasone treatment of human tracheal explants has also been reported to prevent PAF-mediated RGC secretion (Goswami et al., 1989). This action is probably mediated by phospholipase A_2 inhibition which, in turn, reduces the availability of free arachidonic acid for subsequent eicosanoid generation. Furthermore, PAF-evoked MGP secretion can be inhibited using NDGA, whereas cyclooxygenase inhibitors (ibuprofen or indomethacin) failed to suppress the PAF mucous secretory action. (3) A selective 5-lipoxygenase inhibitor L-651,392 inhibited PAF-induced RGC secretion by feline and human airway organ cultures (Lundgren et al., 1990b).

In summary, the mucous secretagogue property of PAF is well established. Although this action could occur in part secondary to recruitment and activation of inflammatory cells by PAF, a substantial amount of data supports the concept that PAF-induced mucous hypersecretion occurs by direct activation of mucus-secreting cells and is mediated by arachidonic acid-derived metabolites.

Mast Cell Products

Large numbers of mast cells reside within the tracheobronchial tree (Guerzon et al., 1979). Mast cell activation results in the release of several mediators that are responsible for type 1 immediate hypersensitivity reactions (e.g., early asthmatic reaction). Mast cell degranulation in cultured human airways increases the release of RGC, thereby supporting the idea that immediate hypersensitivity reaction products can modulate mucous secretion (Shelhamer et al., 1980). Histamine, various eicosanoids (especially sulfidoleukotrienes), prostaglandin-generating factor of anaphylaxis (PGF-A), platelet-activating factor, and chymase are among the mast cell-derived mediators that can cause mucous hypersecretion.

Histamine has been reported to enhance glycoconjugate secretion from human airways (Shelhamer et al., 1980), ferret trachea (Webber and Widdicombe, 1987), and cultured bovine airway gland serous cells (Sommerhoff et al., 1989). In human tracheal organ cultures and in bovine airway gland serous cells, this effect was prevented by cimetidine, an H_2 receptor antagonist. Activated mast cells also release PGF-A, a 2-kD peptide that causes mucous secretion when added to human airway organ cultures (Marom et al., 1984c). Concomitant stimulation of airway eicosanoid metabolism is likely to be the mechanism by which PGF-A exerts its secretagogue activity. Caughey has recently reported (1991) that more than 70% of the mast cells within 20 μm of bronchial submucosal glands contain chymase, a serine protease. Chymase has been reported to cause the release of radiolabeled glycoconjugates from the cell surface of canine tracheal epithelial cells (Varsano et al., 1987) and from the secretory granules of bovine tracheal gland serous cells (Sommerhoff et al., 1989). Thus, mast cells, through a vast array of mediators, are capable of influencing airway mucous secretion.

Eosinophil Products

Eosinophils present within asthmatic airways may contribute to mucous hypersecretion by at least two mechanisms. First, eosinophil activation leads to the release of preformed and newly generated products that can stimulate mucous secretion. Newly generated lipid mediators, such as PAF and eicosanoids, are potent mucous secretagogues. Activated eosinophils also release granule-associated proteins, such as major basic protein (MBP), eosinophil cationic protein (ECP), eosinophil-derived neurotoxin, and eosinophil peroxidase. A recent study (Lundgren et al., 1991) demonstrated that crude extracts from isolated eosinophil granules stimulated the release of RGC from feline tracheal organ cultures. Furthermore, this study also revealed that purified eosinophil cationic protein caused a dose-dependent increase in RGC release from both feline and human airway organ cultures, whereas major basic protein inhibited RGC release. Eosinophil-derived neurotoxin and eosinophil peroxidase had no effect.

Second, major basic protein (MBP) may be cytotoxic to superficial epithelium and may indirectly provoke mucous hypersecretion. This may occur as a result of airway surface epithelial damage and shedding, with resultant exposure of C fiber endings. As previously described, stimulation of exposed C fiber ends by various inflammatory stimuli can result in submucosal gland cell stimulation through transspinal and intra-airway reflexes.

Neutrophil Products

Neutrophils are recruited to the airway in acute and chronic bronchitis (Thomson et al., 1989), cystic fibrosis (Bedrossian et al., 1976), the late asthmatic response (Metzger et al., 1987), and after exposure to environmental stimuli, such as ozone (Murlas and Roum, 1985) and sulfur dioxide (Seltzer et al., 1984). Neutrophil products may contribute to airway mucous hypersecretion associated with these disorders. The ability of neutral serine proteinases, such as elastase and cathepsin G, to stimulate airway mucin release is well documented. Previous studies have described two mechanisms by which neutrophil proteinases can induce the release of glycoconjugates from mucus-secreting cells. Some studies have suggested that neutrophil proteinases can increase the release of glycoconjugates associated with the mucus-secreting cell surface (Kim et al., 1987; Varsano et al., 1987), whereas others have demonstrated direct degranulation (Breuer et al., 1987; Sommerhoff et al., 1990). A 115-kD peptide, isolated from degranulated human neutrophils, also stimulates the release of RGC from human tracheal organ cultures (Logun et al., 1988).

Adler and colleagues have demonstrated that toxic oxygen metabolites, which can be released by neutrophils and macrophages, can stimulate airway mucous secretion (Adler et al., 1990). They demonstrated that the mechanism of oxygen metabolite-induced secretion is likely to involve airway epithelial production of cyclooxygenase products (mainly $PGF_{2\alpha}$) within the airway epithelium (Adler et al., 1990). Finally, neutrophils can also produce eicosanoids and PAF, thereby influencing the secretion of mucus.

Macrophage–Monocyte Products

Macrophages infiltrate the airway mucosa of patients with chronic bronchitis. Mononuclear phagocytes are also present in the mucosal inflammatory cell infiltrate in chronic asthma. There is definite evidence of macrophage activation in both chronic bronchitis and asthma. It has been reported that the number of activated macrophages recovered by bronchoalveolar lavage increases after allergen challenge of asthmatic airways in vivo (Metzger et al., 1987). Some of the mediators released after macrophage activation can influence airway mucous secretion (see Table 3). Human monocyte–macrophage-derived mucous secretagogue (MMS) is a 2-kD oligopeptide synthesized and released following cell surface activation of human pulmonary macrophages or peripheral monocytes. Synthesis and release of MMS is completely inhibited by cyclohexamide, confirming that it is a newly synthesized peptide. When added to human airways in culture or to Ishikawa cells, MMS stimulates the release of mucous glycoproteins (Marom et al., 1984b, 1985a). Clone 63, an MMS-producing macrophage line, has recently been generated from the fusion of an hypoxanthine guanine phosphoribosyltransferase-deficient promonocytic line (U937) with macrophages (Sperber et al., 1991). The MMS produced by this clone possesses biological activity capable of inducing RGC release from human airways and Ishikawa secretory cells.

B. Plasma-Derived Mediators

The influence of plasma-derived inflammatory mediators on airway mucous secretion has also been studied. The anaphylatoxin C3a, generated during complement system activation, and bradykinin, a product of the kinin pathway, have both influenced mucous secretion in vitro. Biologically active products of complement activation may be present in inflamed airways. Among them, C3a is a low M_r fragment that can be generated following activation of either the classic or alternative complement pathways. Exposure of human tracheal organ cultures to C3a results in a dose-related increase in RGC release (Marom et al., 1985b). The mechanism of C3a-induced mucous secretion is unknown, but seems to be independent of mast cell activation or eicosanoid generation within the tracheal explant.

Bradykinin, a nine-amino acid peptide, is produced as a consequence of the proteolytic actions of kallikreins and other kininogenases on tissue and plasma kininogens. Autoradiographic examinations of the lower respiratory tract (Mak and Barnes, 1991) and nasal mucosa (Baraniuk et al., 1990c) have demonstrated that bradykinin-binding sites are located primarily on blood vessels. In contrast, submucosal gland- and epithelial-binding sites for bradykinin were identified at a very low density within the lower respiratory tract and were absent in the nasal mucosa.

Some of the biological effects of bradykinin might be mediated by its ability to stimulate bronchial C fibers, with consequent axonal or transspinal vagal reflexes. Such transspinal reflexes mediate bradykinin-induced secretion from canine tracheal glands (Davis et al., 1982). In a series of experiments, Baraniuk and associates (1990c) examined the secretory response to bradykinin in respiratory mucous membranes. Bradykinin, when applied to the luminal surface of ferret tracheal segments mounted in a Ussing chamber, slightly increased the flux of ^{35}S-glycoconjugates. Bradykinin also increased the release of RGC from human nasal mucosal explants, an effect prevented by coincubation with NDGA or ibuprofen. This suggests that bradykinin acts primarily by causing release of eicosanoids which, in turn, mediate glycoprotein secretion. However, when added to feline tracheal organ cultures, bradykinin failed to increase the release of RGC. Furthermore, secretions obtained from bradykinin nasal provocations in guinea pigs revealed an increase in albumin concentration (a measure of vascular permeability), without any change in total protein concentration (a measure of glandular secretion plus vascular transudation). Thus, it is possible that bradykinin affects the secretion of airway glycoproteins mainly by indirect mechanisms (sensory nerve stimulation or eicosanoid production). This is further supported by the low density of binding sites found on submucosal glands or surface epithelium.

Leakage of serum proteins into the airway lumen is a feature that often characterizes inflamed airways and can directly increase the volume of airway secretions. As a result of this leakage, mucus-secreting cells may be exposed to secretagogues present in serum. Mucous secretagogue activity has been identified in the sera of cats (Peatfield et al., 1982a), normal humans, and patients with cystic fibrosis (Boat et al., 1982).

C. Bacterial Products

The respiratory tract of patients with cystic fibrosis or chronic bronchitis is frequently colonized or infected with bacteria. Some studies have addressed the possibility that bacteria and their products could contribute to mucous hypersecretion by directly stimulating mucus-secreting cells. Adler and colleagues demonstrated that bacteria-free filtrates from certain strains of *Pseudomonas aeruginosa*, *Streptococcus pneumoniae*, and *Haemophilus influenzae* stimulated the release of radiolabeled macromolecules from guinea pig tracheal organ cultures (Adler et al., 1983, 1986). Another group (Klinger et al., 1986) characterized the products of *P. aeruginosa* that were capable of increasing mucin release from rabbit tracheal surface epithelium. Purified elastase and alkaline proteinase from *P. aeruginosa* induced mucin release, whereas other pseudomonal products, such as lipopolysaccharide, alginate, and exotoxin A did not affect mucin release. Thus, similar to neutrophil elastase, bacterial proteolytic enzymes can increase airway mucous secretion.

We have recently demonstrated that lipopolysaccharide (LPS) or endotoxin, a cell wall component of gram-negative bacteria, can stimulate the release of MGP from primary cultures of feline tracheal epithelial cells. Interestingly, unlike other rapidly acting secretagogues, a significant increase in MGP secretion was not observed until 48 h after endotoxin (*Escherichia coli* 0111:B4 at 20 ng/ml) exposure. Additionally, LPS-induced MGP secretion was prevented by coincubation with cycloheximide, an inhibitor of protein synthesis. The possibility that the LPS-mediated MGP secretion could occur as a consequence of a mitogenic effect on epithelial cells is currently under investigation. Alternatively, LPS exposure may enhance either mucin gene transcription or mucin mRNA translation, thereby increasing production and secretion of mucus. Consequently, studies on mucin gene expression are currently in progress to better define the level of control of LPS-mediated MGP secretion.

The effect of erythromycin, an antibiotic often used in the treatment of acute bronchitis, on mucous secretion has also been studied (Goswami et al., 1990). Erythromycin (10^{-4}–10^{-7} M) decreased the baseline release of RGC when added to human airway organ cultures. The inhibitory effect on mucous secretion was nontoxic and peaked after 16 h of erythromycin treatment. Interestingly, other antibiotics, such as penicillin, ampicillin, cephalosporin, and tetracycline, did not exert an effect on mucous secretion. Thus, these in vitro data suggest that erythromycin, in addition to its antibacterial properties, may also directly reduce the mucous hypersecretion that accompanies bacterial bronchitis.

VI. Inflammation and Secretory Cell Hyperplasia

Submucosal gland hypertrophy and goblet cell hyperplasia constitute important pathological changes seen in the airways of patients with asthma, chronic bronchitis, and cystic fibrosis. *Goblet cell hyperplasia* describes an increase in the number of goblet cells in large airways. In contrast, the presence of goblet cells in the peripheral airways (bronchioles), where they are not normally present, is referred to as *goblet cell metaplasia*. The mechanisms governing the number of goblet cells present in normal and pathological states are still not well characterized. However, it is becoming apparent that multiple polypeptide growth factors and cytokines may be implicated in the regulation of proliferation and differentiation of the tracheobronchial epithelium (for review, see Jetten, 1991).

Some airway irritants are known to induce goblet cell hyperplasia. Inhalants, such as tobacco smoke (Lamb and Reid, 1969) and sulfur dioxide (Lamb and Reid, 1968), and products from neutrophils (Snider et al., 1984), in particular elastase (Breuer et al., 1985a), have induced goblet cell hyperplasia. Recently, Harkema and Hotchkiss reported that endotoxin exposure in vivo may cause similar changes in rat airways (Harkema and Hotchkiss, 1991). They found that repeated intranasal instillations of endotoxin induced a marked bronchiolar epithelial cell hypertrophy or hyperplasia with increased amount of stored intraepithelial mucosubstances.

Exposure of the airway epithelium to injurious agents is often characterized by the recruitment of inflammatory cells. The hypothesis that a causal relation exists between the accumulation of inflammatory cells and the development of secretory cell hyperplasia, has been examined, with special attention given to neutrophils. For example, instillation of a crude neutrophil extract into the trachea of hamsters (Snider et al., 1984) and rats (Lundgren et al., 1988b) can produce goblet cell hyperplasia. These changes were also observed with purified neutrophil elastase (Snider et al., 1984; Breuer et al., 1985a; Lundgren et al., 1988b). Treatment of human neutrophil elastase with Suc-Ala-Ala-Pro-Val chloromethyl ketone (an elastase inhibitor), before intratracheal instillation to hamsters, prevented the development of bronchial secretory cell metaplasia (Breuer et al., 1985b). When given intratracheally to hamsters before human neutrophil elastase, both Eglin-C (Snider et al., 1985) and α_1 proteinase inhibitor (Stone et al., 1990) can moderate or suppress the elastase-induced secretory cell metaplasia. However, coadministration of Suc-Ala-Ala-Pro-Val chloromethyl ketone with crude extract of human neutrophils failed to prevent the development of bronchial secretory cell metaplasia (Snider et al., 1984). Consequently, it has been suggested that other neutrophil products could also contribute to the production of secretory cell metaplasia. To explore this possibility, Lucey and co-workers (1985) studied the effect of cathepsin G on induction of secretory cell metaplasia. They found that purified human neutrophil cathepsin G is a weak inducer of bronchial cell metaplasia in hamsters and that it failed to potentiate the secretory cell metaplasia induced by human neutrophil elastase. Little is known about the specific mechanisms by which elastase and neutrophil extracts cause bronchial secretory cell metaplasia. These products may directly alter the mitotic rate or differentiation of epithelial cells, resulting in hyperplasia or metaplasia of goblet cells. Another alternative is that neutrophil-derived products could damage the airways and promote an inflammatory response characterized by proliferative and differentiation changes. Airway inflammatory changes following administration of neutrophil products have been observed in rats (Lundgren et al., 1988b), but not in hamsters (Snider et al., 1984).

The ability of anti-inflammatory agents to prevent the development of irritant-induced secretory cell hyperplasia also suggests a pathogenic role for inflammation. Dexamethasone has been reported to inhibit the goblet cell hyperplasia induced by neutrophil lysates or purified neutrophil elastase (Lundgren et al., 1988b). Similarly, glucocorticoids, indomethacin (Rogers and Jeffrey, 1986), and phenylmethyloxadiazole (Jones and Reid, 1978) can inhibit tobacco smoke-induced secretory cell hyperplasia. The mechanisms by which nonsteroidal and steroidal anti-inflammatory agents exert this protective effect is unknown. It may be related to their effects on arachidonic acid metabolism. Anti-inflammatory agents may also prevent the influx of inflammatory cells in the airways, thereby limiting the development of secretory cell hyperplasia. This hypothesis has been supported by Lundgren and associates (1988b), who found that rats treated with neutrophil lysates plus dexamethasone developed neither goblet cell hyperplasia nor inflammatory cell infiltration of the submucosa. In contrast, these changes were observed in rats treated with neutrophil lysates alone. The protective effect of glucocorticoids is likely to be multifactorial and could involve regulation of the autocrine or paracrine growth factors, or both, that influence the proliferation of the tracheobronchial epithelial cells. Although there is evidence suggesting that airway inflammation may lead to the development of secretory cell hyperplasia following exposure to airway irritants, more studies are needed to examine the precise mechanisms by which these proliferative changes arise.

VII. Summary

Inflammatory processes arising in the airways are often accompanied by the hypersecretion of mucous glycoproteins. Figure 3 illustrates a proposed sequence of events leading to mucous hypersecretion in airways from patients with asthma, chronic bronchitis, cystic fibrosis, and bacterial bronchitis. This schematic summary is based on the observations mentioned previously in this chapter. Numerous mediators released by the inflammatory response have been identified as mucous secretagogues. The list is extensive and includes lipid mediators, proteinases, oxygen metabolites, and other cell-specific products (i.e., macrophage-derived secretagogue, eosinophil cationic protein). Bacterial products may also be impor-

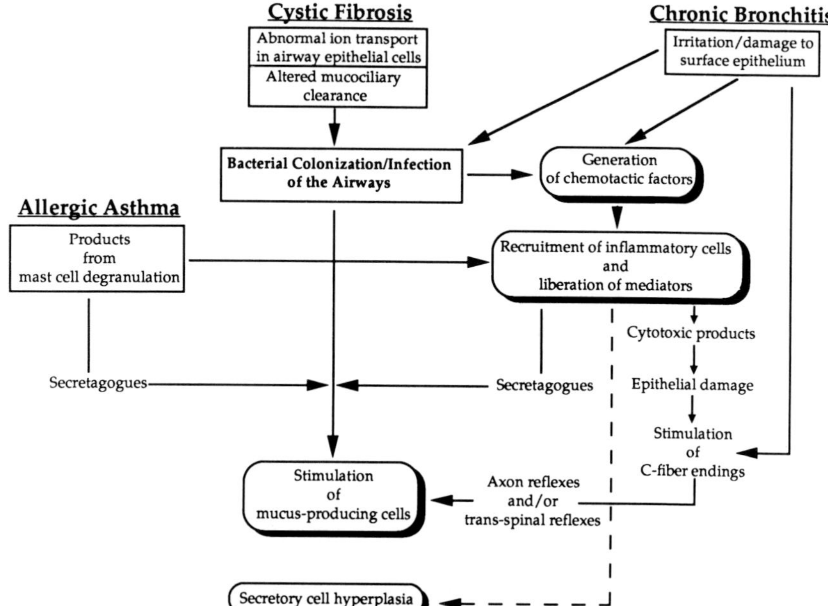

Figure 3 Schematic summary. Proposed sequence of events culminating in mucous hypersecretion in asthma, chronic bronchitis, and cystic fibrosis. The recruitment of inflammatory cells in the airways represents a central event in these disorders. Some of the inflammatory cell products can stimulate airway mucous secretion, enhance epithelial damage, and perhaps also stimulate secretory cell hyperplasia.

tant contributors of mucous hypersecretion seen in chronic bronchitis or cystic fibrosis. Some bioactive peptides released from C fiber afferents in response to airway irritants may also have a pathogenic role in airway inflammation (neurogenic inflammation) and mucous hypersecretion. However, further studies are needed to ascertain the role of these neural mediators in the pathogenesis of mucous hypersecretion associated with inflammatory disorders of human airways. The active role of airway epithelium in inflammatory reactions and cell–cell interactions has recently received more attention. The airway epithelium can assume dynamic functions, such as generation of chemoattractants, production of arachidonate metabolites and neutral endopeptidase which, in turn, can modulate both the inflammatory response and the secretion of airway mucus. Finally, airway inflammation can also contribute an increased quantity of airway secretions by increasing microvascular permeability and, possibly, by contributing to the development of secretory cell hyperplasia.

References

Adler, K. B., Winn, W. C. Jr., Alberghini, T. V., and Craighead, J. E. (1983). Stimulatory effect of *Pseudomonas aeruginosa* on mucin secretion by respiratory epithelium. *JAMA* 249: 1615–1617.

Adler, K. B., Hendley, D. D., and Davis, G. S. (1986). Bacteria associated with obstructive pulmonary disease elaborate extracellular products that stimulate mucin secretion by explants of guinea pig airways. *Am. J. Pathol.* 125: 501–514.

Adler, K. B., Schwartz, J. E., Anderson, W. H., and Welton, A. F. (1987). Platelet activating factor stimulates secretion of mucin by explants of rodent airways in organ culture. *Exp. Lung Res.* 13: 25–43.

Adler, K. B., Holden, Stauffer, W. J., and Repine, J. E. (1990). Oxygen metabolites stimulate release of high-molecular-weigh glycoconjugates by cell and organ cultures of rodent respiratory epithelium via an arachidonic acid-dependent mechanism. *J. Clin. Invest.* 85: 75–85.

Adler, K. B., Akley, N. J., Glascow, W. C. (1992). Platelet-activating factor provokes release of mucin-like glycoprotein from guinea pig respiratory epithelial cells via a lipoxygenase dependent mechanism. *Am. J. Resp. Cell Mol. Biol.* 6: 550–556.

Amin, D. N., Goswami, S., Klein, T., Maayani, and Marom, Z. (1991). Functional antagonism between hormone receptor systems: Modulation of glycoprotein secretion in secretory epithelial cells. *Am. J. Respir. Cell Mol. Biol.* 4: 135–139.

Amitami, R., Wilson, R., Rutman, A., Read, R. Ward, C. Burnett, D., Stockley, R. A., and Cole, P. J. (1991). Effects of human neutrophil elastase and *Pseudomonas aeruginosa* proteinases on human respiratory epithelium. *Am. J. Respir. Cell Mol. Biol.* 4: 26–32.

Annesi, I., and Kauffmann, F. (1986). Is respiratory mucus hypersecretion really an innocent disorder? *Am. Rev. Respir. Dis.* 134: 688–693.

Azzawi, M., Bradley, B., Jeffery, P. K., Frew, A. J., Wardlaw, A. J., Knowles, G. Assoufi, B., Collins, J. V., Durham, S., and Kay, A. B. (1990). Identification of activated T-lymphocytes and eosinophils in bronchial biopsies in stable atopic asthma. *Am. Rev. Respir. Dis.* 142: 1407–1413.

Baraniuk, J. N., Lundgren, J. D., Goff, J., Mullol, J., Castellino, S., Merida, M., Shelhamer, J. H., and Kaliner, M. A. (1990a). Calcitonin gene-related peptide in human nasal mucosa. *Am. J. Physiol.* 258: L81–L88.

Baraniuk, J. N., Lundgren, J. D., Goff, J., Peden, D., Merida, M., Shelhamer, J., and Kaliner, M. (1990b). Gastrin-releasing peptide in human nasal mucosa. *J. Clin. Invest.* 85: 998–1005.

Baraniuk, J. N., Lundgren, J. D., Mizoguchi, H., Peden, D., Gawin, A., Merida, M., Shelhamer, J. H., and Kaliner, M. A. (1990c). Bradykinin and respiratory mucous membranes. Analysis of bradykinin binding site distribution and secretory responses in vitro and in vivo. *Am. Rev. Respir. Dis.* 141: 706–714.

Baraniuk, J. N., Okayama, M., Lundgren, J. D., et al. (1990d). Vasoactive intestinal polypeptide (VIP) in human nasal mucosa. *J. Clin. Invest.* 86: 825–831.

Baraniuk, J. N., Lundgren, J. D., Okayama, M., Goff, J., Mullol, J., Merida, M., Shelhamer, J. H., and Kaliner, M. A. (1991). Substance P and neurokinin A in human nasal mucosa. *Am. J. Respir. Cell Mol. Biol.* 4: 228–236.

Baraniuk, J., Lundgren, J., Shelhamer, J., and Kaliner, M. (1992). Gastrin-releasing peptide (GRP) binding sites in human tracheobronchial mucosa. *Neuropeptides* 21: 81–84.

Barnes, P. J. (1986). Neural control of human airways in health and disease. *Am. Rev. Respir. Dis.* 134: 1289–1314.

Barnes, P. J. (1989). A new approach to the treatment of asthma. *N. Engl. J. Med.* 321: 1517–1527.

Barnes, P. J., and Basbaum, C. B. (1983). Mapping of adrenergic receptors in the trachea by autoradiography. *Exp. Lung Res.* 5: 183–192.

Barnes, P. J., Chung, K. F., and Page, C. P. (1988). Platelet-activating factor as a mediator of allergic disease. *J. Allergy Clin. Immunol.* 81: 919–934.

Barnes, P. J., Kuo, H.-P., Rogers, D. F., Rohde, J. A. L., and Tokuyama, K. (1990). Effect of sensory neuropeptides on goblet cell secretion in guinea pig trachea in vivo. *J. Physiol. (Lond.)* 422: 100P.

Basbaum, C. B., Mann, J. K., Chow, A. W., and Finkbeiner, W. E. (1984). Monoclonal antibodies as probes for unique antigens in secretory cells of mixed exocrine organs. *Proc. Natl. Acad. Sci. USA* 81: 4419–4423.

Basbaum, C., Chow, A., Macher, B., Finkbeiner, W., Veissiere, D., and Forsberg, L. (1986). Tracheal carbohydrate antigens identified by monoclonal antibodies. *Arch. Biochem. Biophys.* 249: 363–373.

Beasley, R., Roche, W. R., Roberts, J. A., and Holgate, S. T. (1989). Cellular events in the bronchi in mild asthma and after bronchial provocation. *Am. Rev. Respir. Dis.* 139: 806–817.

Bedrossian, C. W. M., Greenberg, S. D., Singer, S. B., Hansen, J. J., and Rosenberg, H. S. (1976). The lung in cystic fibrosis. A quantitative study including prevalence of pathologic findings among different age groups. *Hum. Pathol.* 2: 195–204.

Bigby, T., Goetzl, E. J., and Holtzman, M. J. (1985). Epithelial cells from canine trachea generate leukotriene B_4 in response to calcium ionophore. *Clin. Res.* 33: 76A.

Boat, T. F., and Kleinerman, J. I. (1975). Human respiratory tract secretions: Effect of cholinergic and adrenergic agents on in vitro release of protein and mucous glycoprotein. *Chest* 67: 32S–34S.

Boat, T. F., Polony, I., and Cheng, P. V. (1982). Mucin release from rabbit tracheal epithelium in response to sera from normal and cystic fibrosis subjects. *Pediatr. Res.* 16: 792–797.

Borson, D. B., Charlin, M., Gold, B. D., and Nadel, J. A. (1984). Neural regulation of $^{35}SO_4$-macromolecule secretion from tracheal glands of ferrets. *J. Appl. Physiol.* 57: 457–466.

Borson, D. B., Corrales, R., Varsano, S., Gold, M., Viro, N., Caughey, G., Ramachandran, J., and Nadel, J. A. (1987). Enkephalinase inhibitors potentiate substance P-induced secretion of $^{35}SO_4$-macromolecules from ferret trachea. *Exp. Lung Res.* 12: 21–36.

Boyd, M. R. (1977). Evidence for the Clara cell as a site of cytochrome P-450–dependent mixed-function oxidase activity in the lung. *Nature* 269: 713–715.

Breuer, R., Christensen, T. G., Lucey, E. C., Stone, P. J., and Snider, G. L. (1985a). Quantitative study of secretory cell metaplasia induced by human neutrophil elastase in the large bronchi of hamsters. *J. Lab. Clin. Med.* 105: 635–640.

Breuer, R., Lucey, E. C., Stone, P. J., Christensen, T. G., and Snider, G. L. (1985b).

Proteolytic activity of human neutrophil elastase and porcine pancreatic trypsin causes bronchial secretory cell metaplasia in hamsters. *Exp. Lung Res.* 9: 167–175.

Breuer, R., Christensen, T. G., Lucey, E. C., Stone, P. J., and Snider, G. L. (1987). An ultrastructural morphometric analysis of elastase-treated hamster bronchi shows discharge followed by progressive accumulation of secretory granules. *Am. Rev. Respir. Dis.* 136: 698–703.

Burnstock, G. (1972). Purinergic nerves. *Pharmacol. Rev.* 24: 509–581.

Burnstock, G., and Kennedy, C. (1985). Is there a basis for distinguishing two types of P_2-purinoceptor? *Gen. Pharmacol.* 16: 433–440.

Carstairs, J. R., and Barnes, P. J. (1986a). Autoradiographic mapping of substance P receptors in lung. *Eur. J. Pharmacol.* 127: 295–296.

Carstairs, J. R., and Barnes, P. J. (1986b). Visualization of vasoactive intestinal peptide receptors in human and guinea pig lung. *J. Pharmacol. Exp. Ther.* 239: 249–255.

Caughey, G. H. (1991). The structure and airway biology mast cell proteinases. *Am. J. Respir. Cell Mol. Biol.* 4: 387–394.

Chase, K. V., Flux, M., and Sachdev, G. P. (1985). Comparison of physicochemical properties of purified mucus glycoproteins isolated from respiratory secretions of cystic fibrosis and asthmatic patients. *Biochemistry* 24: 7334–7338.

Cheng, P. W., Sherman, J. M., Boat, T. F., and Bruce, M. (1981). Quantitation of radio-labeled mucous glycoproteins secreted by tracheal explants. *Anal. Biochem.* 117: 301–306.

Cheng, P. W., Levin, S., Chen, G., Ropp, P., and Boat, T. F. (1986). Corticosteroid inhibition of the synthesis and release of ferret tracheal glycoconjugates. *Am. Rev. Respir. Dis.* 133: A295.

Chodosh, S. (1979). Examination of sputum cells. *N. Engl. J. Med.* 282: 854–857.

Coles, S. J., Said, S. I., and Reid, L. (1981). Inhibition by vasoactive intestinal peptide of glycoconjugate and lysozyme secretion by human airways in vitro. *Am. Rev. Respir. Dis.* 124: 531–536.

Coles, S. J., Bhaskar, K. R., O'Sullivan, D. D., Neill, K. H., and Reid, L. M. (1984a). Airway mucus: Composition and regulation of its secretion by neuropeptides in vitro. In *Mucus and Mucosa. Ciba Found. Symp.* 109: 40–60.

Coles, S. J., Neill, K. H., and Reid, L. M. (1984b). Potent stimulation of glycoprotein secretion in canine trachea by substance P. *J. Appl. Physiol.* 57: 1323–1327.

Cosio, M. G., Ghezzo, H., Hogg, J. C., Corbin, R., Loveland, M., Dosman, J., and Macklem, P. T. (1978). The relations between structural changes in small airways and pulmonary function tests. *N. Engl. J. Med.* 298: 1277–1281.

Cosio, M. G., Hale, K. A., and Niewoehner, D. E. (1980). Morphologic and morphometric effects of prolonged cigarette smoking on the small airways. *Am. Rev. Respir. Dis.* 122: 265–271.

Culp, D. J., Penney, D. P., and Marin, M. G. (1983). A technique for the isolation of submucosal gland cells from cat trachea. *J. Appl. Physiol.* 55: 1035–1041.

Cushley, M. J., Tattersfield, A., and Holgate, S. T. (1984). Adenosine-induced broncho-constriction in asthma. Antagonism by inhaled theophylline. *Am. Rev. Respir. Dis.* 129: 380–384.

Cuss, F. M., Dixon, C. M. S., and Barnes, P. J. (1986). Effect of inhaled platelet-activating factor on pulmonary function and bronchoresponsiveness in humans. *Lancet* 2: 189–192.

Davis, B., and Nadel, J. A. (1980). New methods used to investigate the control of mucus secretion and ion transport in airways. *Environ. Health Perspect.* 35: 121–130.

Davis, B., Marin, M., Fischer, S., Graf, J., Widdicombe, J., and Nadel, J. A. (1976). New method for study of canine mucous gland secretion in vivo. Cholinergic regulation. *Am. Rev. Respir. Dis.* 113: 257.

Davis, B., Roberts, A. M., Coleridge, H. M., and Coleridge, J. C. G. (1982). Reflex tracheal gland secretion evoked by stimulation of bronchial C-fibers in dogs. *J. Appl. Physiol.* 53: 985–991.

Djukanovic, R., Roche, W. R., Wilson, J. W., Beasley, C. R. W., Twentyman, O. P., Howarth, P. H., and Holgate, S. T. (1990). Mucosal inflammation in asthma. *Am. Rev. Respir. Dis.* 142: 434–457.

Dulfano, M. J., Adler, K., and Phillipoff, W. (1971). Sputum viscoelasticity in chronic bronchitis. *Am. Rev. Respir. Dis.* 104: 88–98.

Dunnill, M. S. (1960). The pathology of asthma, with special reference to changes in the bronchial mucosa. *J. Clin. Pathol.* 13: 27–33.

Durham, S. R., and Kay, A. B. (1985). Eosinophils, bronchial hyperreactivity and late-phase asthmatics reactions. *Clin. Allergy* 15: 411–418.

Dusser, D. J., Djokic, T. D., Borson, D. B., and Nadel, J. A. (1989). Cigarette smoke induces bronchoconstrictor hyperresponsiveness to substance P and inactivates airway neutral endopeptidase in the guinea pig. Possible role of free radicals. *J. Clin. Invest.* 84: 900–906.

Eling, T. E., Danilowicz, R. M., Henke, D. C., Sivarajah, K., Yankaskas, J. R., and Boucher, R. C. (1986). Arachidonic acid metabolism by canine tracheal epithelial cells. Product formation and relationship to chloride secretion. *J. Biol. Chem.* 261: 12841–12849.

Fels, A. O. S., Pawlowski, N. A., Cramer, E. B., et al. (1982). Human alveolar macrophages produce leukotriene B_4. *Proc. Natl. Acad. Sci. USA* 79: 7866–7870.

Finkbeiner, W. E., and Basbaum, C. B. (1988). Monoclonal antibodies directed against human airway secretions. *Am. J. Pathol.* 131: 290–297.

Finkbeiner, W. E., Nadel, J. A., and Basbaum, C. B. (1986). Establishment and characterization of a cell line derived from bovine tracheal glands. *In Vitro* 22: 561–567.

Florey, H. W. (1962). The secretion of mucus and inflammation of mucous membranes. In *General Pathology*. Edited by H. W. Florey. London, Lloyd-Luke, pp. 167–196.

Frigas, E., and Gleisch, G. J. (1986). The eosinophil and the pathophysiology of asthma. *J. Allergy Clin. Immunol.* 77: 527–537.

Gallagher, J. T., Kent, P. W., Passatore, M. Phipps, R. J., and Richardson, P. S. (1975). The composition of tracheal mucus and the nervous control of its secretion in the cat. *Proc. R. Soc. Lond.* 192: 49–76.

Gashi, A. A., Borson, D. B., Finkbeiner, W. E., Nadel, J. A., and Basbaum, C. B. (1986). Neuropeptides degranulate serous cells of ferret tracheal glands. *Am. J. Physiol.* 251: C223–229.

Gashi, A. A., Nadel, J. A., and Basbaum, C. B. (1987). Autoradiographic studies on the distribution of [35]sulfate label in ferret trachea: Effects of stimulation. *Exp. Lung Res.* 12: 83–86.

Glasgow, W., Akley, N. J., and Adler, K. B. (1991). Platelet-activating factor provokes release of mucin-like glycoproteins from guinea pig tracheal epithelial cells via a lipoxygenase-dependent mechanism. *Am. Rev. Respir. Dis.* 143: A147.

Godard, P., Chaintreuil, J., Damon, M., Coupe, M., Flandre, O., Crastes de Paulet, A., and Michel, F. B. (1982). Functional assessment of alveolar macrophages: Comparison of cells from asthmatics and normal subjects. *J. Allergy Clin. Immunol.* 70: 88–93.

Goldyne, M. E., Burrish, G. F., Poubelle, P., and Borgeat, P. (1984). Arachidonic acid metabolism among human mononuclear leukocytes. Lipoxygenase-related pathways. *J. Biol. Chem.* 259: 8815–8819.

Goswami, S. K., Ohashi, M., Stathas, P., and Marom, Z. M. (1989). Platelet-activating factor stimulates secretion of respiratory glycoconjugate from human airways in culture. *J. Allergy Clin. Immunol.* 84: 726–734.

Goswami, S. K., Kivity, S., and Marom, Z. (1990). Erythromycin inhibits respiratory glycoconjugate secretion from human airways in vitro. *Am. Rev. Respir. Dis.* 141: 72–78.

Guerzon, G. M., Pare, P. D., Michoud, G. C., and Hogg, J. C. (1979). The number and distribution of mast cells in monkey lungs. *Am. Rev. Respir. Dis.* 119: 59–66.

Hamid, G., Azzawi, M., Ying, S., Moqbel, R., Wardlaw, A. J., Corrigan, C. J., Bradley, B., Durham, S. R., Collins, J. V., Jeffery, P. K., Quint, D. J., and Kay, A. B. (1991). Expression of mRNA for interleukin-5 in mucosal bronchial biopsies from asthma. *J. Clin. Invest.* 87: 1541–1546.

Hahn, H.-L., Purnama, I., Lang, M., and Sannwald, U. (1986). Effects of platelet activating factor on tracheal mucus secretion, on airway mechanics and on circulating blood cells in live ferrets. *Eur. J. Respir. Dis.* 69: S277–S284.

Harkema, J. R., and Hotchkiss, J. A. (1991). In vivo effects of endotoxin on intraepithelial mucosubstances in rat pulmonary airways. *Am. Rev. Respir. Dis.* 143: A136.

Henderson, W. R., and Klebanoff, S. J. (1983). Leukotrienes production and inactivation by normal, chronic granulomatous disease and myeloperoxidase-deficient neutrophils. *J. Biol. Chem.* 258: 13522–13527.

Henderson, W. R., Jr. (1991). Eicosanoids and platelet-activating factor in allergic respiratory diseases. *Am. Rev. Respir. Dis.* 143: S86–S90.

Holtzer, P. (1988). Local effector functions of capsaicin-sensitive sensory nerve endings: Involvement of tachykinins, calcitonin-gene related peptide and other neuropeptides. *Neuroscience* 24: 739–768.

Holtzman, M. J. (1991). Arachidonic acid metabolism. Implications of biological chemistry for lung function and disease. *Am. Rev. Respir. Dis.* 143: 188–203.

Holtzman, M. J., Aizawa, H., Nadel, J. A., and Goetzl, E. J. (1983). Selective generation of leukotriene B_4 by tracheal epithelial cells from dogs. *Biochem. Biophys. Res. Commun.* 114: 1071–1076.

Hutson, P. A., Varley, J. G., Sanjar, S., Kings, M., Holgate, S. T., and Church, M. K. (1990). Evidence that neutrophils do not participate in the late phase airway response provoked by ovalbumin inhalation in conscious, sensitized guinea pigs. *Am. Rev. Respir. Dis.* 141: 535–539.

Irvine, R. F. (1982). How is the level of free arachidonic acid controlled in mammalian cells? *Biochem J.* 204: 3–16.

Jacoby, D. B., Tamaoki, J., Borson, D. B., and Nadel, J. A. (1988). Influenza infection causes airway hyperresponsiveness by decreasing enkephalinase. *J. Appl. Physiol.* 64: 2653–2658.

Jetten, A. M. (1991). Growth and differentiation factors in tracheobronchial epithelium. *Am. J. Physiol.* 260: L361–L373.

Joad, J. P. (1990). Characterization of the human peripheral lung adenosine receptor. *Am. J. Respir. Cell Mol. Biol.* 2: 193–198.

Johnson, H. G., and McNee, M. L. (1985). Adenosine-induced secretion in the canine trachea: Modification by methylxanthines and adenosine derivatives. *Br. J. Pharmacol.* 86: 63–67.

Johnson, H. G., Chinn, R. A., Chow, A. W., Bach, M. K., and Nadel, J. A. (1983). Leukotriene C_4 enhances mucus production from submucosal glands in canine trachea in vivo. *Int. J. Immunopharmacol.* 5: 391–396.

Johnson, C. W., Rieves, R. D., Logun, C., and Shelhamer, J. H. (1990). Muscarinic stimulation of human submucosal gland secretion is mediated at least in part by M_1 receptor. *Clin. Res.* 38: 273A.

Johnson, C. W., Rieves, R. D., Logun, C., and Shelhamer, J. H. (1991). Endothelin-1 stimulates secretion of respiratory mucous glycoproteins from human airways in vitro. *Am. Rev. Respir. Dis.* 143: A138.

Jones, R., and Reid, L. (1978). Secretory cell hyperplasia and modification of intracellular glycoprotein in rat airways induced by short periods of exposure to tobacco smoke and the effect of the anti-inflammatory agent phenylmethyloxadiazole. *Lab. Invest.* 39: 41–49.

Joseph, M., Tonnel, A. B., Torpier, G., Capron, A., Arnoux, B., and Benveniste, J. (1983). Involvement of immunoglobulin E in the secretory processes of alveolar macrophages from asthmatic patients. *J. Clin. Invest.* 71: 221–230.

Kaliner, M. A., Shelhamer, J. H., Borson, D. B., Patow, C. A., Marom, Z., and Nadel, J. A. (1988). Respiratory mucus. In *The Airways. Neural Control in Health and Disease.* Edited by M. A. Kaliner, and P. J. Barnes. New York, Marcel Dekker, pp. 575–595.

Kay, A. B. (1991). Asthma and inflammation. *J. Allergy Clin. Immunol.* 5: 893–910.

Kim, K. C. (1985). Possible requirement of collagen gel substratum for production of mucin-like glycoproteins by primary rabbit tracheal epithelial cells in culture. *In Vitro* 21: 617–621.

Kim, K. C., and Brody, J. S. (1989). Use of primary cell culture to study regulation of airway surface epithelial mucus secretion. In *Mucus and Related Topics.* Edited by E. N. Chantler, and N. A. Ratcliffe. Cambridge, Company of Biologists Limited, pp. 231–239.

Kim, K. C., and Lee, B. C. (1991). P_2 purinoceptor regulation of mucin release by airway goblet cells in primary culture. *Br. J. Pharmacol.* 103: 1053–1056.

Kim, K. C., Wasano, K., Niles, R. M., Schuster, J. E., Stone, P. J., and Brody, J. S. (1987). Human neutrophil elastase releases cell surface mucins from primary cultures of hamster tracheal epithelial cell. *Proc. Natl. Acad. Sci. USA* 84: 9304–9308.

Kim, K. C., Nassiri, J., and Brody, J. S. (1989). Mechanisms of airway goblet cell mucin release: Studies with cultured tracheal surface epithelial cells. *Am. J. Respir. Cell Mol. Biol.* 1: 137–143.

Klinger, J. D., Tandler, B., Liedtke, C. M., and Boat, T. F. (1984). Proteinases of *Pseudomonas aeruginosa* evoke mucin release by tracheal epithelium. *J. Clin. Invest.* 74: 1669–1678.

Koshino, T., Bhaskar, K. R., Reid, M., et al. (1990). Recovery of an epitope recognized by a novel monoclonal antibody from airway lavage during experimental induction of chronic bronchitis. *Am. J. Respir. Cell Mol. Biol.* 2: 453–462.

Kuo, H. P., Rohde, J. A. L., Tokuyama, K., Barnes, P. J., and Rogers, D. F. (1990). Capsaicin and sensory neuropeptide stimulation of goblet cell secretion in guinea pig trachea. *J. Physiol. (Lond.)* 431: 629–641.

Lam, S., LeRiche, J., Phillips, D., and Chan-Yeung, M. (1987). Cellular and protein changes in bronchial lavage fluid after late asthmatic reaction in patients with red cedar asthma. *J. Allergy Clin. Immunol.* 80: 44–50.

Lamb, D., and Reid, L. (1968). Mitotic rates, goblet cell increase and histochemical changes in mucus in rat bronchial epithelium during exposure to sulfur dioxide. *J. Pathol. Bacteriol.* 96: 97–111.

Lamb, D., and Reid, L. (1969). Goblet cell increase in rat bronchial epithelium after exposure to cigarette and cigar tobacco smoke. *Br. Med. J.* 1: 33–35.

Lang, M., Hansen, D., and Hahn, H. L. (1987). Effects of the PAF-antagonist CV-3988 on PAF-induced changes in mucus secretion and in respiratory and circulatory variables in ferrets. *Agents Actions* 21: S245–S252.

Laviolette, M., Chang, J., and Newcombe, D. S. (1981). Human alveolar macrophages: A lesion in arachidonic acid metabolism in cigarette smokers. *Am. Rev. Respir. Dis.* 124: 397–401.

Lazarus, S. C., Basbaum, C. B., Barnes, P. J., and Gold, W. M. (1986). Cyclic AMP immunocytochemistry provides evidence for VIP receptors in trachea. *Am. J. Physiol.* 251: C115–C119.

Lee, T. C., Wu, R., Brody, A. R., Barrett, J. C., and Nettesheim, P. (1984). Growth and differentiation of hamster tracheal epithelial cells in culture. *Exp. Lung Res.* 6: 27–45.

Leikauf, G. D., Ueki, I. F., and Nadel, J. A. (1984). Autonomic regulation of viscoelasticity of cat tracheal gland secretions. *J. Appl. Physiol.* 56: 426–430.

Lietdke, C. M., Rudolph, S. A., and Boat, T. F. (1983). β-Adrenergic modulation of mucin secretion in cat trachea. *Am. J. Physiol.* 244: C391–C398.

Lin, H., Carlson, D. M., St. George, J. A., Plopper, C. G., and Wu, R. (1989). An ELISA method for the quantitation of tracheal mucins from human and nonhuman primates. *Am. J. Respir. Cell Mol. Biol.* 1: 41–48.

Logun, C., Rieves, R. D., Lundgren, J. D., Marom, Z., Kaliner, M., and Shelhamer, J. H. (1988). Activated human neutrophils release a high molecular weight protein which stimulates respiratory glycoconjugates release from human airways in vitro. *Am. Rev. Respir. Dis.* 137: A14.

Logun, C., Mullol, J., Rieves, D., Hoffman, A., Johnson, C., Miller, R., Goff, J., Kaliner, M., and Shelhamer, J. H. (1991). Use of a monoclonal antibody enzyme-linked immunosorbent assay to measure human respiratory glycoprotein production in vitro. *Am. J. Respir. Cell Mol. Biol.* 5: 71–79.

Lucey, E. C., Stone, P. J., Breuer, R., Christensen, T. G., Calore, J. D., Cantanese, A., Franzblau, C., and Snider, G. L. (1985). Effect of combined human neutrophil cathepsin G and elastase on induction of secretory cell metaplasia and emphysema in hamsters, with in vitro observations on elastolysis by these enzymes. *Am. Rev. Respir. Dis.* 132: 362–366.

Lundberg, J. M., and Saria, A. (1982). Capsaicin-sensitive vagal neurons involved in control of vascular permeability in rat trachea. *Acta Physiol. Scand.* 115: 521–523.

Lundberg, J. M., and Saria, A. (1983). Capsaicin-induced desensitization of airway mucosa to cigarette smoke, mechanical and chemical irritants. *Nature* 302: 251–253.

Lundgren, J. D., and Shelhamer, J. H. (1990). Pathogenesis of airway mucus hypersecretion. *J. Allergy Clin. Immunol.* 85: 399–419.

Lundberg, J. M., Lundblad, L., Anggard, A., Martling, C.-R., Theodorsson-Norheim, E., St. Jarne, P., Hokfelt, T. G., and Saria, A. (1988). Bioactive peptides in capsaicin-sensitive C-fiber afferents of the airways. Functional and pathophysiological implications. In *The Airways. Neural Control in Health and Disease*. Edited by M. A. Kaliner, and P. J. Barnes. New York, Marcel Dekker, 33: 417–445.

Lundgren, J., Kaliner, M. A., Logun, C., and Shelhamer, J. H. (1987). The effects of endorphins on mucous glycoprotein secretion from feline airways in vitro. *Exp. Lung Res.* 12: 303–309.

Lundgren, J. D., Hirata, F., Marom, Z., Logun, C., Steel, L., Kaliner, M., and Shelhamer, J. H. (1988a). Dexamethasone inhibits respiratory glycoconjugate secretion from feline airways in vitro by the induction of lipocortin (lipomodulin) synthesis. *Am. Rev. Respir. Dis.* 137: 353–357.

Lundgren, J. D., Kaliner, M., Logun, C., and Shelhamer, J. H. (1988b). Dexamethasone reduces rat tracheal goblet cell hyperplasia produced by human neutrophil products. *Exp. Lung Res.* 14: 853–863.

Lundgren, J. D., Wiedermann, C. J., Logun, C., Plutchok, J., Kaliner, M., and Shelhamer, J. H. (1989). Substance P receptor-mediated secretion of respiratory glycoconjugate from feline airways in vitro. *Exp. Lung Res.* 15: 17–29.

Lundgren, J. D., Ostrowski, N., Baraniuk, J. N., Shelhamer, J. H., and Kaliner, M. (1990a). Gastrin-releasing peptide stimulates glycoconjugate release from feline tracheal explants. *Am. J. Physiol.* 258: L68–L74.

Lundgren, J. D., Kaliner, M., Logun, C., and Shelhamer, J. H. (1990b). Platelet-activating factor and tracheobronchial respiratory glycoconjugate release in feline and human explants: Involvement of the lipoxygenase pathway. *Agent Actions* 30: 329–337.

Lundgren, J. D., Davey, R. J., Jr., Lundgren, B., Mullol, J., Marom, Z., Logun, C., Baraniuk, J., Kaliner, M. A., and Shelhamer, J. H. (1991). Eosinophils and mucus airway secretion: Eosinophil cationic protein stimulates and major basic protein inhibits secretion from airway organ culture. *J. Allergy Clin. Immunol.* 87: 689–698.

MacGlashan, D. W., Schleimer, R. P., Peters, S. P., Schulman, E. S., Adams, G. K., III, Newball, H. H., and Lichtenstein, L. M. (1982). Generation of leukotrienes by purified human lung mast cells. *J. Clin. Invest.* 70: 747–751.

Mak, J. C. W., and Barnes, P. J. (1988). Autoradiographic localization of calcitonin gene-related peptide binding sites in human and guinea lung. *Peptides* 9: 957–964.

Mak, J. C. W., and Barnes, P. J. (1990). Autoradiographic visualization of muscarinic receptor subtypes in human and guinea pig lung. *Am. Rev. Respir. Dis.* 141: 1559–1568.

Mak, J. C. W., and Barnes, P. J. (1991). Autoradiographic visualization of bradykinin receptors in human and guinea pig lung. *Eur. J. Pharmacol.* 194: 37–43.

Marom, Z., Shelhamer, J. H., and Kaliner, M. (1981). The effect of arachidonic acid, monohydroxyeicosatetraenoic acid and prostaglandins on the release of mucous glycoproteins from human airways in vitro. *J. Clin. Invest.* 67: 1695–1702.

Marom, Z., Shelhamer, J. H., Bach, M. K., Morton, D. R., and Kaliner, M. (1982). Slow-reacting substances, leukotriene C_4 and D_4, increase the release of mucus from human airways in vitro. *Am. Rev. Respir. Dis.* 126: 449–451.

Marom, Z., Shelhamer, J. H., Sun, F., and Kaliner, M. (1983). Human airway mono-hydroxyeicosatetraenoic acid generation and mucus release. *J. Clin. Invest.* 72: 122–127.

Marom, Z., Shelhamer, J. H., Alling, D., and Kaliner, M. (1984a). The effect of cortico-steroids on mucous glycoprotein secretion from human airways in vitro. *Am. Rev. Respir. Dis.* 129: 62–65.

Marom, Z., Shelhamer, J. H., and Kaliner, M. (1984b). Human pulmonary macrophage-derived mucus secretagogue. *J. Exp. Med.* 159: 844–860.

Marom, Z., Shelhamer, J. H., Steel, L., Goetzl, E. J., and Kaliner, M. (1984c). Prostaglandin-generating factor of anaphylaxis induces mucous glycoprotein release and formation of lipoxygenase products of arachidonate from human airways. *Prostaglandin* 28: 79–91.

Marom, Z., Shelhamer, J. H., and Kaliner, M. (1985a). Human monocyte-derived mucus secretagogue. *J. Clin. Invest.* 75: 191–198.

Marom, Z., Shelhamer, J., Berger, M., Frank, M., and Kaliner, M. (1985b). Anaphylatoxin C3a enhances mucous glycoprotein release from human airways in vitro. *J. Exp. Med.* 161: 657–668.

McCormack, D. G., Salonen, R. O., and Barnes, P. J. (1989). Effect of sensory neuropep-tides on canine bronchial and pulmonary vessels in vitro. *Life Sci.* 45: 2405–2012.

McDonald, D. M. (1988). Neurogenic inflammation in the rat trachea. 1. Changes in venules, leukocytes and epithelial cells. *J. Neurocytol.* 17: 583–603.

Metzger, W. J., Zavala, D., Richerson, H. B., Moseley, P., Iwamota, P., Monick, M. Sjoerdsma, K., and Hunninghake, G. W. (1987). Local allergen challenge and bronchoalveolar lavage of allergic asthmatics lungs. Description of the model and local airway inflammation. *Am. Rev. Respir. Dis.* 135: 433–440.

Mullen, J., Brendan, M., Wright, J., Wiggs, B., Pare, P., Hogg, J., (1985). Reassessment of inflammation of the airways in chronic bronchitis. *Br. Med. J.* 291: 1235–1239.

Mullol, J., Ohkubo, K., Rieves, D., Wu, T., Hausfield, J., Shelhamer, J., and Kaliner, M. (1991). Endothelin in human nasal mucosa. *J. Allergy Clin. Immunol.* 87: A217.

Murlas, C. G., and Roum, J. H. (1985). Sequence of pathologic changes in the airway mucosa of guinea pigs during ozone-induced bronchial hyperreactivity. *Am. Rev. Respir. Dis.* 131: 314–320.

Murlas, C. G., Williams, G., Lang, Z., and Chodimella, V. (1990). Aerosolized neutral endopeptidase reverses the increased airway reactivity to substance P caused by ozone. *Am. Rev. Respir. Dis.* 141: A734.

Nadel, J. A., and Borson, D. B. (1991). Modulation of neurogenic inflammation by neutral endopeptidase. *Am. Rev. Respir. Dis.* 143: S33–S35.

Nakamura, H., Yoshimura, K., Jaffe, A., and Crystal, R. G. (1991). Interleukin-8 gene expression in human bronchial epithelial cells. *J. Biol. Chem.* 266: 19611–19617.

Niewoehner, D. E., Kleinerman, J., and Rice, D. B. (1974). Pathologic changes in the peripheral airways of young cigarette smokers. *N. Engl. J. Med.* 291: 755–758.

O'Byrne, P. M., ed. (1990). *Asthma as an Inflammatory Disease.* New York, Marcel Dekker, pp. 1–320.

Palmer, J. B., Cuss, F. M. C., and Barnes, P. J. (1986). VIP and PHM and their role in nonadrenergic inhibitory responses in isolated human airways. *J. Appl. Physiol.* 61: 1322–1328.

Panula, P., Hadjiconstantinou, H. A., and Yang, T. (1983). Immunohistochemical localization of bombesin/gastrin-releasing peptide and substance P in primary sensory neurons. *J. Neurosci.* 3: 2021–2029.

Peachell, P. T., Columbo, M., Kagey-Sobotka, A., Lichtenstein, L. M., and Marone, G. (1988). Adenosine potentiates mediator release from human lung mast cells. *Am. Rev. Respir. Dis.* 138: 1143–1151.

Peatfield, A. C., and Richardson, P. S. (1983). Evidence for noncholinergic, nonadrenergic nervous control of mucus secretion into the cat trachea. *J. Physiol. (Lond.)* 342: 335–345.

Peatfield, A. C., Hall, R. L., Richardson, P. S., and Jeffery, P. K. (1982a). The effect of serum on the secretion of radiolabeled macromolecules into the lumen of the cat trachea. *Am. Rev. Respir. Dis.* 125: 210.

Peatfield, A. C., Piper, P. J., and Richardson, P. S. (1982b). The effect of leukotriene C_4 on mucus release into the cat trachea in vivo and in vitro. *Br. J. Pharmacol.* 77: 391–393.

Peatfield, A. C., Barnes, P. J., Bratcher, C., Nadel, J. A., and Davis, B. (1983). Vasoactive intestinal peptide stimulates tracheal submucosal gland secretion in ferret. *Am. Rev. Respir. Dis.* 128: 89–93.

Phipps, R. J., Williams, I. P., Richardson, P. S., Pell, J., Pack, R. J., and Wright, N. (1982). Sympathomimetic drugs stimulate the output of secretory glycoproteins from human bronchi in vitro. *Clin. Sci.* 63: 23–28.

Plaut, M., Pierce, J. H., Watson, C. J., Hanley-Hyde, J., Nordan, R. P., and Paul, W. E. (1989). Mast cell lines produce lymphokines in response to cross-linkage of FcεRI or to calcium ionophores. *Nature* 339: 64–67.

Puchelle, E., Tournier, J. M., Zahm, J. M., and Sadoul, P. (1984). Rheology of sputum collected by a simple technique limiting salivary contamination. *J. Lab. Clin. Med.* 103: 347–353.

Rahmoune, H., Lamblin, G., Lafitte, J. J., Galabert, C., Filliat, M., and Roussel, P. (1991). Chondroitin sulfate in sputum from patients with cystic fibrosis and chronic bronchitis. *Am. J. Resp. Cell Mol. Biol.* 5: 315–320.

Rearick, J. I., Deas, M., and Jetten, A. M. (1987). Synthesis of mucous glycoproteins by rabbit tracheal cells in vitro. Modulation by substratum, retinoids and cyclic AMP. *Biochem. J.* 242: 19–25.

Rieves, R. D., Lundgren, J. D., Logun, C., Wu, T., and Shelhamer, J. H. (1991). The effect of protein kinase C activating agents upon respiratory glycoconjugate release from feline airways. *Am. J. Physiol.* 261: L415–L423.

Rieves, R. D., Goff, J., Wu, T., Larivee, P., Logun, C., and Shelhamer, J. H. (1992). Airway epithelial cell mucin release: Immunologic quantitation and response to platelet activating factor. *Am. J. Respir. Cell Mol. Biol.* 6: 158–167.

Robinson, N., Widdicombe, J. G., and Xie, C. C. (1983). In vitro collection of mucus from the ferret trachea. *J. Physiol.* 340: 7–8.

Rogers, D. F., and Barnes, P. (1989). Opioid inhibition of nonadrenergic, noncholinergic neural control of mucus secretion in human bronchi in vitro. *Am. Rev. Respir. Dis.* 139: A411.

Rogers, D. F., and Jeffery, P. K., (1986). Inhibition of cigarette smoke-induced airway secretory cell hyperplasia by indomethacin, dexamethasone, prednisolone, or hydrocortisone in the rat. *Exp. Lung Res.* 10: 285–298.

Rogers, D. F., Aursudkij, B., and Barnes, P. J. (1989). Effects of tachykinins on mucus secretion in human bronchi in vitro. *Eur. J. Pharmacol.* 174: 283–286.

Sahu, S., and Lynn, W. (1978). Hyaluronic acid in pulmonary secretions of patients with asthma. *Biochem. J.* 173: 565–568.

Said, S. I. (1991). VIP as a modulator of lung inflammation and airway constriction. *Am. Rev. Respir. Dis.* 143: S22–S24.

Salonen, R. O., Webber, S. E., and Widdicombe, J. G. (1988). Effects of neuropeptides and capsaicin on the canine tracheal vasculature in vivo. *Br. J. Pharmacol.* 95: 1262–1270.

Sasaki, T., Shimura, S., Ikeda, K., Sasaki, H., and Takishima, T. (1989). Platelet-activating factor increases platelet-dependent secretion from tracheal submucosal gland. *Am. J. Physiol.* 257: L373–L378.

Schleimer, R. P., MacGlashan, D. W., Peters, S. P., Pinckard, R. N., Adkinson, N. F., and Lichtenstein, L. M. (1986). Characterization of inflammatory mediator release from purified human lung mast cells. *Am. Rev. Respir. Dis.* 133: 614–617.

Sekizawa, K., Tamaoki, J., Graf, P. D., Basbaum, C. B., and Nadel, J. A. (1987). Enkephalinase inhibitor potentiates mammalian tachykinin-induced contraction in ferret trachea. *J. Pharmacol. Exp. Ther.* 243: 1211–1217.

Seltzer, J., Scanlon, P. D., Drazen, J. M., Ingram, R. H., Jr., and Reid, L. (1984). Morphologic correlation of physiologic changes caused by SO_2-induced bronchitis in dogs: The role of inflammation. *Am. Rev. Respir. Dis.* 129: 790–797.

Serabjit-Singh, C. J., Wolf, C. R., Philpot, R. M., and Plopper, C. G. (1979). Cytochrome P-450 localization in rabbit lung. *Science* 207: 1469–1470.

Shelhamer, J. H., Marom, Z., and Kaliner, M. (1980). Immunologic and neuropharmacologic stimulation of mucus glycoprotein release from human airways. *J. Clin. Invest.* 66: 1400–1408.

Sheppard, D., Thomson, J. E., Scypinski, L., Dusser, D., Nadel, J. A., and Borson, D. B. (1988). Toluene diisocyanate increases airway responsiveness to substance P and decreases airway enkephalinase. *J. Clin. Invest.* 81: 1111–1115.

Shimura, S., Sasaki, T., Sasaki, H., and Takishima, T. (1986). Contractility of isolated single submucosal gland from trachea. *J. Appl. Physiol.* 60: 1237–1247.

Shimura, S., Sasaki, T., Okayama, H., Sasaki, H., and Takishima, T. (1987). Effect of substance P on mucus secretion of isolated submucosal glands from feline trachea. *J. Appl. Physiol.* 63: 646–653.

Shimura, S., Sasaki, T., Ikeda, K., Sasaki, H., and Takishima, T. (1988a). VIP augments cholinergic-induced glucoconjugates secretion in tracheal submucosal glands. *J. Appl. Physiol.* 65: 2537–2544.

Shimura, S., Sasaki, T., Sasaki, H., and Takishima, T. (1988b). The mechanism of glucocorticoid inhibitory action on mucus glycoprotein secretion from isolated tracheal glands. *Am. Rev. Respir. Dis.* 137: A6.

Sigal, E., and Nadel, J. A. (1991). The airway epithelium and arachidonic acid 15-lipoxygenase. *Am. Rev. Respir. Dis.* 143: S71–74.

Smith, L. J. (1991). The role of platelet-activating factor in asthma. *Am. Rev. Respir. Dis.* 143: S100–102.

Snider, G. L., Lucey, E., Christensen, T. G., Stone, P. J., Calore, J. D., Catanese, A., and Franzblau, C. (1984). Emphysema and bronchial secretory cell metaplasia induced in hamsters by human neutrophil products. *Am. Rev. Respir. Dis.* 129: 155–160.

Snider, G. L., Stone, P. J., Lucey, E. C., Breuer, R., Calore, J. D., Seshadri, T., Catanese, A., Maschler, R., and Schnebli, H.-P. (1985). Eglin-C, a polypeptide derived from the medicinal leech, prevents human neutrophil elastase-induced emphysema and bronchial secretory cell metaplasia in the hamster. *Am. Rev. Respir. Dis.* 132: 1155–1161.

Snyder, F., ed. (1987). *Platelet-Activating Factor and Related Lipid Mediators.* New York, Plenum Press, pp. 1–472.

Sommerhoff, C. P., Caughey, G. H., Finkbeiner, W. E., Lazarus, S. C., Basbaum, C. B., and Nadel, J. A. (1989). Mast cell chymase: A potent secretagogue for airway gland serous cells. *J. Immunol.* 142: 2450–2456.

Sommerhoff, C. P., Nadel, J. A., Basbaum, C. B., and Caughey, G. H. (1990). Neutrophil elastase and cathepsin G stimulate secretion from cultured bovine airway gland serous cells. *J. Clin. Invest.* 85: 682–689.

Sperber, K., Goswani, S. K., Gollub, E., Mayer, L., and Marom, Z. (1991). Mucus secretagogue production by a human macrophage hybridoma. *J. Allergy Clin. Immunol.* 87: 490–498.

Stone, P. J., Lucey, E. J., Vinca, G. D., Christensen, T. G., Breuer, R., and Snider, G. L. (1990). alpha 1-Protease inhibitor moderates human neutrophil elastase-induced emphysema and secretory cell metaplasia in hamsters. *Eur. Respir. J.* 3: 673–678.

Sturgess, J., and Reid, L. (1972). An organ culture study of the effects of drugs on secretory activity of human bronchial submucosal glands. *Clin. Sci.* 43: 533–

Thompson, A. B., Daughton, D., Robbins, R., Ghafoury, M. A., Oehlerking, M., and Rennard, S. I. (1989). Intraluminal airway inflammation in chronic bronchitis. Characterization and correlation with clinical parameters. *Am. Rev. Respir. Dis.* 140: 1527–1537.

Tokuyama, K., Kuo, H. P., Rohde, J. A. L., Barnes, P. J., and Rogers, D. F. (1990). Neural control of goblet cell secretion in guinea pig airways. *Am. J. Physiol.* 259: L108–L115.

Tournier, J. M., Merten, M., Meckler, Y., Hinnraski, J., Fuchey, C., and Puchelle, E. (1990). Culture and characterization of human tracheal gland cells. *Am. Rev. Respir. Dis.* 141: 1280–1288.

Ueki, I., and Nadel, J. A. (1981). Differences in total protein concentration in submucosal gland fluid: alpha-Adrenergic vs cholinergic. *Fed. Proc.* 40: 622–62.

Ueki, I., German, V. F., and Nadel, J. A. (1980). Micropipette measurement of airway submucosal gland secretion: Autonomic effects. *Am. Rev. Respir. Dis.* 121: 351–357.

Van Scott, M. R., Yankaskas, J. R., and Boucher, R. C. (1986). Culture of airway epithelial cells: Research techniques. *Exp. Lung Res.* 11: 75–94.

Van Scott, M. R., Cheng, P. W., Henke, D. C., and Yankaskas, J. R. (1991). Cell culture of airway epithelia. In *The Airway Epithelium. Physiology, Pathophysiology and Pharmacology*. Edited by S. G. Farmer, and W. P. Hay. New York, Marcel Dekker, pp. 135–167.

Varsano, S., Basbaum, C. B., Forsberg, L. S., Borson, D. B., Caughey, G., and Nadel, J. A. (1987). Dog tracheal epithelial cells in culture synthesize sulfated macromolecular glycoconjugates and release them from the cell surface upon exposure to extracellular proteinases. *Exp. Lung Res.* 13: 157–184.

Wardlaw, A. J., Dunnette, S., Gleich, G. J., Collins, J. V., and Kay, A. B. (1988). Eosinophils and mast cells in bronchoalveolar lavage fluid in subjects with mild asthma. Relationship to bronchial hyperreactivity. *Am. Rev. Respir. Dis.* 137: 62–69.

Webber, S. E., and Widdicombe, J. G. (1987). The actions of metacholine, phenylephrine, salbutamol and histamine on mucus secretion from the ferret in vitro trachea. *Agents Actions* 22: 82–85.

Weller, P. F., Lee, C. W., Foster, D. W., Corey, E. J., Austen, K. F., and Lewis, R. A. (1983). Generation and metabolism of 5-lipoxygenase pathway leukotrienes by human eosinophils: Predominant production of leukotriene C_4. *Proc. Natl. Acad. Sci. USA* 80: 7626–7630.

Widdicombe, J. G. (1988). Vagal reflexes in the airways. In *The Airways: Neural Control in Health and Disease*. Edited by M. A. Kaliner, and P. J. Barnes. New York, Marcel Dekker, pp. 187–199.

Wu, R., (1986). In vitro differentiation of airway epithelial cells. In *In Vitro Models of Respiratory Epithelium*. Edited by L. J. Schiff. Boca Raton, CRC Press, pp. 1–26.

Wu, R., Martin, W. R., Robinson, C. B., St. George, J. A., Plopper, C. G., Kurland, G., Last, J. A., Cross, C. E., McDonald, R. J., and Boucher, R. (1990). Expression of mucin synthesis and secretion in human tracheobronchial epithelial cells grown in culture. *Am. J. Respir. Cell Mol. Biol.* 3: 467–478.

Wu, T., Rieves, D., Logun, C., and Shelhamer, J. (1991). Platelet activating factor stimulates the production of a variety of eicosanoids in feline tracheal epithelial cells. *Am. Rev. Respir. Dis.* 143: A152.

14

Abnormalities of Airway Epithelial Chloride Transport in Cystic Fibrosis

MICHAEL J. WELSH, MATTHEW P. ANDERSON, DEVRA P. RICH,
HERBERT A. BERGER, GERENE M. DENNING,
LYNDA S. OSTEDGAARD, and DAVID N. SHEPPARD

Howard Hughes Medical Institute
University of Iowa College of Medicine
Iowa City, Iowa

I. Introduction

Cystic fibrosis (CF) is a common lethal genetic disease that affects epithelia. Although several different organs are affected—including the pulmonary airways, pancreas, sweat gland, intestine, and male genital tract—lung disease is the major cause of morbidity and mortality.

Airway epithelia have the capacity for either absorption or secretion; the quantitative aspects of these two processes depend on the species, the airway region, and the neurohumoral environment (Welsh, 1987). Both Cl^- secretion and Na^+ absorption involve two sets of transport processes, one set at the basolateral membrane and one at the apical membrane. For Cl^- secretion, a series of basolateral membrane transport processes accumulate Cl^- intracellularly at a concentration above electrochemical equilibrium. Then, on activation, apical membrane Cl^- channels allow Cl^- to exit passively from the cell, moving down a favorable electrochemical gradient into the airway lumen. Apical Cl^- exit is presumably followed by Na^+ flow through the paracellular pathway, and the secretion of water ensues. For Na^+ absorption, Na^+ enters the cell through apical membrane Na^+ channels, moving down a favorable electrochemical gradient. It is then actively expelled across the basolateral membrane by the basolateral Na,K-ATPase. Presumably counterions and water follow to generate volume flow.

Work from several laboratories has established that epithelia affected by CF are relatively Cl$^-$ impermeable (reviewed in Boat et al., 1989; Frizzell, 1987; Welsh, 1987; Boucher et al., 1983; Quinton, 1990). In airway and several other epithelia, the defect in Cl$^-$ permeability has been localized to the apical cell membrane: an increase in cellular levels of cAMP increases the apical membrane Cl$^-$ conductance of normal, but not CF, airway epithelia. In addition, CF airway epithelia have an increased rate of Na$^+$ absorption (Boucher et al., 1986). The combination of defective Cl$^-$ permeability and, hence, reduced capacity for Cl$^-$ secretion, as well as an increased rate of Na$^+$ absorption, may generate a dehydrated respiratory tract fluid. As a result, the efficiency of the normal mucociliary clearance defense mechanism may be impaired, and the lungs may become more susceptible to bacterial infection. This scenario provides an attractive explanation for how epithelial electrolyte transport abnormalities cause lung disease in CF. However, there is as yet little direct data to support this hypothesis.

Current insight into how CF causes disease is based on a combination of physiological and molecular genetic studies. The physiological studies have been facilitated by the development of powerful electrophysiological techniques (Hamill et al., 1981). Molecular genetic research has accelerated since the discovery of the cystic fibrosis transmembrane conductance regulator (CFTR); mutations in the gene encoding CFTR cause CF (Rommens et al., 1989; Riordan et al., 1989; Kerem et al., 1989; Rich et al., 1990; Drumm et al., 1990). The gene was identified based on three criteria: it mapped to the correct chromosomal region; there was an appropriate pattern of tissue expression (i.e., in the epithelia affected by CF); and a mutation in CFTR was identified that was present on approximately 70% of CF chromosomes and was absent on non-CF chromosomes. Since then, numerous other mutations have been discovered in the CFTR gene (for a review, see Tsui and Buchwald, 1991).

This chapter will focus on the normal function of CFTR and its abnormal function in CF. For further reviews and references on CF, CFTR, Cl$^-$ channels, and electrolyte transport by airway epithelia the reader may turn to several recent reviews (Frizzell et al., 1979; Frizzell, 1987; Welsh, 1987; Gögelein, 1988; Boat et al., 1989; Frizzell and Halm, 1990; Quinton, 1990; Wine, 1991; Tsui and Buchwald, 1991; Cheng et al., 1992; Anderson et al., 1992).

II. Function of the Cystic Fibrosis Transmembrane Conductance Regulator

A. Predictions from the Amino Acid Sequence

From its deduced amino acid sequence, Riordan et al. (1989) suggested that CFTR consists of the following domains (in order from the NH$_2$- to the COOH-terminus;

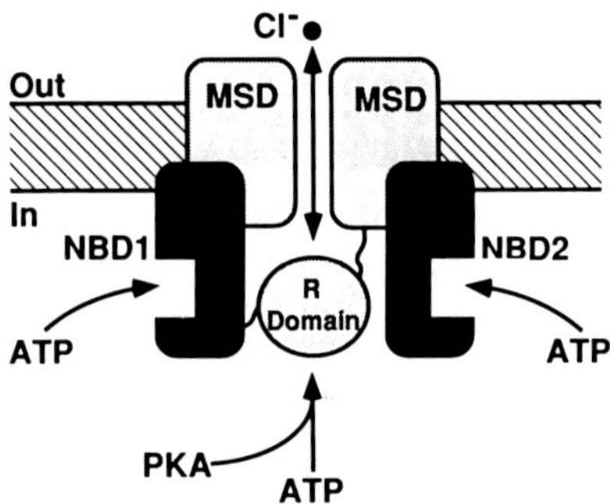

Figure 1   Model of the domain structure of CFTR in the membrane: MSD, membrane-spanning domain; NBD, nucleotide-binding domain, the R domain is indicated; PKA, cAMP-dependent protein kinase. The plasma membrane is represented by the cross-hatched area.

Fig. 1): a membrane-spanning domain (consisting of six membrane-spanning segments), a putative nucleotide-binding domain, a large polar segment called the R domain (which contains multiple potential phosphorylation sites), and then a second membrane-spanning domain, followed by a second nucleotide-binding domain. The predicted topology of CFTR, with the exception of the R domain, resembles that of several other membrane proteins, including the multidrug resistance P-glycoprotein, the yeast *STE6* gene product, and several bacterial periplasmic permeases. This family of membrane proteins has been given several names, such as the ABC transporters (Hyde et al., 1990), traffic ATPases (Ames et al., 1990), and the TM6/NBF family (transmembrane 6/nucleotide-binding fold) (Riordan et al., 1991). The most conserved features in members of this family are the nucleotide-binding domains, in which there is substantial amino acid sequence similarity. The membrane-spanning domains are also an important feature in that there are predicted to be two sets of five or six such membrane-spanning sequences in each family member. The putative membrane-spanning domains do not, however, share amino acid sequence similarity.

These predictions from the amino acid sequence of CFTR and comparison with other members of the family suggested that CFTR was a membrane protein (Riordan et al., 1989). They also suggested that it may hydrolyze ATP, and that it may be regulated by phosphorylation with cAMP-dependent protein kinase. In addition, similarity to other family members suggested that CFTR might be involved in transport. If it were involved in transport of electrolytes across the cell membrane, it would tie together two observations: CFTR is mutated in patients with CF, and electrolyte transport is defective in CF-affected epithelia.

Biochemical studies showed that CFTR could be expressed both in vitro and in vivo (Gregory et al., 1990; Kartner et al., 1991). The resulting protein was membrane-associated and was glycosylated at two sites (asparagine residues 894 and 900) (Cheng et al., 1990). Several polyclonal and monoclonal antibodies were also raised and detected CFTR produced both in vitro and in vivo.

B. Localization

The observations that CFTR is a membrane protein and that the electrolyte transport defect in CF is in the apical membrane, suggested that CFTR would be located in the apical membrane of secretory epithelia. Evidence supporting this hypothesis came from several studies. In the human pancreas, antibodies raised against CFTR peptides immunocytochemically localized CFTR to small branching tubular structures. These results suggested that proximal duct epithelial cells expressed CFTR at the apical region of the cell (Marino et al., 1991; Crawford et al., 1991). The CFTR was also observed immunocytochemically in the sweat gland duct epithelium (Cohn et al., 1991; Crawford et al., 1991). Staining of CFTR was most prominent at the apical domain, but was also detected near the basolateral surface. Antibodies have also identified CFTR in the jejunum; again it appeared to be localized near the apical region of the cells (Crawford et al., 1991). In intestinal Cl^--secreting epithelial cell lines (T84, CaCo2, and HT29 clone 19A), CFTR was located in the apical region of the cell by confocal immunofluorescence microscopy (Denning et al., 1992). An extracellular domain antibody stained the apical surface of nonpermeabilized epithelial cells, indicating that CFTR was actually present within the apical membrane (Denning et al., 1992).

The conclusion that CFTR is located in the apical membrane indicates that it is in a position where it might directly mediate Cl^- movement across the apical membrane. These results do not exclude the possibility that CFTR is also present beneath the apical membrane, perhaps in intracellular vesicles, where it might have additional functions. It will be particularly important to localize CFTR in the airway epithelia. This goal, however, may be difficult, because CFTR is present at very low levels in airway epithelia. One immunofluorescent study was unable to identify CFTR in the airway epithelia (Crawford et al., 1991). Attempts to measure CFTR mRNA levels in airway epithelia have suggested that the number of copies is very low, in the range of a few per cell (Trapnell et al., 1991).

C. Evidence That This Receptor Forms Cyclic AMP-Regulated Chloride Channels

After the full-length CFTR-coding sequence was constructed, the first functional studies were directed at expressing CFTR in CF epithelial cells. Expression of normal CFTR cDNA in CF airway epithelial cells (Gregory et al., 1990; Rich et al., 1990) and in a CF pancreatic carcinoma cell line (Drumm et al., 1990) corrected the CF defect in Cl^- permeability. Addition of cAMP agonists to CF cells expressing recombinant CFTR generated a cAMP-regulated anion permeability. Studies using the patch–clamp technique demonstrated that CFTR generated a Cl⁻ current that had a linear current–voltage (I–V) relationship and little time-dependent voltage effects.

To probe its function, CFTR was expressed in a wide variety of nonepithelial cells with little or no endogenous CFTR. It has been expressed in HeLa cells (Anderson et al., 1991c; Berger et al., 1991), CHO cells (Anderson et al., 1991c; Tabcharani et al., 1991), NIH 3T3 fibroblasts (Anderson et al., 1991b; Berger et al., 1991), mouse L cells (Rommens et al., 1991), Vero cells (Dalemans et al., 1991), Sf9 insect cells (Kartner et al., 1991), and Xenopus oocytes (Drumm et al., 1991; Bear et al., 1991). In each case, expression of CFTR generated a unique Cl⁻ current that was activated by cAMP agonists (forskolin, 3-isobutyl-1-methylxanthine, and membrane-permeant cAMP analogues). Such Cl⁻ currents were not observed in mock-transfected cells.

The whole-cell Cl⁻ currents generated by expression of recombinant CFTR in these different cells displayed similar regulatory properties. They were all regulated by cAMP agonists or, in excised, inside-out, cell-free membrane patches, by cAMP-dependent protein kinase. Membrane potential had little effect on channel activity, and channel activation did not require an elevation of intracellular Ca^{2+}. An examination of the biophysical properties of the channel revealed an I–V relationship that was linear in the presence of symmetric Cl⁻ concentrations. The anion permeability sequence has usually been Br⁻ > Cl⁻ > I⁻. The channel was blocked by high concentrations of diphenylamine-2-carboxylate (DPC), and micromolar concentrations of the sulfonylurea glibenclamide, but not by 4,4′-dinitrostilbene-2,2′-disulfonic acid (DIDS). Single-channel studies revealed properties that were predicted from the whole-cell patch–clamp studies. In addition, they showed a single-channel conductance of approximately 8–10 pS; Figure 2 shows an example of single-channel currents from CFTR.

More direct evidence supporting the conclusion that CFTR is a Cl⁻ channel came from studies that examined the effect of mutations on the anion selectivity (Anderson et al., 1991b). In wild-type CFTR, the anion selectivity sequence is Br⁻ > Cl⁻ > I⁻. Mutation of basic residues in the membrane-spanning domains of CFTR to acidic residues (lysine 95 mutated to aspartic acid or lysine 335 mutated to glutamic acid) changed the anion permeability sequence to I⁻ > Br⁻ > Cl⁻. In contrast, mutation of two other basic amino acids in the putative membrane-spanning sequences (arginine 347 and arginine 1030 mutated to glutamic acid) did not alter the selectivity sequence. These results provide the most compelling evidence that CFTR itself forms a Cl⁻ channel.

The interpretation that CFTR is itself a Cl⁻ channel does not, however, exclude the possibility that it might have additional, as yet undiscovered, functions. It belongs to a family of proteins, many of which use the energy of ATP hydrolysis to actively transport substrates across the cell membrane (Ames et al.,

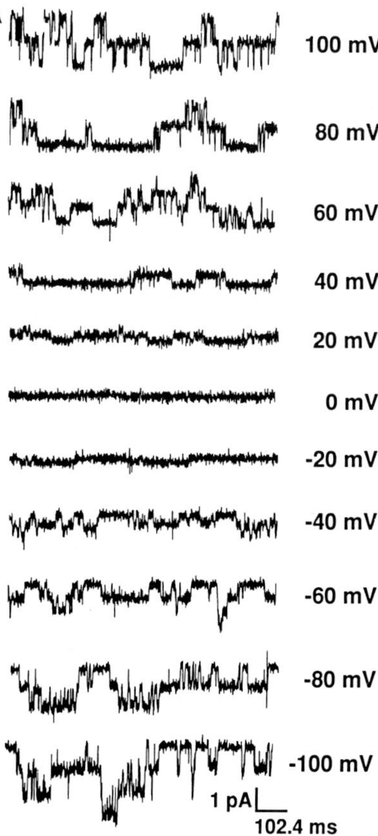

Figure 2 Single channel current tracings from a CFTR Cl⁻ channel that had been activated by PKA and ATP in an excised, inside-out patch of membrane. (From Berger et al., 1991.)

1990; Hyde et al., 1990; Riordan et al., 1991). Accordingly, it has been suggested that CFTR might also function as a pump. Short of the sequence homology with other active transporters, there is no evidence to support such a conjecture. Nevertheless, it is possible that such a function will be discovered. If it is, such a discovery may help explain some of the other phenotypic manifestations of the disease. It also seems likely that CFTR will be associated with other membrane proteins or possibly with the cytoskeleton, as are other channels and transporters. The detection of such relationships may provide new insight into the complex regulation, function, and localization of CFTR.

D. Regulation of CFTR Chloride Channels

From an analysis of the amino acid sequence and the observation that CF epithelia lack a cAMP-regulated Cl^- permeability, Riordan et al. (1989) predicted that CFTR would be regulated by phosphorylation. Several studies have provided direct evidence that the CFTR Cl^- channel is regulated by phosphorylation with the cAMP-dependent protein kinase. In the cell-attached and whole-cell patch–clamp configurations, the channel is reversibly activated by cAMP agonists. In excised, inside-out patches CFTR is opened by phosphorylation with the catalytic subunit of cAMP-dependent protein kinase (Tabcharani et al., 1991; Berger et al., 1991). Biochemical studies have also demonstrated that CFTR is a phosphoprotein (Gregory et al., 1990): protein kinase A (PKA) phosphorylates CFTR in vitro on seven serine residues (Cheng et al., 1991). In vivo studies have shown that four serine residues located within the R domain are substrates for PKA-dependent phosphorylation. Evidence that the four sites are important for regulation of the channel came from the observation that concomitant mutation of those serines to alanines prevents cAMP-dependent activation (Cheng et al., 1991). Further evidence indicating that the R domain regulates the CFTR Cl^- channel came from the observation that deletion of most of the R domain produced a channel that was constitutively open, even without an increase in cAMP (Rich et al., 1991).

More recent studies have shown that the CFTR Cl^- channel is also regulated by nucleoside triphosphates such as ATP (Anderson et al., 1991a). After phosphorylation by PKA, the channel required cytosolic ATP to remain open. The ATP opened the channel by a mechanism that was both independent of PKA and the R domain. Although ATP was proposed to act through the nucleotide-binding domains of CFTR, direct evidence for this hypothesis has not yet been obtained. That speculation is, however, supported by the observation that in other members of the traffic ATPase/ABC transporters, hydrolysis of ATP occurs in the nucleotide-binding domains.

E. Cyclic AMP Regulation of Apical Membrane Chloride Conductance

Several studies have clearly shown that the apical membrane of airway epithelia contains cAMP-regulated Cl^- channels. Thus, it is important to consider whether the properties of the apical membrane Cl^- conductance match the properties of CFTR. Several studies now suggest this is true (for a review see Anderson et al., 1992). (1) Both conductances are regulated by cAMP. (2) The I–V relationship is linear for both. (3) Neither show time-dependent voltage effects on current. (4) The anion permeability sequence for each is $Cl^- > I^-$. (5) The Cl^- current for both is insensitive to DIDS, but is inhibited by DPC. These properties of the epithelial apical membrane are also identical with those of cAMP-activated Cl^- currents studied with the whole-cell patch–clamp technique in cells expressing endogenous CFTR (Cliff and Frizzell, 1990; Anderson and Welsh, 1991; Wagner et al., 1991).

These results indicate that CFTR is a cAMP-regulated Cl⁻ channel located in the apical membrane of Cl⁻ secreting epithelia.

III. Mutations in the Cystic Fibrosis Transmembrane Conductance Regulator Cause Defective Chloride Permeability

Several studies have demonstrated that in native and primary cultures of CF airway epithelia, cAMP fails to increase the apical membrane Cl⁻ conductance. This observation, plus the conclusion that CFTR is a cAMP-activated Cl⁻ channel, raises the question of how CF-associated mutations lead to the characteristic Cl⁻ impermeability of CF epithelia. Mutations in CFTR could result in a loss of Cl⁻ permeability in one of two general ways: the mutated protein may not reach the apical membrane at which it normally mediates Cl⁻ permeability, or the mutated Cl⁻ channel might reach the plasma membrane, but have little or no function. It is also possible that some mutations could lead to a defect in both delivery to the apical membrane and in function.

Studies in which CFTR was expressed in heterologous cells suggest that several CF-associated mutations, including the most common (deletion of phenylalanine at position 508; CFTRΔF508), are incompletely processed (Gregory et al., 1991; Cheng et al., 1990). This inference was based on the finding that wild-type CFTR underwent two stages of glycosylation: core glycosylation (endoglycosidase H-sensitive) characteristic of processing in the endoplasmic reticulum, and a more extensive glycosylation characteristic of processing in the Golgi. In contrast, CFTRΔF508 only underwent core glycosylation. The results suggested that the mutant protein did not reach the Golgi. Instead, it was speculated that CFTRΔF508 was retained in the endoplasmic reticulum and was not delivered to the plasma membrane. Of nine CF-associated mutants that were studied, six were incompletely glycosylated, and all six failed to generate a cAMP-stimulated anion permeability, as assessed using a halide-sensitive fluorophore, 6-methoxy-*N*-(3-sulfopropyl)quinolinium. Incomplete glycosylation alone did not cause Cl⁻ impermeability, because a site-directed mutant that lacked sites for glycosylation was present in the plasma membrane and had normal Cl⁻ channel activity. In addition, CFTR expressed in the Sf9 insect cell line is not completely glycosylated, yet retains its channel function (Kartner et al., 1991). Three of the nine CF-associated mutants studied were processed appropriately, but still failed to generate a cAMP-regulated anion permeability. These results suggested that in those cases the protein was transported to the plasma membrane normally, but had little or no channel function. Because the incompletely glycosylated mutants represent well over 70% of all CF chromosomes, it was proposed that defective trafficking of CFTR is the molecular basis for most cases of CF.

Another recent study of CFTR overexpressed in heterologous cells (Dalemans et al., 1991) suggested that the most common mutant, CFTRΔF508, retained some Cl⁻ channel activity: CFTRΔF508 channels had approximately 25% of the activity of wild-type channels. The investigators also found that there were fewer channels in the plasma membrane of cells expressing CFTRΔF508. The combination of lower single-channel activity and a reduced number of channels suggests a low level of channel activity. In previous studies of Cl⁻ currents in cells expressing CFTRΔF508, no cAMP-stimulated activation was observed (Anderson et al., 1991c). In the latter study, the difference in expression system, recording method, and cell type could have resulted in an inability to detect such a level of activity. Another study suggested that when CFTRΔF508 was expressed in Xenopus oocytes, a cAMP-regulated Cl⁻ current was generated (Drumm et al., 1991). However, in oocytes the current was much larger, approximately 62% of that observed with wild-type CFTR. The increased current in Xenopus oocytes may reflect differences in protein processing by amphibian oocytes, compared with mammalian cells.

Further studies are required to learn how CF-associated mutations of CFTR lead to a Cl⁻-impermeable apical membrane in native CF epithelia. If CFTR mutants retain Cl⁻ channel activity and are present in the apical membrane, one might design a therapeutic strategy to increase the activity of these CFTR Cl⁻ channels. If mutant CFTR is not present in the apical membrane, it is unlikely that such therapeutic maneuvers will be successful. In addition, an understanding of CFTR processing may increase our understanding of how mutations in the protein produce other aspects of the clinical CF phenotype; for example, other associated proteins might also fail to reach the apical membrane.

IV. Implications for Abnormal Epithelial Function

We can now describe both the clinical phenotype of patients with CF and some of the properties of CFTR; however, there is a large gap in our understanding of the processes that lie between these two. We do not yet understand how mutations in CFTR produce the clinical phenotype (i.e., What is the pathogenesis of the lung disease, the infection, and the inflammation?). Our current lack of rigorous data is emphasized by consideration of the multiple abnormalities observed in CF. On the one hand, it appears to be easy to explain why there is a defect in cAMP-regulated Cl⁻ permeability. It is, however, much more difficult to explain other manifestations at the cellular or clinical level. For example, we do not currently understand why CF airway epithelia have an increased rate of Na$^+$ absorption (Boucher et al., 1986), nor do we understand the basis of the increased protein sulfation that occurs in CF airway epithelia (Cheng et al., 1989). An understanding of how the multiple phenotypic manifestations are produced is of central importance in the development and assessment of new therapeutic strategies. It is interesting to recall that some forms of myotonia are caused by a defect in a single gene encoding a muscle Cl$^-$ channel (Steinmeyer et al., 1991). Yet despite that single-gene defect, there have been several phenotypic abnormalities reported in the membrane of affected cells. Cystic fibrosis would not be the first example in which a single-gene defect produces multiple phenotypic manifestations.

The pulmonary airways are the site of repeated infections in CF. Can the pathogenesis and pathophysiology of lung disease be attributed entirely to a failure of transepithelial Cl$^-$ secretion and an increase in Na$^+$ absorption? A recent hypothesis has been put forward that proposes defective acidification of intracellular compartments in CF airway epithelial cells (Barasch et al., 1991). It was proposed that such a defect may be responsible for some of the CF abnormalities of protein modification. Intracellular vesicles are acidified by a proton pump and a Cl$^-$ channel, located in parallel on the vesicular membrane. The proton pump provides the driving force for acidification and the Cl$^\times$ channel provides a pathway for anion movement (to maintain electroneutrality) as well as a means to regulate acidification. Recent work suggests defective acidification of the *trans*-Golgi, endosomes, and prelysosomes in CF airway epithelia (Barasch et al., 1991) caused by a defective vacuolar Cl$^-$ channel. If CFTR can be localized to intracellular vesicles and if defective acidification leads to abnormal processing of several surface proteins, then the results may have important implications for understanding how the defect in CFTR produces the CF phenotype.

Most attention has focused on defective electrolyte transport by the surface epithelium of CF airways. However, altered electrolyte transport by the epithelium of the submucosal glands might also alter the respiratory tract fluid and mucus. Recent data, suggesting that Cl$^-$ secretion is defective in the submucosal glands of CF trachea (Yamaya et al., 1991a,b), point to the potential effect that dysfunctional glands might have on the mucociliary transport process. They also serve to emphasize the limitations of our understanding of how mutations in CFTR lead to disease.

Acknowledgments

We thank Theresa Mayhew for secretarial assistance. Work from the author's laboratory was supported in part by grants from the Howard Hughes Medical Institute, the National Heart Lung and Blood Institute, and the Cystic Fibrosis Foundation.

References

Ames, G. F., Mimura, C. S., and Shyamala, V. (1990). Bacterial periplasmic permeases belong to a family of transport proteins operating from *Escherichia coli* to human: Traffic ATPases. *FEMS Microbiol. Rev.* 6: 429–446.

Anderson, M. P., and Welsh, M. J. (1991). Calcium and cAMP activate different chloride channels in the apical membrane of normal and cystic fibrosis epithelia. *Proc. Natl. Acad. Sci. USA* 88: 6003–6007.

Anderson, M. P., Berger, H. A., Rich, D. P., Gregory, R. J., Smith, A. E., and Welsh, M. J. (1991a). Nucleoside triphosphates are required to open the CFTR chloride channel. *Cell* 67: 775–784.

Anderson, M. P., Gregory, R. J., Thompson, S., Souza, D. W., Paul, S., Mulligan, R. C., Smith, A. E., and Welsh, M. J. (1991b). Demonstration that CFTR is a chloride channel by alteration of its anion selectivity. *Science* 253: 202–205.

Anderson, M. P., Rich, D. R., Gregory, R. J., Smith, A. E., and Welsh, M. J. (1991c). Generation of cAMP-activated chloride currents by expression of CFTR. *Science* 251: 679–682.

Anderson, M. P., Sheppard, D. N., Berger, H. A., and Welsh, M. J. (1992). Chloride channels in the apical membrane of normal and cystic fibrosis airway and intestinal epithelia. *Am. J. Physiol.* 263: L1–L14.

Barasch, J., Kiss, B., Prince, A., Saiman, L., Gruenert, D., and Al-Awqati, Q. (1991). Acidification of intracellular organelles is defective in cystic fibrosis. *Nature* 352: 70–73.

Bear, C. E., Duguay, F., Naismith, A. L., Kartner, N., Hanrahan, J. W., and Riordan, J. R. (1991). Cl$^-$ channel activity in Xenopus oocytes expressing the cystic fibrosis gene. *J. Biol. Chem.* 266: 19142–19145.

Berger, H. A., Anderson, M. P., Gregory, R. J., Thompson, S., Howard, P. W., Maurer, R. A., Mulligan, R., Smith, A. E., and Welsh, M. J. (1991). Identification and regulation of the CFTR-generated chloride channel. *J. Clin. Invest.* 88: 1422–1431.

Boat, T. F., Welsh, M. J., and Beaudet, A. L. (1989). Cystic fibrosis. In *The Metabolic Basis of Inherited Disease*. Edited by C. R. Scriver, A. L. Beaudet, W. S. Sly, and D. Valle. New York, McGraw-Hill, pp. 2649–2680.

Boucher, R. C., Knowles, M. R., Stutts, M. J., and Gatzy, J. T. (1983). Epithelial dysfunction in cystic fibrosis lung disease. In *Lung*. 161: 1–17.

Boucher, R. C., Stutts, M. J., Knowles, M. R., Cantley, L., and Gatzy, J. T. (1986). Na$^+$ transport in cystic fibrosis respiratory epithelia. Abnormal basal rate and response to adenylate cyclase activation. *J. Clin. Invest.* 78: 1245–1252.

Cheng, P. W., Boat, T. F., Cranfill, K., Yankaskas, J. R., and Boucher, R. C. (1989). Increased sulfation of glycoconjugates by cultured nasal epithelial cells from patients with cystic fibrosis. *J. Clin. Invest.* 84: 68–72.

Cheng, S. H., Gregory, R. J., Marshall, J., Paul, S., Souza, D. W., White, G. A., O'Riordan, C. R., and Smith, A. E. (1990). Defective intracellular transport and processing of CFTR is the molecular basis of most cystic fibrosis. *Cell* 63: 827–834.

Cheng, S. H., Rich, D. P., Marshall, J., Gregory, R. J., Welsh, M. J., and Smith, A. E. (1991). Phosphorylation of the R domain by cAMP-dependent protein kinase regulates the CFTR chloride channel. *Cell* 66: 1027–1036.

Cheng, S. H., Gregory, R. J., Amara, J. F., Rich, D. P., Anderson, M., Welsh, M. J., and Smith, A. E. (1993). Intracellular processing of CFTR as the molecular basis of cystic fibrosis. In *Current Topics in Cystic Fibrosis*. Edited by J. Dodge, D. J. Brock, and J. M. Widdicombe, Chichester, John Wiley, Chapter 8, pp. 175–189.

Cliff, W. H., and Frizzell, R. A. (1990). Separate Cl⁻ conductances activated by cAMP and Ca^{2+} in Cl⁻-secreting epithelial cells. *Proc. Natl. Acad. Sci. USA* 87: 4956–4960.

Cohn, J. A., Melhus, O., Page, L. J., Dittrich, K. L., and Vigna, S. R. (1991). CFTR: Development of high-affinity antibodies and localization in sweat gland. *Biochem. Biophys. Res. Commun.* 181: 36–43.

Crawford, I., Maloney, P. C., Zeitlin, P. L., Guggino, W. B., Hyde, S. C., Turley, H., Gatter, K. C., Harris, A., and Higgins, C. F. (1991). Immunocytochemical localization of the cystic fibrosis gene product CFTR. *Proc. Natl. Acad. Sci. USA* 88: 9262–9266.

Dalemans, W., Barbry, P., Champigny, G., Jallat, S., Dott, K., Dreyer, D., Crystal, R. G. Pavirani, A., Lecocq, J., and Lazdunski, M. (1991). Altered chloride ion channel kinetics associated with Δ F508 cystic fibrosis mutation. *Nature* 354: 524–528.

Denning, G. M., Ostedgaard, L. S., Cheng, S. H., Smith, A. E., and Welsh, M. J. (1992). Localization of cystic fibrosis transmembrane conductance regulator in chloride secretory epithelia. *J. Clin. Invest.* 89: 339–349.

Drumm, M. L., Pope, H. A., Cliff, W. H., Rommens, J. M., Marvin, S. A., Tsui, L.-C., Collins, F. C., Frizzell, R. A., and Wilson, J. M. (1990). Correction of the cystic fibrosis defect in vitro by retrovirus-mediated gene transfer. *Cell* 62: 1227–1233.

Drumm, M. L., Wilkinson, D. J., Smit, L. S., Worrell, R. T., Strong, T. V., Frizzell, R. A., Dawson, D. C., and Collins, F. S. (1991). Chloride conductance expressed by ΔF508 and other mutant CFTRs in *Xenopus* oocytes. *Science* 254: 1797–1799.

Frizzell, R. A. (1987). Cystic fibrosis: A disease of ion channels? *Trends Neurosci.* 10: 190–193.

Frizzell, R. A., and Halm, D. R. (1990). Chloride channels in epithelial cells. In *Current Topics in Membranes and Transport*. New York, Academic Press, pp. 247–282.

Frizzell, R. A., Field, M., and Schultz, S. G. (1979). Sodium-coupled chloride transport by epithelial tissues. *Am. J. Physiol.* 236: F1–F8.

Gögelein, H. (1988). Chloride channels in epithelia. *Biochim. Biophys. Acta* 947: 521–547.

Gregory, R. J., Cheng, S. H., Rich, D. R., Marshall, J., Paul, S. Hehir, K., Ostedgaard, L., Klinger, K. W., Welsh, M. J., and Smith, A. E. (1990). Expression and characterization of the cystic fibrosis transmembrane conductance regulator. *Nature* 347: 382–386.

Gregory, R. J., Rich, D. P., Cheng, S. H., Souza, D. W., Paul, S. Manavalan, P., Anderson, M. P., Welsh, M. J., and Smith, A. E. (1991). Maturation and function of cystic fibrosis transmembrane conductance regulator variants bearing mutations in putative nucleotide-binding domains 1 and 2. *Mol. Cell Biol.* 11: 3886–3893.

Hamill, O. P., Marty, A., Neher, E. Sakmann, B., and Sigworth, F. J. (1981). Improved patch–clamp techniques for high-resolution current recording from cells and cell-free membrane patches. *Pfleugers Arch.* 391: 85–100.

Hyde, S. C., Emsley, P., Hartshorn, M. J., Mimmack, M. M., Gileadi, U., Pearce, S. R., Gallagher, M. P., Gill, D. R., Hubbard, R. E., and Higgins, C. F. (1990). Structural model of ATP-binding proteins associated with cystic fibrosis, multidrug resistance and bacterial transport. *Nature* 346: 362–365.

Kartner, N., Hanrahan, J. W., Jensen, T. J., Naismith, A. L., Sun, S., Ackerley, C. A., Reyes, E. F., Tsui, L.-C., Rommens, J. M., Bear, C. E., and Riordan, J. R. (1991). Expression of the cystic fibrosis gene in non-epithelial invertebrate cells produces a regulated anion conductance. *Cell* 64: 681–691.

Kerem, B., Rommens, J. M., Buchanan, J. A., Markiewicz, D., Cox, T. K., Chakravarti, A., Buchwald, M., and Tsui, L. C. (1989). Identification of the cystic fibrosis gene: Genetic analysis. *Science* 245: 1073–1080.

Marino, C. R., Matovcik, L. M., Gorelick, F. S., and Cohn, J. A. (1991). Localization of the cystic fibrosis transmembrane conductance regulator in pancreas. *J. Clin. Invest.* 88: 712–716.

Quinton, P. M. (1990). Cystic fibrosis: A disease in electrolyte transport. *FASEB J.* 4: 2709–2717.

Rich, D. P., Anderson, M. P., Gregory, R. J., Cheng, S. H., Paul, S., Jefferson, D. M., McCann, J. D., Klinger, K. W., Smith, A. E., and Welsh, M. J. (1990). Expression of cystic fibrosis transmembrane conductance regulator corrects defective chloride channel regulation in cystic fibrosis airway epithelial cells. *Nature* 347: 358–363.

Rich, D. P., Gregory, R. J., Anderson, M. P., Manavalan, P., Smith, A. E., and Welsh, M. J. (1991). Effect of deleting the R domain on CFTR-generated chloride channels. *Science* 253: 205–207.

Riordan, J. R., Rommens, J. M., Kerem, B. Alon, N., Rozmahel, R., Grzelczak, Z. Zielenski, J., Lok, S., Plavsic, N., Chou, J. L., Drumm, M. C., Iannuzzi, M. C., Collins, F. S., and Tsui, L.-C. (1989). Identification of the cystic fibrosis gene: Cloning and characterization of complementary DNA. *Science* 245: 1066–1073.

Riordan, J. R., Alon, N., Grzelczak, Z., Dubel, S., and Sun, S.-Z. (1991). The CF gene product as a member of a membrane transporter (TM6-NBF) super family. In *The Identification of the CF Gene*. Edited by L.-C. Tsui. New York, Plenum Press, pp. 19–29.

Rommens, J. M., Iannuzzi, M. C., Kerem, B.-S., Drumm, M. L., Melmer, G., Dean, M., Rozmahel, R., Cole, J. L., Kennedy, D., Hidaka, N., Zsiga, M., Buchwald, M., Riordan, J. R., Tsui, L.-C., and Collins, F. S. (1989). Identification of the cystic fibrosis gene: Chromosome walking and jumping. *Science* 245: 1059–1065.

Rommens, J. M., Dho, S., Bear, C. E., Kartner, N., Kennedy, D., Riordan, J. R., Tsui, L., and Foskett, J. K. (1991). cAMP-inducible chloride conductance in mouse fibroblast lines stably expressing the human cystic fibrosis transmembrane conductance regulator. *Proc. Natl. Acad. Sci. USA* 88: 7500–7504.

Steinmeyer, K., Kocke, R. Ortland, C. Gronemeier, M. J., Jockusch, H., Grunder S., and Jentsch, T. J. (1991). Inactivation of muscle chloride channel by transposon insertion in myotonic mice. *Nature* 354: 304–308.

Tabcharani, J. A., Chang, X.-B., Riordan, J. R., and Hanrahan, J. W. (1991). Phosphorylation-regulated Cl^- channel in CHO cells stably expressing the cystic fibrosis gene. *Nature* 352: 628–631.

Trapnell, B. C., Chu, C. S., Paakko, P. K., Banks, T.C., Yoshimura, K., Ferrans, V. J., Chernick, M. S., and Crystal, R. G. (1991). Expression of the cystic fibrosis transmembrane conductance regulator gene in the respiratory tract of normal individuals and individuals with cystic fibrosis. *Proc. Natl. Acad. Sci. USA* 88: 6565–6569.

Tsui, L.-C., and Buchwald, M. (1991). Biochemical and molecular genetics of cystic fibrosis. In *Advances in Human Genetics*. Edited by H. Harris, and K. Hirschhorn. New York, Plenum Press, pp. 153–266.

Wagner, J. A., Cozens, A. L., Schulman, H., Gruenert, D. C., Stryer, L., and Gardner, P. (1991). Activation of chloride channels in normal and cystic fibrosis airway epithelial cells by multifunctional calcium/calmodulin-dependent protein kinase. *Nature* 349: 793–796.

Welsh, M. J. (1987). Electrolyte transport by airway epithelia. *Physiol. Rev.* 67: 1143–1184.

Wine, J. J. (1991). Basic aspects of cystic fibrosis. *Clin. Rev. Allergy* 9: 1–28.

Yamaya, M., Finkbeiner, W. E., and Widdicombe, J. H. (1991a). Ion transport by cultures of human tracheobronchial submucosal glands. *Am. J. Physiol.* 261: L485–L490.

Yamaya, M., Finkbeiner, W. E., and Widdicombe, J. H. (1991b). Altered ion transport by tracheal glands in cystic fibrosis. *Am. J. Physiol.* 261: L491–L494.

15

Airway Hypersecretion in Bronchial Asthma and Chronic Obstructive Pulmonary Disease

TAMOTSU TAKISHIMA and SANAE SHIMURA

Tohoku University School of Medicine
Sendai, Japan

I. Introduction

Airway hypersecretion is one of the characteristic features of chronic obstructive lung disease (COPD), and *chronic bronchitis* has been defined by the Ciba guest symposium of 1959 and American Thoracic Society (1962) as a disease marked by chronic and recurrent excessive secretion of mucus in the bronchial tree. Thus, airway hypersecretion is a principal clinical feature in chronic bronchitis. Mucous hypersecretion also accompanies bronchial asthma, especially during the attack; a large amount of mucous plugging in airways is frequently observed in the autopsied lungs of patients with bronchial asthma. In this chapter, we discuss the following items: (1) Structural alteration of secretory cells, (2) chemical and rheological properties of sputum, (3) airway hypersecretion and hyperresponsiveness, (4) airway hypersecretion and obstructive impairment, and (5) airway hypersecretion and mortality.

II. Structural Alteration of Secretory Cells

Secretory cells in the airways consist of submucosal glands and superficial epithelial mucous cells (goblet cells). Chronic inflammation produces hyperplasia or hypertrophy of these secretory cells in the airways, resulting in airway hypersecretion. The increase in total volume of these cells in the airways seems to be due to hyperplasia, rather than hypertrophy, although there has been no direct evidence for which is responsible.

A. Submucosal Glands

The fundamental morphological alteration in chronic bronchitis is enlargement of the tracheobronchial glands brought about by hyperplasia of the acinar secretory cells (Reid, 1954, 1960). Methods of morphologically estimating or quantifying tracheobronchial gland size or volume have been developed to investigate chronic obstructive pulmonary disease, particularly chronic bronchitis. Reid (1960) described a measurement of the gland/wall ratio, which is generally referred to as the Reid index (Fig. 1), and its increase in chronic bronchitis has been confirmed by most observers. Reid (1960) reported that the ratio ranges is 0.14–0.36 (mean 0.26) normally, 0.41–0.79 (mean 0.59) in bronchitis, and 0.28–0.43 (mean 0.33) in emphysema.

There are inherent problems with this assessment of gland size, since the glands lie not only between the epithelium and cartilage, but also between the plates of cartilage external to them and the membranous portion. Some investigators have cited this as the reason there is some overlap between normal and bronchitis groups and that the Reid index is not significantly related to sputum volume (Thurlbeck and Angus, 1964; McKenzie et al., 1969; Jamal et al., 1984). Some attempts have been made by several investigators to overcome this criticism. A radial intercepts method (Alli, 1975), the point-count technique (Hale et al., 1968; Dunnill et al., 1969; Macleod and Heard 1969; Wheeldon and Pirie,

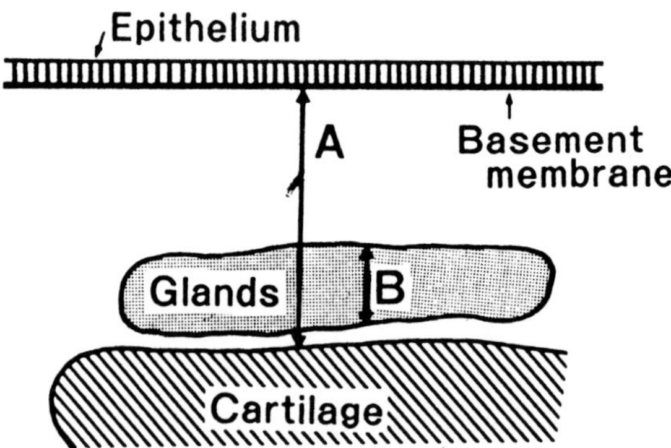

Figure 1   Illustration of the method used for measuring the gland/wall ratio (Reid index). See text for detail. (From Reid, 1960.)

1974; Lennox, 1975; Oberholzer et al., 1978; Berend et al., 1979; Hayashi et al., 1979), and weighing of paper cutouts of drawings (Restrepo and Heard, 1963a,b), all reflecting two-dimensional attempts at greater precision, have been applied to glandular and other bronchial constituents. More recently, absolute glandular area and volume proportion measurements have been made by projecting images onto a computer-assisted graphics tablet (Jamal et al., 1984; Nagai et al., 1985; Aikawa et al., 1989, 1992). In the central airways of lungs afflicted with chronic bronchitis, the volume proportion of submucosal glands to bronchial wall are reported to be 10–30% and that of controls is 7–10% (Takizawa and Thurlbeck, 1971; Aikawa et al., 1989). Nevertheless, the Reid index has been recommended by several investigators because it requires less skill and offers a significant saving in time and cost. The Reid index retains a useful place both as a quick method of measurement for routine hospital use and in epidemiological (Scott, 1973) or experimental studies (Phipps et al., 1986).

In addition to the measurements of whole-gland size or volume, gland acinar counts per light microscopic field (Reid, 1960) and the ratio of mucous to serous acini (Glynn and Michaels, 1960) have also been suggested as indices of bronchial glandular hypertrophy. Glynn and Michaels reported that both the acinar portion and the ratio of mucous to serous acini increased in chronic bronchitis. Serous cells contain and secrete lysozyme and lactoferrin, which are antibacterial agents (Bowes and Corrin, 1977; Tom-Moy et al., 1983). Thus, a decrease in serous cells relative to mucous cells in submucosal glands might produce some disturbance in the airway defense mechanisms. Furthermore, the presence of both neutral and acid glycoprotein has been demonstrated in mucous cells of the submucosal glands. Kollerstrom et al. (1977) examined the percentage area of acid glyco-protein in bronchial glands. The amount of acid glycoprotein in submucosal glands increases in chronic bronchitis, resulting in a decrease of mucociliary transport in the airways.

Submucosal gland hypertrophy is also known to be one of pathological characteristics of bronchial asthma in both biopsy specimens (Cutz et al., 1978; Glynn and Michaels, 1960) and autopsied lungs (Cardell and Pearson, 1959; Dunnill, 1960; Messer et al., 1960; Houston et al., 1953; Dunnill et al., 1969). Meanwhile, Sobonya (1984) reported that the size of submucosal glands from the lungs of bronchial asthma patients did not significantly differ from those of nonsmoking controls. Aikawa et al. (1992) found that the submucosal gland hypertrophy or hyperplasia from autopsied lungs of patients with bronchial asthma is similar to that seen in chronic bronchitis (Dunnill et al., 1969; Takizawa and Thurlbeck, 1971; Aikawa et al., 1989). In addition to the differences among patients with bronchial asthma, there is a heterogeneity of bronchial asthma that may be due to duration, smoking habits, medication, or treatment. For example, a β-adrenergic stimulant is frequently used for the treatment of bronchial asthma, and it is experimentally known to induce increases in both the size of the tracheal glands and the number of goblet cells throughout the airways in rats and pigs (Sturgess and Reid, 1973; Jones and Reid, 1979).

In addition to chronic bronchitis and bronchial asthma, tracheobronchial gland hyperplasia is associated with some conditions or diseases of the lung. These include mainly tobacco smoke (Ryder et al., 1971), air or environmental pollution (Hayes, 1969; Scott, 1973), pneumoconiosis (McKenzie, et al., 1969; Douglas, 1980; Douglas et al., 1982), and cryptogenic fibrosing alveolitis (Edwards and Carlile, 1982; Andoh et al., 1992a). Smoking has been identified as the major risk factor in the development of chronic obstructive pulmonary disease, and prolonged smoking induces the mucous hypersecretion associated with enlargement of the mucus-secreting tissue and mucosal inflammation of the airways (Mullen et al., 1987; Cosio et al., 1980). Andoh et al. (1992a) have found some patients with idiopathic pulmonary fibrosis with chronic hypertrophy and mucus accumulation in the airways to a degree similar to that shown in chronic bronchitis (Aikawa et al., 1989).

B. Epithelial Goblet Cells

Superficial epithelial mucous cells, goblet cells, are known to increase in response to chronic airway inflammation, and goblet cell hyperplasia or metaplasia are one of the indexes of chronic bronchitis, in addition to submucosal gland hyperplasia. In the airways of bronchial asthma and chronic bronchitis, goblet cell hyperplasia has been observed, and the increase is up to two- or threefold, compared with controls (Cutz et al., 1978; Glynn and Michaels, 1960). Similar goblet cell hyperplasia is also observed in animal experiments: human neutrophil product-induced and cigarette smoke-induced goblet cell hyperplasia has been demonstrated in the rat (Lundgren et al., 1988b; Snider et al., 1984; Rogers and Jeffery, 1986). However, goblet cell hyperplasia is not always accompanied by chronic bronchitis. For example, Aikawa et al. (1989) reported that goblet cell hyperplasia was not significant in the autopsied lungs from severe obstructive chronic bronchitis patients.

Goblet cell hyperplasia is also one of the characteristics of bronchial asthma (Cutz et al., 1978; Dunnill et al., 1969). Aikawa et al. (1992) have found marked goblet cell hyperplasia in the airways of patients who died of severe acute asthma attack. Markedly significant increases in goblet cells were more prominent in the peripheral airways: a 30-fold increase compared with controls. In bronchioles, submucosal glands are absent, and goblet cells have a principal role in the secretion. Additionally, the site of increased airway resistance in patients with chronic obstructive impairment has been shown to be the small airways including the bronchioles (Hogg et al., 1968; Sekizawa et al., 1986). Possibly, the goblet cell metaplasia produces impairments of mucociliary transport and ion transport across the epithelium. In contrast, Lozewics et al. (1990) and Jeffery et al. (1989)

reported that there were no significant differences in the morphological features of the bronchial epithelium in biopsy specimens between the mild asthmatic and the healthy groups.

Goblet cells in the superficial epithelium are sometimes difficult to identify, as they contain no mucin after acute secretion. Acute bronchial inflammation is known to induce a decrease or disappearance of goblet cells or intracellular mucin (Holtzman et al., 1983; Breuer et al., 1987). β-Adrenergic agonists have been reported to produce goblet cell hyperplasia in animals (Sturgess and Reid, 1973; Jones and Reid, 1979). In contrast, some animal experiments (Lundgren et al., 1988b; Rogers and Jeffery, 1986) have shown that glucocorticoids can reduce airway goblet cell hyperplasia induced by neutrophil products or smoking. These may be responsible for some of the conflicting reports concerning goblet cell hyperplasia in diseased lungs.

III. Enhanced Secretion

A. Mucous Secretion

In addition to the increase in the number and size of the plural mucus-producing structures, accumulation of inflammatory cells in the airway wall and lumen is one of the characteristic features in the pathological background of chronic bronchitis and bronchial asthma. These migratory cells release various chemical mediators and substances that are capable of inducing airway secretion.

Neutrophils are greatly increased in the purulent sputum of patients with chronic bronchitis and neutrophil accumulation in the airway lumen and wall is a pathological finding characteristic of chronic bronchitis. Neutrophils are a source of a variety of potentially important mediators of inflammation, including neutral proteinases (Baggiolini et al., 1978). Prominent among these are the lysosomal proteinases, cathepsin G and elastase, which are released from neutrophils during phagocytosis and cell death. Cathepsin G and elastase are potent stimulants of both goblet cell and submucosal gland secretion (Breuer et al., 1987; Kim et al., 1987; Sommerhoff et al., 1990). For example, neutrophil elastase causes an increase in secretion of 1800% over baseline and the response is tenfold or more larger than that caused by other agonists, such as prostaglandins, histamine, and neurotransmitters in glycoconjugate secretion from bovine airway gland cells (Sommerhoff et al., 1990). Recent studies (Sommerhoff et al., 1989) have also shown that mast cells contain a chymase, the magnitude of which in secretory response is equipotent to neutrophil elastase in causing glycoconjugate secretion from airway gland cells.

An acute asthmatic attack is usually composed of an acute reaction caused by mast cell or basophil activation and a late-phase reaction that occurs 4–8 h later. The late-phase reaction is accompanied by an accumulation of eosinophils, neutrophils, and macrophages in the airways. The inflammatory cells may produce and release various compounds and substances that also may stimulate airway secretion. These include histamine, prostaglandins, leukotrienes, and platelet-activating factor (PAF) all of which are capable of stimulating airway secretion (Adler et al., 1987; Kaliner et al., 1984; Lundgren et al., 1985; Marin et al., 1977; Marom et al., 1981, 1982, 1983, 1984a,b; Rees et al., 1985; Rich et al., 1984; Sasaki et al., 1989; Shelhamer et al., 1980). Eosinophil granules contain one or more proteins that are capable of releasing mucus from cultured airways. For example, Lundgren et al. (1991) have reported that eosinophilic cationic protein stimulates glycoconjugate secretion from feline tracheal explants. A recent study by Poston et al. (1992) has shown macrophage accumulation in the airway walls of bronchial asthma. Macrophages and monocytes also secrete a mucous secretagogue—macrophage-derived mucous secretagogue (MMS) (but only after the cells are activated), which has a relative molecular mass (M_r) of approximately 2 kd (Marom et al., 1984c, 1985). Various chemical mediators, including prostaglandins and leukotrienes, augment neural reflex secretion by acting on ganglions (Johnson et al., 1983) or on neurocellular junctions (Shimura et al., 1987b; 1992).

Clinically, pseudomonas infection induces airway hypersecretion. *Pseudomonas aeruginosa* produces numerous substances that can induce airway secretion in vitro (Somerville et al., 1991, 1992). Some harmful substances from *P. aeruginosa* can damage airway epithelium (Stutts et al., 1986), resulting in an increase in airway mucosal permeability to albumin (Ishihara et al., 1991). Serum itself is known to induce airway secretion (Peatfield et al., 1982). Some investigators have discussed the ways in which inflammatory cells might alter the eipithelium, leading to the activation of C fiber reflexes and, perhaps, to the induction of mucous hypersecretion. Pathological evidence indicates that inflammatory changes in chronic bronchitis and bronchial asthma include epithelial injury and damage. Epithelial damage and detachment produce an exposure of nerve endings of sensory nerves or C fibers, resulting in an augmentation of neural reflex secretion in the airways. Cough receptors and sensory nerve C fibers are localized superficially, just below the tight junctions of the epithelium (Schultz et al., 1985). Chronic irritation of these receptors may cause reflex-increased airway secretion (Davis et al., 1982). Tachykinins, including substance P, are localized in C-type neurons of nerve endings in the airways of many species, including human, and are released by the axonal reflex by various stimulations (Lundberg and Saria, 1983; Barnes, 1986; Saria et al., 1988). These tachykinins are known to stimulate airway secretion (Coles et al., 1984; Borson et al., 1987; Gashi et al., 1986; Lundgren et al., 1989a; Shimura et al., 1987a; Tamaoki et al., 1988). Inflammatory change could also result in the production of bradykinin, which can stimulate mucous secretion directly or indirectly by activating sensory bronchial C fibers, thereby producing a reflex stimulation of submucosal gland secretion (Davis et al., 1982).

Goblet cell secretion is not under pharmacological control (Kim et al., 1989), but mechanical strain can cause mucin release from airway epithelial cells (Kim and Brody, 1992). Such a mechanism may be operative in the physiological regulation of goblet cell mucin secretion for which mechanical strains may be induced on epithelial cells by underlying smooth muscles. This is an important finding for the understanding of mucous plugging in the airways of bronchial asthma.

B. Fluid Secretion

Airway secretion consists of a 95% or more fluid component and a small amount of mucin. Airway fluid comes from both superficial epithelial cells and submucosal gland cells. Active chloride secretion with water to the airway lumen is observed in superficial epithelial cells and submucosal gland cells (Frizell, 1988; Marin et al., 1977; Sasaki et al., 1990; Tamaoki et al., 1988). Almost all agonists and chemical mediators that are stimulants of airway mucin secretion are also known to stimulate chloride secretion in both epithelial cells and submucosal gland cells. Therefore, in diseased lungs, an increase in mucin secretion is thought to be accompanied by an increase in fluid secretion. Although the mechanism is unknown, it is clinically observed that enhanced fluid secretion is not necessarily associated with an increase in mucin secretion. For example, *Bronchorrhea* is defined as more than 100 ml of watery sputum produced per day and is only occasionally associated with chronic bronchitis and bronchial asthma, in addition to alveolar cell carcinoma (Lopez-Vidriero et al., 1975b, 1979). Shimura et al. (1988a) have reported that bronchorrhea was seen in 8.7% patients with bronchial asthma during an attack. Its origin is believed to be fluid movement into the lumen by active ion transport in superficial epithelial cells or in submucosal gland cells, since the Na^+/Cl^- ratio of bronchorrhea sputum during an asthmatic attack showed a decrease, compared with that of mucoid sputum (Table 1) (Shimura et al., 1988a).

C. Mucosal Exudation

Although it is not really secretion from airway secretory cells, mucosal exudation to the airway lumen plays an important role in hypersecretion or sputum production in patients with bronchial asthma and chronic obstructive pulmonary disease. *Exudation* is defined as serum leakage from microvessels in the airway submucosa to the airway lumen. For exudation, both microvascular and epithelial leakages are necessary, and epithelial leakage is a determinant in airway exudation, since the epithelial barrier is much tighter than the endothelial barrier. Namely, it is necessarily accompanied by epithelial damage, especially to the tight junction between superficial epithelial cells. Thus, the exudation depends on the paracellular permeability of macromolecules in the airway epithelium. Chronic airway

Table 1 Chemical Properties of Saliva, Bronchorrhea and Mucoid Sputum in Bronchial Asthma

Property	Saliva	Bronchorrhea	Mucoid sputum
Dry weight (%)	0.76 ± 0.47	1.70 ± 0.60*[§§]	3.18 ± 1.08
Albumin (g/dl)	0.03 ± 0.06	0.20 ± 0.20*[§§]	0.51 ± 0.24
pH	7.16 ± 0.61	6.69 ± 0.96	7.50 ± 0.69
Na⁺/Cl⁻ ratio	0.89 ± 0.40	0.86 ± 0.10[§§]	0.99 ± 0.08
Histamine (μg/ml)	0.68 ± 0.05	3.15 ± 1.40**[§]	2.08 ± 0.82

Mean ± SE; *$p < 0.05$; **$p < 0.01$; compared with saliva; [§]$p < 0.05$; [§§]$p < 0.01$, compared with mucoid sputum.
Source: Shimura et al., 1988a.

inflammation, with some epithelial injury and damage, is characteristic not only of chronic bronchitis, but also of bronchial asthma.

Many studies of airway mucosal permeability have now been performed using inhaled tracers that have been believed to diffuse from the lungs into the bloodstream. In human lungs, the isotope count in peripheral blood after isotope ([99mTc]-DTPA) inhalation has been detected by examining the relationship between absorption and clearance of isotopes from the lung (Borland et al., 1985; Elwood et al., 1983; Gellert et al., 1985; Kennedy et al., 1984; Rees et al., 1985). With these methods of estimating airway mucosal permeability, it is now considered that large variations, both in the area and volume of initial deposition and in the penetration rate across the airway mucosa, are present in chronic obstructive pulmonary disease with hypersecretion. Furthermore, there has been no direct evidence that permeability examined by the inhaled isotope method is bidirectional. The permeability from blood flow to airway lumen must play an important role in increased mucous secretion as well as in bronchial hyperreactivity. The method used in Honda et al.'s study (1988) was to measure the radioactivity of sputum after injection of [131I]-albumin, which is especially advantageous when the role of airway mucosal permeability contributing to the mucous hypersecretion is to be examined. Their method provides an estimate of the permeability from the bloodstream to the airway lumen, whereas the inhalation method assesses the permeability from the airway lumen to the bloodstream. However, the possibility that these two methods measure different processes involved in solute movement cannot be ruled out because of the difference in size of [99mTc]-DTPA (492 Da) and albumin (69,000 Da), even if the permeability measured is bidirectional.

To determine airway mucosal permeability, Honda et al. (1988) examined radiolabeled albumin in sputum on the basis of sputum collection every 2 h for as long as 8 h after [131I]-labeled human serum albumin injection in patients with chronic bronchitis and stable bronchial asthma with hypersecretion. Between the bronchitic and asthmatic groups, there was no significant difference in sputum production or in obstructive impairment. The ratio of radiocount in sputum to that in serum (permeability) in the bronchitic group was significantly higher than that in the asthmatic group at each sampling period (Fig. 2). Thus, these authors found that airway mucosal permeability is much greater in bronchitics than in asthmatics. One possible cause of airway hyperreactivity may be that the respiratory mucosa is abnormally permeable to antigens and mediators of allergic responses (Hogg, 1984). However, Rees et al. (1985) examined the effects of histamine on permeability in normal and asthmatic subjects and suggested that there is no direct relation between bronchoconstriction and permeability. Elwood et al. (1983) showed that permeability was no greater in subjects with stable asthma than it was in normal subjects. In addition, Kennedy et al. (1984) examined the permeability in smokers and reported that there is no evidence of increased airway reactivity, despite increased permeability. Because these investigators examined the permeability from the airway lumen to the bloodstream, their results

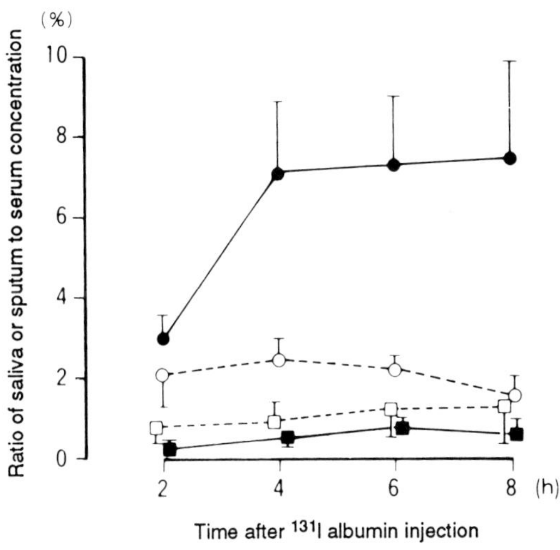

Figure 2   Ratio of saliva or sputum to serum concentration (cpm/ml) of ^{131}I-albumin at each sampling period. Saliva samples from all patients (asthmatic group, open squares; bronchitic group, closed squares) show much lower ratios than do those of sputum samples (asthmatic group, open circles; bronchitic group, closed circles) at each sampling period. Sputum samples in bronchitic group show significantly higher ratios than did those in asthmatic group ($p < 0.05$, two-way analysis of variance) and the ratio of bronchitic group reached a plateau at 4 h in the sampling period (bars indicate SEM). (From Honda et al., 1988.)

do not necessarily conflict with those of Honda et al. (1988) (i.e., from the bloodstream to the airway lumen). This suggests that an increase in mucosal permeability in chronic bronchitis is due to mucosal epithelial damage by chronic inflammation, which is not a primary underlying abnormality in stable asthma. However, it is possible that bronchial asthmatic attack produces an increase in the permeability across airway mucosa, playing a role in airway hypersecretion during the asthmatic attack. In fact, recent animal experiments (Ohrui et al., 1991, 1992) have shown that an asthmatic attack induces microvascular leakage in the airway wall and, possibly, also epithelial damage. Moreover, Fick et al. (1987) reported that the concentrations of total proteins and albumin in the bronchoalveolar lavage fluid in allergic asthmatics exhibited no significant differences from those of healthy subjects before exposure, but after exposure, these concentrations rose. They also reported that an increase in microvascular permeability to plasma protein was found in local regions exposed to the antigen solution before the occurrence of bronchial constriction. Persson and Svensjö (1983), based on their results in studies with guinea pigs, stated that most chemical mediators involved in the induction of bronchial constriction caused vascular leakage of plasma protein, and also that a larger amount of plasma protein leaked from blood vessels into the airway within a few minutes after the challenge of mediator to airway mucosa (Persson and Erjefält, 1986).

In the study of Honda et al. (1988) bronchitics showed significantly higher values than asthmatics, both in radiolabeled albumin concentration and in the ratio of sputum to serum concentration, suggesting that increased permeability is a result of inflammatory changes in the airways. The change in permeability is related to changes in the tight junctions that join the epithelial cells together, and damage to the tight junctions can increase the airway mucosal permeability to macromolecules (Schneeberger and Lynch, 1984). Furthermore, Peatfield et al. (1982) reported that serum or albumin promotes the secretion of mucous glycoproteins in the cat trachea, and this mechanism may also involve mucous hypersecretion in chronic bronchitis. Hypersecretion in bronchitics must involve increased permeability—exudate or transudate—as well as increased secretion from secretory cells in the airways.

Chronic *P. aeruginosa* infection is frequently seen in patients with cystic fibrosis, a common disease among the white population, and in patients with chronic bronchitis with severe obstruction, which is common in Japanese (Homma et al., 1983). During chronic infection, *P. aeruginosa* produces numerous substances that can damage airway epithelium, including exotoxin A, proteineases, elastases, leukocidin, phospholipase C, exoenzyme S, and several hemolysins (Liu, 1966; Morihara et al., 1965). In fact, an in vitro experiment by Stutts et al. (1986) has demonstrated that *P. aeruginosa* increases the solute flow around cells in both canine and human bronchial epithelium, suggesting that toxic substances from the bacteria impair the tight junctions between cells. Ishihara et al. (1991)

examined the effect of *P. aeruginosa* infection on the barrier function of airway epithelium in pulmonary diseases. They examined airway mucosal permeability by measuring radiolabeled albumin in sputum from patients (Honda et al., 1988) suffering from chronic bronchitis with chronic *P. aeruginosa* infection, and compared it with that from patients without *P. aeruginosa* infection. The pseudomonas-infected group showed significantly higher values in the ratio of sputum to serum radiocounts than did the group without pseudomonas infection at all sampling times up to 24 h (Fig. 3). Furthermore, the ratios significantly correlated with sputum volume per day (Fig. 4), whereas they did not correlate with any other factors (age, obstructive impairment, and duration of disease). These findings suggest that chronic *P. aeruginosa* infection produces an increase in airway mucosal permeability to albumin, in addition to the direct stimulation of airway secretion by pseudomonas products (Somerville et al., 1991, 1992).

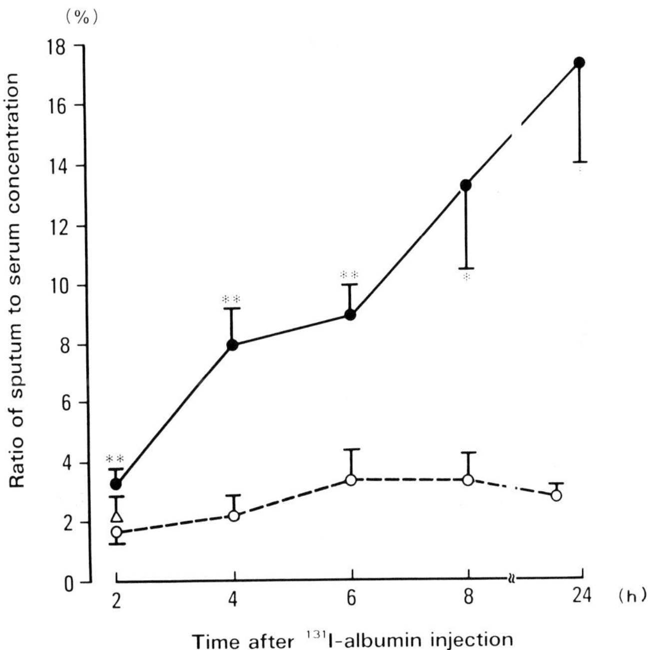

Figure 3 Ratio of sputum to serum concentration (cpm/ml) of ^{131}I-albumin at each sampling period. Sputum samples from patients with *Pseudomonas aeruginosa* infection (group A, closed circles) show significantly higher ratios than do those from patients without *P. aeruginosa* infection (group B, open circles). Differences between groups A and B were statistically significant in each sampling period; one asterisk, $p < 0.05$; two asterisks, $p < 0.01$; bars indicate SEM. (From Ishihara et al., 1991.)

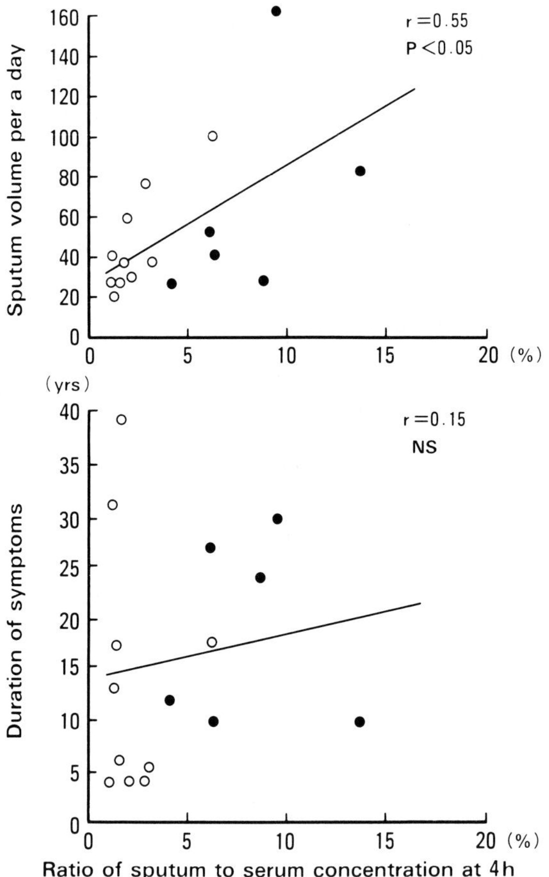

Figure 4   Relationships between ratio of sputum to serum [31]I-albumin concentration 4 h after injection and sputum volume (ml/day) (upper panel), and between the ratio and duration of symptoms (lower panel). Sputum volume significantly correlates with the ratio of sputum to serum concentration (upper panel), whereas the duration of symptom does not (lower panel). Closed circles indicate group A (pseudomonas infection group) and open circles indicate group B (no pseudomonas infection group). (From Ishihara et al., 1991.)

IV.   Chemical and Rheological Properties of Sputum

Most of the information concerning changes in the composition of mucus in diseased lungs is derived from the examination of sputum. However, to understand the alterations in mucous production in the airways, sputum alone may not be representative for several reasons. Sputum is a mixture of molecules with origins from several cell sources. Saliva inevitably will be mixed with the tracheobronchial mucus and can potentially alter the chemical and rheological properties. After sputum is expectorated, its biophysical properties may change within hours. Parameters measured or found in sputum cannot be compared with normal values, since healthy people do not produce sputum. This presents a problem, especially when comparing results from different laboratories. Therefore, mucus collected from laryngectomized patients and sputum induced in normal persons by inhalation of mucous secretagogues have been used as "controls."

A. Variation with Diseases

Sputa from patients with bronchial asthma are reported to show a higher viscosity, compared with sputa from patients with chronic bronchitis, bronchiectasis, cystic fibrosis, and normal persons in whom its production has been artificially induced (controls) (Charman and Reid, 1972; Chase et al., 1985; Lopez-Vidriero et al., 1973, 1977, 1978). The dry weight of asthmatic sputum is increased threefold compared with controls. This increase in dry weight probably is caused by enhanced secretion from mucus-producing cells in the airways, since the markers of mucous glycoprotein (fucose and sulfate) are increased in concentration (Lundgren et al., 1989b). Exudation of plasma proteins from vessels may also contribute, since the concentration of N-acetylneuraminic acid (NANA; marker of mucous glycoprotein as well as plasma proteins) increases relatively more than the fucose concentration (Lopez-Vidriero and Reid, 1978), and two other plasma proteins (albumin and transferrin) are also increased (Brogan et al., 1975). The concentration of lactoferrin and lysozyme does not differ between asthmatic patients and those with chronic bronchitis (Harbitz et al., 1984), whereas the levels of IgA in asthmatic sputum is twice as high as in controls, but fivefold less than sputum from chronic bronchitis (Lundgren et al., 1989b).

We routinely differentiate between mucoid and purulent sputum macroscopically as a tentative means of judging whether bacterial infection is involved. Purulent sputum from chronic bronchitis contains a large number of neutrophils, whereas some purulent or yellow sputum from bronchial asthma contains a large number of eosinophils (May, 1954). However, purulence of sputum is usually evidence of the presence of deoxyribonucleic acid (DNA) derived from neutrophils and other disintegrated cells. Neutrophils, which are present in large numbers in purulent sputum, contain a considerable amount of elastase, a substance that is a potent stimulant for both submucosal gland and goblet cell secretion and is also injurious to the epithelium of airways (see Sec. II). If sputum samples are left to stand, the viscosity of purulent sputum is reduced more quickly than that of mucoid sputum, which is attributed to the action of the proteolytic enzymes from neutrophils.

Because of mast cell degranulation, the histamine concentration in airways increases during an acute attack, whereas the concentration in the stable phase of asthma corresponds with levels measured in the sputa from patients with chronic bronchitis (Bryant and Pui, 1982). Eosinophils are found in high numbers in asthamtic sputum. Major basic protein and Charcot–Leyden crystals are two proteins derived from the eosinophil granule. Major basic protein is a protein, with an Mr of 9300, that constitutes about 50% of the protein content of the eosinophil granule. Charcot–Leyden crystal is the crystal precipitate of the lyso-phospholipase (phospholipase B) also found in the eosinophil. Radioimmuno-assays have been developed to estimate their concentrations in sputum (Dor et al., 1984). Both proteins are found in increased amounts in asthmatic sputum compared with the value in sputum from chronic bronchitis. Levels of these proteins are further increased during the acute asthmatic attack when compared with asymptomatic asthmatics. Neutrophils and their products are also increased in the asthmatic airway mucus as well as in the sputum, but not to the same degree as in chronic bronchitis. Two other formations are traditionally described to be present in asthamtic sputum. Creola bodies are conglomerates of hundreds of airway surface epithelial cells, probably resulting from the detachment of the airway epithelium that occurs in severe asthmic attacks (Naylor, 1962). Curschmann's spirals consist of mucoid material infiltrated with whole eosinophils and Charcot–Leyden crystals. Curschmann's spirals are also found in the distal bronchioli (Dunnill, 1960), and are probably mucous casts of these bronchioli.

In addition to changes in the composition of asthmatic mucus, the amount or volume of secretion is greater than in normal persons, even though there seems to be great variability in mucous production among different asthma patients. Shimura et al. (1988a) reported that during an asthmatic attack 18 out of 207 patients (8.7%) fulfilled the criteria for bronchorrhea (over 100 ml/day of watery sputum). From an epidemiological questionnaire, 100 of 130 asthmatics (77%) had increased sputum production during an acute attack (Turner-Warwick, 1987). The increased volume and viscosity of the mucus, results in the accumulation of mucus in the asthmatic airways. In addition to mucous hypersecretion, this retention of mucus is also partly the result of a decrease in mucociliary clearance (Ahmed et al., 1981; Bateman et al., 1983; Mezey et al., 1978; Pavia et al., 1985; Wanner, 1977). The mucociliary clearance in the trachea of asthmatics may be decreased by as much as 60% compared with normal controls, and some abnormality in the mucociliary clearance may also be seen after allergen challenge (Mezey et al., 1978).

B. Bronchorrhea in Bronchial Asthma

Bronchorrhea has been defined as the copious (over 100 ml/day) production of nonpurulent sputum, the appearance of which suggests diluted uncooked egg white (Fig. 5; Keal, 1971). Bronchorrhea may be idiopathic or associated with lung diseases such as tuberculosis, alveolar cell carcinoma, chronic bronchitis, or bronchial asthma (Lopez-Vidriero et al., 1975a,b). Bronchorrhea was seen in 18

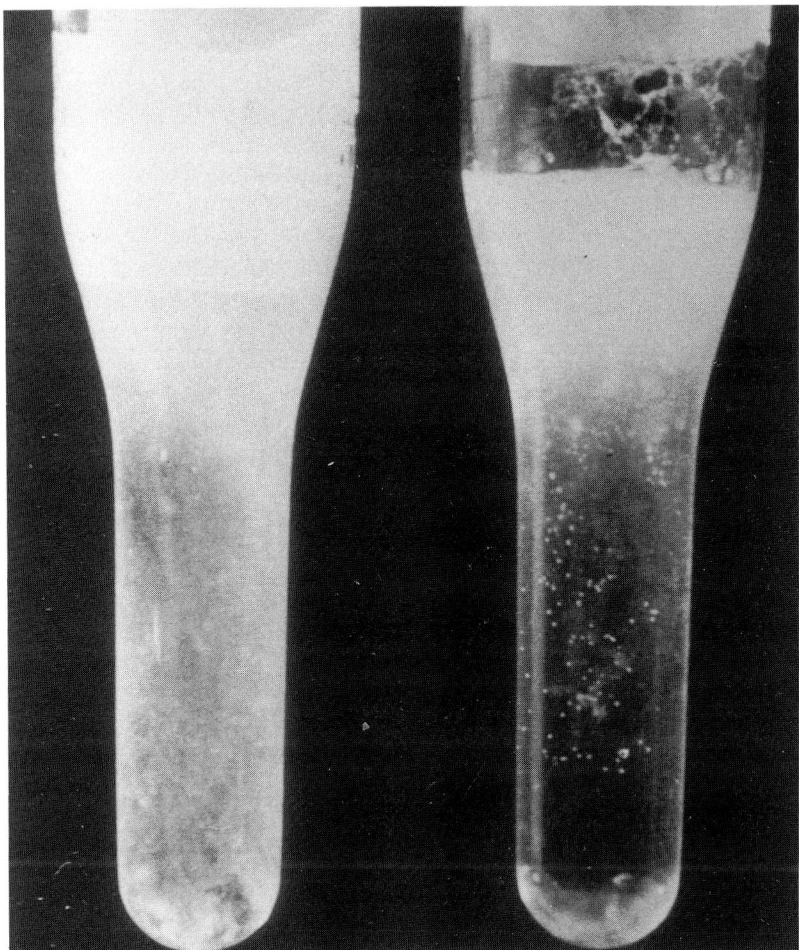

Figure 5 Bronchorrheal sputum obtained from a patient with bronchial asthma (30 yr, female) during asthmatic attack. Immediately after expectoration, the bronchorrheal sputum was macroscopically similar to saliva (left container). However, separation into two layers with formation of clot in the upper layer occurred, as shown in right container, 4–6 h after collection. (From Shimura et al., 1988b.)

of 207 patients (8.7%) during an attack (Shimura et al., 1988a). Bronchorrhea sputa samples were chemically examined using ten parameters: dry weight and albumin, IgA, pH, Na^+, Cl^-, K^+, prostaglandins E and F, and histamine concentrations, and compared with saliva samples and mucoid sputa samples during clinical remission (see Table 1; Shirmura et al., 1988a). Bronchorrhea sputum differed from saliva in its chemical profile. This sputum exhibited values intermediate between those of saliva and mucoid sputum, except for two: The pH of bronchorrhea sputum was significantly lower than that of mucoid sputum, and the histamine concentration, expressed as weight per dry weight of sample, was significantly higher in bronchorrhea than in mucoid sputum. This study shows that bronchorrhea sputum differs chemically from saliva, indicating that it does not result from hypersalivation. The viscoelastic properties of this sputum also differ from saliva: bronchorrheal sputum increased in viscoelasticity over a period of some hours, whereas saliva never increased (Fig. 6; Shimura et al., 1989b).

It is possible that bronchorrhea in an asthmatic attack has its origin in the following: (1) fluid movement into the lumen by active ion transport in the epithelium or in the submucosal gland, and (2) increased permeability in the epithelium. Between the two possibilities, the latter seems unlikely because albumin concentration in bronchorrhea, which is known to be an indicator of permeability, is much lower than in mucoid sputum (see Table 1). Although there is no direct evidence suggesting which is the main source—superficial epithelial cells or submucosal gland cells—one can speculate on the role of "active ion

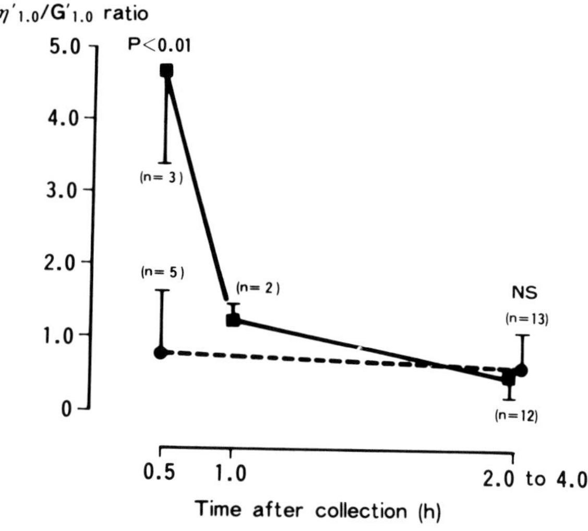

Figure 6   Changes with time after collection in relation to the viscosity to elasticity ratio at 1.0 rad/s ($\eta'_{1.0}/G'_{1.0}$) in bronchorrhea (continuous line) and mucoid sputum (dotted line). Thirty minutes after expectoration, a much higher ratio was seen for bronchorrhea sputum, compared with that for mucoid sputum, and 2–4 h after collection, no differences in ratio between bronchorrhea and mucoid sputum were found. (From Shimura et al., 1988b.)

transport in the epithelium or submucosal gland" in the formation of bronchorrhea sputum. Histamine concentration, expressed as weight per dry weight of sample, in bronchorrhea sputum is significantly higher than that in mucoid sputum, which is compatible with Bryant and Pui's report (1982). Although the bronchorrhea sputum had a histamine concentration similar to mucoid sputum when expressed as weight per volume of sample, the total histamine in the secretion must be considerably greater in bronchorrhea, since patients with bronchorrhea expectorated three times more than those with mucoid sputum. In Shimura et al.'s study (1988a), a histamine H_1-blocker reduced significantly the amount of bronchorrhea, although histamine, acting through stimulation of H_2 receptors, increases airway mucous glycoprotein secretion in humans (Shelhamer et al., 1980). In in vitro experiments, histamine is known to increase secretion of the fluid component of airway secretion. Marin et al. (1977) have shown that histamine significantly increases the net flux of chloride toward the lumen in canine trachea (Cl^- secretion) and that H_1-type receptors mediate the increase of ion flux toward the lumen, which is associated with the water or fluid movement. Shimura et al.'s (1988a) study showed a significant decrease in the Na^+/Cl^- ratio of bronchorrhea sputum, compared with that of mucoid sputum. Furthermore, administration of corticosteroids also reduced bronchorrhea (Fig. 7), and glucocorticosteroids are known to inhibit the release of chemical mediators including histamine (Schleimer et al., 1982) and to directly reduce submucosal gland secretion (Marom et al., 1984a; Lundgren et al., 1988a; Shimura et al., 1990; Satoh et al., 1992). These

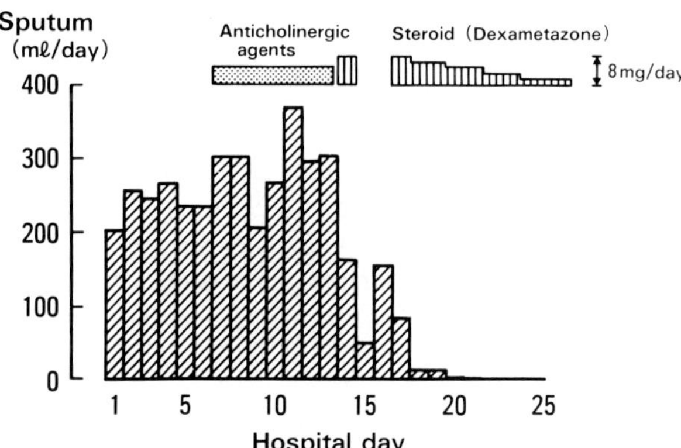

Figure 7 A typical example of bronchorrhea from patient during asthmatic attack (30 yr, female). She expectorated 200–300 ml/day of watery sputum with asthmatic dyspnea on admission. Inhaled or intramuscular anticholinergic agents (ipratropium bromide or atropine sulfate) did not alter the volume, but intravenously or orally administered corticosteroid (dexamethasone) abolished expectoration. (From Shimura et al., 1988a.)

facts suggest that histamine released during an asthamtic attack may play a role in the formation of bronchorrhea sputum in the airways by the increased water movement across airway mucosa into the airway lumen. In human airways, sputum produced after inhalation of histamine contains relatively more transudate than sputum produced after inhalation of prostaglandin $F_{2\alpha}$ (Lopez-Vidriero et al., 1977). Therefore, it is speculated that bronchorrhea during the asthmatic attack is not under cholinergic nervous control, since the volume did not alter with either inhaled or injected anticholinergic agents. Lopez-Vidriero et al. (1975a) studied the effect of atropine and found no significant change in bronchorrhea sputum volume and no changes in the sputum dry weight, neuraminic acid, or fucose context in patients with bronchial asthma.

Compared with mucoid sputum (pH 6.69), bronchorrhea sputum obtained during an asthmatic attack had significantly lower pH (pH 7.16) (see Table 1; Shimura et al., 1988a). The pH of mucus in the normal rat trachea is reported to range from 7.42 to 7.57 (average 7.52; Gatto, 1981) which is similar to that from mucoid sputum samples in the present study. Homma et al. (1977) have reported that ciliary inhibition is seen in bovine trachea at low pH, especially near 6.5. Thus, both low pH and viscoelasticity much lower than the optimal range for mucociliary velocity in bronchorrhea (Chen and Dulfano, 1978; Shimura et al., 1988b) during the asthmatic attack may result in a lower mucociliary transport rate in the airways than that of mucoid sputum, probably leading to the formation of mucous plugs. Dulfano and Luk (1982) have found a ciliary inhibitory factor in watery sputum obtained from a patient with bronchial asthma during an attack. It remains to be determined how the chemical and viscoelastic properties peculiar to bronchorrhea are related to the ciliary inhibitory factor.

V. Airway Hypersecretion and Hyperresponsiveness

Airway hyperresponsiveness is one of the characteristic features of bronchial asthma and an occasional feature in patients with chronic obstructive pulmonary disease and chronic bronchitis. Several mechanisms by which airway hyper-responsiveness occurs have been postulated, and some of them have been confirmed. Among the known mechanisms, there is the presence of excessive airway secretion, which is a common pathological feature of bronchial asthma and chronic obstructive pulmonary disease. Here, we discuss possible roles of airway hypersecretion in airway responsiveness or reactivity.

A. Hyporesponsiveness by Excessive Mucus

Several factors contribute to airway responsiveness or reactivity, as defined by the usual criteria for assessing the response to an inhaled bronchoconstrictor aerosol.

Airway responsiveness or reactivity is influenced by the distribution of the aerosol within the lung and by factors limiting the accessibility of the bronchoconstrictive agent to the target site (smooth muscle) once it has been deposited in the airways. It is possible that the mucous lining of the airway might modify the bronchoconstrictor response. Mucus could potentially modify the response by diluting the pharmacoactive agent or by delaying its passage to the target site, or perhaps even by binding or inactivating it. Delayed passage of the agent (reduced permeability) would produce an effect similar to dilution, since the concentration of the bolus of the pharmacoactive agent reaching the target site would attain a lower peak value, thereby shifting the classic dose–response curve to the right. Several investigators have speculated on the possible inhibitory role of mucus in modifying airway reactivity. In a study of chronic sulfur dioxide exposure in dogs, Drasen et al. (1982) reported that the exposed dogs developed chronic airway obstruction and mucous hypersecretion. They found that the airway responsiveness to inhaled mediators (histamine, $PGF_{2\alpha}$, and carbacol) decreased after exposure, whereas it remained unchanged when the mediators were administered intravenously. They suggested that this might be attributable to the apparent increase in mucous production. Seltzer et al. (1984), Scanlon et al. (1987), Shore et al. (1987), and Desanctis et al. (1987) also found a decreased airway responsiveness to aerolized histamine or methacholine with mucous hypersecretion in sulfur dioxide-induced bronchitis in dogs. In sheep exposed to ozone, Abraham et al. (1983) also found findings similar to Drasen et al. (1982). King et al. (1985) investigated whether mucous influx (secretion) is related to the alteration in airway reactivity to inhaled aerosols in dogs with permanent tracheostomies. They found that dogs with elevated secretion levels are relatively unresponsive to aerosolized, as opposed to infused, methacholine (i.e., there was a strong association between pulmonary resistance and mucous depth). Later, the same group reported hyporesponsiveness to aerosolized methacholine, but not to infused methacholine in cigarette-smoking dogs (Desanctis et al., 1987). Consequently, to the extent that infusion reactivity reflects innate airway reactivity, the reactivity to inhaled aerosol may underestimate the true value when mucous hypersecretion occurs. Therefore, it is possible that, if chronic bronchitis develops in a person with bronchial asthma, the chronic mucous hypersecretion will be associated with a loss of airway responsiveness, similar to that observed in these studies.

The hyporesponsiveness with airway hypersecretion possibly involves the inactivation of inhaled bronchoconstrictive agents, although we have yet no direct evidence supporting this idea. For example, cholinesterase and histamine methyltransferase are found to exist in airway epithelium and are known to modulate smooth-muscle function (Ohrui et al., 1991, 1992). Therefore, it is possible that the amount of these enzymes in airway secretions may influence the inactivation of inhaled acetylcholine and histamine by airway mucus.

B. Hyperresponsiveness by Excessive Mucus

In contrast, if mucous accumulation is limited to a certain region of the lungs, the resulting uneven flow resistance within the airway system will direct aerosol into the region of least resistance (i.e., normal airways; Kim and Eldridge, 1985). A consequent increase in aerosol deposition in the normal airways, therefore, may cause an enhanced airway responsiveness to inhaled aerosols. These opposing effects of excessive airway mucus on airway responsiveness to inhaled aerosols were examined in sheep by Kim et al. (1988, 1989). They measured airway responsiveness to carbacol by inhalation or by intravenous injection and the cumulative aerosol deposition in awake sheep in association with the injection of artificial mucus into both lungs or into the right lung only. They found that excessive airway mucus has at least two effects on airway responsiveness to an inhaled bronchoconstrictor agent: reduction in airway responsiveness by providing a protective layer over the mucosa when injected into both lungs and an increase in airway responsiveness owing to enhanced aerosol deposition when injected into only the right lung. Chronic obstructive impairment will also result in a central shift of aerosol deposition, and increased concentrations of bronchoconstrictors in the airways will contribute more strongly to this resistance (Strohl et al., 1981).

If sufficient mucus is present to alter luminal space occupation, it could also alter airway responsiveness because of its structural change. Concerning the effect of luminal space occupation, Suzuki et al. (1992) examined whether luminal space occupation induces airway hyperresponsiveness and how luminal space occupation changes dose–response curves to bronchoconstrictors in anesthetized cats. After small plastic beads (2.2 mm OD) were put into the right and left lobar bronchi, serotonin inhalation and serotonin infusion challenges were performed. Although the baseline pulmonary resistance values were not significantly increased, there were leftward shifts in dose–response curves to serotonin inhalation or infusion challenges after the insertion of beads in all cats. In fact, there are significantly larger amounts of intraluminal mucus in the airways of patients with bronchial asthma than in normal controls (Aikawa et al., 1992). These facts suggest that luminal space occupation amplifies airway response, and that it is an important mechanical factor of airway hyperresponsiveness.

Thus, experimentally induced or clinically observed hyperresponsiveness and hyporesponsiveness can be due to combinations of many factors. These include the pattern of aerosol deposition (Wanner et al., 1985), epithelial permeability, number and affinity of receptors for bronchoconstrictors, quantities of circulating and locally released chemical mediators and substances, and modulating reflexes.

C. Airway Lining Fluid and Airway Responsiveness

A wide variety of chemically distinct mediators are known to be produced by inflammatory cells. These mediators induce smooth-muscle contraction and also alter fluid balance in the airways. Airway fluid balance in asthma is largely determined by ion transport, with fluid and plasma exudation from mucosal microvessels into the luminal space. The exudated plasma is a fluid source rich in protein and cell mediators capable of inhibiting airway surfactant function (Phang and Keough, 1986; Fuchimukai et al., 1987). A decrease in the surfactant function in the small airways possibly induces an increase in the collapsibility (Macklem et al., 1970). This mechanism is also responsible for the increased airway responsiveness.

When airway mucosa is compressed, the internal airway lumen collapses to form epithelial ridges that protrude into the luminal space. Luminal perimeter and airway wall cross-sectional areas have been determined to remain constant during bronchoconstriction (James et al., 1988, 1989). However, these epithelial projections form pockets or interstices in which liquids can collect, as shown by Yager et al. (1989; Fig. 8). Liquid-filled interstices could amplify the degree of luminal compromise in at least two distinct ways (Fig. 9). First, luminal cross-sectional area will be reduced from that before the presence of liquid. Second, if the pressure tension of the liquid lining the airway is greater than zero, the additional pressure drop across the airway–liquid interface will produce an additional inward force that can compromise the airway lumen. Therefore, the presence of liquid can act to amplify the bronchoconstrictor response by causing edema of the airway wall itself, by filling airway interstices, and by creating an additional inward force because of surface tension, which further constricts and possibly closes the airways, thereby significantly increasing airway resistance (Yager et al., 1989, 1991).

There is an increase in the number of mast cells and basophils in the airway lumens of patients with bronchial asthma (Tomioka et al., 1984). These mast cells and basophils are present in the fluid lining the epithelial layer, and the environmental effects on these cells have recently received much attention. There have been some reports suggesting that a change of osmolarity induces instability and activation of these cells, initiating the first step of asthmatic attack. Allegra and Bianco (1980) reported that airway resistance of asthmatic subjects could be abnormally increased by inhaling an aerosol of distilled water. Additionally, Schoeffel et al. (1981) described the effect on the forced expiratory volume in 1s (FEV_1) of changing the osmolarity of inhaled aerosols of saline in asthmatic subjects. They found that there was a progressive increase in sensitivity to these aerosols as the osmolarity was increased or decreased from that of normal saline. Unlike aerosols of methacholine and histamine, nonisotonic aerosols do not act directly on smooth muscle to cause contraction (Finney et al., 1987). Rather, they appear to invoke an intermediate event, which is currently thought to be the release of mediators from mast cells in the airway lumen and submucosa (Eggleston et al., 1987). The release of mast cell mediators is thought to be associated with activation and recruitment of cells to the airways and the subsequent develop-

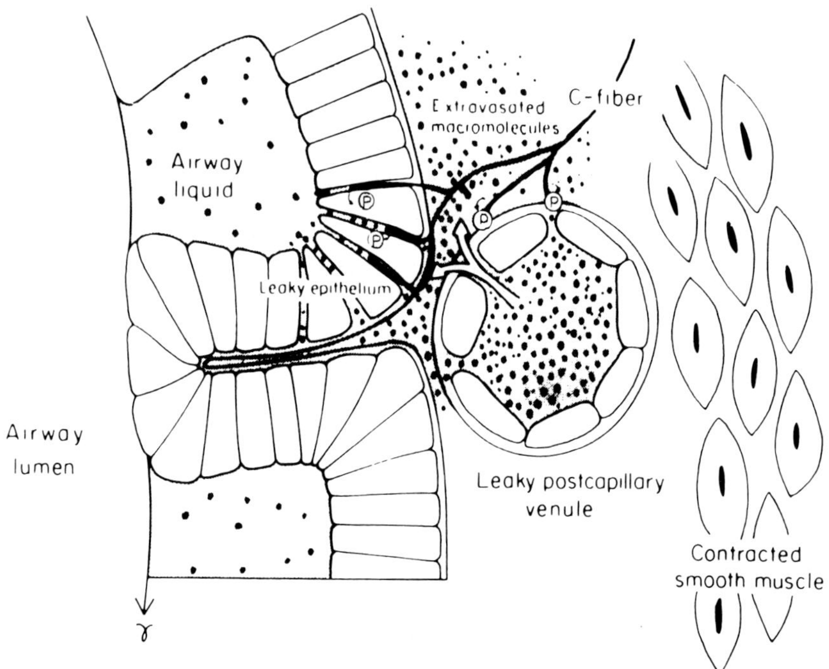

Figure 8 Inflammatory mediator-induced microvascular leakage results in extravasation of plasma and plasma macromolecules into the airway mucosa. Tachykinins such as substance P(P) released by sensory C fibers also increases endothelial as well as epithelial permeability. Epithelial leakage results in exudation of liquid and macromolecules into the airway lumen; this liquid further compromises airway patency by filling interstices between epithelial projections and providing a source of inward recoil because of the surface tension (γ) of the air–liquid interface. (From Yager et al., 1991.)

ment of mucosal inflammation, one of the hallmarks of asthma (Holgate, 1987). In addition, Bianco et al. (1988, 1989) reported that inhalation of furosemide prevented exercise-induced bronchoconstriction and allergen-induced early and late asthmatic reactions. In vitro, furosemide inhibits the secretion of chloride ion into the bronchial lumen by blocking the cotransport of sodium and chloride ions on the basolateral membrane of epithelial cells (Frizzel, 1988; Welsh, 1983). Therefore, it seems possible that the mechanism of furosemide involves the control of the osmotic or ionic environment of epithelial cells which, in turn, may affect the activation of mast cells and other inflammatory cells (Hook and Siraganian, 1981; Naccache et al., 1977).

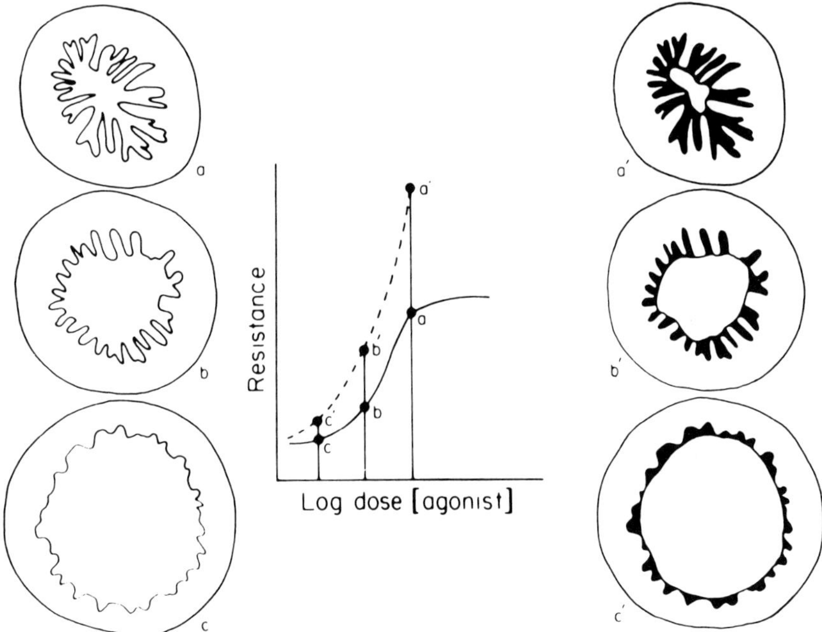

Figure 9   The effects of increasing degrees of airway smooth-muscle contraction on luminal cross-sectional area are schematically shown, and a plot of airflow resistance as a function of dose of agonist is presented for the case of no airway luminal liquid (a, b, c; solid line) and in the presence of liquid-filled interstices (a', b', c'; dashed line). (From Yager et al., 1991.)

VI.   Airway Hypersecretion and Obstructive Impairment

A.   Sputum Production and Airway Obstruction

Mucous hypersecretion is one of the characteristic features of chronic obstructive pulmonary disease. This hypersecretion is now estimated by expectorated sputum volume or by glandular or goblet cell hypertrophy in the airway wall. Hyperplasia of bronchial glands in proximal airways is the main diagnostic histological criteria of chronic bronchitis and has been reported to correlate with sputum volume in chronic bronchitis by Reid (1960) and Jamal et al. (1984). The common association of chronic bronchitis and chronic limitation of airflow leads us to assume that hypersecretion of mucus results in limitation of airflow (Reid, 1954). Chest physiotherapy, which consists of several maneuvers combining postural drainage, clapping, mechanical percussion, breathing excess, vibration, and cough, has been shown to facilitate sputum expectoration and, therefore, improvement in pulmonary functions (Cochrance et al., 1977; May and Munt, 1979). Samios (1975) and Cochrance et al. (1977) have reported increases in the post-expectoration forced FEV_1 and decreases in the airway resistance resulting from physiotherapy methods. Clarke et al. (1973) reported that, after physiotherapy of patients with chronic bronchitis and bronchiectasis, airway resistance decreased as a result of expectoration of sputum, but that no correlation was found between the amount of sputum expectorated and the reduction in airway resistance.

Some epidemiological studies have suggested that chronic bronchitis and chronic obstructive impairment may be considered as separate entities, rather than as manifestations of a single disease (Bates, 1973; Fletcher and Peto, 1977; Peto et al., 1983), whereas an epidemiological report by Annesi and Kauffmann (1986) is in conflict with this assumption. Epidemiological studies have depended mainly on the presence of symptoms (sputum, wheezing, and dyspnea during exercise) and spirometric abnormalities for diagnosis of chronic airway obstruction. These findings are nonspecific and do not differentiate between airway obstruction caused by airway diseases and those caused by pulmonary emphysema. In fact, in the study of Mitchell et al. (1976) of lungs from 242 subjects, the severity of emphysema was overwhelmingly the most important correlate of the clinical state of chronic airway obstruction. Hale et al. (1984) also compared the involvement of bronchial gland enlargement, bronchial abnormality, and emphysema. They found that emphysema was the major determinant of severe airflow limitation, and it was uncommon to find severe airflow limitation in patients with little or no emphysema. Thus, it is difficult to estimate the degree of emphysema in chronic obstructive pulmonary disease by the epidemiological studies. Variation in the degree of emphysema in subjects in these studies might possibly make it difficult to clarify the role of chronic hypersecretion in the obstructive impairment in chronic obstructive pulmonary disease. In addition, there are other factors that have masked important roles of hypersecretion. First, *simple bronchitis* is used to refer to mucous hypersecretion alone, and chronic bronchitis does not always indicate severe airflow limitation. Excess glandular secretion need not be associated with glandular enlargement, and hypersecretion possibly occurs as one of the airway defense mechanisms. Furthermore, it is believed that most of the abnormal mucous secretion arises from changes in the large airways (Reid, 1960), whereas most of the airflow limitation arises initially from changes in the small airways. The site of increased airway resistance in most patients with obstructive impairments has been shown to be the small airways (Hogg et al., 1968; Pride, 1984). One can speculate that slight airway hypersecretion does not cause airway obstruction in the absence of a disturbance in airway clearance, mucociliary transport, and cough (Camner et al., 1973; Thompson and Short, 1969; Wanner, 1977).

In Japan, chronic bronchitis with severe obstruction is observed in non-smokers as well as smokers (Homma et al., 1983). In spite of severe obstruction (about 30% in $FEV_{1\%}$), no emphysematous lesions are found in these cases of chronic bronchitis, and sputum production, even during clinical remission, reaches 200 ml/day (Andoh et al., 1992b; Akai et al., 1992; Aikawa et al., 1989; Homma et al., 1983; Honda et al., 1988; Ishihara et al., 1991; Nagaki et al., 1992). Such chronic bronchitis is a good model for examining the role of hypersecretion in airway obstructive impairment, and it has been shown that mucous hypersecretion results in mucous accumulation in the airways and is parallel with airway obstruction (Aikawa et al., 1989).

Clinically, it is often observed that patients with bronchial asthma expectorate a significant amount of sputum, especially during an asthmatic attack, and are subsequently released from dyspnea after the expectoration of a large amount of sputum. Moreover, a large amount of mucous plugging in airways with an increase in secretory cells (submucosal glands and goblet cells) is frequently observed in autopsied lungs of patients with bronchial asthma (Aikawa et al., 1992; Cardell and Pearson, 1959; Dunnill, 1960; Houston et al., 1953; Messer et al., 1960). These suggest that mucous accumulation (mucous plugging) in airways resulting from mucous hypersecretion contribute to airway obstruction in addition to broncho-constriction and mucosal edema.

B. Luminal Mucus in the Airways in Chronic Obstructive Pulmonary Disease

Smoking has been identified as the major risk factor in the development of chronic obstructive pulmonary disease (Thurlbeck et al., 1963), and prolonged smoking induces mucous hypersecretion associated with enlargement of the mucus-secreting tissue and mucosal inflammation of the airways (Cosio et al., 1980; Mullen et al., 1987). Airway hypersecretion is a principal clinical feature characteristic of chronic obstructive pulmonary disease, and it has been suggested that mucous plugging in the airways produces airway narrowing and corresponds with functional abnormalities (Anthonisen et al., 1967; Woolcock et al., 1969). A study of Mullen et al. (1987) has shown that ex-smokers in whom mucous hypersecretion persisted after they had stopped smoking had mucosal inflammation in both central and peripheral airways and also produced abnormal results in the nitrogen washout test.

Despite speculation that hypersecretion results in mucous accumulation in the airways and contributes to obstructive impairment by occupying the airway lumen, there have been very few reports on the presence or amount of mucus in the airway lumen in patients with chronic obstructive pulmonary disease. Matsuba and Thurlbeck (1973) have estimated the amount of mucus in small airways of autopsied lungs from patients with chronic bronchitis without pulmonary dysfunction and from patients with pulmonary emphysema by the point-counting method. They observed a significant amount of luminal mucus not only in chronic bronchitis, but also in pulmonary emphysema, but with no difference between the former and the latter, although they have found more peripheral airway mucous plugging in pulmonary emphysema with chronic bronchitis than in pulmonary emphysema or chronic bronchitis alone. Later, Cosio et al. (1977) measured mucus and cells in the peripheral airway lumen in surgical specimens and reported that occlusion of the lumen by mucous plugs was not a determinant of pulmonary function or other pathological scores. Almost all of these investigators used lungs fixed by intrabronchial instillation of formalin. Although the fixation through the bronchus is suitable for morphometry of alveolar regions, it may be inadequate for estimation of luminal mucus. It is possible that fixation through the bronchus washes out and decreases the amount of mucus, resulting in changes in its distribution in the airways.

For the measurements of intraluminal mucus, Aikawa et al. (1989) employed fixation by immersion, to prevent its washout from the airways. They have shown, in fact, a reduction in the amount of intraluminal mucus in lungs fixed by the intrabronchial route compared with that in the opposite lung fixed by immersion. As shown in Figure 10, first, the length of the basement membrane (L_1), inside area of the airway (Sb_1), and the mucous area (Sm) were measured with a digitalizing tablet coupled to a computer, using a video image obtained directly from a microscope. To exclude variations caused by differences in collapsibility among samples fixed by immersion, the area Sb_2 was estimated by assuming a circular airway of circumference L_1. Diameter (Br) was also estimated by assuming a round airway. The volume proportion of mucus was determined as the ratio of mucus to airway lumen, that is, the ratio of the sum of Sm to the sum of Sb_2 in each patient was regarded as the mucus-occupying ratio (MOR).

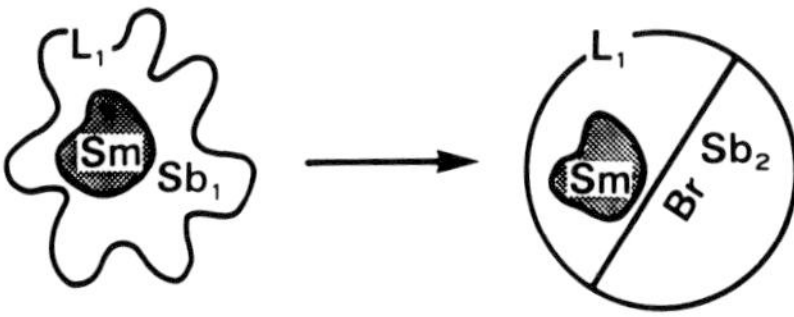

Mucus occupying ratio

Sm/Sb₂

Figure 10   Length of basement membrane (L_1), inside area of the airway (Sb_1), and area of the mucus (Sm) were measured using a digitalizing computer. The area Sb_2 and diameter Br are estimated by assuming a circular airway of circumference L_1. Sm/Sb_2 is regarded as the mucus-occupying ratio (MOR). (From Aikawa et al., 1989.)

Aikawa et al. (1989) showed a significant increase in the volume of mucus in the airway lumen, especially in the bronchioles, in chronic bronchitis, and there was no increase in pulmonary emphysema, despite the presence of an obstructive impairment similar to chronic bronchitis (Figs. 11 and 12). They showed no significant difference in luminal area of airways among the chronic bronchitis, pulmonary emphysema, and control groups, suggesting that narrowing of the airways was mainly due to mucous plugs in the patients with chronic bronchitis chosen for their study. On the basis of several in vitro experiments (Petty et al., 1981, 1984), it is well known that the mechanism of obstructive impairment in moderate or advanced pulmonary emphysema is a loss of elastic recoil caused by destruction of the alveolar regions. These findings suggest that airway hypersecretion results in accumulation of mucus, especially in the peripheral airways, which could be an important contributing factor to obstructive impairment in chronic bronchitis, but not in pulmonary emphysema. Such differences in the fixation procedure seem to be a major reason for the differences between the results of previous workers (Matsuba and Thurlbeck, 1973; Cosio et al., 1977) and those of Aikawa et al. (1989). In addition, case selection procedures used by the previous workers may also contribute to the differences. Matsuba and Thurlbeck (1973) used the lungs from patients with slight or no pulmonary dysfunction and point-counting methods that may be inaccurate when the component under investigation is only a small percentage of the whole. Cosio et al. (1977) applied a semiquantitative method, pathological scores, to estimate intraluminal mucus. In Aikawa et al.'s study (1989), patients with pulmonary emphysema had moderate or severe obstructive impairment, similar to chronic bronchitis, but without significant mucous hypersecretion, as supported by morphometric data from submucosal glands and goblet cells. Aikawa et al. (1989) also obtained the volume proportion by measuring the area, using a computer-assisted tablet, and measured intraluminal mucus, excluding definitely fresh exudate and clusters of migrating cells, whereas Matsuba and Thurlbeck (1973) and Cosio et al. (1977) included these into the intraluminal mucous assessment. It is possible that cell infiltration and fresh exudate into airway lumen occurred just before death and, therefore, does not represent a chronic state.

Although submucosal glands are abundant in the central airways and absent in the peripheral airways, the mucus-occupying ratio (MOR) in the peripheral airways is larger than that in the central airways. These facts suggest that goblet cells in the epithelium are the source of intraluminal mucus in the peripheral airways and that mucus that may be hypersecreted in the peripheral airways is difficult to transport toward the central airways, contributing to the obstructive impairment. Impairment of the mucociliary transport system has been reported in chronic obstructive pulmonary disease (Wanner, 1977). Glandular hypertrophy in the central airways may relate to sputum production and not directly to obstructive impairment, as pointed out by Jamal et al. (1984). However, in the study by

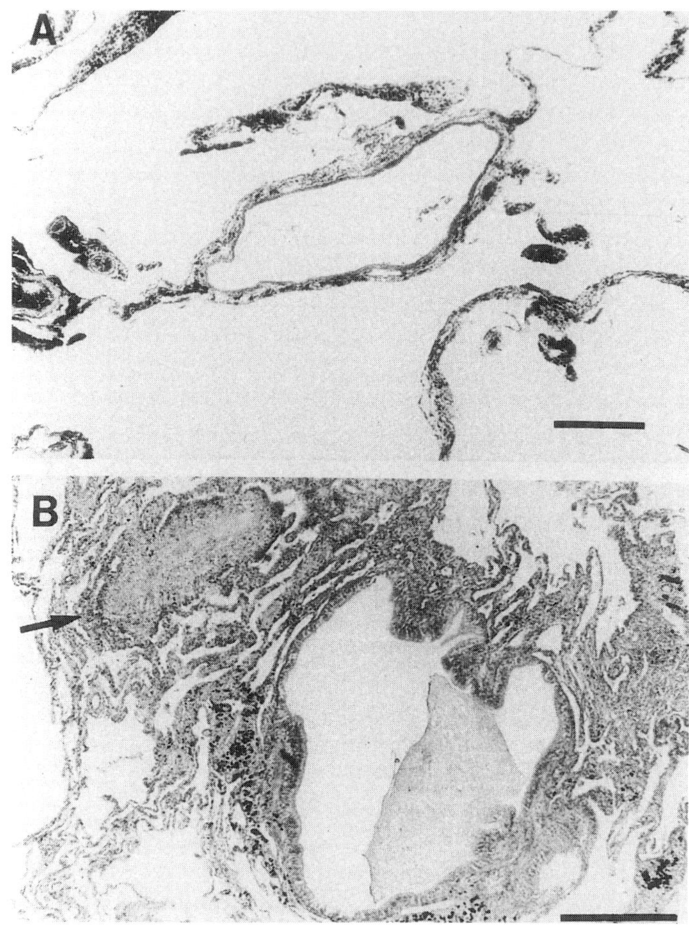

Figure 11   (A) Light micrograph of peripheral airway from a male patient, 79 years of age, with pulmonary emphysema. Note the absence of intraluminal mucus, except for some cell debris. Surrounding alveoli show some destruction. (Elastica Goldner stain, bar = 0.5 mm). (B) Light micrograph of peripheral airways from a male patient, 80 years of age, with chronic bronchitis. A large amount of mucous obstruction is seen in the airway lumen of a bronchiole in the center and completely obstructs the lumen of a bronchiole in the left upper corner (arrow). Peribronchiolar cell infiltration and pigmentation are also seen (Elastica Goldner stain; bar = 0.5 mm). (From Aikawa et al., 1989.)

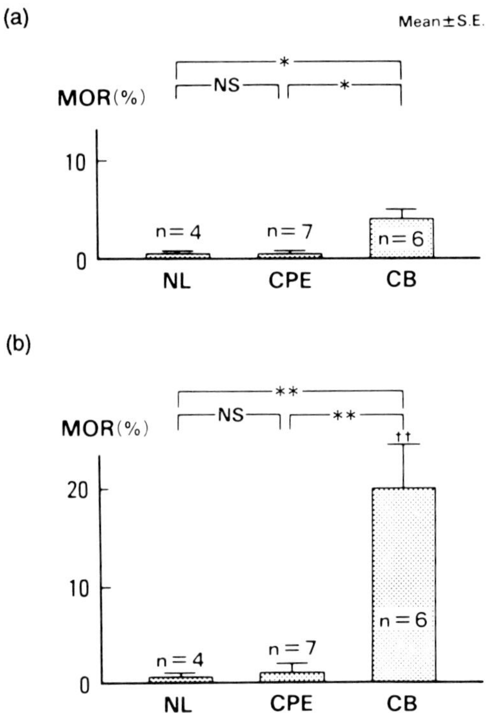

Figure 12 Mucus-occupying ratio (MOR) of each group in (a) central and (b) peripheral airways. MOR values of (a) central or (b) peripheral airways in chronic bronchitis (CB) are significantly higher than those of normal (control) lung (NL) or chronic pulmonary emphysema (CPE). MOR in peripheral airways in CB is also significantly higher than that in central airways in CB (NS, not significant; single asterisk, $p < 0.05$; double asterisks, $p < 0.01$, differences between CB and NL or CPE. (From Aikawa et al., 1989.)

Aikawa and colleagues (1989), gland volume proportion was correlated with MOR in central or peripheral airways (Fig. 13); also, the increase in goblet cell mucous volume proportion in chronic bronchitis was not significant when compared with that in pulmonary emphysema or controls. The data of Aikawa et al. (1989) showed the presence of inflammation, judged by cell infiltration, pigmentation, and fibrosis, in not only the central airways, but also in the peripheral airway walls of patients with chronic bronchitis, but not in patients with pulmonary emphysema. Repeated or persistent inflammation of airways (from central bronchi to bronchioles) would induce hyperplasia of mucous secretory tissues causing accumulation of mucus in the airways, especially in small airways, by producing

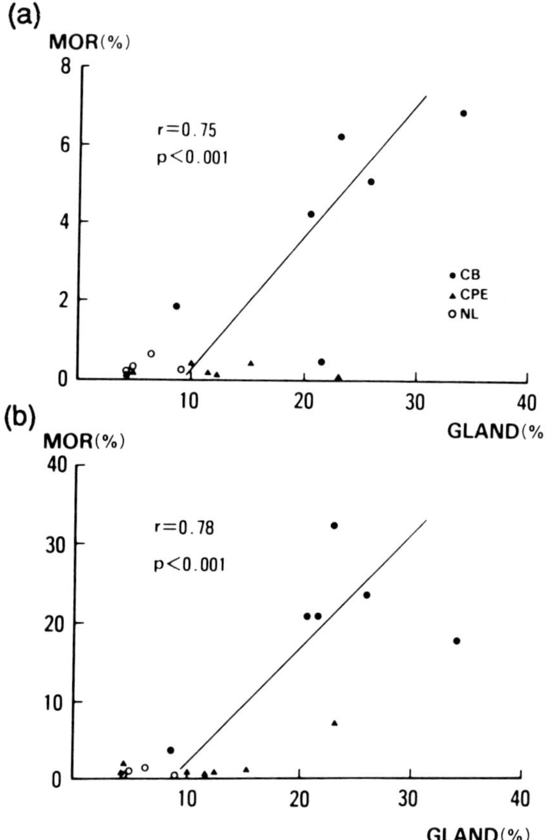

Figure 13   Relationship between submucosal glands in central airways (gland%) and mucus-occupying ratio (MOR) in (a) central airways or in (b) peripheral airways. Not only MOR in central airways and gland% but also MOR in peripheral airways and gland% are significantly correlated ($p < 0.001$ each) (closed circles, chronic bronchitis; closed triangles, chronic pulmonary emphysema; open circles, control lungs). (From Aikawa et al., 1989.)

mucous hypersecretion and also by inducing impairment of mucociliary transport by a loss or reduction of ciliary epithelium (Anthonisen et al., 1967).

There are inherent problems in the assessment of autopsied lung. The postmortem finding—the increase in mucus in the small airways—needs to be related to the situation before death; there is reasonably good bronchographic evidence that the mucous plugs in the airways of chronic bronchitis do occur in life (Gregg and Trapnell, 1969). The other factors (i.e., airway smooth-muscle spasms and mucosal edema) are also important determinants of obstructive impairment in life. Mucosal edema caused by inflammation contributes to airway obstruction, as has been reported by Laitinen et al. (1986).

In conclusion, Aikawa et al.'s morphometric data (1989) from autopsied lungs fixed by immersion show a large amount of mucus in the airways in chronic bronchitis, especially in the peripheral airways, but not in pulmonary emphysema, despite the presence of obstructive impairment similar to that seen in chronic bronchitis. These findings suggest that mucous accumulation in the airways contributes to obstructive impairment in chronic bronchitis, but not in pulmonary emphysema. But because almost all patients with chronic obstructive pulmonary disease show the pathological features of both pulmonary emphysema and chronic bronchitis, the role of mucous hypersecretion is usually an important clinical feature.

C. Mucous Plugging in Airways in Bronchial Asthma

The pathological changes seen in asthmatic airways are striking and are helpful for understanding the mechanisms causing mucous accumulation. Mucous plugging, goblet cell hyperplasia, smooth-muscle hypertrophy, submucosal gland hyperplasia, thick basement membrane, eosinophilic infiltration, or combinations thereof, are known to be pathological characteristics of bronchial asthma in both biopsy specimens (Cutz et al., 1978; Glynn and Michael, 1960) and autopsied lungs (Sobonya et al., 1984; Cardell and Pearson, 1959; Dunnill, 1960; Messer et al., 1960; Houston et al., 1953; Dunnill et al., 1969). It is possible that, in addition to bronchoconstriction and mucosal edema, mucous plugs contribute to airway obstruction and death in bronchial asthma, since a large amount of mucous plugging in airways is frequently observed in the autopsied lungs of bronchial asthma (Fig. 14) (Aikawa et al., 1992; Cardell and Pearson, 1959; Dunnill, 1960; Houston et al., 1953; Messer et al., 1960). In some areas, the airway mucosa is denuded of the surface epithelium, thereby impairing ciliary function, allowing inhalants to diffuse more easily to the submucosa and exposed sensory nerves (Laitinen et al., 1985), which in turn, augments mucous secretion. It has been suggested that major basic protein from eosinophil granules is a factor contributing to these alterations in the surface cell structure, since major basic protein is found in the asthmatic mucosa (Filley et al., 1982) and because major basic protein, in isolated form, is toxic to airway epithelium in vitro (Frigas et al., 1980). The submucosal loose connective tissue is edematous and infiltrated with eosinophils, neutrophils, and macrophages. Furthermore, various chemical mediators released from these migrating cells are potent in stimulating airway secretion (see Sec. III). The submucosal glands are enlarged and the number and size of the gland cells are increased in bronchial asthma (Aikawa et al., 1992; Dunnill, 1975). In fatal asthmatic cases, it has been demonstrated that major parts of the airways

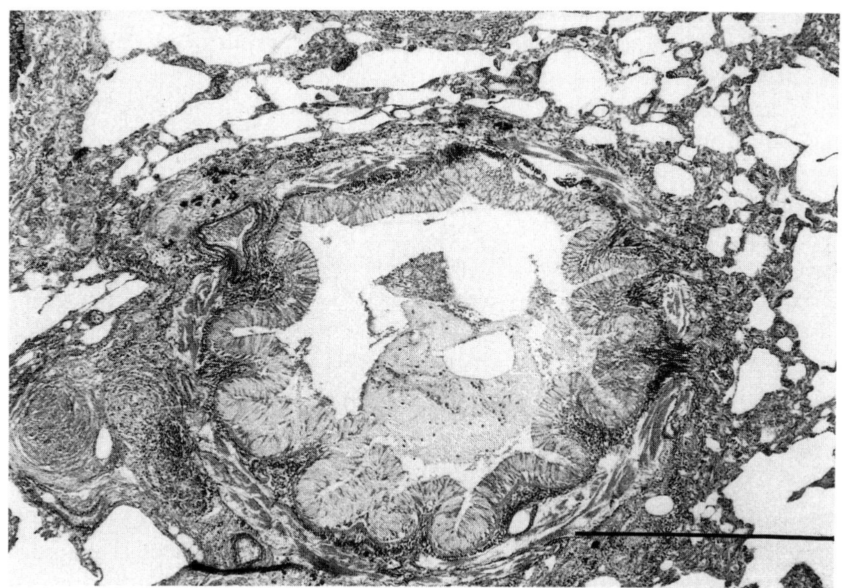

Figure 14   Light micrograph of peripheral airway from a female patient, 73 years of age, who died of severe asthmatic attack. Marked goblet cell hyperplasia, with intraluminal accumulation of mucus was observed in addition to smooth-muscle contraction, peribronchiolar cell infiltration, and fibrosis (bar = 0.5 mm; Elastica-Goldner stain). (From Aikawa et al., 1992.)

may be blocked by mucous plugs, contributing to the respiratory insufficiency characteristic of this condition. Thus, asthmatic airways show definite signs of abnormalities in the production and clearance of mucus.

Meanwhile, it is also known that some asthmatic patients show an absence of excessive bronchial mucus in autopsied lungs (Reid, 1987). For example, Sobonya (1984) reported that mucous plugs, the size of submucosal glands, and the smooth muscles in the airways from the lungs in bronchial asthmatic patients, not dying in status asthmaticus, did not significantly differ from those of nonsmoking controls. Likewise, Lozewics et al. (1990) and Jeffery et al. (1989) reported that there were no significant differences in the morphological features of the biopsy specimens from the bronchial epithelium from the mild asthmatic and the healthy groups. The difference in the airway mucus might be caused by differences in the clinical features of asthma; that is, the presence or absence of asthmatic attacks, the severity of asthmatic attacks or their duration, smoking habits, medication, treatment or cause of death. From autopsied lungs, it has been noted that airway mucous plugging seems to be more prevalent in patients who died of severe acute asthmatic attacks. There have been some descriptions on postmortem findings of status asthmaticus (Cardell and Pearson, 1959; Dunnill, 1960; Dunnill et al., 1969; Houston et al., 1953; Messer et al., 1960).

Aikawa et al. (1992) analyzed intraluminal mucus from the autopsied lungs of patients with bronchial asthma and compared their clinical features with the morphometric data of the submucosal glands, goblet cells, and epithelial layer to ascertain which is responsible for accumulation of mucus in the airways and whether mucous plugging in the airways is related to death caused by an asthmatic attack. They performed morphometric analysis of autopsied lungs from outpatients who died of severe acute asthma and compared these with patients who died of chronic asthma. Area proportion of bronchial glands to bronchial wall (gland%), goblet cells to total epithelial layer (goblet%) and intraluminal amount of mucus in the airways (MOR) were measured in a paraffin section. There were no significant differences in age, sex, smoking history, duration of bronchial asthma history, and dosage of glucocorticoids received between the two groups. Although both groups showed significantly larger values in gland percentage in central airways or inflammatory cell numbers in the airway walls than did the control group (patients who died of nonrespiratory-related causes), no significant differences were observed between the two asthmatic groups. In contrast, marked significant increases in both goblet percentage and MOR from the sudden-death group were observed compared with those from the other bronchial asthma or control group: 30-fold and 3-fold increases compared with the non-status–asthmaticus group in goblet percentage (Fig. 15) and MOR (Fig. 16), respectively. The origin of excessive mucus, especially in the peripheral airway, is thought to be hyperplastic or hypertrophic goblet cells, since MOR significantly correlated with goblet percentage. These findings suggest that a marked increase in goblet cells of the airways is a feature characteristic of bronchial asthma patients who die of a severe acute attack.

The possibility that mucus secreted by submucosal glands in the central airway was aspirated to peripheral airway seems remote because there was no significant difference in gland percentage between the two groups, in spite of the glandular hyperplasia in asthmatic patients in both groups, which was similar to that seen in chronic bronchitis (Aikawa et al., 1989; Lozewicz et al., 1990). Furthermore, gland percentage in the central airways did not correlate with goblet percentage in the peripheral airways. Mucous retention is enhanced by a decrease in the number and length of the cilia at small airways and a reduction in the rate of mucous transport with increasing airway branching (Iravani and Van, 1972; Wanner, 1977). The site of increased airway resistance in patients with chronic obstructive impairment has been shown to be the small airways (Hogg et al., 1968; Sekizawa et al., 1986). Possibly, in addition, the goblet cell metaplasia produces impairments of mucociliary and ion transport across epithelium by a few ciliary cells, epithelial damage, and large amounts of intraluminal mucus in the small

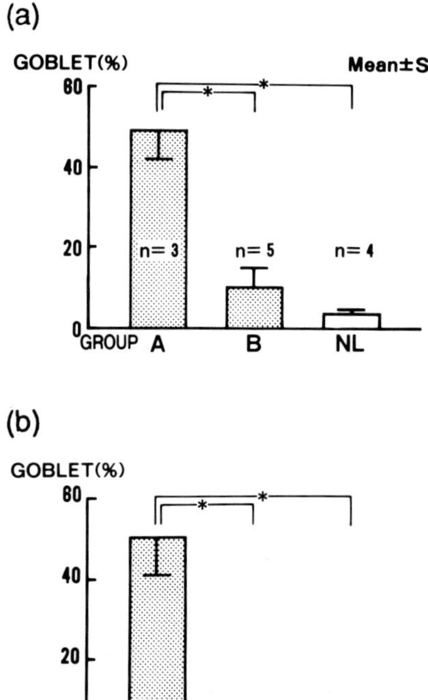

Figure 15 Goblet cell area ratio (goblet%) of three groups in (a) central and (b) peripheral airways. Group A: bronchial asthma patients who died of severe acute attack; group B: bronchial asthma patients who died of non–status asthmaticus; group NL: controls. Group A showed much higher values than group B both in the central and the peripheral airways. The marked goblet% increase was more dominant in peripheral airways (b). (*$p < 0.05$). (From Aikawa et al., 1992.)

airways. Furthermore, mucosal edema and bronchoconstriction may accelerate the impairment of mucociliary clearance.

Goblet cell mucin secretion is not under any pharmacological control (Kim et al., 1989), which is different from glandular secretion. Furthermore, some differences exist between secretions from submucosal glands and those from goblet cells (i.e., goblet cells are thought to secrete a more acidic mucous glycoprotein than do submucosal glands; Stahl and Ellis, 1973). Such conditions facilitate mucous plug formation and hinder the removal of the obstructive impairments, resulting in an accumulation of mucus in the small airways in death caused by an acute asthmatic attack.

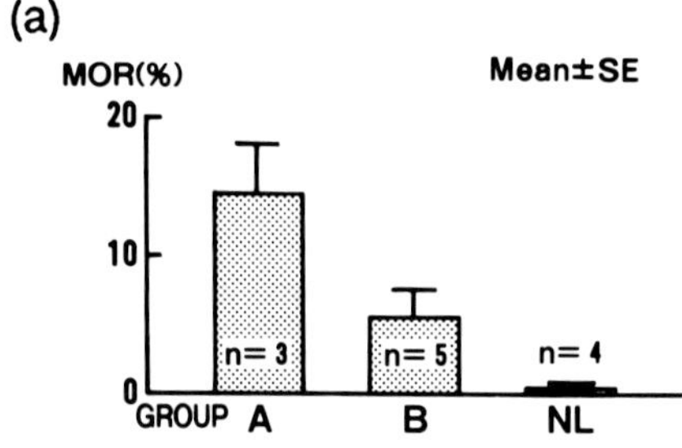

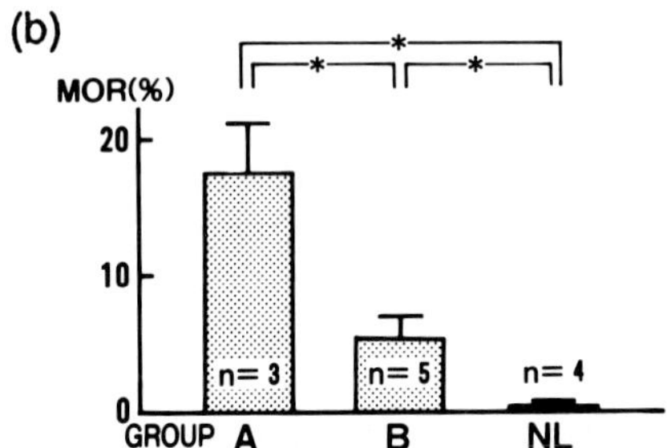

Figure 16 Mucus-occupying ratio (MOR) of the same three groups as in Figure 15 in (a) central and (b) peripheral airways; MOR in peripheral airways of group A was significantly higher than that of group B or NL; MOR in central airways of group A tended to be higher than that of group B, but did not reach statistical significance. Asterisks indicate $p < 0.05$. (From Aikawa et al., 1992.)

VII.   Airway Hypersecretion and Mortality

A.   Bronchial Asthma

The heterogeneity of the asthma population is also reflected in the postmortem findings. Although increased production of viscous mucus causing airway plugging is known to be a common pathological feature of deaths caused by asthma (Cardell and Pearson, 1959; Dunnill, 1960; Messer et al., 1960; Houston et al., 1953), in some patients, sudden death occurs with an absence of excessive bronchial mucus (Reid, 1987; Robin and Lewiston, 1989). Thus, empty airways could be found if the cause of death is cardiac dysfunction or the result of drug sensitivity. Cardiac arrhythmia could cause sudden death without major airway symptoms (Lehr, 1972). However, a recent study by Saetta et al. (1991) has reported that asthmatic patients who died suddenly and unexpectedly showed lumen occlusion by mucous plugs, plasma exudate, and inflammatory cells in the peripheral airways of autopsied lungs. The classic descriptions of the pathological findings in fatal cases of bronchial asthma are mainly from patients who died in the hospital after some days (or months) of treatment. Therefore, it is possible that many factors other than an asthmatic attack affect the pathological findings, producing the heterogeneity in the postmortem findings of bronchial asthma. To exclude this possibility, Aikawa et al. (1992) selected only outpatients with bronchial asthma, who suddenly died of severe acute asthmatic attacks, for their study, as compared with patients with bronchial asthma who died of chronic asthma. In their patients, definite asthmatic attacks were confirmed clinically before death, which also differed from the patients with cardiac asthma by clinical and pathological findings. The degree of goblet cell hyperplasia has been shown to be up to a two- or threefold increase, compared with controls in animal experiments and studies of diseased lung (Ahlstedt and Enander, 1987; Cutz et al., 1978; Glynn and Michael, 1960; Larsen et al., 1989; Lundgren et al., 1988b; Rogers and Jeffery, 1986). To our knowledge, Aikawa et al. (1992) is the first report showing marked goblet cell hyperplasia, a 30-fold increase, in patients with bronchial asthma who died of a severe acute asthmatic attack, when comparing with bronchial asthma patients who died of a nonacute asthmatic attack. If the patient is known to have asthma and to have died during a sudden, severe attack, asthma may be accepted as the cause of death, and no autopsy is performed. This may be one of the explanations for the scarcity of reports similar to Aikawa et al.'s report (1992).

From the findings by Aikawa et al. (1992), it is possible that the marked goblet cell hyperplasia in the peripheral airways is characteristic of death caused by an acute asthmatic attack. Until now, endobronchial biopsy specimens have usually been obtained from central airways of asthmatics. If small-airway specimens come to be frequently obtained by transbronchial biopsies, the finding of goblet cell hyperplasia could be used as a marker to identify bronchial asthma patients at risk for severe attacks.

B. Chronic Obstructive Pulmonary Disease

Some epidemiological reports (Fletcher and Peto, 1977; Peto et al., 1983) indicated that, after controlling for the degree of lung function, airway hypersecretion or phlegm was not significantly associated with death caused by chronic obstructive pulmonary disease, and they suggested that the hypersecretory disorder is an innocent disease. Very few studies included analyses on both respiratory symptoms and lung function, partly because mucous hypersecretion, initially believed to be the first step of airway obstruction, was considered a symptom of minor importance after the longitudinal study of Fletcher and Peto (1977). Nevertheless, other investigators observed a significant association between phlegm (or airway hypersecretion) and all causes of mortality (Annesi and Kauffmann, 1986). In a survey also conducted in a general population, Petty et al. (1976) reported that for subjects with FEV_1/FVC greater than 75%, the observed 6-year death rate was 1.74-fold for those with chronic bronchitis versus those without, and 1.47-fold for men with a FEV/FVC 60–75%, but they did not adjust for age and smoking. An epidemiological report by Annesi and Kauffmann (1986) confirmed this finding. The relation of chronic airflow limitation and airway hypersecretion to all causes of mortality was studied in a population of 1061 men working in the Paris area, surveyed initially in 1960 and 1961, and followed for 20 years. They found that besides the obstructive disorder, the hypersecretory disorder (chronic phlegm) was significantly associated with mortality. Controlling for age, obstructive impairment, smoking habits, and dust exposure, all factors associated with chronic mucous hypersecretion and mortality, showed that phlegm production remained significantly related to death.

C. Pulmonary Fibrosis with Airway Hypersecretion

Idiopathic pulmonary fibrosis has been characterized by a recurrent or chronic inflammation in the alveolar regions that progresses to interstitial fibrosis. Much attention has been paid to the abnormalities of alveolar or peripheral lung regions in studying the pathophysiology of idiopathic pulmonary fibrosis. However, there have been few studies concerning the airway lesions, despite the speculation of their being one of the factors determining the clinical features of this condition. Turner-Warwick et al. (1980) found that half the idiopathic pulmonary fibrosis patients from their study expectorated a significant amount of sputum. Hiwatari et al. (1991) revealed that 44% of idiopathic pulmonary fibrosis patients who survived over 1 year had mucous hypersecretion, even in the early period without any definite respiratory infections, and that idiopathic pulmonary fibrosis patients who suffer from mucous hypersecretion have a shorter survival rate than do those without mucous hypersecretion (Table 2) (Fig. 17). Edwards and Carlile (1982) observed hyperplasia of bronchial glands in a morphometric analysis of autopsied lungs from idiopathic pulmonary fibrosis patients. Later, Andoh et al.'s study (1992) indicated that idiopathic pulmonary fibrosis patients with mucous hypersecretion have airway glandular hyperplasia with intraluminal mucous accumulation, whereas idiopathic pulmonary fibrosis patients without sputum do not. Preexisting chronic bronchitis as a factor seems unlikely, since there was no history of this condition before the onset of idiopathic pulmonary fibrosis in any of the patients in their study. Furthermore, postmortem examination also revealed no histological findings that indicated fibrosis caused by chronic bronchitis, that is, peribronchial fibrosis. Smoking is known to induce bronchial gland hyperplasia, resulting in mucous hypersecretion (Cosio et al., 1980), and there has

Table 2 Clinical and Laboratory Data in Idiopathic Pulmonary Fibrosis Patients with Hypersecretion (Group A) and Without Hypersecretion (Group B)

	Group A (n = 11)	Group B (n = 14)
Sex	2F/9M	7F/7M
Age at onset (yr)	65 ± 3	55 ± 4
Duration of survival (yr)	5.8 ± 0.6**	9.7 ± 0.9
Grade of dyspnea[a]	2.8 ± 0.3	2.0 ± 0.2
Dyspnea (%)	100	79
Cough (%)	100	86
Sputum volume (ml/d)	24 ± 5**	0.7 ± 0.5
Smokers (%)	36 (1F/3M)	43 (2F/4M)
Laboratory		
Sedimentation rate (mm/1 h)	61 ± 11	52 ± 11
LDH (IU/L)	401 ± 25	399 ± 29
C-reactive protein positive (%)	73	43
VC (%)	63 ± 5	78 ± 9
FEV_1 (%)	84 ± 1	84 ± 2
Pao_2 (mm Hg)	59 ± 4	66 ± 3
D_{LCO} (%)	47 ± 10	62 ± 6
Radiographic findings		
Types I or II (%)	91	100
Types III or IV (%)	73	57
Bronchoalveolar lavage		
Recovery of fluid (%)	52 ± 11	46 ± 5
Cell differentials		
Macrophage (%)	72 ± 12	91 ± 4
Lymphocyte (%)	6 ± 2	7 ± 4
Neutrophil (%)	17 ± 9*	1 ± 0.3
Eosinophil (%)	5 ± 2*	0.6 ± 0.3

Data are shown as mean ± SE.
[a]Based on the classification of Hugh-Jones.
*$p < 0.05$; **$p < 0.001$; significant difference between groups A and B.
Source: Hiwatari et al., 1991.

been a recent report that the prognosis is significantly poorer in cigarette smokers than in nonsmokers with idiopathic pulmonary fibrosis, but the report lacks descriptions concerning sputum production (Smith et al., 1990).

These findings indicate that idiopathic pulmonary fibrosis is sometimes accompanied by a persistent mucous hypersecretion and bronchial gland hyperplasia. In a morphometric study of the large bronchi of autopsied lungs from

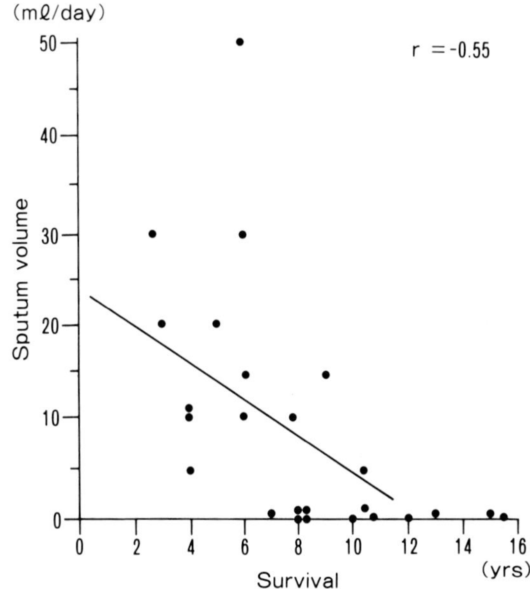

Figure 17 Relationship between sputum volume (ml/day) and the duration of survival (yr) in 25 patients with idiopathic pulmonary fibrosis. Sputum volume is significantly correlated with the duration of survival ($r = -0.55$; $p < 0.01$). (From Hiwatari et al., 1991.)

idiopathic pulmonary fibrosis patients, Edwards and Carlile (1982) reported that the quantity of submucosal glands is significantly greater than that of normal control subjects, and similar to that of patients with chronic bronchitis. Although the clinical features, especially mucous hypersecretion, of the patients are uncertain in their report, the degree of gland hyperplasia is similar to that of Andoh et al.'s patients with idiopathic pulmonary fibrosis who showed mucous hypersecretion. Idiopathic pulmonary fibrosis with mucous hypersecretion showed a significant correlation between gland hyperplasia and the amount of intraluminal mucus in central and peripheral airways (Andoh et al., 1992a), as shown in chronic bronchitis (Aikawa et al., 1989).

Currently, the precise mechanisms responsible for increased production of mucus with gland hyperplasia in idiopathic pulmonary fibrosis is unclear, but we can consider some possibilities. One possibility is that some idiopathic pulmonary fibrosis patients have abnormalities in various defense mechanisms in the airways: cough, mucociliary transport, local immunology, structural deformities, and others, and recurrent and persistent respiratory infection may produce gland hyperplasia with mucous hypersecretion. Another is that inflammations from noninfectious causes that localize in alveolar regions extend to the airways, resulting in glandular hyperplasia, since various inflammations are known to induce mucous hypersecretion and bronchial gland hyperplasia. In conclusion, their study shows the presence of a subtype of idiopathic pulmonary fibrosis patients who have bronchial gland hyperplasia with mucous hypersecretion, resulting in the accumulation of mucus in the airways. The accumulation of mucus in the airways may cause uneven ventilation under the restrictive impairment that takes part in hypoxia and frequent airway infections.

Acknowledgments

We thank Ms Kumiko Shibuya for typing the manuscript. This study was in part supported by scientific grants from the Ministry of Education, Science and Culture of Japan (No. 59570321, 60570342, 62570340, 01570422, and 04454249).

References

Abraham, W. M., Chapman, C. A., and Marchette, B. (1983). Differences between inhaled and intravenous carbacol in detecting O_3-induced airway effects. *Environ. Res.* 35: 430–438.

Adler, K. B., Schwartz, J. E., Anderson, W. H., and Welton, A. F. (1987). Platelet activating factor stimulates secretion of mucin by explants of rodent airways in organ cultures. *Exp. Lung Res.* 13: 25–43.

Ahlstedt S., and Enander I. (1987). Immune regulation of goblet cell development. *Int. Arch. Allergy Appl. Immunol.* 82: 357–360.

Ahmed, T., Greenblatt, D. W., Birch, S., Marchette, B., and Wanner, A. (1981). Abnormal mucociliary transport in allergic patients with antigen-induced bronchospasm: Role of slow-reacting substance of anaphylaxis. *Am. Rev. Respir. Dis.* 124: 110–114.

Aikawa, T., Shimura, S., Sasaki, H., Takishima, T., Yaegashi, H., and Takahashi, T. (1989). Morphometric analysis of intraluminal mucus in airways in chronic obstructive pulmonary diseases. *Am. Rev. Respir. Dis.* 140: 477–482.

Aikawa, T., Shimura, S., Sasaki, H., Ebina, M., and Takishima, T. (1992). Marked goblet cell hyperplasia with mucus accumulation in the airways of patients who died of severe acute asthma attack. *Chest* 101: 916–921.

Akai, S., Okayama, H., Shimura, S., Tanno, Y., Sasaki, H., and Takishima, T. (1992). Delta F508 mutation of cystic fibrosis gene is not found in chronic bronchitis with severe obstruction in Japan. *Am. Rev. Respir. Dis.* 146: 781–783.

Allegra, L., and Bianco, S. (1980). Non-specific bronchoreactivity obtained with an ultrasonic aerosol of distilled water. *Eur. J. Respir. Dis.* 61: 41–49.

Alli, A. F. (1975). The radial intercepts method for measuring bronchial mucous gland volume. *Thorax* 30: 687–692.

American Thoracic Society. (1962). Chronic bronchitis, asthma and pulmonary emphysema. A statement by the Committee on Diagnostic Standards for Nontuberculous Respiratory Diseases. *Am. Rev. Respir. Dis.* 85: 762–768.

Andoh, Y., Aikawa, T., Shimura, S., Sasaki, H., and Takishima, T. (1992a). Morphometric analysis of airways in idiopathic pulmonary fibrosis patients with mucous hypersecretion. *Am. Rev. Respir. Dis.* 145: 175–179.

Andoh, Y., Shimura, S., Aikawa, T., Sasaki, H., and Takishima, T. (1992b). Perivascular fibrosis of muscular pulmonary arteries in chronic pulmonary disease. *Chest* 102: 1645–1650.

Annesi, I., and Kauffmann, F. (1986). Is respiratory mucus hypersecretion really an innocent disorder? A 22-year mortality survey of 1061 working men. *Am. Rev. Respir. Dis.* 134: 688–693.

Anthonisen, N. R., Bass, H., Heckscher, T., Oriol, A., and Bates, D. V. (1967). Recent observations on the measurement of regional V/Q ratios in chronic lung disease. *J. Biol. Nucl. Med.* 11: 73–76.

Baggiolini, M., Bretz, U., and Dewald, B. (1978). Subcellular localization of granulocyte enzymes. In *Neutral Proteases of Human Polymorphonuclear Leukocytes*. Edited by K. Havemann, and A. Janoff. Baltimore-Munich, Urban and Schwarzenberg, pp. 3–17.

Barnes, P. J. (1986). Asthma as an axon reflex. *Lancet* 1: 242–245.

Bateman, J. R. M., Pavia, D., Sheahan, N. G., Agnew, J. E., and Clark, S. W. (1983). Impaired tracheobronchial clearance in patients with mild stable asthma. *Thorax* 38: 463–467.

Bates, D. V. (1973). The fate of the chronic bronchitis. *Am. Rev. Respir. Dis.* 108: 1043–1065.

Berend, N., Woolcock, A. J., and Marlin, G. E. (1979). Correlation between the function and structure of the lung in smokers. *Am. Rev. Respir. Dis.* 119: 695–705.

Bianco, S., Vaghi, A., Robushi, M., and Pasargiklian, M. (1988). Prevention of exercise-induced bronchoconstriction by inhaled furosemide. *Lancet* 2: 252–255.

Bianco, S., Pieroni, M. G., Refini, R. M., Rottoli, L., and Sestini, P. (1989). Protective effect of inhaled furosemide on allergen-induced early and late asthmatic reactions. *N. Engl. J. Med.* 321: 1069–1073.

Borland, C., Chamberlain, A., Barber, B., and Higenbotam T. (1985). Pulmonary epithelial permeability after inhaling saline, distilled water "fog" and cold air. *Chest* 87: 373–376.

Borson, D. B., Corrales, R., Varsano, S., Gold, M., Viro, N., Gaughey, G., Ramachandran, J., and Nadel, J. A. (1987). Enkephalinase inhibitors potentiate substance P-induced secretion of $^{35}SO_4$-macromolecules from ferret trachea. *Exp. Lung Res.* 12: 21–36.

Bowes, D., and Corrin, B. (1977). Ultrastructural immunocytochemical localization of lysozyme in human bronchial glands. *Thorax* 32: 163–170.

Breuer, R., Christensen, T. G., Lucey, E. C., Stone, P. J., and Snider, G. L. (1987). An ultrastructural morphometric analysis of elastase-treated hamster bronchi shows discharge followed by progressive accumulation of secretory granules. *Am. Rev. Respir. Dis.* 136: 698–703.

Brogan, T. D., Ryley, H. C., Neale, L., and Yassa, J. (1975). Soluble proteins of bronchopulmonary secretions from patients with cystic fibrosis, asthma, and bronchitis. *Thorax* 30: 72–79.

Bryant, D. H., and Pui, A. (1982). Histamine content of sputum from patients with asthma and chronic bronchitis. *Clin. Allergy* 12: 19–27.

Camner P., Mossberg B., and Philipson K. (1973). Tracheobronchial clearance and chronic obstructive lung disease. *Scand. J. Respir. Dis.* 54: 272–281.

Cardell, B. S., and Pearson, R. S. B. (1959). Death in asthmatics. *Thorax* 14: 341–352.

Chase, J. V., Flux, M., and Sachdey, G. P. (1985). Comparison of physicochemical properties of purified mucus glycoproteins isolated from respiratory secretion of cystic fibrosis and asthmatic patients. *Biochemistry* 24: 7334–7341.

Charman, J., and Reid, L. (1972). Sputum viscosity in chronic bronchitis, bronchiectasis, asthma and cystic fibrosis. *Biorheology* 9: 185–199.

Chen, T. M., and Dulfano, M. (1978. Mucus viscoelasticity and mucociliary transport rate. *J. Lab. Clin. Med.* 91: 423–431.

Ciba Guest Symposium. (1959). Terminology, definitions and classifications of chronic pulmonary emphysema and related conditions. *Thorax* 14: 286–299.

Clarke, S. W., Cochrance, G. W., and Webber, B. (1973). Effects of sputum on pulmonary function. *Thorax* 28: 262.

Cochrance, G. M., Webber, B., and Clarke, S. W. (1977). Effects of sputum on pulmonary function. *Br. Med. J.* 2: 1181–1183.

Coles, S. J., Neil, K. H., and Reid, L. M. (1984). Potent stimulation of glycoprotein secretion in canine trachea by substance P. *J. Appl. Physiol.* 57: 1323–1327.

Cosio, M., Ghezzo, H., Hogg, J. C., Corbin, R., Loveland, M., Dosmaan, J., and Macklem, P. T. (1977). The relations between structural changes in small airways and pulmonary-function tests. *N. Engl. J. Med.* 298: 1277–1281.

Cosio, M. G., Hale, K. A., and Niewoehner, D. E. (1980). Morphologic and morphometric effects of prolonged cigarette smoking on the small airways. *Am. Rev. Respir. Dis.* 122: 265–271.

Cutz, E., Levison, H., and Cooper, D. M. (1978). Ultrastructure of airways in children with asthma. *Histopathology* 2: 407–421.

Davis, B., Roberts, A. M., Coleridge, H. M., and Coleridge, J. C. G. (1982). Reflex tracheal gland secretion evoked by stimulation of bronchial C-fibers in dogs. *J. Appl. Physiol.* 53: 985–991.

Desanctis, G. T., Kelly, S. M., Saettam, M. P., et al. (1987). Hyporesponsiveness to aerosolized but not to infused methacholine in cigarette-smoking dogs. *Am. Rev. Respir. Dis.* 135: 338–344.

Dor, P. J., Acerman, S. J., and Gleich, G. J. (1984). Charcot–Leyden crystals and eosinophil granule major basic protein in sputum of patients with respiratory diseases. *Am. Rev. Respir. Dis.* 130: 1072–1077.

Douglas, A. M. (1980). Quantitative study of bronchial mucous gland enlargement. *Thorax* 35: 198–201.

Douglas, A. N., Lamb, D., and Ruckley, V. A. (1982). Bronchial gland dimensions in coalminers: Influence of smoking and dust exposure. *Thorax* 37: 760–764.

Drasen, J. M., O'Cain, C. F., and Ingram, R. H., Jr. (1982). Experimental induction of chronic bronchitis in dogs: Effects on airway obstruction and responsiveness. *Am. Rev. Respir. Dis.* 126: 75–79.

Dulfano, M. J., and Luk, C. K. (1982). Sputum and ciliary inhibition in asthma. *Thorax* 37: 646–651.

Dunnill, M. D. (1960). The pathology of asthma with special reference to changes in the bronchial mucosa. *J. Clin. Pathol.* 13: 27–33.

Dunnill, M. D., Massarella, G. R., and Anderson, J. A. (1969). A comparison of the quantitative anatomy of the bronchi in normal subjects, in status asthmaticus, in chronic bronchitis and in emphysema. *Thorax* 24: 176–179.

Dunnill, M. S. (1975). The morphology of the airways in bronchial asthma. In: *New Directions in Asthma*. Edited by M. Stein. Park Ridge, Ill., American College of Chest Physicians, pp.213–221.

Edwards, C. W., and Carlile, A. (1982). The larger bronchi in cryptogenic fibrosing alveolitis: A morphometric study. *Thorax* 37: 828–833.

Eggleston, P. A., Kagey-Sobotka, A., and Lichtenstein, L. M. (1987). A comparison of the osmotic activation of basophils and human mast cells. *Am. Rev. Respir. Dis.* 135: 1043–1048.

Elwood, R. K., Kennedy, S., Belzberg, A., Hogg, J. C., and Pare, P. D. (1983). Respiratory mucosal permeability in asthma. *Am. Rev. Respir. Dis.* 128: 523–527.

Fick, R. B., Jr., Richardson, H. B., Zavala, D. C., and Hunninghake, G. W. (1987). Bronchoalveolar lavage in allergic asthmatics. *Am. Rev. Respir. Dis.* 135: 1204–1209.

Filley, W. V., Holley, K. E., Kephart, B. M., and Gleich, G. J. (1982). Identification by immunofluorescence of eosinophil granule major basic protein in lung tissue of patients with bronchial asthma. *Lancet* 2: 11–15.

Finney, M. J. B., Anderson, S. D., and Black, J. L. (1987). The effect of non-isotonic solutions on human isolated airway smooth muscle. *Respir. Physiol.* 69: 277–286.

Fletcher, C., and Peto, R. (1977). The natural history of chronic airflow obstruction. *Br. Med. J.* 1: 1645–1648.

Florey, H., Carleton, H. M., and Wells, A. Q. (1932). Mucus secretion in the trachea. *Br. J. Exp. Pathol.* 13: 269–284.

Frigas, E., Loegering, D. A., and Gleich, G. J. (1980). Cytotoxic effects of the guinea pig eosinophil major basic protein on tracheal epithelium. *Lab. Invest.* 42: 35–43.

Frizzel, R. A. (1988). 1. Molecular biology. Role of absorptive and secretory process in hydration of the airway surface. *Am. Rev. Respir. Dis.* 138: S3–S6.

Fuchimukai, T., Fujiwara, T., Takahashi, A., and Enhorning, G. (1987). Artificial pulmonary surfactant inhibited by proteins. *J. Appl. Physiol.* 62: 429–437.

Gashi, A. A., Borson, D. B., Finkbeiner, W. E., Nadel, J. A., and Basbaum, C. B. (1986). Neuropeptides degranulate serous cells of ferret tracheal glands. *Am. J. Physiol.* 251: C223–C229.

Gatto, L. A. (1981). pH of mucus in rat trachea. *J. Appl. Physiol.* 50: 1224–1228.

Gellert, A. R., Lewis, C. A., Langford, J. A., Tolfree, S. E. J., and Rudd, R. M. (1985). Regional distribution of pulmonary epithelial permeability in normal subjects and patients with asbestosis. *Thorax* 40: 734–740.

Glynn, A. A., and Michaels, L. (1960). Bronchial biopsy in chronic bronchitis and asthma. *Thorax* 15: 142–153.

Gregg, I., and Trapnell, D. H. (1969). The bronchographic appearances of early chronic bronchitis. *Br. J. Radiol.* 42: 132–139.

Hale, F. C., Olsen, C. R., and Mickey, M. R., Jr. (1968). The measurement of bronchial wall components. *Am. Rev. Respir. Dis.* 98: 978–987.

Hale, K. A., Ewing, S. L., Gosnell, B. A., and Niewoehner, D. E. (1984). Lung disease in long-term smokers with and without chronic air-flow obstruction. *Am. Rev. Respir. Dis.* 130: 718–721.

Harbitz, O., Jenssen, A. O., and Smildsrød, O. (1984). Lysozyme and lactoferrin in sputum from patients with chronic obstructive lung disease. *Eur. J. Respir. Dis.* 65: 512–520.

Hayashi, M., Sornberger, G. C., and Huber, G. L. (1979). Morphometric analysis of tracheal gland secretion and hypertrophy in male and female rats after experimental exposure to tobacco smoke. *Am. Rev. Respir. Dis.* 119: 67–73.

Hayes, J. A. (1969). Distribution of bronchial gland measurements in a Jamaican population. *Thorax* 24: 619–622.

Hiwatari, N., Shimura, S., Sasaki, T., Aikawa, T., Ando, H., Ishihara, H., Sekizawa, K., Sasaki, H., and Takishima, T. (1991). Prognosis of idiopathic pulmonary fibrosis with mucus hypersecretion. *Am. Rev. Respir. Dis.* 143: 182–185.

Hogg, J. C. (1984). Bronchial mucosal permeability and its relationship to airways hyperreactivity. *Am. Rev. Respir. Dis.* 129: 143–148.

Hogg, J. C., Macklem, P. T., and Thurlbeck, W. M. (1968). Site and nature of airway obstruction in chronic obstructive lung disease. *N. Engl. J. Med.* 278: 1355–1360.

Holgate, S. T. (1987). Contributions of inflammatory mediators to the immediate asthmatic reaction. *Am. Rev. Respir. Dis.* 135: 557–562.

Holtzman, M. J., Fabbri, L. M., O'Byrne, P. M., Gold, B. D., Aizawa, H., Walters, E. H., Alpert, S. E., and Nadel, J. A. (1983). Importance of airway inflammation for the hyperresponsiveness induced by ozone. *Am. Rev. Respir. Dis.* 127: 686–690.

Holma, B., Kinderrgren, M., and Andersen, J. M. (1977). pH effects of ciliomotilty and morphology of respiratory mucosa. *Arch. Environ. Health* 32: 216–226.

Homma, H., Yamanaka, A., Tanimoto, S., et al. (1983). Diffuse panbronchiolitis: A disease of the transitional zone of the lung. *Chest* 83: 63–69.

Honda, I., Shimura, S., Sasaki, T., Sasaki, H., Takishima, T., and Nakamura, M. (1988). Airway mucosal permeability in chronic bronchitics and bronchial asthmatics. *Am. Rev. Respir. Dis.* 137: 866–871.

Hook, W. A., and Siraganian, R. P. (1981). Influence of anions, cations and osmolarity on IgE-mediated histamine release from human basophils. *Immunology* 43: 723–731.

Houston, J. C., De Navasquez, S., and Thoimce, J. R. (1953). A clinical and pathological study of fatal cases of status asthmaticus. *Thorax* 8: 207–213.

Iravani, J., and Van As, A. (1972). Mucus transport in the tracheobronchial tree of normal and bronchitic rats. *J. Pathol.* 106: 81–93.

Ishihara, H., Honda, I., Shimura, S., Sasaki, H., and Takishima, T. (1991). Role of chronic *Pseudomonas aeruginosa* infection in airway mucosal permeability. *Chest* 100: 1607–1613.

Jamal, K., Cooney, T. P., Fleetham, J. A., and Thurlbeck, W. M. (1984). Chronic bronchitis. Correlation of morphologic findings to sputum production and flow rates. *Am. Rev. Respir. Dis.* 129: 719–722.

James, A. L., Paré, P. D., and Hogg, J. C. (1988). Effect of lung volume, bronchoconstriction, and cigarette smoke on morphometric airway dimension. *J. Appl. Physiol.* 64: 913–919.

James, A. L., Paré, P. D., and Hogg, J. C. (1989). The mechanics of airway narrowing in asthma. *Am. Rev. Respir. Dis.* 139: 242–246.

Jeffery, P. K., Wardlaw, A. J., Nelson, F. C., Collins, J. V., and Kay, A. B. (1989). Bronchial biopsies in asthma. An ultrastructural, quantitative study and correlation with hyperreactivity. *Am. Rev. Respir. Dis.* 140: 1745–1753.

Johnson, H. G., Chinn, R. A., Chow, A. W., Bach, M. K., and Nadel, J. A. (1983). Leukotriene C_4 enhances the release of mucus from submucosal glands in canine trachea in vivo. *Int. J. Immunopharmacol.* 5: 391–396.

Jones, R., and Reid, L. (1979). Beta-agonists and secretory cell number and intracellular glycoprotein in airway epithelium: The effect of isoproterenol and salbutamol. *Am. J. Pathol.* 95: 407–422.

Kaliner, M., Marom, Z., Patow, C., and Shelhamer, J. (1984). Human respiratory mucus. *J. Allergy Clin. Immunol.* 73: 318–323.

Keal, E. E. (1971). Biochemistry and rheology of sputum in asthma. *Postgrad. Med. J.* 47: 171–177.

Kennedy, S. M., Elwood, R. K., Wiggs, B. J. R., Par, P. D., and Hogg, J. C. (1984). Increased airway mucosal permeability of smokers. Relationship to airway reactivity. *Am. Rev. Respir. Dis.* 129: 143–148.

Kim, C. S., and Eldridge, M. A. (1985). Aerosol deposition in the airway model with excessive mucus secretions. *J. Appl. Physiol.* 59: 1766–1772.

Kim, C. S., Eldridge, M. A., and Wanner, A. (1988). Airway responsiveness to inhaled and intravenous carbachol in sheep: Effect of airway mucus. *J. Appl. Physiol.* 65: 2744–2754.

Kim, C. S., Abraham, W. H., Garcia, L., and Sacker, M. A. (1989). Enhanced aerosol deposition in the lung with mild airway obstruction. *Am. Rev. Respir. Dis.* 139: 422–426.

Kim, K. C., and Brody, J. S. (1992). Mechanical strain causes release of mucins from airway epithelial cells. *Am. Rev. Respir. Dis.* 145: A617.

Kim, K. C., Wasano, K., Niles, R. M., Schuster, J. E., Stone, P. J., and Brody, J. S. (1987). Human neutrophil elastase releases cell surface mucins from primary cultures of hamster tracheal epithelial cells. *Proc. Natl. Acad. Sci. USA* 84: 9304–9308.

Kim, K. C., Nassiri, J., and Brody, J. S. (1989). Mechanisms of airway goblet cell mucin release: Studies with cultured tracheal surface epithelial cells. *Am. J. Respir. Cell Mol. Biol.* 1: 137–143.

King, M., Kelly, S., and Cosis, S. (1985). Alteration of airway reactivity by mucus. *Respir. Physiol.* 62: 47–59.

Kollerstrom, N., Lord, P. W., and Whimster, W. F. (1977). Distribution of acid mucus in the bronchial mucous glands. *Thorax* 32: 160–162.

Laitinen, L. A., Heino, M., Laitinin, A., Kava, T., and Haahtels, T. (1985). Damage of the epithelium and bronchial reactivity in patients with asthma. *Am. Rev. Respir. Dis.* 131: 599–606.

Laitinen, L. A., Robinson, M. P., Laitinen, A., and Eiddicombe, J. G. (1986). Relationship between tracheal mucosal thickness and vascular resistance in dogs. *J. Appl. Physiol.* 61: 2186–2193.

Larsen, P. K., Lundgren, J. D., and Egeberg, J. (1989). The whole-mount method as a technique for measuring experimental changes in airway goblet cell number. *Acta Pathol. Microbiol. Immunol. Scand.* 97: 1141–1145.

Lennox, B. (1975). Observations on the accuracy of point counting including a description of a new particle. *J. Clin. Pathol.* 28: 99–103.

Lehr, D. (1972). Isoproterenol and sudden death of asthmatic patients in ventricular fibrillation. *N. Engl. J. Med.* 287: 987–988.

Liu, P. V. (1966). The roles of various fractions of *Pseudomonas aeruginosa* in its pathogenesis. III: Identify of the lethal toxin produced in vitro and in vivo. *J. Infect. Dis.* 116: 481–489.

Lopez-Vidriero, M. T., and Reid, L. (1978). Chemical markers of mucous and serum glycoproteins and their relation to viscosity in mucoid and purulent sputum from various hypersecretory disease. *Am. Rev. Respir. Dis.* 117: 465–477.

Lopez-Vidriero, M. T., Charman, J., Keal, E., and Reid, L. (1973). Sputum viscosity: Correlation with chemical and clinical features in chronic bronchitis. *Thorax* 28: 401–408.

Lopez-Vidriero, M. T., Costello, J., Clark, T. J., Das, I., Keal, E., and Reid, L. (1975a). Effect of atropine on sputum production. *Thorax* 30: 543–547.

Lopez-Vidriero, M., Charman, J., Keal, E., and Reid, L. (1975b). Bronchorrhoea. *Thorax* 30: 624–630.

Lopez-Vidriero, M. T., Das, I. Smith, A. P., Picot, R., and Reid, L. (1977). Bronchial secretion from normal human airways after inhalation of prostaglandin $F_{2\alpha}$, acetylcholine, histamine, and citric acid. *Thorax* 32: 734–739.

Lopez-Vidriero, M. T., Das, I., and Reid, L. (1979). Bronchorrhea—separation of mucus and serum components in sol and gel phases. *Thorax* 34: 512–517.

Lozewics, S., Wells, C., Gomez, E., Ferguson, H., Richman, P., Davalia, J., and Davies, R. J. (1990). Morphological integrity of the bronchial epithelium in mild asthma. *Thorax* 45: 12–15.

Lundberg, J. A. M., and Saria, A. (1983). Capsaicin induced desensitization of the airway mucosa to cigarette smoke, mechanical and chemical irritants. *Nature* 302: 251–253.

Lundgren, J. D., Shelhamer, J., and Kaliner, M. (1985). The role of eicosanoids in respiratory mucus hypersecretion. *Ann. Allergy* 55: 5–12.

Lundgren, J. D., Hirata, F., Marom, Z., Logun, C., Steel, L., Kaliner, M., and Shelhamer, J. (1988a). Dexamethasone inhibits respiratory glycoconjugate secretion from feline airways in vitro by the induction of lipocortin (lipomodulin) synthesis. *Am. Rev. Respir. Dis.* 137: 353–357.

Lundgren, J. D., Kaliner, M., Logun, C., and Shelhamer, J. H. (1988b). Dexamthasone reduces rat tracheal goblet cell hyperplasia produced by human neutrophil products. *Exp. Lung Res.* 14: 853–863.

Lundgren, J. D., Wiederman, C. J., Logun, C., Plutchok, J., Kaliner, M., and Shelhamer, J. H. (1989a). Substance P receptor-mediated secretion of respiratory glycoconjugate from feline airways in vitro. *Exp. Lung Res.* 15: 17–29.

Lundgren, J. D., Kaliner, M. A., and Shelhamer, J. H. (1989b). Respiratory mucus production in bronchial asthma. In *What Can We Learn With the Analysis of Sputum?* Edited by S. Nagaoka. Tokyo, Life Science Publishing, pp.116–155.

Lundgren, J. D., Davey, R. T., Jr., Lundgren, B., Mullol, J., Marom, Z., and Logun, C. (1991). Eosinophil cationic protein stimulates and major basic protein inhibits airway mucus secretion. *J. Allergy Clin. Immunol.* 87: 689–698.

Macklem, P. T., Proctor, D. F., and Hogg, J. C. (1970). The stability of peripheral airways. *Respir. Physiol.* 8: 191–203.

Macleod, L. J., and Heard, B. E. (1969). Area of muscle in tracheal wall in bronchitis, measured by point-counting. *J. Pathol.* 97: 157–161.

Marin, M. G., Davis, B., and Nadel, J. A. (1977). Effect of histamine on electrical and ion transport properties of tracheal epithelium. *J. Appl. Physiol.* 42: 735–738.

Marom, Z., Shelhamer, J. H., and Kaliner, M. (1981). Effects of arachidonic acid, monohydroxyeicosatetraenoic acid and prostaglandins on the release of mucous glycoproteins from human airways in vitro. *J. Clin. Invest.* 67: 1695–1702.

Marom, Z., Shelhamer, J. H., Bach, M. K., Morton, D. R., and Kaliner, M. (1982). Slow-reacting substances, leukotriene C_4 and D_4, increase the release of mucus from human airways in vitro. *Am. Rev. Respir. Dis.* 126: 449–451.

Marom, Z., Sun, F., Shelhamer, J. H., and Kaliner, M. (1983). Human airway mono-hydroxyeicosatetraenoic acid generation and mucus release. *J. Clin. Invest.* 72: 122–127.

Marom, Z., Shelhamer, J., Alling, D., and Kaliner, M. (1984a). The effect of corticosteroids on mucus glycoprotein secretion from human airways in vitro. *Am. Rev. Respir. Dis.* 129: 62–65.

Marom, Z., Shelhamer, J. H., Steel, L., Goetzl, E. J., and Kaliner, M. (1984b). Prosta-glandin-generating factor of anaphylaxis induces mucous glycoprotein release and the formation of lipoxygenase products of arachidonate from human airways. *Prostaglandins* 28: 79–91.

Marom, Z., Shelhamer, J. D., and Kaliner, M. (1984c). Human pulmonary macrophage-derived mucus secretagogue. *J. Exp. Med.* 159: 844–860.

Marom, Z., Shelhamer, J. H., and Kaliner, M. (1985). Human macrophage-derived mucus secretagogue. *J. Clin. Invest.* 75: 191–198.

Matsuba, K., and Thurlbeck, W. M. (1973). Disease of the small airways in chronic bronchitis. *Am. Rev. Respir. Dis.* 107: 552–558.

May, R. J. (1954). Pathogenic bacteria in chronic bronchitis. *Lancet* 2: 839–842.

May, D. B., and Munt, P. W. (1979). Physiologic effects of chest percussion and postural drainage in patients with stable chronic bronchitis. *Chest* 75: 29–32.

McKenzie, H. I., Glick, M., and Outhred, K. G. (1969). Chronic bronchitis in coal miners: Ante-mortem/post-mortem comparisons. *Thorax* 24: 527–535.

Messer, J. W., Peters, G. A., and Bennett, W. A. (1960). Cause of death and pathologic findings in 304 cases of bronchial asthma. *Dis. Chest* 38: 616–624.

Mezey, R. J., Chohn, M. A., Fernandex, R. J., Januszkiewicx, A. J., and Wanner, A. (1978). Mucociliary transport in allergic patients with antigen induced bronchospasm. *Am. Rev. Respir. Dis.* 118: 667–684.

Mitchell, R. S., Stanford, R. E., Johnson, J. M., Silvers, G. W., Dart, G., and George, M. S. (1976). The morphologic features of the bronchi, bronchioles and alveoli in chronic airway obstruction: A clinicopathologic study. *Am. Rev. Respir. Dis.* 144: 137–145.

Morihara, K., Tsuzuki, H., Oka, T., Inoue, H., and Ebata, M. (1965). *Pseudomonas aeruginosa* elastase: Isolation, crystallization and preliminary characterization. *J. Biol. Chem.* 240: 3295–3304.

Mullen, J. B. M., Wright, J. L., Wiggs, B. R., Pare, P. D., and Hogg, J. C. (1987). Structure of central airways in current smokers and ex-smokers with and without mucus hypersecretion: Relationship to lung function. *Thorax* 42: 843–884.

Naccache, P. H., Showell, H. J., Becker, E. L., and Sháafi, R. I. (1977). Transport of sodium, potassium, and calcium across rabbit polymorphonuclear leukocyte membranes: Effect of chemotactic factor. *J. Cell Biol.* 73: 428–444.

Nagai, A., West, W. W., Paul, J. L., and Thurlbeck, W. M. (1985). The National Institute of Health intermittent positive pressure breathing trial: Pathology studies. I. Interrelationships between morphologic lesions. *Am. Rev. Respir. Dis.* 132: 937–945.

Nagaki, M., Shimura, S., Tanno, Y., Ishibashi, T., Sasaki, H., and Takishima, T. (1992). Role of chronic *Pseudomonas aeruginosa* infection in the development of bronchiectasis. *Chest* 102: 1464–1469.

Naylor, B. (1962). The shedding of the mucosa of the bronchial tree in asthma. *Thorax* 17: 69–72.

Oberholzer, M., Dalquen, P., Wyss, M., and Rohr, H. P. (1978). The applicability of the gland/wall ratio (Reid index) to clinico-pathological correlation studies. *Thorax* 33: 779–784.

Ohrui, T., Sekizawa, K., Yamauchi, K., Ohkawara, Y., Hakazawa, H., Aikawa, T., Sasaki, H., and Takishima, T. (1991). Chemical oxidant potentiates electrically and acetylcholine-induced contraction in rat trachea: Possible involvement of cholinesterase inhibition. *J. Pharmacol. Exp. Ther.* 259: 371–376.

Ohrui, T., Sekizawa, K., Aikawa, T., Yamauchi, K., Sasaki, H., and Takishima, T. (1992). Vascular permeability and airway narrowing during late asthmatic response in dogs treated with metopirone. *J. Allergy Clin. Immunol.* 89: 933–943.

Pavia, D., Bateman, J. R. M., Sheahan, M. F., Agnew, J. E., and Clarke, S. W. (1985). Tracheobronchial mucociliary clearance in asthma; impairment during remission. *Thorax* 40: 171–175.

Peatfield, A. C., Hall, R. L., Richardson, P. S., and Jeffery, O. J. (1982). The effect of serum on the secretion of radiolabeled mucus macromolecules into the lumen of the cat trachea. *Am. Rev. Respir. Dis.* 125: 210–215.

Persson, C. G. A., and Svensjö, E. (1983). Airway hyperreactivity and microvascular permeability to large molecules. *Eur. J. Respir. Dis.* 64(Suppl. 131): 181–214.

Persson, C. G. A., and Erjefält, I. (1986). Inflammatory leakage of macromolecules from the vascular compartment into the tracheal lumen. *Acta Physiol. Scand.* 126: 615–616.

Peto, R., Speizer, F. E., and Cochrane, A. L. (1983). The relevance in adults of airway-flow obstruction, but not of mucus hypersecretion, to mortality from chronic lung disease. *Am. Rev. Respir. Dis.* 128: 491–500.

Petty, T. L., Pierson, D. J., Dick, N. P., Hudson, L. D., and Walker, S. H. (1976). Follow-up evaluation of a prevalence study for chronic bronchitis and chronic airway obstruction. *Am. Rev. Respir. Dis.* 114: 881–890.

Petty, T. L., Silvers, G. W., and Stanford, R. E. (1981). Functional correlations with mild and moderate emphysema in excised human lungs. *Am. Rev. Respir. Dis.* 124: 700–704.

Petty, T. L., Silvers, G. W., and Stanford, R. E. (1984). Small airway disease is associated with elastic recoil changes in excised human lungs. *Am. Rev. Respir. Dis.* 130: 42–45.

Phang, P. T., and Keough, M. W. (1986). Inhibition of pulmonary surfactant by plasma from normal adults and from patients having cardiopulmonary bypass. *J. Thorac. Cardiovasc. Surg.* 91: 248–251.

Phipps, R. K., Denas, S. M., Sielczak, M. W., and Wanner, A. (1986). Effect of 0.5 ppm ozone on glycoprotein secretion, ion and water fluxes in sheep trachea. *J. Appl. Physiol.* 60: 918–927.

Poston, R. N., Chanez, P., Lacoste, J. Y., Litchfield, Lee, T. H., and Bousquest, J. (1992). Immunohistochemical characterization of the cellular infiltration in asthmatic bronchi. *Am. Rev. Respir. Dis.* 145: 918–921.

Pride, N. B. (1984). Definitions of emphysema, chronic bronchitis, asthma, and airflow obstruction: 25 year on from the Ciba symposium. *Thorax* 39: 81–85.

Rees, P. J., Shelton, D., Chan, T. B., Eiser, N., Clark, T. J. H., and Maisey, M. N. (1985). Effects of histamine on lung permeability in normal and asthmatic subjects. *Thorax* 40: 603–606.

Reid, L. (1954). Pathology of chronic bronchitis. *Lancet* 256: 275–278.

Reid, L. (1960). Measurement of the bronchial mucous gland layer: A diagnostic yardstick in chronic bronchitis. *Thorax* 15: 132–141.

Reid, L. M. (1987). The presence or absence of bronchial mucus in fatal asthma. *J. Allergy Clin. Immunol.* 80: 415–416.

Restrepo, G. L., and Heard, B. E. (1963a). The size of bronchial glands in bronchitis. *J. Pathol. Bacteriol.* 95: 305–310.

Restrepo, G. L., and Heard, B. E. (1963b). Mucous gland enlargement in chronic bronchitis: Extent of enlargement in the tracheo-bronchial tree. *Thorax* 18: 334–339.

Rich, B., Peatfield, A. C., Williams, I. P., and Richardson, P. S. (1984). Effects of prostaglandings E_1, E_2 and $F_2\alpha$ on mucin secretion from human bronchi in vitro. *Thorax* 39: 420–423.

Robin, E. D., and Lewiston, N. (1989). Unexpected, unexplained sudden death in young asthmatic subjects. *Chest* 96: 790–793.

Rogers, D. F., and Jeffery, P. K. (1986). Inhibition of cigarette smoke-induced airway secretory cell hyperplasia by indomethacin, dexamethasone, prednisolone, or hydrocortisone in the rat. *Exp. Lung Res.* 10: 285–298.

Ryder, R. C., Dunnill, M. S., and Anderson, J. A. (1971). A quantitative study of bronchial mucous gland volume, emphysema and smoking in a necropsy population. *J. Pathol.* 104: 59–71.

Saetta, M., Stefano, A. D., Rosina, C., Thiene, G., and Fabbri, L. M. (1991). Quantitative structural analysis of peripheral airways and arteries in sudden fatal asthma. *Am. Rev. Respir. Dis.* 143: 138–143.

Samios, R. (1975). Relationship of sputum quantity to pulmonary function. *Physicotherapy* 61: 336.

Saria, A., Martling, C. -R., Yan, Z., Theodorsson-Norhteim, E., Ganse, R., and Lundberg, J. M. (1988). Release of multiple tachykinins from capsaicin sensitive, sensory nerves in the lung by bradykinin, histamine, dimethylphenyl piperazinium, and vagal nerve stimulation. *Am. Rev. Respir. Dis.* 137: 1330–1335.

Sasaki, T., Shirmura, S., Ikeda, K., Sasaki, H., and Takishima, T. (1989). PAF increases platelet-dependent glycoconjugate secretion from tracheal submucosal glands. *Am. J. Physiol.* 257: L373–L378.

Sasaki, T., Shimura, S., Ikeda, K., Sasaki, H., and Takishima, T. (1990). Sodium efflux from isolated submucosal gland in feline trachea. *Am. J. Physiol.* 258: L112–L117.

Satoh, M., Shimura, S., Ishihara, H., Yamada, K., Masuda, T., Sasaki, T., Sasaki, H., and T. Takishima (1992). Effect of glucocorticoid on fluid secretion across airway mucosa. *Am. J. Physiol.* (in press).

Scanlon, P. D., Seltzer, J., Ingram, R. H., Jr., Reid, L., and Drasen, J. M. (1987). Chronic exposure to sulfur dioxide. Physiologic and histologic evaluation of dogs exposed to 50 or 15 ppm. *Am. Rev. Respir. Dis.* 135: 831–839.

Schleimer, R. P., MacGlashan, D. W., Gillespie, E., Jr., and Lichtenstein, L. M. (1982). Inhibition of basophil histamine release by anti-inflammatory steroids: II. Studies on the mechanism of action. *J. Immunol.* 129: 1632–1636.

Schneeberger, E. E., and Lynch, R. D. (1984). Tight junctions. Their structure, composition and function. *Circ. Res.* 55: 723–733.

Schoeffel, R. E., Anderson, S. D., and Altounyan, R. E. C. (1981). Bronchial hyperreactivity in response to inhalation of ultrasonically nebulized solutions of distilled water and saline. *Br. Med. J.* 283: 1285–1287.

Schultz, H. D., Roberts, A. M., Bratcher, C., Coleridge, H. M., Coleridge, J. C. G., and Davis, B. (1985). Pulmonary C-fibers reflexively increase secretion by tracheal submucosal glands in dogs. *J. Appl. Physiol.* 58: 907–910.

Scott, K. W. M. (1973). An autopsy study of bronchial mucous gland hypertrophy in Glasgow. *Am. Rev. Respir. Dis.* 107: 239–245.

Sekizawa, K., Sasaki, H., Shimizu, Y., and Takishima, T. (1986). Dose-response effects of methacholine in normal and asthmatic subjects: Relationship between the site of airway response and overall airway hyperresponsiveness. *Am. Rev. Respir. Dis.* 133: 593–599.

Seltzer, J., Scanlon, P. D., Drasen, J. M., Ingram, R. H., Jr., and Reid, L. (1984). Morphologic correlation of physiologic changes caused by SO_2-induced bronchitis in dogs. The role of inflammation. *Am. Rev. Respir. Dis.* 129: 790–797.

Shelhamer, J. H., Marom, Z., and Kaliner, M. (1980). Immunologic and neuropharmacologic stimulation of mucus glycoprotein release from human airways. *J. Clin. Invest.* 66: 1400–1408.

Shimura, S., Sato, S., Takishima, T., Otsubo, T., and Umeya, K. (1980). Relaxation behavior of sputum studied using the raised cosine pulse method. *Biorheology* 17: 363–375.

Shimura, S., Sasaki, T., Okayama, H., Sasaki, H., and Takishima, T. (1987a). Effect of substance P on mucus secretion of isolated gland from feline trachea. *J. Appl. Physiol.* 63: 646–653.

Shirmura, S., Sasaki, T., Okayama, H., Sasaki, H., and Takishima, T. (1987b). Neural control of contraction in isolated submucosal gland from feline trachea. *J. Appl. Physiol.* 62: 2404–2409.

Shirmura, S., Sasaki, T., Sasaki, H., and Takishima, T. (1988a). Chemical properties of bronchorrhea sputum in bronchial asthma. *Chest* 94: 1211–1215.

Shimura, S., Sasaki, T., Sasaki, H., Takishima, T., and Umeya, K. (1988b). Viscoelastic properties of bronchorrhea sputum in bronchial asthmatics. *Biorheology* 25: 173–179.

Shimura, S., Sasaki, T., Ikeda, K., Yamauchi, K., Sasaki, H., and T. Takishima (1990). Direct inhibitory action of glucocorticoid on glycoconjugate secretion from airway submucosal glands. *Am. Rev. Respir. Dis.* 141: 1044–1049.

Shimura, S., Sasaki, T., Ishihara, H., Satoh, M., Sasaki, H., and Takishima, T. (1992). Autonomic innervation to feline tracheal submucosal glands for mucus glycoprotein. *Am. J. Physiol.* 262: L15–L20.

Shore, S. A., Kariya, S. T., Anderson, K., Skornik, W., Feldman, H. A., Pennington, J., Goldleski, J., and Drasen, J. M. (1987). Sulfur-dioxide-induced bronchitis in dogs. *Am. Rev. Respir. Dis.* 135: 840–847.

Smith, C., Feldman, C., Levy, H., Kallenbach, J. M., and Zwi, S. (1990). Cryptogenic fibrosing alveolitis. A study of an indigenous African population. *Respiration* 57: 364–371.

Snider, G. L., Lucey, E., Christensen, T. G., Stone, P. J., Calore, J. D., Catanese, A., and Flanzblau, C. (1984). Emphysema and bronchial secretory cell metaplasia induced in hamsters by human neutrophil products. *Am. Rev. Respir. Dis.* 129: 155–160.

Sobonya, R. E. (1984). Quantitative structural alterations in long-standing allergic asthma. *Am. Rev. Respir. Dis.* 130: 289–292.

Somerville, M., Richardson, P. S., Rutman, A., Wilson, R., and Cole, P. J. (1991). Stimulation of secretion into human and feline airways by *Pseudomonas aeruginosa* proteases. *J. Appl. Physiol.* 70: 2259–2267.

Somerville, M., Taylor, G. W., Watson, D., Rendell, N. B., Rutman, A., Todd, H., Davies, J. R., Wilson, R., Cole, P., and Richardson, P. S. (1992). Release of mucus glycoconjugates by *Pseudomonas aeruginosa* rhamnolipids into feline trachea in vivo and human bronchus in vitro. *Am. J. Respir. Cell Mol. Biol.* 6: 116–122.

Sommerhoff, C. P., Caughy, C. H., Finkbeiner, W. E., Lazarus, S. C., Basbaum, C. B., and Nadel, J. A. (1989). Mast cell chymase: A potent secretagogue for airway gland serous cells. *J. Immunol.* 142: 2450–2456.

Sommerhoff, C. P., Nadel, J. A., Basbaum, C. B., and Caughey, G. H. (1990). Neutrophil elastase and cathepsin G stimulate secretion from cultured bovine airway gland serous cells. *J. Clin. Invest.* 85: 682–689.

Stahl, G. H., and Ellis, D. B. (1973). Biosynthesis of respiratory-tract mucins: A comparison of canine epithelial goblet-cell and submucosal-gland secretions. *Biochem. J.* 136: 845–850.

Strohl, K. P., O'Cain, C. F., Ingram, R. H., Jr., Yanta, M. A., Kaplan, W. D., and MacFadden, E. R., Jr. (1981). Inhalation patterns and predominant site of bronchoconstriction in healthy subjects. *J. Appl. Physiol.* 50: 575–579.

Sturgess, T., and Reid, L. (1973). The effect of isoprenaline and pilocarpine on (a) bronchial mucus-secreting tissue and (b) pancreas, salivary glands, heart, thymus, liver and spleen. *Br. J. Exp. Pathol.* 54: 388–403.

Stutts, M. J., Sckwab, J. H., Chen, M. G., Knowles, M. R., and Boucher, R. C. (1986). Effects of *Pseudomonas aeruginosa* on bronchial epithelial ion transport. *Am. Rev. Respir. Dis.* 134: 17–21.

Suzuki, T., Inoue, H., Lin, J.-T., and Takishima, T. (1992). Intraluminal space occupying substance induces airway hyperresponsiveness. *Am. Rev. Respir. Dis.* 145: A50.

Takizawa, T., and Thurlbeck, W. M. (1971). Muscle and mucous gland size in the major bronchi of patients with chronic bronchitis, asthma and asthmatic bronchitis. *Am. Rev. Respir. Dis.* 104: 331–336.

Tamaoki, J., Ueki, I. F., Widdicombe, J. H., and Nadel, J. A. (1988). Stimulation of Cl$^-$ secretion by neurokinin A and neurokinin B in canine tracheal epithelium. *Am. Rev. Respir. Dis.* 137: 899–902.

Thompson, M. L., and Short, M. D. (1969). Mucociliary function in health, chronic obstructive airway disease, and asbestosis. *J. Appl. Physiol.* 26: 535–539.

Thurlbeck, W. M., Angus, G. E., and Pare, J. A. P. (1963). Mucus gland hypertrophy in chronic bronchitics and its occurrence in smokers. *Br. J. Dis. Chest.* 57: 73–78.

Thurlbeck, W. M., and Angus, G. E. (1964). A distribution curve in chronic bronchitis. *Thorax* 19: 436–442.

Tom-Moy, M., Basbaum, C. B., and Nadel, J. A. (1983). Localization and release of lysozyme from ferret trachea: Effect of adrenergic and cholinergic drugs. *Cell Tissue Res.* 228: 549–562.

Tomioka, M., Ida, I., Shindoh, Y., Ishihara, T., and Takishima, T. (1984). Mast cells in bronchoalveolar lumen of patients with bronchial asthma. *Am. Rev. Respir. Dis.* 129: 1000–1005.

Turner-Warwick, M., and Openshaw, P. (1987). Sputum in asthma. *Postgrad. Med. J.* 63(Suppl. 1): 79–82.

Turner-Warwick, M., Burrows, B., and Johnson, A. (1980). Cryptogenic fibrosing alveolitis: Clinical features and their influence on survival. *Thorax* 35: 171–180.

Wanner, A. (1977). Clinical aspects of mucociliary transport. *Am. Rev. Respir. Dis.* 116: 73–125.

Wanner, A., Brodnan, J. M., Perez, J., Henke, K. G., and Kim, C. S. (1985). Variability of airway responsiveness to histamine aerosol in normal subjects: Role of deposition. *Am. Rev. Respir. Dis.* 131: 3–7.

Welsh, M. J. (1983). Inhibition of chloride secretion by furosemide in canine tracheal epithelium. *J. Membr. Biol.* 71: 219–226.

Wheeldon, E. B., and Pirie, H. M. (1974). Measurement of bronchial wall components in young dogs, adult normal dogs, and adult dogs with chronic bronchitis. *Am. Rev. Respir. Dis.* 110: 609–615.

Woolcock, J. A., Vincent, N. J., and Macklem, P. T. (1969). Frequency dependence of compliance as a test for obstruction in the small airways. *J. Clin. Invest.* 48: 1097–1106.

Yager, D., Butler, J. P., Bastacky, J., Israel, E., Smith, G., and Drasen, J. M. (1989). Amplification of airway constriction due to liquid-filling of airway interstices. *J. Appl. Physiol.* 66: 2873–2884.

Yager, D., Shore, S., and Drasen, J. M. (1991). Airway luminal liquid. Sources and roles as an amplifier of bronchoconstriction. *Am. Rev. Respir. Dis.* 143: S52–S54.

16

Sputum Production and Chronic Bronchitis

SANFORD CHODOSH

Veterans Administration Outpatient Clinic
and Boston University School of Medicine
Boston, Massachusetts

I. Introduction

The sputum expectorated by chronic bronchitic patients serves as a mirror of the ongoing pathological process in the bronchial tree. Evaluation of the various components that make up this complex material can provide important information to describe the current clinical status of the individual patient, as well as insight concerning the basic pathophysiology of the disease itself. However, description of the sputum in chronic bronchitis is confounded by several factors. From the clinical perspective, the definition of chronic bronchitis is based on simple, nondifferential symptoms. The presence of chronic productive cough on most days for 3 months in each of 2 successive years does not separate chronic bronchial asthma, tuberculosis, or cystic fibrosis from chronic bronchitis. The nature of the airway obstruction, when present, is also not diagnostic of the specific broncho-pulmonary disease process. Most investigations of sputum do not describe the criteria used to establish that the material examined actually came from patients with chronic bronchitis. The frequent concurrence of chronic bronchitis and bronchial asthma in the same patient further compounds the dilemma. Authors who describe the population studied as chronic obstructive pulmonary disease (COPD) at least are acknowledging that their investigations failed to specify which of the diseases that constitute COPD were included. Chronic bronchitics also vary considerably in severity of illness so that either stratification for this factor should be considered, or large numbers of patients need to be studied.

Additional problems exist because of the nature of the expectorated sputum itself. There is almost a universal admixture with oral secretions, with occasional contamination with nasopharyngeal material. Few investigators describe whether, or how, they separated out the bronchial material from the contaminating secretions from other sources. Assumptions that such separation can be made based on the physical appearance of the material are invalid. Even when careful selection of bronchial material is performed, the homogeneity may be questioned, particularly in clinically stable subjects. Descriptions of the pathology suggest that different levels of infection, inflammation, and stasis of secretions are going on in different areas of the chronic bronchitic's bronchial system, resulting in different kinds of sputum being produced, with the expectorated material being a conglomerate of these.

Despite all of these problems, the study of the sputum can reveal much about the disease called chronic bronchitis and about other bronchopulmonary disease. Sputum has the unique attribute of being repetitively and noninvasively available from the same patient so that the dynamics of naturally occurring and imposed changes can be observed.

II. Chronic Bronchitis

Understanding the nature of the sputum in chronic bronchitis requires a perspective of the characteristics of the disease itself. Chronic bronchitis has likely always affected mankind, since the causative factors have been present throughout human history. The historical significance is difficult to ascertain, since it shares a similar set of symptoms with many other diseases. Laennec first provided a useful clinical description in the early 1800s, calling it *catarrhe muqueux*. Biermer, in 1855, first recognized the value of sputum examination in differentiating chronic bronchitis from other lung diseases in which sputum is produced. The importance of bacterial infection in chronic bronchitis was noted in the early 1900s. However, it was not until the middle of the 20th century that chronic bronchitis again received attention as a separate disease entity. Despite its social and economic importance, the basic information concerning etiology, pathophysiology, natural course, and management remains incomplete. Even the standard definition of *chronic bronchitis* reflects the lack of definitive criteria (American Thoracic Society, 1962); namely, chronic productive cough that lasts for at least 3 months of the year for 2 successive years. This assumes the exclusion of other causes of this symptom complex, such as asthma, tuberculosis, carcinoma of the lung, cystic fibrosis, congestive heart failure, and pulmonary mycosis.

The incidence of chronic bronchitis has been estimated from a number of epidemiological studies and health statistics data. These data likely underestimate the incidence, since many individuals consider their cough and sputum production to be normal. Despite this, studies in the United States suggest that 30–60% of adults who smoke cigarettes have the symptoms of chronic bronchitis. Ferris and Anderson (1962) estimated that chronic bronchitis, with or without emphysema, occurred in 15–30% of adults in a small town. Medical survey data indicate that, of the large number with symptoms, only 7.5 million Americans seek medical care for these symptoms. The economic impact on individual patients and society in terms of morbidity, mortality, and dollars is immense.

The societal factors responsible for the high worldwide incidence of chronic bronchitis include cigarette smoking, air pollution, and bronchopulmonary infections. The epidemic proportions of cigarette smoking in this century may well be most important. Inhaled cigarette smoke contains a large load of particulates that increase mucociliary clearance demands, as well as gas-phase cell toxins. The severity of chronic bronchitis is directly related to the number of cigarettes that an individual smokes. There is strong evidence that children secondarily exposed to cigarette smoke in the home are predisposed to chronic bronchopulmonary problems. Industrialization has exposed more workers to a large variety of toxic dusts and fumes and increased air pollution in many of the urban areas. This persists as a problem, despite environmental and health policies aimed at decreasing these risks. Bronchopulmonary infection is a frequent etiological factor in the initiation of the chronic bronchitis syndrome. Although definitive preventive and therapeutic means exist to minimize the effect of such infections, inadequate health care in many parts of the world work against the advantage such measures could provide. Decreasing cigarette smoking results in measurable gains in decreasing the incidence of chronic bronchitis and carcinoma of the lung. The results of reducing air pollution is less easily measured, but is biologically sensible. Providing prompt and appropriate treatment of the common "chest cold" would clearly slow the progression of existing chronic bronchitis and could be preventative in many instances. Decreasing the incidence and severity of chronic bronchitis would be a worthy worldwide goal.

Understanding the composition and origins of the sputum produced in chronic bronchitis requires a comprehension of the known and possible pathophysiological mechanisms operative in this disease (Chodosh, 1980a). Individual susceptibility to the development of chronic bronchitis is at least partially determined by host factors that may be either inherited or acquired, or both. Host defense mechanisms are dependent on cellular, immunological, nonspecific humoral, and mucociliary functions, as well as pathological changes of anatomical structure. Additionally, compromise of host defense function may be compounded by dysfunctions associated with other concurrent diseases, such as tuberculosis, bronchiectasis, or asthma; or because of unusual exposures to toxic bronchial stimuli.

No single specific cause of chronic bronchitis has been identified. It would appear that numerous toxic stimuli may be involved and affect the susceptible bronchi through their inhalation and their inherent toxic or stimulating action. These inhaled toxic stimuli include gases, particles, and infectious agents. Some of the gases commonly implicated are sulfur dioxide, oxidant air pollutants, cyanide, and anesthetic agents. Besides containing toxic gases, cigarette smoke supplies the major load of particulates that impinge on the bronchopulmonary system. Dusty work environments and hydrocarbon particles in air pollution are also sources of potentially noxious particles. Viral, bacterial, mycobacterial, and fungal infections of the lung are frequent initiating stimuli. It is unclear how these various factors interact, but histories of chronic bronchitics often suggest that more than one factor is operative. For example, an acute infectious bronchitis in a cigarette smoker appears to be more likely to lead to chronic bronchitis than the same acute infection in a nonsmoker. Variations in host defense mechanisms also seems important in that the symptoms of chronic bronchitis may appear within months of initiating cigarette smoking in one individual, but may never develop in another who has smoked for decades.

The bronchial response to toxic stimuli may be separated into at least four categories: inflammation, hypersecretion, increased vagal (cholinergic) discharge, and ciliary dysfunction. The level of response of each of these factors probably varies from one individual to the next. Some of the interrelationships of these responses that result in the clinical picture called chronic bronchitis are known, but others still remain hypotheses. It is likely that increased vagal activity and the inflammatory response become additional stimuli to hypersecretion (Florey, 1970). Mediators such as histamine, leukotrienes, prostaglandins, and other agents from inflammatory cells may contribute to mucous secretion (Raphael and Metcalfe, 1986). There is little doubt that, once hypersecretion becomes established, the excessive and abnormal interluminal material plays an important role in the clinical features that characterize chronic bronchitis (Chodosh, 1980b). The increase of secretions mixed with the products of inflammation would adversely affect mucociliary clearance. The excessive coughing associated with attempts to clear secretions may further cause more vagal discharge. With the delayed clearance of bacteria, infection of the bronchial tissue occurs with establishment of a resident population of pathogens. This low-grade infectious process now can act as an internal toxic stimulus to elicit more of all four types of bronchial response. This may explain, in part, why some chronic bronchitics persist with symptoms even when they eliminate some of the external toxic stimuli (e.g., cigarette smoking).

The pathological changes in the bronchial tissue support the concept of chronic bronchitis as a distinct disease entity and of the pathophysiological mechanisms involved. Reid (1960) described the mucous gland hypertrophy and hyperplasia which, along with proliferation of the goblet cells in the ciliated bronchial epithelium, have become key diagnostic features of chronic bronchitis. These changes have been noted before the development of the characteristic symptoms of chronic productive cough, and clearly are the anatomical correlate for the hypersecretion response. Less striking, but perhaps more significant changes in the bronchial epithelium were described by Auerbach et al. (1961) in chronic cigarette smokers. They noted scattered areas of shallow mucosal ulcerations interspersed with normal ciliated or metaplastic epithelium, suggesting that the pathological changes are not uniform throughout the bronchial tree. There is also hyperplasia of the basal cell layer of the bronchial epithelium, which may contribute to metaplasia. Although the development of metaplasia is disadvantageous to ciliary function, it is possible that metaplastic epithelium may be more resistant to infection or damage. These abnormalities decline in severity in exsmokers, and the epithelium becomes indistinguishable from that of nonsmokers after 5–10 years of smoking cessation. This strongly suggests that chronic bronchitis is a curable disease. Each area of damaged bronchial epithelium elicits a typical inflammatory response unique to the temporal onset and etiology of that injury; the acute response is characterized by an initial preponderance of neutrophils followed by an influx of monocytes and macrophages as resolution of each local process occurs. The ratio of neutrophils to mononuclear cells observed in the expectorated sputum reflects the balance between the number of areas with acute inflammation versus the number of areas recovering from the injury. These ulcerated areas may heal with regrowth of normal ciliated epithelium, but may be replaced with metaplasia. Such nonciliated areas likely contribute to chronically inadequate ciliary clearance of secretions. Medici and Chodosh (1973) estimated the average extent of bronchial epithelial damage in the stable chronic bronchitic and during acute bacterial exacerbations of the disease at a loss of 5.26 cm^2 and 10.10 cm^2 of surface epithelium per day, respectively. A chronic bronchitic who remained free of acute bacterial exacerbations would denude approximately one-third of the bronchial epithelium in 1 year. This figure obviously would vary considerably with different severities of chronic bronchitis. There are several pathological and physiological changes in chronic bronchitis that contribute to a chronic inadequacy of ciliary clearance of secretions. Pathologically, metaplasia replaces normal ciliated epithelium in localized areas subjected to recurrent injury. The proliferation of goblet cells crowds out ciliated epithelial cells. Physiologically, normal ciliary function is adversely affected by exposure to cigarette smoke, other toxic inhalants, and viral infection. The thickened layer of abnormal and excessive exudate that covers the ciliated epithelial surface makes it impossible for even normally beating cilia to move secretions. This set of circumstances leads the individual patient to use cough as the means of expelling these secretions.

More subtle influences on the pathophysiology of chronic bronchitis relate to defects in the immunological, cellular, and nonspecific host defense mechanisms. It is unclear if the defects of these systems in chronic bronchitis are inherited, acquired, or both. The submucosa in established chronic bronchitis has increased accumulations of lymphocytes and plasma cells (Hers, 1961; Salvato, 1968). Immunoglobulins A, M, G, and E are found in these cells. Secretory IgA, which is locally produced, is of prime importance in protection of the respiratory tract against infection (Tomasi, 1971; Chanock, 1971). Medici and Bürgi (1971) found that the amount of IgA in the sputum decreased as the severity of the chronic bronchitis increased. It is not clear whether a decreased production of secretory IgA leads to a more severe disease state or vice versa.

There is also evidence that the reticuloendothelial system cells in the inflammatory response in chronic bronchitis is deficient, particularly the polymorphonuclear neutrophil (PMN) and macrophage. The PMN is essential in the protection of the host against microbial invaders (Hirsch, 1965). Medici and Chodosh (1972) observed that PMNs were excreted daily in the sputum of stable chronic bronchitics in hundreds of millions, and that this increased significantly during acute bacterial exacerbations. The numbers of PMN with phagocytosed bacteria also increased with acute infection. However, the percentage of PMN with ingested bacteria was low when the patients were stable (4.06 ± 3.35) and did not increase in the face of acute bacterial infection (4.08 ± 3.52). Eichel and Chodosh (1976) observed that cigarette-smoking chronic bronchitics have less sputum myeloperoxidase than ex-smokers, and that the amount of myeloperoxidase per PMN did not increase in smokers during acute bacterial exacerbations. Sputum myeloperoxidase is almost totally derived from the PMN in chronic bronchitis, for which it is important in the bactericidal activity of the PMN. These defects in response to bacterial infection in chronic cigarette smokers may partially explain why this subgroup of chronic bronchitics appear to have difficulty in managing this toxic insult. There is also evidence that the macrophage in chronic bronchitis is inadequate in the sputum in maintaining cellular host defense. The macrophage seen in the sputum in chronic bronchitis is likely derived from circulating blood lymphocytes or monocytes and tissue histiocytes, which are attracted to the necrotic ulcerated areas of bronchial mucosa as a normal part of the inflammatory process. These bronchial macrophages (BM), which provide antimicrobial action, appear to be morphologically and functionally distinct from alveolar macrophages (Truitt and Mackaness, 1971; Mackaness, 1971). Observations by Medici and Chodosh (1972) of changes in sputum from chronic bronchitics suggest that the number of macrophages is decreased during acute bacterial exacerbations, with increases during recovery, although the timing of these changes varies with each event. This may imply a deficiency of cellular host defense, but it may merely reflect the predominant role of the PMN during the acute inflammatory response. The bactericidal function of BM may be compromised in cigarette-smoking chronic bronchitics (Eichel and Chodosh, 1976). Sputum catalase activity is considerably less in smokers than in ex-smokers when they are clinically stable, and there is tenfold less activity in the face of acute bacterial infection. These bits of evidence suggest that chronic bronchitic smokers have less than adequate cellular host defense capability.

Chronic vagal stimulation results in increased cholinergic activity, which increases the bronchomotor tone of the bronchial smooth muscle and reduces the diameter of the bronchi. The airway obstruction seen in chronic bronchitis is likely related to this abnormality, along with the excessive bronchial secretions and exudate. Complete plugging of smaller bronchi may well lead to increased levels of carbon dioxide in the airways, retrograde to the obstruction, a condition that may be conducive for the growth of certain microorganisms.

Although little is known about the initial pathophysiological events in chronic bronchitis, the widely accepted theory is that the initial event is hypersecretion of mucus, which leads to hypertrophy and hyperplasia of the mucus-producing cells in the bronchial mucosa. Knauss et al. (1976) presented data from the sulfur dioxide-exposed rat model, suggesting that the earliest change is an exudation of inflammatory cells that occurs before there is evidence of hypersecretion. The increase of material in the bronchi after 9 h of exposure to sulfur dioxide was entirely due to cell mass. The first increase of non-cell–mass was noted only after 30 h of exposure. Considering the temporal relation of events, it is unclear if the sulfur dioxide eventually resulted in the hypersecretion, or if the inflammatory response was the essential precursor event. Since most toxic stimuli implicated in chronic bronchitis result in cell death, it is not surprising that the inflammatory response appears to be the logical next event. Evidence of the importance of inflammation of cartilaginous airways in human chronic bronchitis was reported by Mullen et al. (1985). They noted that those with chronic bronchitis had significantly greater inflammation on mucosal surfaces and around glands and gland ducts than did a group without chronic bronchitis; whereas, the two groups did not differ in Reid's indexes, pulmonary function, condition of small airways, or emphysema. Indeed, "chronic" bronchitis is likely a misnomer. Data to be noted later demonstrates that the neutrophil is usually the main inflammatory cell seen in active chronic bronchitis. The clinical picture that is most commonly seen suggests that it should be renamed so that the recurrent, overlapping, acute bronchitis aspects are taken into consideration.

III. Sputum

Sputum is the abnormal material produced by, or expectorated from, the bronchopulmonary system. Production of sputum by a patient is indicative of an ongoing pathological process in the lung. Evaluation of its constituents provides an opportunity to define the nature of the pathological process that it reflects and is useful for investigations of the inflammatory process in humans. Sputum is the frequently neglected "biopsy" material that is repetitively available without the aid of invasive procedures. Observations of chronic bronchitic sputum can reveal important clinical information concerning the type and level of the inflammatory process, the physical properties of the material, the extent of bronchial mucosal damage, and the identification of pathogenic microorganisms that may be present. Assessment of the nature of the inflammatory response can provide key information for the differential diagnosis between chronic bronchitis and chronic bronchial asthma, for which the clinical presentation may be very similar. In known chronic bronchitics, the same methods can be applied to determining the likely cause of acute exacerbations and for evaluating the efficacy of many of the treatment modalities used in this disease.

The ultimate value of any of the stated evaluations depends on obtaining a valid collection of sputum from the bronchopulmonary tree (Chodosh, 1988). The common method of collection in chronic bronchitis is by spontaneous expectoration; although noninvasive passage through the oropharynx often leads to admixture with oral and nasopharyngeal secretions. Other methods of obtaining sputum may also suffer from this problem. However, microscopic assessment of selected aliquots can determine the bronchopulmonary versus oropharyngeal origin of the specimen. The collection method employed should be dictated by clinical judgment in each case. Factors that should be considered include the seriousness of the disease state, the need to establish a definitive diagnosis, the risks of the procedure, the ability of a given technique to provide the needed information, and the ability of the patient to cooperate with the procedure. Collecting expectorated sputum is noninvasive and is repetitively available for following the course of the disease process. Any random specimen can provide qualitative information that is useful. However, quantitative assessment of the severity of the inflammatory response and the extent of bronchial damage becomes possible only when sputum is collected over a set period. A 24-h collection is particularly useful in patients whose expectoration is variable throughout the day. Patients often need to be instructed to collect material produced by deep cough, but secretions expectorated after throat clearing also may have come from the lung. The true origin can readily be determined by microscopic examination. Induction of sputum expectoration can be useful in patients not spontaneously expectorating when clinical assessment suggests the presence of secretions. Teaching the patient more efficient cough maneuvers, repetitive chest percussion with cupped hands or externally applied vibrators, and appropriate postural drainage techniques are useful methods. Inhalation of aerosols of bronchodilators, saline, or irritative materials may stimulate a more productive cough. The combination of an inhaled aerosol followed by mechanical induction methods may be successful. Invasive methods should not be used if satisfactory specimens can be obtained by either spontaneous or induced expectoration. Occasionally, in children or debilitated adults, gastric contents containing swallowed mucous plugs can be obtained through gastric aspiration or in vomitus. This possible source of sputum should not be ignored.

In chronic bronchitis, the invasive procedures that can be used to obtain sputum include tracheobronchial aspiration, bronchoscopy, and transtracheal aspiration. The use of these methods becomes important when the patient cannot cooperate because of depressed mental status or inability to develop an effective cough. With tracheobronchial aspiration, a wide-bore catheter is passed through the nose or mouth and secretions obtained with gentle and intermittent suctioning. Accomplishing this in alert patients requires their understanding and cooperation. Irritation from the catheter usually induces cough, which can move secretions closer to the catheter tip. The instillation of a bolus of a few milliliters of sterile saline may induce productive cough and loosen secretions, although this introduces a variable dilution factor. Advantages are that removal of secretions may be therapeutically indicated anyway, more invasive procedures can be avoided, professionals specially trained to perform bronchoscopy or transtracheal aspiration are not required, thicker secretions are more likely to be obtained through the catheter's large bore, and the procedure can be easily repeated. Disadvantages include damage to mucosa, with possible bleeding from unnecessarily vigorous suctioning; induction of vomiting, with subsequent bronchopulmonary aspiration; apnea secondary to neural reflex stimulation; and hypoxemia if oxygen-enriched ventilation is not provided during the procedure. The use of this procedure is quite simple in patients with an endotracheal tube or tracheostomy. The specimens obtained may be contaminated by aspiration of upper respiratory secretions into the tracheobronchial tree. The flexible fiber-optic bronchoscope provides a useful means of obtaining secretions under direct visualization. Contamination with upper respiratory secretions can be minimized if a protected catheter tip is used. The disadvantages of this procedure are that highly trained professionals are required and, in chronic bronchitis, samples should be obtained from several different areas to be representative of the processes in the various parts of the bronchopulmonary system. Obtaining such samples usually requires use of variable amounts of lavage fluid, which needs to be considered (Thompson and Rennard, 1988). Transtracheal aspiration by direct, percutaneous cricothyroid puncture should not be a routine procedure for obtaining secretions. Although relatively safe in the hands of experienced professionals, it has been associated with serious complications. The stated advantage of minimizing upper respiratory secretion admixture is lost if the catheter tip is inadvertently directed toward the larynx, or is coughed into that position by the patient. Aspiration of thick secretions through the small-bore catheter used in this procedure is difficult. Transtracheal aspiration is contraindicated if the patient has a bleeding diathesis, severe cough, or active hemoptysis. With all of these invasive procedures, microscopic examination of the obtained material should be used to ascertain that the material is of bronchopulmonary origin.

The techniques of handling the specimen during and after collection may be just as important as the method used for collection. The type of examination to be carried out should be kept in mind to determine the appropriate methodology. A common misunderstanding is that it is essential to deal only with freshly collected specimens, with particular emphasis on the first of the morning expectoration. Numerous evaluations in my laboratory have demonstrated that the 24-h collection of sputum from chronic bronchitics is at least as valid as fresh specimens when the evaluations are concerned with the cellular constituents, microbiology, biochemical, and even measurement of physical properties. The mucins in the sputum gel appear to be an excellent milieu for maintaining the integrity of the specimen. If bacterial flora is to be evaluated by cultures, the inhibiting effect of local anesthetics or the bacteriostatic additives in sterile saline used for lavage, as well as inadvertent contamination by secretions from the upper airways, must be avoided. Specimens being aspirated should be directed into sterile Lukens traps without the use of any solution. Mechanical homogenization leads to destruction of cells and enzymatic lysis of the mucous gel may destroy cells and microorganisms (Medici et al., 1988).

Ascertaining that the specimen originated in the lung and the selection of valid aliquots for evaluation requires a simple, but essential step. The specimen should be placed in a petri dish and examined macroscopically for areas most likely to be true sputum. Such areas should be transferred to a glass slide and scanned microscopically under low power. Reducing the transmitted light makes identification of the cells easier. If there are significant numbers of large, irregularly shaped oropharyngeal squamous cells noted, the aliquot is not representative of the process in the lung. The presence of even a rare macrophage identifies that the aliquot is from the lung. This latter type of material should be used in all subsequent examinations.

A. Composition and Characteristics of Sputum

The composition of the sputum that is coughed up in pure chronic bronchitis is a complex mixture of mucous secretions from the bronchial system and exudative products from the mucosal ulcerations and the inflammatory response to these lesions. In addition, there are elements that have been inhaled or aspirated into the bronchopulmonary system. If there is any associated pulmonary edema, then substances related to the transudation may also be present. The interrelations of the various elements in the individual's sputum determine the gross appearance of the sputum and its physical properties. The composition may vary in the same chronic bronchitic depending on the current diseased state when the specimen is collected. Even greater variations in composition may be observed when comparing one bronchitic's sputum with others. Descriptions of composition should be considered in the context of such variability. The clinical circumstances at the time specimens are obtained should be carefully defined. The existing literature in this area generally has not stratified results based on such criteria. Clinical categorizations should consider the duration and severity of the bronchitic state, the presence or absence of acute inflammatory events, the cigarette-smoking status at the time of collection, and the association with other diseases that could influence the composition of the sputum being produced.

Description of the constituents of sputum may best be divided into cellular, noncellular, and nonpulmonary elements. The cellular composition can be further divided into cells that are exfoliated from the bronchial tissue, those originated in the alveolar areas, and inflammatory cells from the circulation. The noncellular material originates from the mucus-producing cells of the lung, the noncellular exudate or transudate, and cellular breakdown products. Nonpulmonary elements include microorganisms and inhaled or aspirated materials.

The mixture of these components determines the gross appearance of the sputum in terms of the volume expectorated, the color, and the rheological properties of the material. The information that most clinicians obtain from sputum examination is often limited to these gross physical characteristics. A useful general principle is that the volume of sputum expectorated usually reflects the severity of the chronic bronchitis. The volume should be obtained over a set period. A routine collection that includes a 24-h period is most valuable, since this accommodates the variability among bronchitics in terms of when each raises their sputum. Less representative is the common practice of measuring only that sputum that is raised shortly after the patient arises in the morning. The premise that this morning collection is fresher or more representative is not substantiated by critical data (Medici et al., 1988).

Daily sputum volume measurements provide a useful and simple parameter for following the course of the chronic bronchitic process in a single patient and for comparisons between different subgroups of chronic bronchitics. Quantitative sputum investigations absolutely require a timed period of collection. Weighing the specimen in a preweighed collection container makes the measurement simple. Patients must be repetitively instructed to collect only sputum raised from the lungs by means of deep cough to maintain a consistency of specimens. The volume of sputum may need to be adjusted if microscopic evaluation of the specimen reveals that some portion of the material was nonpulmonary in origin. The patient often misjudges the amount of sputum being expectorated; thus, historical estimates often do not correlate with actual measurements. The range of volumes expectorated in chronic bronchitis varies from 1 to 100 ml/day, with a rare individual producing more. The average range is 5–40 ml/day when patients are clinically stable, and may double or triple when acute infection is present (Medici and Chodosh, 1973). Individual chronic bronchitic patients tend to expectorate similar daily volumes, as long as their clinical status remains stable. One must assume that not all of the sputum produced in the bronchopulmonary tree is expectorated, since some portion often is swallowed. However, individual patients tend to have a consistent pattern. Changes in their clinical status can markedly alter their daily sputum volume. The patient who decreases their cigarette smoking significantly can easily demonstrate a tenfold decrease in sputum volume, and some may even stop sputum expectoration. Increases of daily sputum volume are most commonly associated with increases of bronchial infection or of cigarette smoke inhalation, although an increased exposure to any toxic stimulus may be implicated.

The color and estimations of the specimen's degree of purulence can also provide some valuable information concerning the pathology in the bronchopulmonary system. As with all other aspects of sputum evaluation, it is essential that the areas described originated in the lung. Contaminating saliva may look mucoid and expectorated sinonasal drainage may look purulent. Mucoid sputum resembles fresh egg white, but varies from this clear translucency to a whitish or opalescent appearance as more intact cells are concentrated in the specimen. Secretions with this appearance have usually been cleared quickly from the airways following their excretion into the bronchi and are not a reflection of the cellularity of the specimen. The purulence of the specimen depends on the degree of yellow to green coloration. The usual implication of purulence in the literature is that this finding is synonymous with the presence of bronchopulmonary infection. Robertson (1952) clearly related this green coloration to the presence of myeloperoxidase released from degenerated PMN, an enzyme also prevalent in eosinophils. This coloration strongly suggests stasis in the airways of secretions containing polymorphonuclear leukocytes, which allows time for these cells (either neutrophils or eosinophils) to break down and release their peroxidases. The more peroxidases released, the greener the specimen. The clinical implication of purulent sputum is that secretions are not being promptly cleared and, as such, is important information. Expectorated mucoid sputum containing significant numbers of polymorphonuclear leukocytes will show this same change to purulence if sufficient time passes. Sputum that has a gray or brownish color usually suggests excessive dust or tobacco smoke in the specimen. Patients exposed to smoke from a fire can have almost black sputum. Pink- or reddish-colored sputum suggests the presence of red blood cells, although certain inhaled adrenergic bronchodilators may also cause this coloration. Red blood cell breakdown products give a brownish coloration to the sputum. Chronic bronchitis is the most common cause of overt hemoptysis, and there is often microscopic evidence of red blood cell extravasation in the specimens. Certain foods can impart different colors to sputum, but are usually the result of contamination during passage of the expectorated material through the mouth. Coffee, chocolate, and tea are common here.

The rheology of airway mucus is discussed at length elsewhere in this book. Assessment of these physical properties of chronic bronchitic sputum is of considerable clinical importance. Dulfano and Philippoff (1973) described many of the problems inherent in the systematic characterization of the physical properties of sputum. The standard rheological principles, as derived from knowledge of newtonian substances, are difficult to directly apply to sputum, with its heterogeneous composition. The complex interactions between the large and small molecules, particles, and intact cellular elements provide the basis for a physicist's nightmare. When sputum is placed in a glass dish and examined against a dark background, it is apparent that it is composed of strands and plugs of varying sizes and densities. Characterization in the standard terms of viscosity, adhesiveness, elasticity, shearing forces, and stress relaxation may have little clinical or practical value. It is likely that measurements of sputum made in equipment developed for newtonian fluids provides results that cannot be interpreted on sound physicochemical principles. Studies carried out by Chodosh et al. (1973a) compared the results obtained using five different methods for measuring physical properties from 169 fresh sputum samples from bronchitics. The methods included the Chodosh inclined tube, Brookfield plate-cone (Lieberman, 1968), Visco-Consistometer (Hirsch, et al., 1966), Haake plate-cone, and Haake couette. Although there was a scattering of significant correlations between most of the techniques, there was considerable nonuniformity of relation between methods and within measurements from the same methods. Even when correlations were found, the level of significance made it unlikely that the results from one method could be predictive of those from the other. The conclusion was that different techniques measure different, and possibly unrelated, physical properties of the sputum.

Despite these methodological problems, some relationships between measured physical properties and other sputum characteristics and clinical measurements have been observed. Sturgess et al. (1970) found that purulent sputum had a higher viscosity than mucoid sputum; whereas, Dulfano et al. (1971) observed that elastic recoil values were lower in purulent sputum than in mucoid sputum. Sputum viscosity also appears to be directly related to the DNA content (Bürgi et al., 1968), a factor that could explain the relationship of viscosity with sputum purulence. The major source of both myeloperoxidase and DNA is lysed PMN. Viscosity in chronic bronchitic sputum is also likely related to the amount of mucoproteins or mucopolysaccharides, since sputum viscosity can be dramatically decreased by the action of N-acetylcysteine (Chodosh, 1971). The contribution of intrabronchial secretions to airway obstruction in chronic bronchitis is based on both clinical and pathological observations. Several investigations have demonstrated that the degree of airway obstruction is inversely related to the physical properties of the sputum (i.e., the thicker the sputum, the greater the decrease of ventilatory capacity; Chodosh et al., 1973b; Keal and Reid, 1973; Lopez-Vidriero, 1973; Pham et al., 1973).

In general, a causal relation between these various characteristics and the physical properties of the sputum remains somewhat conjectural. However, the nature of the bondings that can exist between the large molecular structures, such as DNA and mucoproteins, with small ions and molecules are the likely basis for the rheological characteristics. However, for practical purposes in the clinical setting, a great deal can be deduced about the physical properties from a few simple maneuvers. Inverting the sample in the collection container provides an estimate of the thickness; thin specimens flow like water and the thickest ones do not change shape. The adhesive nature of the sputum can be simultaneously described as the degree to which the specimen sticks to the wall of the container. Grades of thickness between the extremes can be estimated by how the specimen holds together when a wooden applicator stick is used to pull out a portion of the sample. The surface tension of the specimen may also be estimated by noting the extent to which air bubbles are trapped in the specimen. This may be noted microscopically when tiny bubbles are noted in the background matrix of the sputum. However, these bubbles are often seen macroscopically, and the number can be sufficiently great to give a foamlike appearance at the surface of the specimen. These bubbles are usually very resistant to being broken.

When one considers the difficulty in measuring the rheological properties of sputum and the incomplete understanding of how the various components of sputum contribute to the physical characteristics, it is not surprising that our ability to therapeutically alter sputum remains somewhat empirical. Some insight into the physical properties of sputum has been achieved from studies of therapeutic agents used in chronic bronchitis. There is no doubt, from the clinical perspective, that clearance of the excessive secretions from the tracheobronchial tree is of great therapeutic importance in chronic bronchitis. In addition, little is known about how to control the production of these secretions. It is clear that measures that decrease the toxic stimuli (e.g., treatment of bacterial infection or decreased cigarette smoking) have a dramatic beneficial effect. Therapy for existing secretion problems are often empirical and less than ideal. A few of these measures may modify production and others clearly act on the already formed interluminal secretions. Adequate hydration is recommended as an essential measure, although the evidence for efficacy of oral or parenteral water is limited. Chodosh (1973) demonstrated that extra oral water increased the water content and decreased the apparent viscosity of sputum in chronic bronchitis, without increasing the volume expectorated. In vivo evidence that modifying the humidification of the inspired air affects sputum physical properties has not been demonstrated, but is commonly advocated on the basis of benefit noted clinically. Inhaled aerosolized saline appears to increase sputum thickness (Chodosh, 1980c), contrary to the belief by many clinicians that this is useful therapy. Definitive evidence of how drugs considered to be expectorants, (e.g., guaifenesin, iodides, and ammonium chloride) affect the production of secretions is minimal. Despite their common use, there remains considerable controversy concerning mechanisms of action and clinical efficacy. Chodosh (1973) demonstrated that large oral doses of guaifenesin significantly decreased the adhesiveness of sputum, with minimal effect on apparent viscosity or sputum volume. There was suggestive evidence that there was an effect on the water-binding capacity of the sputum gel. Thomson et al. (1973) demonstrated that guaifenesin increased mucociliary clearance. There is other evidence that guaifenesin may decrease platelet adhesiveness and have a protective action on maintaining alveolar surfactant in the face of toxic challenge. The general conclusion from these various studies is that guaifenesin may work on surface adhesiveness. Animal studies with iodides also suggest a protective effect on pulmonary surfactant. However, there is no objective evidence that iodides exert a beneficial effect when used therapeutically in chronic bronchitis. Clinical efficacy has been demonstrated using subjective parameters. The widespread use of these expectorants with apparent clinical benefit suggests that methods to describe the underlying mechanisms of their actions have not yet been developed.

The mechanisms of action of pharmacological agents that are active on the preformed secretions already in the bronchi are more precisely known. The mucolytic N-acetylcysteine is clearly effective in decreasing apparent viscosity when directly applied to sputum. Dulfano and Philippoff (1973) demonstrated a marked decrease of both sputum viscosity and elastic recoil in in vitro experiments. This has a direct clinical correlation with the evidence of efficacy when N-acetylcysteine solution is directly instilled by bronchoscopy to loosen mucous plugs in the bronchi. Sheffner (1963) demonstrated that the sulfhydryl group of N-acetylcysteine splits the disulfide bonds of mucoproteins, resulting in mucolysis. Evidence that inhaling aerosolized solutions of N-acetylcysteine is as immediately effective in chronic bronchitis is less definitive. This is undoubtedly because of difficulty in delivering the active agent to areas of the bronchial tree that are poorly ventilated because of obstruction by the very secretions that are the objectives of the therapy. Although several investigations of short-term (7 days) therapy showed decreases of apparent viscosity without clinical improvement, this could not be confirmed in a double-blinded and crossover study of Chodosh (1980c). The gross estimation of sputum thickness showed a significant decrease with N-acetylcysteine, but measured apparent viscosity did not show a significant decrease. Chodosh et al. (1975) did demonstrate dramatic decreases in sputum viscosity and volume in a few patients after 30–45 days of daily inhalation therapy; effects that were reversed when aerosolized saline was then substituted for the N-acetylcysteine. There is little evidence to support a mucolytic action of N-acetylcysteine administered in low-dose orally, although this is advocated in several countries. Other agents, such as S-carboxymethylcysteine, bromhexadine (Bisolvon), N-acetyl-L-cysteine (Mucosolvin), or bromhexine have little objective evidence of efficacy. Agents active in breaking the DNA molecules in sputum have been used therapeutically. Deoxyribonuclease (DNase) derived from bovine pancreas was too allergenic and insufficiently effective. The recent development of human recombinant DNase may be a safer agent. Preliminary studies in cystic fibrosis have demonstrated clinical efficacy (Hubbard et al., 1992), and in vitro studies with sputum from cystic fibrosis patients demonstrate decreases of sputum thickness (Shak et al., 1990). The mechanism of action appears to be the fragmentation of the DNA molecules. Although decreases of apparent viscosity should improve the ability of patients with chronic bronchitis to clear secretions, this is not always the result. Sputum that is made too thin may still maintain significant elastic recoil. Patients often find it easier to move a thicker bolus of secretions with cough than a thin material that may be easily deformed by cough, but not significantly moved. A great deal still remains to be clarified about the physical properties of sputum and the therapeutic modalities used to affect these characteristics.

B. Cellular Constituents

Cells are a major constituent of sputum in chronic bronchitis. Evaluation of these cells can provide valuable information about the function of cells, the nature and extent of bronchial mucosal damage, the severity of the chronic bronchitis, and serve as a useful means of differentiating the various chronic bronchial diseases, and help ascertain the etiology of the various types of acute exacerbations that occur in chronic bronchitis. With the exceptions of studies carried out by European investigators in the beginning of this century, there have been few applications of sputum cell examination, except for cancer screening. The earlier work has been reviewed and reported by Bezançon and De Jong (1913), von Hoesslin (1926), and Clifford (1932), and these texts are still the most comprehensive reviews of this field. The application of sputum cell examination was stimulated when Papanicolaou (1954) published his excellent studies on exfoliative cytology. Although the prime use has been for diagnosis of cancer of the lung, it was not generally appreciated that this same approach can be useful in the investigation of the bronchopulmonary system in chronic bronchial diseases and other nonmalignant disorders. Chodosh et al. (1961) first described methods for the qualitative and quantitative determination of the bronchial epithelial and inflammatory cells exfoliated into the sputum in various bronchial disorders. It was obvious that the number and relative frequency of the various cells exuded into the bronchial lumen and expectorated in sputum reflect the nature, extent, and severity of the bronchial inflammatory process in the specific diseases. Bertalanaffy (1968) used this information to study the turnover of specific cell types in the lung. The availability of this biopsy material over time also provided a technique for serial observations of pathological change associated with different, identifiable clinical conditions in humans. Advantages of this approach are that naturally occurring disease can be observed, sequential sampling of the product of inflammation is available, and the dynamics of spontaneous or therapeutically induced changes can be noted in individual subjects. The use of animals for such investigations is notably different, since the model pathological state is usually induced, and cohorts of animals are often required to mimic sequential observations.

Methods

Freshly expectorated sputum or 24-h sputum specimens may be used for qualitative sputum cytological studies. Quantitative sputum investigations require a specific-timed period of collection. Sputum presents certain problems when used for investigative work. There is concern for admixture with nonbronchopulmonary material, for nonhomogeneity of content from one area of the lung to another, and for the effects of cellular lysis. The use of microscopic selection of aliquots is absolutely essential, since macroscopic judgment has been unreliable in the selection of bronchopulmonary material (Medici et al., 1970). Chodosh (1970) found it possible to avoid adverse effects on cells caused by homogenization and to maintain the structural integrity of the mucous strands with the entrapped bronchopulmonary cells by examining selected portions of the intact specimen. This provided consistency of results, but was dependent on maintaining strict criteria for avoiding nonbronchopulmonary material. Individual subjects with chronic bronchitis produce qualitatively and quantitatively similar cell populations from day to day during periods of clinical stability (Chodosh, 1963). Gibson et al. (1989) confirmed the reproducibility of the qualitative and quantitative cell population measurements using different plugs from the same specimen and in the same patient from day to day. Deviations from stable levels were usually indicative of clinical change. Contrary to a widely held opinion, there is a remarkable preservation of cells in these sputum samples. Epithelial mucins, in which the sputum cells are imbedded and the cell membranes themselves are protected and fairly resistant to the proteolytic enzymes in sputum. The methodology for the qualitative and quantitative evaluation of sputum cell populations has been fully described by Medici and Chodosh (1973).

Cellular Constituents

Sputum cells can be divided into those exfoliated from the bronchopulmonary parenchyma and those inflammatory cells that appear in response to specific stimuli. Cells of the bronchopulmonary parenchyma are those originating from the bronchial epithelium and those from the alveolar areas. The cells of the bronchial epithelium can be specifically identified in their differentiation, and their exfoliation reflects the nature and extent of involvement of the bronchial mucosa. These represent most of the parenchymal lung cells seen in chronic bronchitis. The inflammatory cells are all representatives of the reticuloendothelial system, which function primarily as phagocytes or as elements of the immunological defense mechanisms or as both. These cells are a reflection of the cellular host defense capability of the bronchopulmonary system.

Bronchial Epithelial Cells

The numbers, types, and characteristics of the exfoliated bronchial epithelial cells (BEC) reflect the state of the bronchial mucosa. Cells are exfoliated from the three chief layers of the bronchial epithelium, representing degrees of differentiation from the basal through the intermediate, and to the columnar cell layer lining the bronchial lumen. The nuclei of BEC from all three layers remain morphologically similar, and it is the cytoplasm and cell shape that changes during differentiation. The nuclei are ovoid to round with a definite chromatin structure. Two nuclei may be seen in occasional cells. The cytoplasm generally has a fine granular reticular texture. Normal, nondegenerated BEC have the following appearances: The basal BEC are about the size of a lymphocyte and have the greatest nucleus/ cytoplasmic ratio. Intermediate-layer BEC have a greater cytoplasmic mass, with an irregular and more polygonal shape. The columnar BEC that line the lumen are either ciliated BEC or nonciliated goblet cells with their variably sized mucopoly-saccharide vacuoles. Both are approximately rectangular, often tapering to a long tail at one end. The nucleus often bulges out the cell membrane in tapered cells. The ciliated brush border of the ciliated BEC faces the bronchial lumen, and the origins of the cilia just beneath the cell membrane are seen as a dark line. The cilia themselves are very delicate, hairlike structures about 5–7 μm long in unfixed preparations, but are shorter after fixation. The secretory system of the goblet cells is at the broader lumenal end and may bulge out the cell with its mucinous product. The exfoliated bronchial epithelial cell types in chronic bronchitis rarely have the normal appearances just described and generally show various degrees of degeneration or metaplastic change, or have intracellular bacteria. Degenerated basal or ciliated BEC are usually pyknotic, with clumped chromatin in the nuclei. Cilia are rarely noted on the columnar cells. Metaplastic BEC either have abnormalities of the nucleus or an orange-red cytoplasm on hematoxylin and eosin (H&E) type stains, generally with features suggesting keratinization. The BEC with bacteria have an intracellular body that possesses the distinct morphological characteristics of a bacterium.

The mucosal layer of the trachea and the bronchi extends to the terminal bronchioles (14–16 generations) and is covered by a functionally highly specialized pseudostratified epithelium. Calculations based on Weibel's (1963) figures for the dimensions of the bronchi indicate a total mucosal surface area of 6261 cm^2 (Chodosh and Medici, 1971). Regeneration occurs with division of basal layer cells giving rise to additional basal cells, with further differentiation into ciliated and secretory cells replacing desquamated BEC. Animal studies of cellular turnover of the respiratory epithelium demonstrate different cell turnover rates varying from 34 to 59 days for the different sites of the air-conducting systems (Bertalanaffy, 1968).

The columnar cells that line the lumen of the bronchus are represented in the sputum by ciliated, goblet, and degenerated columnar cell types. The BEC types that are preponderant in the sputum of chronic bronchitics are the basal and degenerated basal cells. Together, they constitute from 67.4 to 76.8% of all exfoliated BEC. This includes the indistinguishable degenerated intermediate layer cells and cells from hyperplastic areas. The estimation of the extent of mucosal damage using these cells as an index would be rather difficult. They do provide an estimate of damage to the bronchial epithelium and suggest that denudation or ulceration must often extend to the basement membrane. The basal layer is absolutely necessary for renewal of functional surface mucosa by regeneration of epithelial lesions resulting from infection by viruses and bacteria or from inhaled pollutants. Hyperplasia of the basal cell layer is a prominent feature in chronic bronchitis and may progress to metaplasia as a failure of the normal regenerative differentiation to normal columnar cells under the repetitive insults to this tissue. Metaplasia may represent a protective measure on the part of the host to present an epithelial surface that may be more resistant to infection or damage, although less functional as respiratory epithelium. There is evidence that basal cell hyperplasia is an early and frequent response of bronchial epithelium to a variety of nonspecific stimuli and is not unique to chronic bronchitis. Metaplasia of the bronchial epithelium in humans has been described in a wide variety of pathological conditions and in subjects without evidence of pulmonary disease, children, nonsmokers, wind instrument players, and singers. Small areas of metaplasia are a frequent finding in chronic bronchitis and may represent a type of focal atypical regeneration of the superficial epithelial lesions (Sanderud, 1956; Hers, 1961).

Any extensive loss of ciliated columnar bronchial epithelial cells interferes with mucociliary function. During acute infection in chronic bronchitis, increased numbers of both ciliated and degenerated ciliated BEC are exfoliated into sputum compared with an individual's stable state. In patients with chronic bronchitis, the bronchial epithelium characteristically exfoliates as individual cells and ciliated types lose their cilia. These findings suggest that the BEC seen in the sputum of chronic bronchitics is the result of sloughing of damaged and degenerated cells. The millions of damaged bronchial epithelial cells exfoliated daily by chronic bronchitics suggest a necrotizing process. However, the calculated daily loss of surface epithelium, even during acute exacerbations, represents only 0.16% of the available mucosal surface (Chodosh and Medici, 1971). It is not surprising that these lesions may have been overlooked in the examination of morbid tissues. Indeed, Hers and Mulder (1953) specifically commented on the intactness of the mucosa in chronic and acute bronchitis. Auerbach et al. (1961), however, did describe ulcerations and denudation in their extensive examinations of bronchi in smokers. The process in chronic bronchitis is quite different from the exfoliation of swollen individual and clustered bronchial epithelial cells (Creola bodies) with intact cilia in sputum of chronic bronchial asthma and acute viral bronchitis.

Reid (1960) emphasized that hyperplasia or hypertrophy of the mucus-secreting cells of the bronchi are essential structural changes in chronic bronchitis, with measurable change in the mucous glands of the submucosa, as well as of the goblet cells in the mucosal epithelium. Goblet cells constitute 20–50% of the columnar cells in the in situ epithelium in chronic bronchitis. The increase of goblet cells is nonuniform in large and small bronchi. The changed proportion of mucinous-secreting cell types is responsible for the altered proportions of mucopolysaccharide components in the sputum of chronic bronchitis. The number of goblet cells seen in sputum are underestimated, since it is difficult to recognize degenerated forms. Chodosh and Medici (1971) noted that 2.39 million goblet cells are exfoliated per day when chronic bronchitics are stable, and this more than doubles during acute bacterial exacerbations.

The number of BEC with intracytoplasmic bacteria demonstrates the ability of microorganisms to invade these cells. However, definite pathogenicity and virulence of these bacteria in this particular setting are not proved by this evidence. Hers and Mulder (1953) demonstrated *Haemophilus influenzae* between the columnar cells and below the basement membrane in tissue sections, but intracellular organisms were not described. Chodosh and Medici (1971) found bacteria inside BEC in the sputum. They noted an increase of these bacteria-infected cells during acute infection, with a decrease during therapy with antibiotics. The relative frequency, when compared with all of the sputum cell types in the specimen, is the same during stable state and acute infection and only decreases during treatment. Bacteria-infected cells are not completely eliminated by antibiotic therapy.

The techniques for assessing the qualitative and quantitative nature of the exfoliated cells in sputum in chronic bronchitis affords an opportunity to examine changes in the bronchial epithelium occurring during life. Calculation of the surface area of exfoliated columnar cells provides a means of estimating the extent of denudation of the mucosal surface. By using 6 μm as the mean diameter (Rhodin, 1966), the luminal surface area of each columnar cell would be 28.27 μm^2. During the stable state of chronic bronchitis, the mean total number of columnar cells exfoliated is 18.6 $\times$ 10^6/day, representing a loss of 5.26 cm^2 of surface epithelium a day. The average daily loss is 10.10 cm^2 during acute infection, and this loss extends well into the recovery phase. If these calculations are valid, the average stable chronic bronchitic would denude approximately one-third of his or her bronchial epithelium in the period of 1 year. This criterion can be used to classify the severity of chronic bronchitis in individual patients on the basis of the area of bronchial epithelium involved. Long-term damage could be estimated by the addition of a time factor. These measurements could serve as objective criteria for the extent of damage against which other biological variables could be examined.

Reticuloendothelial System Cells

The reticuloendothelial system (RES) cells seen in the inflammatory process have intrigued investigators since Metchnikoff (1893). Sputum is an exudate resulting from specific stimuli imposed on the respiratory surface. Its critical examination can delineate characteristics of the inflammatory response in various bronchopulmonary disorders, since most of the cellular elements of the RES are represented. The characteristics of the host's cellular defense mechanisms can be assessed. Observation of the RES in a naturally occurring inflammatory process provides a unique opportunity that is not often used. The relative frequency and quantities of the RES cells excreted in the sputum can be determined in either wet or fixed preparations. Wet preparation examination provides immediate information relative to the clinical situation at hand. Fixed preparations permits more extensive differential counts of cell types.

Polymorphonuclear Neutrophils

Leukocytes from the circulating blood constitute most of all cells seen in sputum in chronic bronchitis and directly reflect the nature of the inflammatory process. The polymorphonuclear neutrophils (PMNs) are usually multilobed, but often appear multinucleated because the interlobe bridges are not easily seen. They usually appear round or ovoid in sputum, with a size varying from 10 to 15 μm. In wet preparations, their granules appear as fine specks and may manifest brownian movement. Conglomeration of granules, toxic granulation, and phagocytosed material are easily seen. The granules of very fresh PMN often have an eosinophilic cast in the presence of aqueous buffered crystal violet or similar metachromatic stains. In fixed smears stained by Papanicolaou's method, PMNs are primarily identified by their size and the lobed nature of the nucleus. Cytoplasmic granules are not well delineated, and the cytoplasm often appears to be clear. The size of PMN may vary considerably from one preparation to another owing to degeneration and fixation. Intracellular bacteria and toxic granulation are identifiable.

The PMN have been extensively studied. The early diapedesis of PMN in response to an acute inflammatory stimulus is normal and desired. Phagocytosis and destruction of pathogenic bacteria is their common function, and the role of the PMN in the protection of the host against microbial invaders is well established (Hirsch, 1965).

In chronic bronchitis, the number of PMNs in sputum indicates the level of the inflammatory process in the bronchial system. Thompson and Rennard (1988), using selective bronchoalveolar lavage, provide excellent evidence that these PMNs come preponderantly from the bronchi in chronic bronchitics. Increases of these cells during episodes of acute clinical worsening is indicative of a greater level of inflammation. During acute infection, PMNs markedly increase, suggesting an appropriately responsive host cellular defense. In acute bacterial infection, there is a concomitantly significant increase of PMNs having phagocytosed bacteria. However, evaluation of the percentage of PMNs with demonstrable ingested bacteria (in vivo phagocytic index) suggests that the PMNs are not as adequate in host defense in chronic bronchitis as the total number implies. In bacterial pneumonia occurring in patients without chronic bronchitis, a high percentage of PMNs demonstrate phagocytic activity. However, this index is low in the bronchitic, with mean values of 4–8% during both stable state and acute infection and even lower values during recovery (Medici and Chodosh, 1972). Therefore, the increased number of neutrophils with ingested bacteria during acute infection does not imply a qualitatively increased effectiveness. The PMNs seen in the sputum gel are round and show no evidence of pseudopod activity. This suggests that phagocytosis of bacteria occurs in the tissue of the mucosa and not after the PMN enters the bronchial lumen as part of the exudate. Occasionally, chronic bronchitics may show an increase of neutrophils associated with an increase of the neutrophil phagocytic index or in numbers of bronchial macrophages without the symptoms usually noted with acute clinical exacerbations. When this is associated with an increase of bacteria in the sputum, this can be termed a subclinical exacerbation with successful host defense (Chodosh, 1963). In contrast, clinically evident exacerbations may be considered as examples of at least partial failures of cellular host defense.

In chronic bronchitics with viral infections or chemical insults to the lung, it is usual to see a marked neutrophilic response. An adequate neutrophilic response to inflammation may be seen in the sputum, despite many of the conditions characterized by inadequate numbers of PMNs in blood or bone marrow. The practical assessment of the role of PMNs in cellular host defense is possible from sputum examination and is valuable in determining the severity of the chronic bronchitis, evaluating exacerbations, and in planning therapy.

Macrophages

The macrophage (or histiocyte) cells range in size from 10 to 40 μm. The nucleus is usually single, somewhat elliptoid, and is located eccentrically. Multinucleated macrophages are not uncommon. The nucleus is pale, with delicate chromatin, and two nucleoli are usually visible. The cytoplasm varies from a uniform, finely reticulated appearance to one completely filled with ingested materials, such as dust, bacteria, lipids, cells, and such. Macrophages with ingested red blood cells or hemosiderin are called heart failure cells. The cytoplasm avidly takes up metachromatic stain and makes identification easy. The morphology in Papanicolaou-stained smears is similar to that described for the wet preparations. In unstained, wet preparations the cytoplasm is often pigmented, with color ranging from yellowish to rather dark brown. Some of these pigments have fluorescent qualities (Vassar et al., 1960).

The monocyte, which is the precursor of the macrophage, is identified by its typically indented nucleus, with fine reticular chromatin, and its relatively clear cytoplasm. The transitional monocytic–macrophage has maintained the typical monocyte nucleus, but the cytoplasm has assumed the characteristics noted in macrophages. Simple morphological characteristics are not distinctive enough to distinguish between alveolar macrophages and macrophages derived from circulating mononuclear cells.

Examination of macrophages in the sputum presents an opportunity to observe a vital part of the RES that is not otherwise easily accessible in humans. Systematic observations of the occurrence of macrophages in bronchopulmonary diseases has provided some information concerning host defense mechanisms of the lung. High levels of macrophages in sputum in chronic bronchitis, as well as in chronic bronchial asthma and pneumonia, indicate adequate host cellular defenses and usually suggest a favorable prognosis. Absence or low levels of macrophages are usually associated with acute exacerbations of these diseases and may often be noted before the clinical manifestations of such episodes. The functional capability of macrophages can be assessed in sputum by their in vivo phagocytic activity. An increased bacterial phagocytic activity of macrophages has been observed during the resolution of acute infectious episodes in chronic bronchitis.

Macrophages have several important functional capabilities. As scavenger cells, a prime function is intracellular breakdown and disposal of phagocytosed particulate and soluble material (Cohn, 1965; Pearsall and Weiser, 1970). Their role in immunological reactions is well documented. Antigen processing by macrophages is an essential step in the induction of the immune response (Feldman, 1969). Antigen placed in the alveoli is quickly ingested and cleared away by phagocytic cells, which may disperse into the local lymphatic tissue, be expectorated, or gain access to the circulation (Holub and Hauser, 1969). Alveolar macrophages are also a significant reservoir of antibodies and are the primary effector cells in antimicrobial and tissue immunity (Makaness and Blanden, 1967).

Macrophages, or histiocytes, are the second most frequently occurring cells in chronic bronchitics' sputum involved in the nonspecific cellular defenses. These highly specialized RES cells are likely responsible for sterility of the lower airways (Laurenzi et al., 1963; Green and Kass, 1964a). Short-term experiments in animal models suggest a possible relation between functional inhibition of macrophages by certain substances (e.g., ethanol, cigarette smoke, hypoxia, acidosis, azotemia) and the recurrent infections seen in chronic bronchitis (Green and Kass, 1964b; Green and Carolin, 1967). Eichel and Chodosh (1976) demonstrated an inhibition of catalase activity in the sputum from chronic bronchitics who were active cigarette smokers. This may represent one explanation for a reduced bactericidal activity of macrophages in this setting, since catalase is primarily found in macrophages.

Although alveolar macrophages likely come from bone marrow elements that may mature locally in the pulmonary tissue, macrophages found in new inflammatory foci are derived from circulating lymphocytes or monocytes (Bowden et al., 1969; Spector et al., 1965; Van Furth and Cohn, 1968). Blood-borne histiocytes in the lung of immune mice are morphologically and functionally distinct from alveolar macrophages and provide antimicrobial resistance (Mackaness, 1971). Medici and Chodosh (1972), in sputum studies in chronic bronchitis (Table 1), present data that support the presumption that most macrophages in sputum are derived from monocytes at the site of inflammation. This suggests that the use of the term *histiocyte*, rather than *macrophage* (implying alveolar macrophage), would be more appropriate for these phagocytes seen in the sputum of chronic bronchitics. During acute infectious exacerbations of chronic bronchitis, histiocytes do not increase in number, whereas monocytes are increased over stable-state levels. The number of monocytic histiocytes are unchanged. During clinical recovery, the number of histiocytes increases, whereas the monocyte level decreases toward that observed in the stable state. In addition, cells transforming from monocytes to histiocytes occur more frequently than during the acute phase. Chodosh et al. (1982) noted that the average size of mononuclear cells was small during acute bacterial exacerbations and increased in size during effective antimicrobial therapy. This also supports an influx of the smaller monocytes during the acute phase of inflammation, with the maturing into large histicocytes with recovery. This sequence of events strongly suggests that the bacterial stimulus resulted in a monocyte influx at the site of bronchial inflammation, with subsequent maturation into histiocytes. Besides tissue histiocytes, it is likely that some alveolar macrophages must be present in chronic bronchitics' sputum (Spritzer et al., 1968).

The in vivo phagocytic activity of histiocytes for a number of different particles can also be assessed in sputum. The patterns of phagocytosis by histiocytes in chronic bronchitics is different from that seen with neutrophils. During acute infection, bacterial phagocytosis by histiocytes is qualitatively and quantitatively higher than during stable state, increasing further during the recovery phase (see Table 1). Ingestion of nucleated cellular material by histiocytes follows a similar pattern, suggesting a common phagocytic mechanism, as seen with bacteria. Phagocytosis of dust and particulate matter by histiocytes appears to be suppressed during acute bacterial exacerbations and rebounds to stable-state levels by the recovery phase. Whether this is the result of competition, overloading, or decreased presence of particles is unclear. Individual sputum histiocytes may show phagocytosis of more than one type of material. The significance of vacuolated histiocytes is not clear. Vacuolization is a frequent finding in histiocytes expectorated in sputum. It is usually associated with phagocytosis and pinocytosis, and these vacuoles probably represent phagolysosomes containing a great variety of exogenous and autologous substances. Medici and Chodosh (1982), in Papanicolaou-stained preparations, demonstrated that, in chronic bronchitis, these

Table 1 RES Cells in Sputum in Chronic Bronchitis During Phases of Clinical Stability, Acute Infection, and Recovery[a]

Cells	Stable state (SS)	Acute infection (AI)	Recovery (R)	p values ≤ 0.05 ($\times$)		
				SS vs AI	AI vs R	SS vs R
Polymorphonuclear neutrophils	254 ± 234	1,119 ± 818	231 ± 195	×	×	
Polymorphonuclear neutrophils with bacteria	11.1 ± 15.5	49.3 ± 69.0	6.8 ± 9.1	×	×	
Macrophages (histiocytes)	30.6 ± 41.9	25.0 ± 31.4	44.2 ± 52.9		×	
Monocytic histiocytes	5.3 ± 11.8	4.4 ± 5.6	5.1 ± 5.3			
Monocytes	5.9 ± 8.5	13.5 ± 19.8	7.2 ± 11.6	×		
Macrophages with bacteria	1.29 ± 3.31	3.22 ± 9.62	4.29 ± 8.97			×

[a]Means and standard deviations of cells per day $\times$ 10^6

cells are influenced by allergy-related stimuli. It is possible that these cells are actually mast cells. Vacuolated histiocytes are not influenced by acute bacterial infection in chronic bronchitics.

Histiocytes or macrophages are important in the overall cellular defense of chronic bronchitics, even though these cells represent only the third most common cell type in their sputum. Their presence in large numbers in sputum in chronic bronchitis usually denotes stability, adequate RES responsiveness, recovery, or a minimal stage of the disease (Chodosh, 1963). An abrupt decrease in the number of sputum histiocytes of an individual patient may precede a clinically evident acute exacerbation by as much as 2 weeks. Nevertheless, all of the implications of histiocyte population changes are not clear. How they interact with other elements of the host defense system in achieving defense of mucous surfaces against infection or other toxic stimuli remains to be critically evaluated.

Eosinophils

The polymorphonuclear eosinophils (PMEs) are quite similar to PMNs in wet preparations, except for the uniformly sized and generally large eosinophilic granules. The granules can vary in size in different specimens. Vacuolelike clear areas can be seen in the cytoplasm. The nucleus is either nonlobed or bilobed. Charcot–Leyden crystals may be seen in wet preparations as elongated rhomboids, varying in size, but not in shape. With aging, the sharp ends become blunted and rounded. Charcot–Leyden crystals can be considered PME equivalents, since they are formed from the coalescence of freed eosinophil cytoplasm and granules (Archer and Blackwood, 1965). The morphology of PMEs in Papanicolaou stains is similar to the PMNs except for the differences of the nuclear lobation and cytoplasmic granules, which are often not as discretely seen as in wet preparations.

The function of PMEs is still unclear, despite numerous clinical and experimental observations. The physiology of these cells resembles that of PMNs in some ways and that of macrophages in others (Hirsch, 1965). They also originate in bone marrow, circulate for a short time, pass into tissue, and are capable of locomotion and phagocytosis. It is evident that PMEs are involved in host defense. Their role in the immune process is substantiated by their interaction with thymus-dependent lymphocytes, chemotaxis and phagocytosis of immune complexes, and their presence in hypersensitivity reactions. Eosinophils are usually present in small numbers in the sputum of chronic bronchitics, their numbers reflecting the immunological condition of the bronchial mucosa. Focal infiltrations of PMEs are regularly found in the bronchial mucosa of patients with chronic bronchitis (Salvato, 1968). Increases of sputum PMEs are often noted during recovery from acute inflammatory processes.

Charcot–Leyden crystals originate from both PMEs and basophils or mast cells. They are readily seen in wet, unfixed preparations. Chemically, the crystals are composed of a single polypeptide of low molecular weight (Hornung, 1962).

Lymphocytes and Plasma Cells

Small numbers of lymphocytes are often present in sputum. The lymphocyte, as seen in sputum, has the familiar water-color blue, round nucleus and only a few cytoplasmic granules. Its appearance is typical in both fresh and fixed preparations. Basal bronchial epithelial cells with lymphocytes can be confused, since their sizes and nucleus/cytoplasm ratios are quite similar. Plasma cells can be recognized in wet sputum preparations by their round, eccentric nucleus, with the characteristically dense chromatin, but without the expected spokewheel effect. In hematoxylin and eosin-stained preparations the appearance is quite classic, with basophilic cytoplasm, eccentric nucleus, and dense spokewheel-configurated chromatin.

Lymphocytes and plasma cells have important roles in the immunological response. Two physiologically and functionally distinct lymphocyte populations are differentiated: one thymus-dependent (T lymphocytes) and one thymus-independent (B lymphocytes) (Roitt et al., 1969). Plasma cells are derived from B lymphocytes, which are the principal producers of antibodies. T lymphocytes function in cell-mediated immunity, including antimicrobial and antitissue immunity, delayed-type hypersensitivity, and humoral antibody response to certain antigens (Mackaness and Blanden, 1967).

Both cells are present in the normal bronchial mucosa and submucosa, and increased accumulations are found in the submucosa in established chronic bronchitis (Salvato, 1968; Hers, 1961; Tada and Ishizaka, 1970; Mullen et al., 1985). Immunologloglobulins A, M, G, and E are found in these cells. Locally produced secretory IgA is a key factor in the resistance of the respiratory tract to infection (Medici and Bürgi, 1971).

Both lymphocytes and plasma cells are present in sputum of chronic bronchitics in small numbers. Medici and Chodosh (1972) found that the number of lymphocytes excreted in the sputum per day is $0.6 \pm 1.3 \times 10^6$ when chronic bronchitics are stable, significantly increase to $2.2 \pm 4.7 \times 10^6$ during acute bacterial exacerbations, and decrease to 1.4 ± 4.5 during recovery. Plasma cells show a similar pattern, with $0.5 \pm 1.0 \times 10^6$ excreted per day during clinical stability, significantly increasing to $2.7 \pm 3.9 \times 10^6$ during infection, and significantly decreasing to $1.2 \pm 2.7 \times 10^6$ during recovery. This increase during acute infection may in part be related to the depth of the bronchial lesions that expose a greater area of submucosa and result in a nonspecific shedding of these cells from these ulcers.

Mast Cells

Mast cells cannot be identified with certainty in sputum in unstained wet sputum or Papanicolaou-stained preparations. They are indistinguishable from macrophages with both techniques. Staining of unfixed sputum with aqueous buffered crystal violet and observations with a polarizing microscope provides a simple method for identification of mast cells that still retain some of their granules. Mast cells are about 15–20 μm in size, with cytoplasm that is usually full of large granules, with a central Maltese cross birefringence in polarized light. The macrophage-like nucleus is often obscured by these granules, which may vary in size from cell to cell. Mast cells that have functionally extruded their granules look like macrophages.

The functions of the mast cell remain somewhat unsettled. Mast cells are commonly distributed through the connective tissue, particularly around small vessels. In the lung, mast cells are usually found beneath the epithelium of the airways and around blood vessels (Salvato, 1968; Tada and Ishizaka, 1970). Their granules contain a variety of highly active substances, such as heparin, histamine, serotonin, and a chymotrypsinlike enzyme (Benditt, 1968), all essential mediators of inflammatory processes. Mast cells and eosinophils have a similar distribution in tissues exposed to the environment and show a parallel fluctuation in inflammatory exudates and necrotic foci (Selye, 1965; Rebuck et al., 1963). Mast cells are frequently found in the submucosa of patients with chronic bronchial diseases. Schmidt (1892) found them in sputum in bronchial asthma, chronic bronchitis and pneumonia. Rare investigations of mast cells in sputum have been pursued in recent years. Chodosh (1978) confirmed that mast cells are present in the sputum of chronic bronchitics and asthmatics. Medici and Chodosh (1982), in studies of sputum from chronic bronchitis with and without allergic rhinitis, evaluated the occurrence of histiocytes with vacuoles, which likely were mast cells. They noted that the number of such cells excreted per day were either $2.1 \pm 2.1 \times 10^6$ or $1.8 \pm 2.7 \times 10^6$ in those with or without allergic rhinitis, respectively, when measured outside of ragweed season. Changes during ragweed season showed an increase to $8.2 \pm 10.1 \times 10^6$ in bronchitics with allergic rhinitis, and a decrease to $0.7 \pm 1.8 \times 10^6$ in those without. Gibson et al. (1989) noted that an average of 0.14% of all of the sputum cells were mast cells in a group of chronic bronchitics with a mild severity of disease. Further studies of the role of mast cells in the inflammatory process of chronic bronchitis is warranted.

Clinical Applications

Evaluation of the sputum cellular populations is of considerable value in differentiating chronic bronchitis from bronchial asthma, and in determining the etiology of acute exacerbations in chronic bronchitics. In both instances, the clinical presentations and the gross physical characteristics of the sputum may be very similar. The microscopic evaluation of the types of cells in the sputum specimen and Gram stain analysis are the simple methods that can quickly assist the clinician in the differential diagnosis of these conditions.

The differential between chronic bronchitis and bronchial asthma can be readily made on the basis of a few simple criteria (Chodosh, 1970, 1988). The

PMNs are the preponderant inflammatory cells in chronic bronchitis, and the frequency of eosinophils rarely exceed 5% during clinically stable periods. In bronchial asthma, PMNs are also usually the preponderant polymorphonuclear cells, but the average percentage of eosinophils ranges from 20 to 40%, depending on corticosteroid dependency, but may be as high as 90%. The characteristics of the exfoliated bronchial epithelial cells is also differential. Chronic bronchitics typically have pyknotic, single bronchial epithelial cells that are devoid of cilia. The bronchial epithelial cells in asthmatic bronchitis are usually swollen, often in clusters (Creola bodies), and have intact ciliated borders. These characteristics of asthmatics' sputa cells may not be seen during acute bacterial exacerbations when sputum eosinophilia is suppressed and the exfoliated bronchial epithelial cells may look more like those seen in chronic bronchitis. In chronic bronchitics who also have asthma, the bronchial epithelial cells are typically bronchitic, but sputum eosinophils may constitute 5–15% of the cells. When the chronic bronchitic is significantly improved, the emergence of typically asthmatic cytological characteristics is frequently seen. Gibson et al. (1989) confirmed the ability to differentiate bronchial asthma from chronic bronchitis using sputum cytological criteria.

Chronic bronchitics, with or without asthma, often have episodic acute worsening of their pulmonary symptoms that represent acute exacerbations of their disease. The clinical syndrome associated with these exacerbations include increases of cough, sputum production, dyspnea, wheezing, and chest congestion. These symptoms do not differentiate which cause was responsible for the acute syndrome. The exacerbations can be initiated by viral or bacterial infection, excessive exposure to inhaled irritants, troublesome secretions, reductions of background therapy, or allergy. The gross sputum characteristics are also nondifferential. With all of these etiologies, there usually is more sputum, which is thicker and more purulent in appearance. The cytological and Gram stain findings can distinguish the likely cause of the exacerbation (Chodosh, 1987, 1992). Table 2 outlines their distinctive characteristics. The use of these criteria can define the appropriate therapeutic approach for managing such troublesome events.

Bacteria

Bacterial microorganisms are usually found as a component of sputum in chronic bronchitis. Their origin is either through inhalation or aspiration from the ambient air or oro-nasopharynx, or as part of the exudate from infected areas of the bronchi. Stable chronic bronchitics have few bacteria, but the numbers can increase remarkably during acute bacterial exacerbations. Baigelman et al. (1979) characterized the qualitative and quantitative bacterial flora in chronic bronchitis with Gram stains and strict morphological criteria. Table 3 shows the mean numbers of morphological bacteria types identified per oil immersion microscopic field during clinically stable state and acute bacterial exacerbations. The mean

Table 2 Sputum Cytological and Bacteriological Patterns of Various Types of Exacerbations in Chronic Bronchitis

Exacerbation	Volume	Neutrophils	Eosinophils	Macrophages	Bronchial epithelial cells	Bacteria (Gram stain)
Acute bacterial infection	I	I	D	D	Pyknotic	I
Acute viral infection	I	I	D	D	Swollen	O
Subclinical bacterial infection (no acute symptoms)	I	I	D	I	Pyknotic	I
Bacterial colonization	O	O	O	O	Pyknotic	I
Acutely increased inhaled irritant	I	I	D	±	Pyknotic	O
Acute secretion problems[a]	D	O	O	O	Pyknotic	O
Acute allergic	I	D	I	D	Swollen	O

[a]Often related to reductions of background therapy.

I, increased; D, decreased; O, no change; ±, variable change.

Table 3 Morphological Bacterial Types per Oil Immersion Field Seen on Gram Stain During Stable-State (207 Cases) and Acute Bacterial Exacerbations (146 cases) in Chronic Bronchitis

Bacterial type	Acute bacterial exacerbation M ± SD	Stable state	
		M ± SD	M ± 3SD
Pleomorphic gram-negative cocco-bacilli	44.3 ± 41.7	1.26 ± 3.38	11.40
Gram-positive diplococci and cocci	24.2 ± 22.1	1.89 ± 1.94	7.71
Gram-negative kidney-shaped diplococci	52.7 ± 62.2	0.94 ± 1.94	17.41
Staphylococcal-like[a]		0.15 ± 0.46	1.53
Diphtheroid-like[a]		0.25 ± 0.73	2.44
Gram-negative bacilli (large)[a]		0.31 ± 1.47	4.72

[a]No infections caused by these bacteria were noted.

plus 3 standard deviation (SD) values derived from the stable-state values for the three common bacterial types provides criteria for defining a significant increase of the bacterial flora. In terms of total protoplasmic mass, these bacteria contribute little to the composition of the sputum, even when present as hundreds per oil immersion field. The inflammatory response and damaged mucosal tissue that they cause does have a profound effect on the sputum characteristics. The common bacterial species recovered from the sputum of chronic bronchitics during acute bacterial exacerbations are *Haemophilus influenzae*, *Moraxella catarrhalis*, *Streptococcus pneumoniae*, and *Haemophilus parainfluenzae*. Less commonly, *Pseudomonas aeruginosa* and *Klebsiella pneumoniae* can be found.

C. Noncellular Formed Components

Besides the Charcot–Leyden crystals, which have already been described, there are several other formed elements found in the sputum of chronic bronchitics.

Curschmann's Spirals

Although usually associated with eosinophils and Charcot–Leyden crystals in asthmatic sputum, they are commonly seen in chronic bronchitis without any evidence of allergy. These are composed of spirally twisted mucinous material around a central thread. They are probably casts of the smaller bronchi containing the usual components of sputum in a more compact form. In sputum, they are rarely macroscopically visible, more often being of microscopic dimensions. Curschmann's spirals were first described by Von Leyden (1872) but Curschmann (1885) described them more extensively. Gerlach (1892) in a simple, but noteworthy, experiment reproduced Curschmann's spirallike formation by blowing through a humidified tube containing threads of different colors. This suggests that abnormal flow patterns in the conducting airways in chronic bronchial diseases are most likely responsible for these unusual formations of compacted secretions.

Acid Mucopolysaccharide Fibers

The acid mucopolysaccharide fibers can be seen in sputum with special-staining procedures. Sputum consists of a network of interwoven filamentous molecules, DNA, and mucoproteins or mucopolysaccharides. Other sputum constituents, such as kinins, immunoglobulins, lactoferrin, lysozyme, and surfactant, may be attached on these fibers, depending on their electrical charge (Havez et al., 1967).

In sputum of chronic bronchitics mucopolysaccharides consist preponderantly of acid mucopolysaccharides containing sulfate or neuraminic acid and a smaller amount of neutral mucopolysaccharides (Reid, 1968; Schultze and Heremans, 1966). Bürgi (1964) reported that these fibers, stained with basic dyes, can be seen distinctly with polarized light in sputum of stable bronchitics. They can be disrupted by bacterial ectoenzymes, hyaluronidase, and pharmacological agents such as *N*-acetylcysteine.

Deoxyribonucleic Acid Fibers

DNA fibers in sputum originate from nuclei of lysed cells. The thinnest of these are 90–120 Å in diameter, and they tend to lie in parallel bundles. A single fine DNA fiber is composed of six fibrils, each 15 μm in diameter (White et al., 1954).

With use of fluorescence microscopy, a simple technique for assessing DNA fibers stained with acridine orange can be used to routinely evaluate sputum DNA content. The number of DNA fibers visualized in sputum correlates with the absolute amount of DNA determined by spectrophotometry (Bürgi et al., 1968). In chronic bronchial diseases, the amount of DNA fibers is directly related to viscosity and they are another objective criteria for bronchial inflammation.

Myelin

Myelin can be seen intracellularly and extracellularly in sputum. It usually appears as round and oval formations of variable size, with soft contours, being distinctly different from more refractile lipid droplets. Schmidt (1898) described its composition to be fatty acids, phosphatides, and cerebrosides containing choline. It seems possible that these formations may be surfactant. Myelin is most commonly seen in sputum of patients with mild chronic bronchitis or asthma and is almost never present when high levels of neutrophilic inflammation is present. It is easily observed in unfixed preparations. Although distinctive, these fibers have been mistaken for yeast pathogens, but the lack of uniform structure differentiates it from microorganisms.

Corpora Amylacea

Corpora amylacea are round to oval structures with a diameter of 0.04–0.12 mm. They have a pigmented center and a homogeneous outer part of irregular concentric laminations with fibers radially arranged between the rings. Their exact chemical nature is unknown. They should be distinguished from equally sized starch granules, which also show concentric laminations, but stain with Lugol's solution, whereas corpora amylacea do not. Corpora amylacea in sputum is not unique to bronchitis, since they are seen in many diseases of the lung.

Crystals

Crystals, other than Charcot–Leyden crystals, that appear in sputum are cholesterol, hematoidin, fatty acids, leucine, tyrosine, oxalic acid, and phosphate (Von Hoesslin, 1926). Cellular and tissue destruction accounts for their presence in sputum, but this is not diagnostic of any specific lung disease.

D. Chemical Composition

Investigations of the chemical composition of the sputum in chronic bronchitis are complicated because the final product is a variable mixture of tracheobronchial secretions, exudate, and transudate from the inflammatory process. The technical problems of separating the intact cells from the rest of the sputum makes it impossible to directly determine how much these cells contribute to the quantitative values of specific substances determined by standard chemical methods. Histochemical techniques, by localizing specific compounds intracellularly, provide useful data relative to the cellular contribution, but these observations are generally qualitative. Admixture with saliva poses an additional problem that needs to be considered in the assessment of results. However, many of these problems can be avoided if aliquots are selected using the criteria noted earlier for assessment of the cellular components. Determining differences between the chemical components in chronic bronchitic sputum and normal tracheobronchial secretions is complicated by the difficulty in obtaining the latter, since artifacts may be introduced by most techniques used. The problems of obtaining valid normal secretions has been thoughtfully reviewed by Boat and Matthews (1973) and Yeager (1971).

Descriptions of the chemical composition of chronic bronchitic sputum is further complicated by the considerable variability among patients. This variability is related to several factors, a few of which are the severity of the disease, the level of inflammation, the current smoking status of the patient, and the occurrence of acute exacerbations of the disease. Investigations that do not define the status of the patients at the time of sputum collection often report results with large ranges of values. Some of the chemical components of bronchitic sputum are listed in Table 4.

Water

Water is the major component of chronic bronchitic sputum. Chodosh (1973) determined that water constituted an average of between 96 and 97% of the sputum in 30 stable chronic bronchitics. Peroral hydration of these patients resulted in less than an average of 0.5% increase of sputum water. This suggests that sputum is well saturated with water in the environment of the bronchi. This is particularly impressive when one examines how quickly expectorated sputum loses water when exposed to 37°C in a drying oven. An average of 27–34% of the water content is lost in the first hour, with somewhat higher rates of loss of the remaining water in the subsequent 1–4 h. Virtually all of the available water is lost by the sixth hour, although the water loss rates are considerably lower in the last 2 h. The physicochemical nature of how the water molecules are bound in the sputum gel is unknown. The variability of sequential water loss rates reported by Chodosh (1973) suggests that it is likely that the strength of water-bonding varies, depending on the site. Although some investigators have reported an association of water content with the physical properties of nonbronchitic sputum, I have noted only a weak and nonpredictive correlation in chronic bronchitic sputum. When one considers that water is the major component of sputum, it is surprising that so little attention has been given to investigating this molecule.

Glycoproteins

Glycoproteins present in chronic bronchitic sputum are mainly secreted by the goblet cells and submucosal mucous glands, with some coming from plasma. There is a great deal of information on respiratory tract glycoproteins in normal persons and in patients with cystic fibrosis, bronchiectasis, asthma, bronchorrhea, and experimental animals. There are few reports concerning glycoproteins in the sputum of chronic bronchitics. Neutral glycoproteins that contain large amounts of fucose are present in nonpurulent chronic bronchitic sputum; the mean plus or minus the standard error (M ± SE) was 97.7 ± 10.7 mg/100 ml (Puchelle et al., 1973). Acidic glycoproteins become more evident as bronchial inflammation increases. Sialic acid-rich glycoprotein has a reciprocal relationship with the neutral fucose glycoprotein, since they both occupy the terminal position on oligosaccharide chains. Atassi et al. (1957) found sialic concentrations in four bronchitic bronchial aspirates to be 0.43–1.36 mg/ml which was almost fourfold greater than noted in normal controls. The highest levels were noted in bronchitics

Table 4 Chemical Composition of Chronic Bronchitic Sputum

Component	Cells and cellular lysis	Transudation	Secretory
Water	X	X	X
Glycoproteins			
Neutral and acidic		X	Goblet cells, submucosal glands
Secretory piece			Mucosal cells
Fibronectin			
Proteins			
Immunoglobulins		X	Plasma cells
Lysozyme	PMN, macrophages		Submucosal glands
Lactoferrin	PMN		Submucosal glands
Histamine	Gram-negative bacteria		Mast cells
Serotonin			Mast cells
Slow-reacting substance of anaphylaxis			Mast cells
Albumin		X	
Kallikrein		X	
Antiproteinases		X	
Transferrin		X	
Myeloperoxidase	PMN, eosinophils		
Lactate dehydrogenase	X		
Catalase	Macrophages		
Proteinases	Leukocytes, macrophages		
Lipids			
Surfactant			Type II pneumonocytes, Clara cells
Glycolipids	X		
Others	X		
Inorganic molecules			
Sodium, potassium, chloride, phosphorus	X	X	

with increased respiratory symptoms. Lamb and Reid (1968) reported similar values (0.2–1.4 mg/ml) in sputum from chronic bronchitics. Reid (1968) also noted a relation between sputum purulence and sialic acid content. Levels of sialic acid glycoprotein of 55.9 ± 10.4 mg/100 ml (M ± SE) were reported by Puchelle et al. (1973) in chronic bronchitic sputum. There is indirect evidence that the amount of more acidic sulfated glycoproteins may be significantly greater in sputum of chronic bronchitics. Sulfated glycoproteins were found to be 9.8 ± 1.5 mg/100 ml (M ± SE) by Puchelle et al. (1973) in sputum from chronic bronchitics. It is not clear why these changes toward more acid glycoproteins occur in chronic bronchitis. Similar changes are noted in other inflammatory diseases of the bronchial system.

Fibronectin

Haag et al. (1986) reported the presence of the glycoprotein fibronectin in the gel subphase of sputum in chronic bronchitics. They found levels of 94.0 ± 17.7 μg/ml in the gel subphase, compared with only 6.4 ± 0.9 μg/ml in the sol subphase, suggesting that fibronectin is concentrated in the former. Fibronectin may be an important determinant of mucous gel structure and function because it interacts and cross-links with other components of the gel.

Proteins

The proteins found in the sputum of chronic bronchitic patients are derived from secretion from mucus-producing cells and mast cells, transudation from serum and intact and lysed cells from the bronchial mucosa, and the inflammatory process. Brogan et al. (1971) reported the average total protein concentration to be 597 ± 208 mg, as albumin, per 100 ml of sol phase sputum in 19 chronic bronchitics. This value was significantly higher in chronic bronchitics with concurrent heart failure. Fields and Chodosh (1970), using micro-Kjeldahl and modified biuret methods in mechanically homogenized sputum from ten chronic bronchitics, reported the average total protein concentration to be 952.8 mg/100 ml, with a range of 589–1271. Marchioni et al. (1990), from morning-collected samples, reported average concentrations of total protein of 1103.5 ± 828.5, 1139.1 ± 472.1, and 1244.4 ± 783.48 μg/dl in different groups and at different times in chronic bronchitics. The higher levels noted may be attributed to the intracellular material being available for measurement after the mechanical homogenization in the latter investigations.

A number of proteins involved in host defense mechanisms against infection occur in both normal tracheobronchial secretions and in chronic bronchitic sputum. These include immunoglobulins, lysozyme, lactoferrin, and secretory piece, all of which are produced in the bronchial system.

Immunoglobulins

Immunoglobulin A (IgA) is the preponderant immunoglobulin in the sputum of chronic bronchitics. It is mainly produced in local plasma cells, although some may come from serum transudation. The secretory piece is synthesized by mucosal cells lining the respiratory tract. This secretory component is added to 7S IgA, resulting in the more active secretory 11S IgA. Merrill et al. (1980) measured secretory component in healthy smokers and nonsmokers using bronchoalveolar lavage sputum. Although the concentrations of IgA were similar in the two groups, 20% of the smokers had a significantly reduced concentration of secretory piece. Medici and Bürgi (1971) reported a range of values for sputum IgA from 52 ± 34 mg/100 ml in bronchitics with minimal inflammation to 105 ± 90 mg/100 ml in patients with severe levels of inflammation. Patients with mild to moderate chronic bronchitis demonstrated significant increases of sputum IgA in the face of acute inflammatory exacerbations, whereas bronchitics with severe disease did not show such a response. Puchelle et al. (1973) reported IgA mean sputum concentrations of 155.7 mg/100 ml, with a standard error of 11.7. Ryley and Brogan (1973) found concentrations of 80.0 ± 41.8 mg/100 ml (M ± SD) in the sol phase of sputum from 30 chronic bronchitics. Marchioni et al. (1990) reported mildly higher concentrations in a group of 20 bronchitics. The importance of IgA in chronic bronchitis rests mainly in its role in host defense against bacterial infection. However, the effectiveness of IgA is dependent on interaction with complement, secretory piece, lysozyme, and kallikrein.

Other immunoglobulins, G, M, and possible E, may also be found in sputum. Ryley and Brogan (1973) reported concentrations of IgG of 13.3 ± 8.2 mg/100 ml (M ± SD) in the sputum of chronic bronchitics. Marchioni et al. (1990) reported levels in morning specimens obtained at different times in 20 patients with chronic bronchitis. These concentrations for three different groups were 38.8 ± 20.4, 47.9 ± 27.8, and 28.1 ± 16.5 µg/dl. Merrill et al. (1980) noted differences in the IgG/albumin ratios between smokers and nonsmokers in bronchial lavage specimens, when compared with serum ratios. The increased ratios noted in some smokers suggested that there was an accumulation or local synthesis of IgG in smokers. Their role in chronic bronchitis is not clear.

Lysozyme

Lysozyme is relatively abundant in the sputum of chronic bronchitics. Lorenz et al. (1957) first described lysozyme in bronchial aspirates. Brogan et al. (1971) reported that lysozyme represented 19.8 ± 8.0% of the total high molecular weight substances in the sputum sol phases of chronic bronchitic sputum. Marchioni et al. (1990) reported sputum concentrations of lysozyme in different groups of chronic bronchitics of 142 ± 45, 151 ± 94, and 143 ± 26 µg/dl. Lysozyme is likely produced by the submucosal glandular acini and is present in large amounts in macrophages and PMNs. Its extracellular role in host defense may depend on acting in association with IgA and complement to lyse bacteria (Adinolfi et al., 1966), although this has not been investigated in human sputum. The intracellular function in sputum phagocytes appears to be the lysis of ingested bacteria.

Lactoferrin

Lactoferrin was first described in sputum by Biserte et al. (1963). It originates from mucus-producing cells in bronchi (Masson et al., 1966) and is present in PMNs (Masson et al., 1969). It is structurally and functionally similar to serum *transferrin*, which is also found in sputum. Marchioni et al. (1990) noted sputum concentrations of lactoferrin in three groups of chronic bronchitics, studied at different times, of 59.3 ± 32.3, 58.1 ± 36.7, and 59.0 ± 17.2 µg/dl. Puchelle et al. (1973) reported mean levels of transferrin in sputum from chronic bronchitics at 38.2 mg/100 ml, with a standard error of 2.0. The role of lactoferrin and, indirectly, transferrin in host defense may be to inhibit the growth of certain potentially pathogenic bacteria, which include *Staphylococcus aureus* and *Pseudomonas aeruginosa*. Although hypothetical, it is of interest that acute bacterial exacerbations in ambulatory chronic bronchitis are rarely caused by *S. aureus* and are infrequent with *P. aeruginosa*. Both of these compounds may be responsible for trapping iron in the bronchial mucosa of chronic bronchitics resulting in the low serum iron levels often observed in patients with severe and long-standing chronic inflammation (Masson and Heremans, 1973).

Chemical Mediators

Mast cells contain *histamine*, *serotonin*, and *slow-reacting substance of anaphylaxis*, all of which are important mediators of the inflammatory process. The latter two mediators have not been investigated in chronic bronchitis, but are found in the sputum of asthmatics (Levy et al., 1961; Harkavy, 1930). Small amounts of histamine have been reported in the sputum from nonallergic cigarette smokers, in the range of 10–40 µg/g dry weight (Thomas and Simmons, 1969). Large amounts of histamine have been reported in sputum collected during acute infectious exacerbation of chronic lung diseases (Turnbull et al., 1977; Bryant and Pui, 1982; Moodley et al., 1984). Sheinman et al. (1986) and Devalia et al. (1989) demonstrated that the gram-negative bacterial pathogens commonly associated with acute bacterial exacerbations of chronic bronchitis all are capable of histamine synthesis. Their measurements of the pH of the sputum were in the range of 6.9–8.0, which would permit this synthesis to progress. It is unclear if the high levels of histamine noted in sputum during infection is due to bacterial synthesis, released from mast cells as part of the inflammatory process, or both. The author and colleagues have noted large numbers of mast cells in the sputum of stable chronic bronchitics, and a paucity of these cells during acute bacterial exacerbations in these same patients.

Albumin, Transferrin, and Kallikrein

A number of plasma proteins are found in sputum of chronic bronchitics as a result of serum transudation during the inflammatory process. The function of some of these proteins is known. *Albumin* is the main serum protein found in sputum. Ryley and Brogan (1973) reported the average concentration in the sol phase of sputum from 30 chronic bronchitics at 29.7 ± a SD of 8.8 mg/100 ml. Puchelle et al. (1973) reported an almost identical average concentration of 28.7 ± 3.4 mg/100 ml SE in 21 chronic bronchitics. Bronchial samples from chronic bronchitics obtained by bronchial lavage were noted by Thompson et al. (1989) to have an average concentration of 102 ± 13.8 μg/ml, which was approximately twice that noted in asymptomatic smokers and normal subjects. The distal or alveolar samples contained only 7.5 ± 1.1 μg/ml. Their data strongly suggests that the transudation occurred in the areas of inflammation at the bronchial level. An interesting and clinically important observation by Bonomo and D'Addabbo (1964) suggests that this transudation of albumin into the sputum of chronic bronchitics could explain the hypoalbuminemia commonly seen in these patients. They calculated that 8–9% intravenously injected radioiodinated albumin appeared in the sputum over a subsequent 10-day period. *Transferrin* transudation has already been discussed in relation to lactoferrin. *Kallikrein* has also been identified in chronic bronchitic sputum (Havez et al., 1966). Masson and Heremans (1973) discuss the possible role that the kinins may play in the inflammatory reaction to toxic stimuli in respiratory diseases. It is also obvious that any serum protein capable of passage through the capillary bed in the areas of inflammation can be found in the sputum.

Proteinases and Antiproteinases

The importance of antiproteinase activity in the inflammatory process of chronic bronchitis is evident in the development of pulmonary emphysema in patients having a deficiency of these enzymes, and is a strongly supported hypothesis (Wewers, 1989). α_1-Antiproteinase is now a more commonly used name for these enzymes. α_1-antitrypsin and α_1-chymotrypsin are both found in the sputum of chronic bronchitics. Ryley and Brogan (1973) reported average sputum concentrations of 2.7 ± 1.6 mg/100 ml and 1.5 ± 1.1 mg/100 ml, respectively. Large amounts of proteinases are released from inflammatory cells in the lungs of patients with chronic bronchitis. Most of the studies in humans have used bronchoalveolar lavage specimens, rather than sputum. The attractive hypothesis is that the emphysema that appears to be the consequence of chronic bronchitis is likely related to inadequate influx or functional activity of antiproteinases to counteract the tissue destructive proteinases.

The other proteins that have been described in chronic bronchitic sputum owe their presence to the intact and lysed cells. The amounts of these proteins in the whole sputum are an index of the magnitude of the cellular inflammatory response beyond that which quantitative measurements of the numbers of intact cells provide, since this includes cells that have already been destroyed. Some insight into the functional integrity of the cells of the inflammatory process in the chronic bronchitic may also be gained from measurements of specific proteins. The physical properties of the sputum also appear to be dependent on the interaction of some of the proteins released from lysed cells with other sputum components.

The *proteinases* that are released from PMNs and macrophages serve the important function in the inflammatory process of breaking down the lung tissues—so that invading bacteria can be attacked—and the fibrous proteins in the exudative gel. These proteinases are also capable of attacking the elastin in the lung parenchyma. Although investigations of these and other proteinases in sputum have been scant, there is considerable evidence to suggest that neutrophils release elastase, collagenase, and gelatinase as part of the inflammatory process in chronic bronchitis. When these proteinases (of which elastase appears to be most important) interact with potent oxidants (hypochlorous acid and chloramines) formed by myeloperoxidase and NADPH oxidase activity, severe tissue destruction can result (Weiss, 1989). These oxidants inactivate α_1-antiproteinase activity, resulting in a proteinase/antiproteinase imbalance. These effects are usually modulated in acute inflammatory processes in normal lungs so that the tissues are not seriously affected. When these effects are not inactivated, the tissue destruction in chronic bronchitics may result in emphysema and bronchiectasis. There is strong evidence that this imbalance is also operative in cystic fibrosis (Wewers, 1989).

Deoxyribonucleic Acid

Deoxyribonucleic acid (DNA) is found in the sputum of chronic bronchitics, and the amount is directly related to the level of tissue destruction and the inflammatory cell response. It can be measured biochemically, and the DNA fibers can be visualized using optical and electron microscopic techniques (White et al., 1954). Bürgi et al. (1968) demonstrated that the number of DNA fibers visualized by optical microscopy correlates with the amount determined by spectrophotometry. They reported a range of DNA concentrations from 1.1 ± 0.8 to 9.9 ± 2.2 mg/ml of sputum in chronic bronchitis, with the higher levels associated with higher levels of inflammation. Marchioni et al. (1990) found average levels of DNA ranging from 79 to 89 μg/dl, with large standard deviations, in the sputum of three groups of chronic bronchitics. Bornstein et al. (1978) reported an average level of 18 mg/gm of dry sputum, with a range of 16–35 in 12 stable chronic bronchitics. There was a significant increase to an average of 42 mg/g of dry sputum during acute exacerbations of their disease. As previously discussed, DNA is an important determinant of the apparent viscosity of the sputum when high levels of inflammation are present and serves as a measure of the inflammatory response.

Lactate Dehydrogenase, Myeloperoxidase, and Catalase

Eichel and Chodosh (1976) reported the enzyme activities of lactate dehydrogenase, myeloperoxidase, and catalase in sputum from chronic bronchitics under various clinical conditions. Since these enzymes reflect various aspects of cellular function, they provide a means of estimating the functional integrity of these proteins. Lactate dehydrogenase and myeloperoxidase were reported as micromoles $NADH_2$ oxidized per minute per milliliter of sputum. Clinically stable cigarette smoking bronchitics had an average of 4.0 of lactate dehydrogenase, compared with 9.9 for ex-smokers. The levels significantly increased during acute bacterial infection to 14.1 and 59.7, respectively, with the difference between these also being significant. This data suggests that smoking chronic bronchitics may have a defect of carbohydrate metabolism, when compared with the ex-smoking bronchitics. Bürgi et al. (1968) reported levels ranging from 168 ± 140 to 984 ± 304 IU/L in chronic bronchitic sputum, with higher levels being associated with increased inflammation. Eichel and Chodosh (1976) also reported that smoking bronchitics had significantly lower levels of myeloperoxidase than those of the ex-smokers, with levels of 9.6 when stable and 24.4 during acute infection for the smokers, when compared with 32.8 and 197.1, respectively, for the ex-smokers. Since the myeloperoxidase in these patients is derived from the PMNs, these data suggest that smokers would have an impairment of the intracellular bactericidal action and a reduction of oxidant production. Sputum catalase, expressed as micromoles H_2O_2 decomposed per minute per milliliter of sputum is largely derived from macrophages. As with the other enzymes, catalase activity was less in the smokers than in the ex-smokers when they were clinically stable; the averages being 273 and 1303, respectively. Average activity increased significantly in both groups during acute bacterial exacerbations to 1089 and 10,697, a difference that was also significant.

Lipids

The lipids found in sputum are the result of synthesis and secretion within the bronchopulmonary system and from breakdown of cells related to the inflammatory process. Reid and Bhaskar (1989), in their review of the lipids constituents in bronchial secretions, reveal the paucity of data relative to chronic bronchitis. Neutral lipids were the preponderant species in bronchial aspirates from normal volunteers, in which alveolar surfactant was not detected. Bronchial aspirates from asymptomatic smokers revealed small amounts of phospholipids and glycolipids. Bhaskar et al. (1987) found that glycolipids were the major types of lipids found in chronic bronchitis and cystic fibrosis. Schmidt (1898) noted that myelin, which can be seen microscopically in the sputum of mild chronic bronchitics, is composed of fatty acids, phosphatides, and choline-containing cerebrosides. It has been suggested that myelin may be, at least in part, pulmonary surfactant. Lewis

(1971) studied the sputum lipids in one chronic bronchitic and noted that 71% of the total lipids were free fatty acids. It is presumed that these are the result of cell destruction.

Inorganic Components

The inorganic components of chronic bronchitic sputum have received little attention. Hoffman and Ebelt (1968) reported the average concentration levels for sodium, chloride, potassium, and calcium in 21 chronic bronchitics as 80, 89, 21, and 5 mEq/L, respectively. Ryley and Brogan (1969) studied a single bronchitic over consecutive days and reported average concentrations of 100 mEq/L for sodium and chloride, 23 mEq/L for potassium, and 37 mEq/L for phosphate in the sol phase of sputum. They also noted a pH range of 6.3–7.9. This is similar to the range of pH of 6.9–8.0 noted by Devalia et al. (1989) in a group of chronic bronchitics. However, the measurement of pH in expectorated sputum is subject to many variables, which can influence the result.

IV. Further Investigations

The prospectives for future investigations of sputum in chronic bronchitis are almost innumerable. Description of the qualitative and quantitative constituents can provide a sound basis for separating out possibly important subgroups of chronic bronchitics. This could delineate groups with specific defects of host defense, particularly if the effects of acute toxic stimuli are examined. The effects of acute bacterial infection have received attention relative to cellular and noncellular aspects of host defense, but considerably more needs to be evaluated. The effects of other types of acute insults to the respiratory tract need to be assessed to determine if the inflammatory process is similar, or if there are distinguishing differences. The systemic effects of the chronic loss of sophisticated cellular and noncellular components have been only superficially investigated, although much has been hypothesized. The replacement of cells, proteins, and inorganic molecules that are excessively excreted in the sputum may strain the limits of the host's synthesizing capability. Some of the defects noted (e.g., the decrease of IgA in relation to severe chronic bronchitis) may represent an inability of body cells to synthesize sufficient replacement molecules. It is also possible that the increased demand for synthesis could result in defective molecules.

Evaluation of sputum components can also provide insight into the mechanisms of specific therapeutic interventions that are successful. Understanding of such mechanisms can provide a sound basis for assessing the value of new therapies. This pertains to physical properties of sputum, as well as to the constituents themselves. Critical evaluations of the efficacy of antimicrobial agents in acute exacerbations of chronic bronchitis are possible when the dynamics of the qualitative and quantitative cell and bacterial changes are objectively measured. Both the toxic stimulus (bacterial load) and the cellular inflammatory response are assessed simultaneously and serially. Gibson et al. (1990) have also noted the potential value of using qualitative and quantitative sputum cell counts as objective criteria in the evaluation of therapeutic agents. The efficacy of expectorant and mucolytic agents should be measurable, based on changes of the physical properties of sputum. However, our knowledge of the possible mechanisms by which such agents may work is mostly hypothetical. Consequently, devising objectively based protocols to determine their efficacy have been thwarted.

Much of the information that has been reviewed in this chapter suffers from the lack of correlation to the clinical status of the subjects. Future investigations should take care to carefully define the clinical characteristics of the patient population. There is substantial data to indicate that sputum components of chronic bronchitics who are smokers differ from those who have stopped. The duration of the illness and the age and sex of the subjects would likely also influence the results.

The sputum of chronic bronchitics, as well as those with other sputum-producing lung diseases, provides excellent material for the investigation of the inflammatory process in humans. What better model of human disease is there than those humans with disease. The opportunities for investigation are legion.

References

Adinolfi, M., Glynn, A., Lindsay, M., and Milne, C. M. (1966). Serological properties of A antibodies to *Escherichia coli* present in human colostrum. *Immunology* 10:517–526.

American Thoracic Society (1962). Chronic bronchitis, asthma, and pulmonary emphysema. A statement by the Committee on Diagnostic Standards for Non-tuberculous Respiratory Disease. *Am. Rev. Respir. Dis.* 85: 762–768.

Archer, G. T., and Blackwood, A. (1965). Formation of Charcot–Leyden crystals in human eosinophils and basophils and study of the composition of isolated crystals. *J. Exp. Med.* 122: 173–180.

Atassi, M. Z., Barker, S. A., Houghton, L. E., and Stacey, M. (1957). Neuraminic acid and its relationship to chronic bronchitis. *Clin. Chim. Acta* 4: 741–747.

Auerbach, O., Stout, A. P., Hammond, E. C., and Garfinkel, L. (1961). Changes in bronchial epithelium in relation to cigarette smoking and in relation to lung cancer. *N. Engl. J. Med.* 265: 253–267.

Baigelman, W., Chodosh, S. and Pizzuto, D. (1979). Quantitative sputum gram stains in chronic bronchial disease. *Lung* 156: 265–270.

Benditt, E. P. (1968). Mast cell function: Chemical and structural aspects. In *Biochemistry of The Acute Allergic Reactions*. Edited by K. F. Austen, and E. L. Becker. Philadelphia, F. A. Davis, pp. 119–130.

Bertalanaffy, F. D. (1968). Dynamics of cellular populations in the lung. In *The Lung*. Edited by A. A. Liebow, and D. E. Smith. Baltimore, Williams & Wilkins, pp. 19–30.

Bezançon, F., and DeJong, S. I. (1913). *Traité de L'Examen des Crachats*. Paris, Masson.

Bhaskar, K. R., O'Sullivan, D. D., Hincman, H. O., and Reid, L. M. (1987). Lipids in airway secretions. *Eur. J. Respir. Dis.* 71(Suppl. 153): 215–221.

Biserte, G., Havez, R., and Cuvelier, R. (1963). Glycoprotéides des sécrétions bronchiques. *Exp. Ann. Biochim. Méd.* 24: 85–120.

Boat, T. F., and Matthews, L. W. (1973). Chemical composition of human tracheobronchial secretions. In *Sputum, Fundamentals and Clinical Pathology*. Edited by M. J. Dulfano. Springfield, Charles C. Thomas, pp. 243–274.

Bonomo, L., and D'Addabbo, A. (1964). ^{131}I-albumin turnover and loss of protein into the sputum in chronic bronchitis. *Clin. Chim. Acta* 10: 214–222.

Bornstein, A. A., Chen, T. -M., and Dulfano, M. J. (1978). Disulfide bonds and sputum viscoelasticity. *Biorheology* 15: 261–267.

Bowden, D. H., Adamson, L. Y. R., Grantham, W. G., and Wyatt, J. P. (1969). Origin of the lung macrophage. *Arch. Pathol.* 88: 540–546.

Brogan, T. D., Ryley, H. C., Allen, L., and Hutt, H. (1971). Relationship between sputum sol phase composition and diagnosis in chronic chest diseases. *Thorax* 26: 418–423.

Bryant, D. H., and Pui, A. (1982). Histamine content of sputum from patients with asthma and chronic bronchitis. *Clin. Allergy* 12: 19–27.

Bürgi, H. (1964). Die Viscositaet des purulenten und sterilen Sputums bei chronischer Asthmabronchits. *Med. Thorac.* 21: 156–167.

Bürgi, H., Wiesmann, U., Richterich, R., Regli, J., and Medici, T. (1968). New objective criteria for inflammation in bronchial secretions. *Br. Med. J.* 2: 654–656.

Chanock, R. M. (1971). Local antibody and resistance to acute viral respiratory tract disease. In *The Secretory Immunologic System*. Edited by D. H. Dayton, Jr., P. A. Small, Jr., R. M. Chanock, H. E. Kaufman, and T. B. Tomasi, Jr. Washington, US Department of Health, Education and Welfare. Public Health Service, National Institutes of Health, pp. 83–92.

Chodosh, S. (1963). The cytology and histochemistry of sputum cells. III. Longitudinal studies in chronic bronchitis. *Am. Rev. Respir. Dis.* 88: 108.

Chodosh, S. (1970). Examination of sputum cells. *N. Engl. J. Med.* 282: 854–857.

Chodosh, S. (1971). Efficacy of aerosolized acetylcysteine, acetylcysteine with isoproterenol, and isoproterenol in stable chronic bronchitis at home: A double-blind, cross-over evaluation. *Am. Rev. Respir. Dis.* 103: 904–905.

Chodosh, S. (1973). Objective sputum changes associated with glyceryl guaiacolate in chronic bronchial diseases. *Bull. Physiopathol. Respir.* 9: 452–456.

Chodosh, S. (1978). Sputum: Observations in status asthmaticus and therapeutic considerations. In *Status Asthmaticus*. Edited by E. B. Weiss. Baltimore, University Park Press, pp. 173–200.

Chodosh, S. (1980a). Pathophysiologic derangements in the chronic obstructive pulmonary diseases and pharmacologic regulation of airway function. In *Drugs Affecting the Respiratory System*. Edited by D. L. Temple, Jr. Washington, American Chemical Society, pp. 217–249.

Chodosh, S. (1980b). Mucus and respiratory disease. Mucus in the bronchi and respiratory pathophysiology. *Eur. J. Respir. Dis.* 61(Suppl. 111): 35–36.

Chodosh, S. (1980c). Acetylcysteine in chronic bronchitis. *Eur. J. Respir. Dis.* 61(Suppl. 111): 90–92.

Chodosh, S. (1987). Acute bacterial exacerbations in bronchitis and asthma. *Am. J. Med.* 82(Suppl. 4A): 154–163.

Chodosh, S. (1988). Sputum examination. In *Pulmonary Diseases and Disorders.* Edited by A. P. Fishman. New York, McGraw-Hill, pp. 411–426.

Chodosh, S. (1992). Acute bacterial exacerbations in chronic bronchitis and asthma. In *Infectious Diseases in Medicine and Surgery.* Edited by S. L. Gorbach, J. G. Bartlett, and N. R. Blacklow. Philadelphia, W. B. Saunders, pp. 476–485.

Chodosh, S. and Medici, T. (1971). The bronchial epithelium in chronic bronchitis. I. Exfoliative cytology during stable, acute bacterial infection and recovery phases. *Am. Rev. Respir. Dis.* 104: 888–898.

Chodosh, S., Zaccheo, C. W., and Segal, M. S. (1961). The cytology and histochemistry of sputum cells. I. Preliminary differential counts in chronic bronchitis. *Am. Rev. Respir. Dis.* 85: 635–648.

Chodosh, S., Medici, T. C., and Enslein, K. (1973a). Comparison of five methods for measuring sputum physical characteristics. *Bull. Physiopathol. Respir.* 9: 127–139.

Chodosh, S., Medici, T. C., Ishikawa, S., and Enslein, K. (1973b). Relationship of physical sputum characteristics and ventilatory capacity in chronic bronchial disease. *Chest* 63: 56S–58S.

Chodosh, S., Baigelman, W., Medici, T. C., and Enslein, K. (1975). Long-term home use of acetylcysteine in chronic bronchitis. *Curr. Ther. Res.* 17: 319–334.

Chodosh, S., Eichel, B., Ellis, C., and Medici, T. C. (1982). Comparison of trimethoprim–sulfamethoxazole with ampicillin in acute infectious exacerbations of chronic bronchitis: A double-blind crossover study. *Rev. Infect. Dis.* 4: 517–527.

Clifford, R. (1932). *The Sputum, Its Examination and Clinical Significance.* New York, Macmillan.

Cohn, Z. A. (1965). The metabolism and physiology of the mononuclear phagocytes. In *The Inflammatory Process.* Edited by B. W. Zweifach, L. Grant, and R. T. McCluskey. New York, Academic Press, pp. 323–353.

Curschmann, H. (1885). Einige Bermerkunger über die im Bronchialsekret vorkommenden Spiralen. *Arch. Klin. Med.* 36: 578–585.

Devalia, J. L., Grady, D., Harmanyeri, Y., Tabaqchali, S., and Davies, R. J. (1989) Histamine synthesis by respiratory tract microorganisms: Possible role in pathogenicity. *J. Clin. Pathol.* 42: 516–522.

Dulfano, M. J., Adler, K., and Philippoff, W. (1971). Sputum viscoelasticity in chronic bronchitis. *Am. Rev. Respir. Dis.* 104: 88–98.

Dulfano, M. J., and Philippoff, W. (1973). Physical properties. In *Sputum, Fundamentals and Clinical Pathology.* Edited by M. J. Dulfano. Springfield, Charles C Thomas, pp. 201–242.

Eichel, B., and Chodosh, S. (1976). Enzyme activities in human sputum from chronic bronchitics as discriminators between stable state vs. acute bacterial exacerbations and cigarette smokers vs. ex-smokers. *Am. Rev. Respir. Dis.* 113: 234.

Feldman, M. (1969). Macrophages, lymphocytes and antibody formation. In *The Immune Response and Its Suppression*. Edited by E. Sorkin. New York, S. Karger.

Ferris, B. G., and Anderson, D. O. (1962). The prevalence of chronic respiratory disease in a New Hampshire town. *Am. Rev. Respir. Dis.* 86: 165-177.

Fields, J. P., and Chodosh, S. (1970). Quantitation of sputum protein by use of the biuret reaction. *Clin. Chem.* 16: 773–775.

Florey, H. W. (1970). The secretion of mucus and inflammation of the mucus membranes. In *General Pathology*. Edited by H. W. Florey. Philadelphia, W. B. Saunders, pp. 195–225.

Gerlach, W. (1892). Über die Künstliche Darstellbarkeit Curschmannscher Spiralen. *Dtsch. Arch. Klin. Med.* 50: 450.

Gibson, P. G., Girgis-Gabardo, A., Morris, M. M., Mattoli, S., Kay, J. M., Dolovich, J., Denburg, J., and Hargreave, F. E. (1989). Cellular characteristics of sputum from patients with asthma and chronic bronchitis. *Thorax* 44: 693–699.

Gibson, P. G., Dolovich, J., Denburg, J. A., Girgis-Gabardo, A., and Hargreave, F. E. (1990). Sputum cell counts in airways disease: A useful sampling technique. In *Inflammatory Indices in Chronic Bronchitis*. Basel, Birkhauser Verlag, pp. 161–172.

Green, G. M., and Kass, E. H. (1964a). The role of alveolar macrophage in clearance of bacteria from lung. *J. Exp. Med.* 119: 167–175.

Green, G. M., and Kass, E. H. (1964b). Factors influencing clearance of bacteria by lung. *J. Clin. Invest.* 43: 769–776.

Green, G. M. and Carolin, D. (1967). Depressant effect of cigarette smoke on in vitro antibacterial activity of alveolar macrophages. *N. Engl. J. Med.* 276: 421–427.

Haag, M., Morin, R., Ertl, R., VonEssen, S., and Rennard, S. (1986). Fibronectin is concentrated in the gel sub-phase of human sputum. *Am. Rev. Respir. Dis.* 133: A256.

Harkavy, J. (1930). Spasm-producing substance in the sputum of patients with bronchial asthma. *Arch. Intern. Med.* 45: 641–646.

Havez, R., Degand, P., Roussel, P., and Biserte, G. (1966). Isolement et caractérisation immunologique de la Kallicréine bronchique humaine. *C. R. Acad. Sci. [D] (Paris)* 262: 309–311.

Havez, R., Roussel, P., Degand, P., and Bizerte, G. (1967). Etude des Structurer fibrillaires de la Sécrétion bronchique humaine. *Clin. Chim. Acta.* 17: 281–295.

Hers, J. F., and Mulder, J. (1953). The mucosal epithelium of the respiratory tract in mucopurulent bronchitis caused by *Haemophilus influenzae*. *J. Pathol. Bacteriol.* 66: 103–108.

Hers, J. F. (1961). The pathology of chronic relapsing mucopurulent bronchitis, with and without brochiectasis. In *Bronchitis*. Edited by N. G. M. Orie, and H. J. Sluiter. Assen, Royal Vangorcum, pp. 149–158.

Hirsch, J. G. (1965). Neutrophil and eosinophil leukocytes. In *The Inflammatory Process*. Edited by B. W. Zweifach, L. Grant, and R. T. McCluskey. New York, Academic Press, pp. 245–280.

Hirsch, S. R., Kory, R. C., and Hamilton, L. H. (1966). Evaluation of changes in sputum consistency with a new instrument. *Am. Rev. Respir. Dis.* 94: 784–789.

Hoffman, Von H., and Ebelt, H. (1968). Der elektrolytgehalt des sputums und des serums bie patienten mit asthma bronchiole und bie patienten mit chronischer bronchitis. *Allerg. Asthma* 14: 227–239.

Holub, M., and Hauser, R. E. (1969). Lung alveolar histiocytes engaged in antibody production. *Immunology* 17: 207–226.

Hornung, M. (1962). Preservation, recrystallization and preliminary biochemical characterization of Charcot–Leyden crystals. *Proc. Soc. Exp. Biol. Med.* 110: 119–124.

Hubbard, R. C., McElvaney, N. G., Birrer, P., Shak, S., Robinson, W. W., Jolley, C., Wu, M., Chernick, M. S., and Crystal, R. G. (1992). A preliminary study of aerosolized recombinant human deoxyribonuclease I in the treatment of cystic fibrosis. *N. Engl. J. Med.* 326: 812–815.

Keal, E., and Reid, L. (1973). Physico-chemical properties of sputum in reversible airways obstruction. *Chest* 63(Suppl.): 58S–59S.

Knauss, H. J., Robinson, W. E., Medici, T. C., and Chodosh, S. (1976). Cell vs. noncell airway temporal response in rats exposed to sulfur dioxide. *Arch. Environ. Health* 31: 241–247.

Lamb, D., and Reid, L. (1968). Histochemistry, autoradiography, tissue culture and biochemical analysis in the study of bronchial epithelial glycoproteins. In *Hypersecretion Bronchique*. Edited by C. L. Gernex-Rieux, and P. Boulanger. Lille, Colloque International de Pathologie Thoracique, pp. 11–21.

Laurenzi, G. A., Guarneri, J. J., Endriga, R. B., and Carey, J. P. (1963). Clearance of bacteria by the lower respiratory tract. *Science* 142: 1572–1573.

Levy, L. H., Mendes, E., and Cintra, A. (1961). Hydroxytryptamine in the sputum of asthmatic patients. *Acta Allergol.* 16: 121–127.

Lewis, R. W. (1971). Lipid composition of human bronchial mucus. *Lipids* 6: 859–861.

Lieberman, J. (1968). Measurement of sputum viscosity in a cone-plate viscometer. I. Characteristics of sputum viscosity. *Am. Rev. Respir. Dis.* 97: 654–661.

Lopez-Vidriero, M. T. (1973). Individual and group correlations of sputum viscosity and airways obstruction. *Bull. Physiopathol. Respir.* 9: 339–346.

Lorenz, T. H., Korst, D., Simpson, E. J. F., and Musser, M. J. (1957). A quantitative method of bronchial lysozyme. I. An investigation of bronchial lysozyme. *J. Lab. Clin. Med.* 49: 145–150.

Mackaness, G. B. (1971). The induction and expression of cell-mediated hypersensitivity in the lung. *Am. Rev. Respir. Dis.* 104: 813–828.

Mackaness, G. B., and Blanden, R. V. (1967). Cellular immunity. *Prog. Allergy* 11: 89–140.

Marchioni, C. F., Moretti, M., Muratori, M., Casadei, M. C., Guerzoni, P., Scuri, R., and Fregnan, G. B. (1990). Effects of erdosteine on sputum biochemical and rheologic properties: Pharmaco-kinetics in chronic obstructive lung disease. *Lung* 168: 285–293.

Masson, P. L., Heremans, J. F., Prignot, J. J., and Wauters, G. (1966). Immunohistochemical localization and bacteriostatic properties of an iron-binding protein from bronchial mucus. *Thorax* 21: 538–544.

Masson, P. L., Heremans, J. F., and Schonne, E. (1969). Lactoferrin, an iron-binding protein in neutrophilic leukocytes. *J. Exp. Med.* 130: 643–658.

Masson, P. L., and Heremans, J. F. (1973). Sputum proteins. In *Sputum, Fundamentals and Clinical Pathology*. Edited by M. J. Dulfano. Springfield, Charles C Thomas, pp. 412–475.

Medici, T., and Bürgi, H. (1971). The role of immunoglobulin A in endogenous bronchial defense mechanisms in chronic bronchitis. *Am. Rev. Respir. Dis.* 103: 784–791.

Medici, T. C., and Chodosh, S. (1972). The reticuloendothelial system in chronic bronchitis. I. Quantitative sputum cell populations during stable, acute bacterial infection, and recovery phases. *Am. Rev. Respir. Dis.* 105: 792–804.

Medici, T. C., and Chodosh, S. (1973). Nonmalignant exfoliative sputum cytology. In *Sputum, Fundamentals and Clinical Pathology*. Edited by M. J. Dulfano. Springfield, Charles C Thomas, pp. 332–381.

Medici, T. C., and Chodosh, S. (1982). Bronchial inflammation and hyperreactivity: A study on sputum cell excretion in stable chronic bronchitis with and without allergic rhinitis. In *Bronchial Hyperreactivity*. Edited by A. Morley. London, Academic Press, pp. 133–141.

Medici, T., Chodosh, S., and Bürgi, H. (1970). Assessing the sputum. *Lancet* 1: 620.

Medici, T. C., von Graevenitz, A., Shang, H., Böhni, E., and Wall, M. (1988). Gram stain and culture of morning and 24 h sputum in the diagnosis of bacterial exacerbation of chronic bronchitis: A dogma disputed. *Eur. Respir. J.* 1: 923–928.

Merrill, W. W., Goodenberger, D., Strober, W., Matthay, R. A., Naegel, G. P., and Reynolds, H. Y. (1980). Free secretory component and other proteins in human lung lavage. *Am. Rev. Respir. Dis.* 122: 156–160.

Metchnikoff, E. (1893). *Lectures on the Comparative Pathology of Inflammation* (1891). Translated by F. Starling. London, Kagan, Paul, Trench and Trubner.

Moodley, I., Zhong, N. S., Morgan, D. J. R., and Davies, R. J. (1984). A comparison of available methods for the measurement of histamine in sputum. *Clin. Allergy* 14: 153–163.

Mullen, J. B. M., Wright, J. L., Wiggs, B. R., Pare, P. D., and Hogg, J. C. (1985). Reassessment of inflammation of airways in chronic bronchitis. *Br. Med. J.* 291: 1235–1239.

Papanicolaou, G. N. (1954). *Atlas of Exfoliative Cytology*. Cambridge, Harvard University Press.

Pearsall, N. N., and Weiser, R. S. (1970). *The Macrophage*. Philadelphia, Lea & Febiger, pp. 71–82.

Pham, Q. T., Peslin, R., Puchelle, E., Salmon, D. Caraux, G., and Benis, A. M. (1973). Fonction respiratoire et état rhéologique des sécrétions recueillies pendant l'expectoration spontanée et dirigée. *Bull. Physiopathol. Respir.* 9: 293–311.

Puchelle, E., Zahm, J. M., and Havez, R. (1973). Biochemical and rheological data in sputum. III. Relationship between biochemical constituents and the rheological properties of sputum. *Bull. Physiopathol. Respir.* 9: 237–256.

Raphael, G. D., and Metcalfe, D. D. (1986). Mediators of airways inflammation. *Eur. J. Respir. Dis.* 69(Suppl. 147): 44–56.

Rebuck, J. W., Hodson, J. M., Priest, R. J., and Barth, C. L. (1963). Basophilic granulocytes in inflammatory tissues of man. *Ann. N. Y. Acad. Sci.* 103: 409–426.

Reid, L. (1960). Measurement of the bronchial mucous gland layer: A diagnostic yardstick in chronic bronchitis. *Thorax* 15: 132–141.

Reid, L. (1968). Bronchial mucous production in health and disease. In *The Lung*. Edited by A. A. Liebow, and D. E. Smith. Baltimore, Williams & Wilkins, pp. 87–108.

Reid, L. M., and Bhaskar, K. R. (1989). Macromolecular and lipid constituents of bronchial epithelial mucus. In *Symposia of the Society for Experimental Biology*. Great Britain, Society for Experimental Biology, pp. 201–219.

Rhodin, J. A. G. (1966). Ultrastructure and function of the human tracheal mucosa. *Am. Rev. Respir. Dis.* 93: 1–15.

Robertson, A. J. (1952). Green sputum. *Lancet* 1: 12–15.

Roitt, I. M., Greaves, M. F., Torrigiani, G., Brostoff, G., and Playfair, J. H. L. (1969). The cellular basis of immunological responses. *Lancet* 2: 367–371.

Ryley, H. C., and Brogan, T. D. (1969). Variation in the composition of sputum in chronic chest diseases. *Br. J. Exp. Pathol.* 49: 625–633.

Ryley, H. C., and Brogan, T. D. (1973). Quantitative immunoelectrophoretic analysis of the plasma proteins in the sol phase of sputum from patients with chronic bronchitis. *J. Clin. Pathol.* 26: 852–856.

Salvato, G. (1968). Some histological changes in chronic bronchitis and asthma. *Thorax* 23: 168–172.

Sanderud, K. (1956). Squamous metaplasia of the respiratory tract epithelium, an autopsy of 214 cases. *Acta Pathol. Microbiol. Scand.* 44: 21–32.

Schmidt, A. (1892). Beitrag zur Kenntnis des Sputums, insbesondere des asthmatischen und zur Pathologie des Asthma bronchiale. *Z. Klin. Med.* 20: 476–501.

Schmidt, A. (1898). Über die Herkunft und chemische Natur der Myelin-formen des Sputums. *Berlin Klin. Wochenschr.* 4: 73–75.

Schultze, H. E., and Heremans, J. F. (1966). The proteins of respiratory secretions. I. Tracheobronchial secretions. In *Molecular Biology of Human Proteins With Special Reference to Plasma Proteins*, Vol. 1. Edited by H. E. Schultze, and J. F. Heremans, New York, Elsevier, pp. 816–828.

Selye, H. (1965). *The Mast Cells*. Washington, Butterworth, p. 364.

Shak, S., Capon, D. J., Hellmiss, R., Marsters, S. A., and Baker, C. L. (1990). Recombinant human DNase I reduces the viscosity of cystic fibrosis sputum. *Proc. Natl. Acad. Sci. USA* 87: 9188–9192.

Sheffner, A. L. (1963). The reduction in vitro in viscosity of mucoprotein solutions by a new mucolytic agent. *Ann. N. Y. Acad. Sci.* 106: 298–310.

Sheinman, B. D., Devalia, J. L., Davies, R. J., Crook, S. J., and Tabaqchali, S. (1986). Synthesis of histamine by *Haemophilus influenzae*. *Br. Med. J.* 292: 857–858.

Spector, W. G., Walters, M., and Willoughby, D. A. (1965). The origin of mononuclear cells in inflammatory exudates induced by fibrinogen. *J. Pathol. Bacteriol.* 90: 181–192.

Spritzer, A. A., Watson, J. A, Auld, J. A., and Guettnoff, M. A. (1968). Pulmonary macrophage clearance. The hourly rates of transfer of pulmonary macrophages to the oropharynx of the rat. *Arch. Environ. Health* 17: 726–730.

Sturgess, J. M., Palfrey, A. J., and Reid, L. (1970). The viscosity of bronchial secretions. *Clin. Sci.* 38: 145–156.

Tada, T., and Ishizaka, K. (1970). Distribution of E-forming cells in lymphoid tissues of the human and monkey. *J. Immunol.* 104: 377–387.

Thomas, H. V., and Simmons, E. (1969). Histamine content in sputum from allergic and non-allergic individuals. *J. Appl. Physiol.* 26: 793–797.

Thompson, A. B., and Rennard, S. I. (1988). Assessment of airways inflammation utilizing bronchoalveolar lavage. *Clin. Chest Med.* 9: 635–642.

Thompson, A. B., Daughton, D., Robbins, R. A., Ghafouri, M. A., Oehlerking, M., and Rennard, S. I. (1989). Intraluminal airway inflammation in chronic bronchitis. *Am. Rev. Respir. Dis.* 140: 1527–1537.

Thomson, M. L., Pavia, D., and McNicol, N. W. (1973). A preliminary study of the effect of guaifenesin on mucociliary clearance from the human lung. *Thorax* 28: 742–747.

Tomasi, T. B., Jr. (1971). The concept of local immunity and the secretory system. In *The Secretory Immunologic System*. Edited by D. H. Dayton, Jr., P. A. Small, Jr., R. M. Chanock, H. E. Kaufman, and T. B. Tomasi, Jr. Washington, US Department of Health, Education and Welfare. Public Health Service, National Institutes of Health, pp. 3–10.

Truitt, G. L., and Mackaness (1971). Cell-mediated resistance to aerogenic infection of the lung. *Am. Rev. Respir. Dis.* 104: 829–843.

Turnbull, L. S., Turnbull, L. W., Leitch, A. G., Crofton, J. W., and Kay, A. B. (1977). Mediators of immediate-type hypersensitivity in sputum from patients with chronic bronchitis and asthma. *Lancet* 1: 526–529.

Van Furth, R., and Cohn, Z. A. (1968). The origin and kinetics of mononuclear phagocytes. *J. Exp. Med.* 128: 415–435.

Vassar, P. S., Culling, C., and Saunders. A. M. (1960). Fluorescent histiocytes in sputum related to smoking. *Arch. Pathol.* 70: 649–656.

Von Hoesslin, H. (1926). *Das Sputum, Zweite Auflage*. Berlin, Veülag von Julius Springer.

Von Leyden, E. (1872). Zur Kenntnis des Bronchial asthma. *Virchows Arch.* [A] 54: 324–344.

Weibel, E. R. (1963). *Morphometry of Human Lung*. New York, Academic Press, p. 139.

Weiss, S. J. (1989). Tissue destruction by neutrophils. *N. Engl. J. Med.* 320: 365–376.

Wewers, M. (1989). Pathogenesis of emphysema. Assessment of basic science concepts through clinical investigation. *Chest* 95: 190–195.

White, J. C., Elmes, P. C., and Walsh, A. (1954). Fibrous proteins of pathological bronchial secretions studied by optical and electron microscopy: Desoxyribonucleoprotein and mucoprotein in bronchial secretions. *J. Pathol. Bacteriol.* 67: 105–108.

Yeager, H., Jr. (1971). Tracheobronchial secretions. *Am. J. Med.* 50: 493–509.

17

Possible Control of Airway Hypersecretion

ADAM WANNER

University of Miami
Miami, Florida

I. Introduction

The total amount of surface liquid (mucus) in the conducting airways is governed by the rate of mucous secretion, on the one hand, and the clearance of mucus by epithelial reabsorption, evaporation, ciliary transport, and cough transport. Under normal conditions, the secretion and clearance of mucus are balanced, resulting in a thin surface liquid layer covering the tracheobronchial tree. Airway hypersecretion of mucus, if not accompanied by increased mucous clearance can lead to the accumulation of airway mucus. Irrespective of whether the buildup of mucus occurs uniformly and leads to an increased depth of the surface liquid layer, or at discrete sites in the airway lumen, the increased volume of airway mucus has several functional consequences. Undesired effects include airflow obstruction (Petty et al., 1965; Wanner, 1979; Dunnill, 1975), enhanced deposition of inhaled particulate matter in the tracheobronchial tree (Kim et al., 1983, 1985, 1988), and cough (Annesi and Kauffmann, 1986). However, the increased amount of airway mucus may also have a protective role by serving as a physical barrier against biologically active inhalants, preventing bacteria colonizing the airways from adhering to the epithelium, and inactivating cytotoxic products released from luminal leukocytes (mechanical, biological, and chemical screen) (King et al., 1985; Vishwanath and Ramphal, 1984; Cross et al., 1984). Interventions that reduce the total volume and change the distribution of lower airway mucus may, therefore, have both desired and undesired effects in patients with a hypersecretory state.

To reduce the amount of luminal mucus in the airways, three major strategies have been employed. The first is to inhibit mucous hypersecretion by pharmacological agents. The second is to stimulate ciliary activity and improve mucociliary interaction, thereby augmenting ciliary clearance; this is generally also accomplished with pharmacological agents. The third approach is to enhance cough clearance, either by changing the rheological properties of luminal mucus by pharmacological means or by moving mucus physically from smaller to larger airways from where it can be eliminated by cough clearance.

II. Inhibition of Hypersecretion

In airway disease, increased production of airway liquid generally results from epithelial hypersecretion, microvascular hyperpermeability, or both; therefore, pharmacological intervention is aimed at one or both of these abnormalities. To inhibit the hypersecretion of ions, maromolecules, and water by epithelial cells, the causes of the hypersecretion ideally should be known. This is required because a common pathway for the secretory processes has not been identified.

It is generally held that airway hypersecretion is mediated by autonomic neurotransmitters, neuropeptides, and inflammatory cell products. Pharmacological agents capable of inhibiting the synthesis, release, and tissue effects of these substances, and of augmenting their breakdown, ought to prevent or reduce hypersecretion.

The roles of autonomic neurotransmitters, neuropeptides, and inflammatory mediators in the control of airway secretion and the experimental use of drugs to demonstrate the actions of these secretagogues are discussed in Chapters 9–15. In the clinical setting, anticholinergic agents and agents inhibiting the formation and actions of lipid mediators have, based on current knowledge, the greatest therapeutic potential.

A. Anticholinergic Agents

Atropine appears to have relatively little or no effect on baseline epithelial secretions. In the dog trachea, for example, atropine does not influence baseline chloride and, hence, water secretion toward the luminal side (Marin et al., 1976). Likewise, atropine does not alter the volume or rheological properties of submucosal gland secretions, as assessed by single-gland duct cannulation in the cat trachea (Leikauf et al., 1984). Similar results were obtained when total secretory material was examined in a canine tracheal pouch preparation; neither the secretory volume nor the viscoelastic properties of the secretions were changed by atropine in those experiments (Giordano et al., 1978). Somewhat different results have been reported by King and co-workers (1979, 1981), who found a decrease in the secretory volume in the canine trachea after atropine administration. This apparent change in secretory rate was not associated with significant changes in the viscosity/elasticity ratios of the secretions (unless the initial elasticity was low) or the transportability of those secretions on the frog palate.

These observations suggest that muscarinic receptor activation by acetylcholine plays a minor role in the control of baseline airway secretory function. In contrast, vagal stimulation clearly increases the rate of glycoconjugates and water secretion in the airways of several species including humans (Phipps, 1984; Pack and Richardson, 1984; Barnes, 1984). The neurotransmitters involved in vagally induced mucous hypersecretion seem to include acetylcholine as well as neuropeptides (Peatfield and Richardson, 1983; Borson et al., 1982). For example, electrical stimulation of the vagus in the cat has been found to increase secretion of radiolabeled glycoconjugates in the airways, and this was not inhibited by the α-adrenergic antagonist phentolamine and the β-adrenergic antagonist propranolol (Peatfield and Richardson, 1983). Atropine afforded only an attenuation, but no complete blockade. By exclusion, nonadrenergic, noncholinergic effects of electrical vagal stimulation (i.e., peptidergic neurotransmission) was implicated as a contributing factor in vagally induced secretions. In a clinical study, Lopez-Vidriero et al. (1975) showed a decrease in sputum volume in several patients with various forms of airway disease (some with bronchorrhea) who were given a single dose of atropine by inhalation, intramuscular injection, or oral administration. However, the authors attributed the observed decrease in the sputum volume mainly to a decrease in salivary secretion; neither viscosity nor several chemical constituents of sputum were consistently altered by atropine. In one patient, long-term administration of atropine by mouth caused a progressive reduction in the daily sputum volume.

From these examinations of expectorated sputum, it cannot be determined whether the decrease in sputum volume was due to a decrease in the production or a decrease in the clearance of lower airway secretions. Indeed, most investigators agree that atropine depresses mucociliary transport and inhibits ciliary activity in the airways when administered by various routes, including inhalation (Blair and Woods, 1969; Bulbring et al., 1953; Burton, 1962; Foster et al., 1976; Inness and Nickerson, 1970; Pavia and Thompson, 1971; Sackner et al., 1977; Berger et al., 1978; Chopra, 1978). The tertiary ammonium compound ipratropium bromide, at therapeutic doses given over weeks, did not reduce the volume or the dry/wet ratio of sputum in patients with chronic bronchitis (Chervinsky, 1977; Krieger and Reitberger, 1975). In contrast, one study has reported beneficial effects of nasally inhaled ipratropium bromide on nasal hypersecretion in patients with perennial rhinitis, as assessed by symptom scores and other clinical criteria (Borum et al., 1979). Unlike atropine, inhaled ipratropium bromide, given in a single dose for long terms, does not depress airway ciliary clearance in normal subjects or in patients with asthma or chronic bronchitis (Pavia et al., 1980).

From the available information, one might conclude that muscarinic antagonists have no effect or no detectable effect on airway hypersecretion in patients with airway disease. However, it is possible that these agents attenuate airway hypersecretion provoked by stimuli that induce vagally mediated airway responses, particularly in individuals without preexisting hypersecretion.

B.   Inhibitors of Lipid Mediators

Several inflammatory mediators are potent secretagogues in the airways. Lipid mediators seem to be of particular importance because they stimulate epithelial secretion. For example, leukotriene C_4 and D_4, and monohydroxyeicosatetranoic acid increase glycoconjugate and water secretion by human and ovine epithelia in vitro (Marom et al., 1981, 1982; Phipps et al., 1983a) and inhaled prostaglandin $F_{2\alpha}$ to induces sputum in normal human subjects (Lopez-Vidriero et al., 1977). Platelet-activating factor (PAF) is also a secretagogue in human airways in vitro, and it probably exerts this effect by amplifying eicosanoid production (Lundgren et al., 1989). If the synthesis and release of these products is induced by an anaphylactic reaction, the resulting increase in glycoconjugate and water secretion can be blocked or attenuated by pretreatment with the mediator secretion inhibitor cromolyn sodium (Phipps et al., 1983a); with glucocorticosteroids, which inhibit phospholipase A_2 and, hence, arachidonic acid generation by inducing lipocortin (Phipps et al., 1983a; Marom et al., 1984; Shimura et al., 1990; Lundgren et al., 1988); and with sulfidopeptide leukotriene receptor antagonists (Phipps et al., 1983a) in vitro. Some of the drugs have also been shown to lower baseline secretion, possibly reflecting eicosanoid activation resulting from the manipulation of the in vitro preparation. These findings suggest that these drugs might inhibit hypersecretion in other forms of airway inflammation as well. Since lower airway secretions are difficult to quantitate in human subjects, objective data on the clinical antisecretory effects of glucocorticosteroids or other drugs interfering with eicosanoid or PAF are scarce. One study has reported a decrease in sputum volume in asthmatic patients after a course of systemic glucocorticosteroid therapy (Keal, 1971).

III.   Stimulation of Ciliary Clearance

From the trachea to the terminal bronchioles, the epithelium is populated with cilia. The density of the cilia is high in the trachea (about 200 cilia per cell) and diminishes toward the peripheral bronchi (Wanner, 1977). Cilia are between 4 and 6 μm long, depending on airway level (shorter in small bronchi; Serafini and Michaelson, 1977), and 0.1 and 0.2 μm in diameter. The ciliary tip terminates in a crown of short claws that engage the overlying mucous gel, either mechanically or biochemically for mucous transport (Foliguet and Puchelle, 1986). Each cilium contains one pair of central microtubules and nine pairs of peripheral microtubules running the length of the ciliary shaft. The doublets are connected by strands of nexin, and one subfiber of each doublet possesses two dynein arms that project toward the next doublet and a radial spoke that attaches to one of the two central microtubules. The microtubules are constructed from tubulin, a cyclic protein, whereas the dynein arms are large proteins containing ATPase (Satir, 1989). Ciliary bending is accomplished by the active sliding of the dynein arm, containing a microtubule of an outer doublet, along the adjacent microtubule of the neighboring doublet. The ATPase–protein dynein is the site of energy used in this process. The ATP is used to form the molecular bridges between adjacent doublet microtubules ("marching" of dynein along the length of the microtubule) (Satir, 1989; Gibbons and Rowe, 1965). Active sliding of doublets on one side of the axoneme bends the cilium in one direction, and active sliding of doublets on the other side bends it in the opposite direction. Airway cilia move mucus by the mechanics of their beat cycle. Ciliary beat frequency has been reported to range between 15 and 18 Hz in humans (Rutland et al., 1982; Iravani and Van As, 1972). The beat cycle consists of an effective stroke (towards the pharynx for lower airway cilia) and a recovery stroke (opposite direction). During the effective stroke, the cilium moves through an arc of about 110° (maximum tip velocity 100 μm/s; Satir, 1989). and interacts with mucus. At the end of the effective stroke, the cilium disengages from the mucus and rests to prevent backward flow of mucus. The cilium then starts its recovery stroke close to the cell surface. Mucociliary transport is determined by a complicated relation between ciliary beating, mucus (epiphase), and periciliary fluid (hypophase).

Given that the mucous epiphase is a nonnewtonian (elastic) fluid and the periciliary hypophase a newtonian fluid, certain mathematical predictions can be made for the effects of ciliary beat frequency, depth of periciliary fluid and mucus, and viscoelastic properties of mucus on mucociliary transport (Sleigh, 1989; Ross and Corrsin, 1974). Mucociliary transport is related directly to the elastic recoil of the epiphase within wide limits, and indirectly to the viscosity of the epiphase and hypophase. Other physical properties, such as surface tension, stickiness, and spinability (thread-forming ability) may be important in determining mucous transport. Mucous transport is also directly related to ciliary beat frequency (at fixed wave speed) and is influenced by the depth of the periciliary fluid. Some of the determinants have been experimentally verified (Puchelle and Zahm, 1984; Puchelle et al., 1983).

The stimulating effect of drugs on ciliary clearance involves intracellular ciliomodulators. To date, adenosine triphosphate (ATP), calcium ion (Ca^{2+}), cyclic adenosine monophosphate (cAMP), and cyclic guanosine monophosphate (cGMP) have been identified as important factors. ATP has been reported to markedly increase the mucociliary transport rate in frog pharyngeal mucosa (Vorhaus and Deyrup, 1953) and to increase the ciliary beat frequency in the amphibian oviduct (23). The ATP-induced ciliostimulation appears to be associated with an increase in the angular velocity of cilia, with a decrease in the duration of the effective and recovery strokes (Weaver and Hard, 1985). In addition to the intracellular effects of ATP, which appear to result from its chemical energy-converting action, extracellular ATP can also stimulate ciliary activity, suggesting a membrane-associated amplification process (Murakami et al., 1974).

The cytosolic concentration of Ca^{2+} has been reported to influence mitochondrial oxidative phosphorylation and to stimulate glycogenolysis, thereby promoting the generation of ATP (Landowne and Ritchie, 1971). This mechanism of ciliostimulation is consistent with the observation that intracellular Ca^{2+} stimulates ciliary activity indirectly through ATP synthesis, and that Mg^{2+} could be the cofactor of the ciliary ATPase (Eckert and Murakami, 1972). Other mechanisms may also be operative. For example, the cilioexcitatory action of Ca^{2+} in dogs is inhibited by a calmodulin antagonist, implicating the Ca^{2+}–calmodulin system (Hidaka and Tanaka, 1982). Extracellular Ca^{2+} could also be a ciliostimulator, as suggested by Lee et al. (1976) and Verdugo (1980), based on rabbit oviduct experiments. Intracellular calcium, however, is more important as a ciliostimulator than extracellular calcium (Girard and Kennedy, 1986). Villalon et al. (1989) have shown that a rapid and brief increase of cytosolic Ca^{2+} concentration, lasting seconds, initiated a sustained increase in ciliary beat frequency; the relation of a transient change in cytosolic calcium concentration to ATP- or calmodulin-dependent sustained ciliostimulation remains to be explored. Interestingly, calcium appears to be cilioinhibitory in the lateral cilia of the *Mytilus* gill, in contrast with the ciliostimulatory effects of calcium in mammalian ciliated cells (Stommel and Stephens, 1985).

CyclicAMP has increased ciliary beat frequency in mammalian airways (Tamaoki et al., 1989; Di Benedetto et al., 1991). It is operative only as an intracellular messenger, since only permeable analogues of cAMP are effective intact cells, and only cAMP is effective in preparations devoid of functional membranes surrounding the axoneme (Murakami et al., 1974; Bonini et al., 1986). The ciliostimulatory effects of intracellular cAMP may be mediated through the generation of ATP by stimulating glycolysis in the Kreb's cycle (Nelson and Wright, 1974), cAMP-dependent protein phosphorylation (Stommel and Stephens, 1985), and hyperpolarization of the ciliary membrane (Hennessey et al., 1985). CyclicGMP is also ciliostimulatory in rabbit airway epithelium (Kobayashi et al., 1991). The mechanism of GMP-induced ciliostimulation is unknown, but it does not appear to involve activation of intracellular cAMP.

Agents that stimulate ciliary activity frequently also stimulate ion and water transport and glycoconjugate secretion into the airway, thereby increasing the volume of periciliary fluid and mucus. Therefore, the enhanced ciliary clearance of lower airway mucus, an effect usually seen after the administration of a ciliostimulatory agent, may not diminish the net volume of lower airway mucus as efficiently because of concomitant hypersecretion. To what extent these agents decrease the volume of lower airway mucus in hypersecretory states depends on the relative magnitudes of the ciliary and secretory effects of the agents.

A. β-Adrenergic Agonists

The β-adrenergic agonists have been shown to stimulate ciliary clearance in normal subjects (Foster et al., 1976; Konietzko et al., 1975) and in patients with chronic bronchitis (Santa Cruz et al., 1974), cystic fibrosis (Wood et al., 1975), and asthma (Mossberg et al., 1976). Stimulating effects have been observed with all forms of administration (oral, sublingual, inhalation) and with different β-agonists, including epinephrine, isoproterenol, and agonists with preferential $β_2$-action (Iravani, 1972; Van As, 1974; Sackner et al., 1976). In normal dogs, a dose-dependent effect of inhaled isoproterenol and carbuterol delivered by metered-dose aerosol has been demonstrated (Sackner et al., 1976). The peak effect (70–100% increase) occurred between 10 and 30 min after drug administration.

B. Cholinergic Agonists

Acetylcholine and other cholinergic agonists stimulate ciliary activity directly (Bulbring et al., 1953) and stimulate mucociliary clearance in vivo (Berger et al., 1978; Camner et al., 1974). Although potent stimulators of ciliary clearance, these agents cannot be administered to patients with airway disease because of their bronchoconstricting effect.

C. Methylxanthines

Theophylline and aminophylline administered intravenously or orally have clear-cut stimulatory effects on mucociliary clearance in intact animals and human subjects (Serafini et al., 1976; Sutton et al., 1981; Matthys et al., 1983). In these studies, the effects were demonstrable in normal airways, as well as in abnormal airways (chronic bronchitis). In one study, a positive correlation was found between the improvement in ciliary clearance and serum theophylline levels after theophylline administration (Matthys et al., 1983). The mechanism by which methylxanthines stimulate ciliary activity and clearance have not been elucidated, but may include inhibition of phosphodiesterases, leading to increased intracellular cAMP levels (Nelson and Wright, 1974; Soliman, 1984).

D. Mucolytic Agents

Ideally, mucolytic agents should exert their beneficial action on luminal mucus without inhibiting ciliary function, causing hypersecretion, or aggravating persisting hypersecretion. The desired effect of mucus is to move its viscoelastic properties into a range that enhances mucociliary interaction and, hence, ciliary clearance. *N*-Acetylcysteine, *S*-carboxymethylcysteine, bromhexine, iodide and iodized compounds, and digestive enzymes have been extensively studied for their ability to change the viscoelastic properties of mucus. *N*-Acetylcysteine is presumed to exert its effect on mucus by breaking disulfide bonds, thereby depolymerizing the glycoconjugate molecule. *N*-Acetylcysteine reduces the viscosity of expectorated sputum in vitro and the elasticity of lower airway mucus, and increases the transportability of that mucus on the frog palate, suggesting improved mucociliary interaction (Puchelle et al., 1980; Martin et al., 1980). Likewise, *S*-carboxymethylcysteine reduces the viscosity of sputum (Edwards et al., 1976). Bromhexine, which can dissolve acidic glycoconjugates contained in mucus, has been reported to decrease both the viscosity and elasticity of lower airway secretions after oral administration in guinea pigs (Martin et al., 1990). Iodides accelerate the digestion of purulent sputum by proteolytic enzymes in vitro, thereby presumably lowering sputum viscosity (Reas, 1963). Finally, pancreatic dornase and trypsin can alter the physical properties of mucus by breaking down DNA and by proteolysis (Lieberman, 1968a,b). Other agents, such as urea and 2-α-thenoylthioproprionylglycine also reduce the viscosity and elasticity of mucus in vitro by unknown mechanisms (Limber et al., 1952; Davis et al., 1985).

Despite these effects on mucous rheology, the actions of mucolytics on ciliary clearance are generally absent, inconsistent, or (at high concentrations) detrimental (e.g., *N*-acetylcysteine) (Millar et al., 1985; Stafanger et al., 1988; Thomson et al., 1975; Ericsson et al., 1987). Clearly, the search for more effective agents must continue.

E. Hydration

Most investigations of the effects of local hydration (inhaled bland aerosols) and systemic hydration on ciliary clearance have not been able to detect stimulation of ciliary clearance by these interventions (Wanner, 1977; Marchette et al., 1985; Wanner and Rao, 1980).

IV. Stimulation of Cough Clearance

Mucus can be cleared from the airways by cough or forced expiration. These maneuvers differ fundamentally from ciliary clearance, because the energy needed to move the mucus is derived from air movement, rather than from cilia.

The efficacy of this process depends mainly on fluid dynamic interactions between the mucous layer and the airflow. The independence from the ciliary activity makes these secondary clearance mechanisms particularly important when ciliary clearance fails.

Air flowing through the airways thickly lined with mucus interacts with the mucous layer and develops a shear force on the interfacial surface of the mucous layer (Clarke et al., 1970). Because the magnitude of the shear force is directly proportional to the *kinetic energy of airflow* (which is defined as a product of the density of air and the square of the mean airflow velocity), the mucous layer can be propelled in the direction of airflow if airflow velocity is sufficiently high to overcome the viscous and gravitational resistance of the mucous layer. Depending on the magnitude of airflow velocity and the physical characteristics of mucus, the mucous layer moves in different patterns (Leith, 1977). When the rate of mucous accumulation exceeds the rate of removal and the airways are thereby plugged with mucus, air may flow through the mucus as small bubbles, pushing the mucous plug slowly (bubble flow; airflow velocity <0.6 ms^{-1}). As the airflow velocity increases, the bubbles grow in size and combine together (slug flow; $0.6-10$ ms^{-1}), and eventually form a continuous channel through the mucus (annular flow; $10-25$ ms^{-1}). At very high airflow velocity, the mucous layer can be blown off the airway surface as droplets (mist flow; >25 ms^{-1}).

There is a critical depth below which the mucous layer cannot be moved by the shear force imparted from the airflow (Clarke et al., 1970; Kim et al., 1986, 1987). The critical depth decreases with an increase in airflow velocity. The critical depth also increases with an increase in viscosity of mucus, and at the same level of viscosity it tends to increase with elasticity. During cough, the critical depth may range between 100 and 400 μm in the viscosity range of 10–600 Poise in the midsized airways (Kim et al., 1986). Thus, normal subjects cannot clear airway mucus by coughing because the normal mucous layer is too thin for effective gas–liquid interaction.

Lowering the viscosity of mucus is essential for improving clearance by two-phase flow mechanisms. However, if the viscosity of mucus is too low (< 10 Poise), gravity flow dominates over two-phase flow and results in flooding of the lower airways. The ideal viscosity for two-phase flow transport appears to be between 10 and 100 Poise, depending on the gravity angle of the airways. The effect of mucous elasticity on cough clearance has not been fully established (King et al., 1985a,b). This is because changes in the elasticity of mucus are generally associated with greater changes in its viscosity, thereby making it difficult to separate the individual effects of viscosity and elasticity.

Cough is characterized by a brief inspiration, followed by an explosive expiration. In the beginning of the expiratory effort, the glottis is closed briefly (about 0.2 s); during this time the intrathoracic pressure is raised to 50–100 mm Hg or more (Leith, 1977). After the sudden opening of the glottis, expiratory flow accelerates rapidly and reaches a peak value of about 10 L/s within 30–50 ms (supramaximal flow). An extremely high airflow velocity is associated with this, often approaching the sonic velocity, because during cough a dramatic narrowing of the central airways occurs.

Forced expiration can also move mucus. The forced expiratory maneuver consists of a forced expiration from midlung volume to low lung volume, followed by a period of relaxed breathing (Pryor et al., 1979). Airway narrowing is an essential part of the forced expiratory maneuver, enhancing airflow velocity, as in cough. The initiation of forced expiratory maneuver from the midlung volume moves the equal-pressure point into more peripheral bronchi, thereby extending the number of bronchial generations with effective air–liquid interaction.

Major requirements for an effective cough or forced expiratory maneuver are a high airflow velocity and a relatively low mucous viscosity. Regardless of which maneuver is used, airflow velocities are insufficient in small bronchi. Therefore, it is the objective of therapeutic interventions to propel mucus from small to large airways, where it encounters higher airflow velocities, and to optimize its rheological properties for air–liquid interaction. Chest physical therapy intends to meet the first objective, whereas hydration and pharmacological agents have been employed in an attempt to meet the second objective.

A. Chest Physical Therapy

The goal of chest physical therapy is to move mucus by gravity, chest vibration (oscillation), or both. Since noninvasive methods that visualize and quantitate tracheal mucous secretions directly are not available, two indirect methods have been employed to determine the role of chest physical therapy: volumetric measurement of expectorated sputum and the determination of mucous clearance in the tracheobronchial tree. A single session of postural drainage (usually 20°– 40° head-down tilt) will increase clearance of central airway secretions and the amount of sputum in patients with cystic fibrosis or chronic bronchitis (Pavia et al., 1976). Most of the patients thus studied had considerable sputum production. This appears to be an important prerequisite for the effectiveness of postural drainage, because the same maneuver does not enhance mucociliary clearance in normal control subjects. Likewise, it has been suggested that postural drainage increases airway clearance only if combined with coughing; if cough is suppressed, a significant effect of postural drainage is not observed. Chest percussion or vibration per se may also stimulate mucociliary clearance or sputum production; however, clinical studies have been controversial, with some suggesting a beneficial effect and others no independent or additive effect of chest vibration to postural drainage (Pavia et al., 1976). The frequency of chest clapping has not always been reported, but with conventional techniques, it can be assumed to have been 4–5 Hz. By using external vibrating devices, the frequencies studied have been as high as 41 Hz. These frequencies may not be optimal for effective chest vibration. Additional experiments have tried to define the specifications of optimal chest physical therapy. The currently 20°–45° head-down tilt appears to be ideal for clearing lower airway secretions, in that it creates a large enough gravitational force without intolerable side effects. However, the efficacy of conventional chest clapping or chest wall vibration has been called into question. Chest wall oscillations at frequencies between 5 and 17 Hz (but not at 3 Hz) have increased transport of mucus in the trachea of dogs, with a peak effect at 15 Hz (King et al., 1983). Other investigators have made similar observations with oscillation applied either to the chest wall or at the airway opening in sheep (Rubin et al., 1989; Freitag et al., 1989a,b). Since air–liquid interaction appears to be the principal mechanism whereby chest oscillations move secretions, one would expect that an expiratory bias in airflow and a high airflow velocity are required for effective mucous propulsion. The observations that mucus indeed moves in the direction of airflow bias during oscillation (cephalad for expiratory bias, caudal for inspiratory bias) and that oscillations applied at the airway opening might be more effective than chest wall oscillations are consistent with this idea (Freitag et al., 1989a; King et al., 1984). In contrast to oscillations at the airway opening where the force is applied close to its desire effect of action, the force applied by chest wall oscillations is partially absorbed by the capacitance of the air volume of the lung interposed between the chest wall and the bronchi. Thus, the ideal method of chest oscillation should use a frequency of about 15 Hz and apply the oscillations close to the large airways (i.e., at the airway opening). One might speculate that the ideal frequency of approximately 15 Hz is near or at the resonant frequency of large airways and that, at this frequency, the amplitude of airway wall oscillations is the greatest, thereby favoring the buildup of mucus and augmenting the gas–liquid interactions. This proposed mechanism remains to be examined.

B. Hydration

As with ciliary clearance, there is no evidence that cough clearance is facilitated by the inhalation of bland aerosols or by systemic hydration (Reas, 1963; Wanner and Rao, 1980). Shim et al. (1987) found no effect of increased oral water intake on sputum production in patients with chronic bronchitis. Sputum volume, sputum elasticity, and the viscosity/elasticity ratio of sputum were not significantly altered by hydration. Since water secretion and hydration of mucus in the lower airways is an active process, the failure of systemic hydration to alter the rheological properties and expectoration of mucus is not entirely surprising. It is less clear why inhalation of bland aerosols, which add water directly to airway mucus, is also ineffective in enhancing cough clearance in patients with hypersecretory states.

C. Pharmacological Agents

Theoretically, mucolytic and other pharmacological agents capable of changing the viscosity of lower airway mucus such that it falls within an optimal range for air–liquid interaction, would be expected to enhance cough clearance of excessive lower airway mucus. Aerosolized mucolytic agents (*N*-acetylcysteine and enzymes) indeed reduce the viscosity of expectorated sputum in patients with hypersecretory states (Marchette et al., 1985; Wanner and Rao, 1980). However, the effects of these agents on cough clearance have been incompletely studied.

References

Annesi, I., and Kauffmann, F. (1986). Is respiratory mucus hypersecretion really an innocent disorder? *Am. Rev. Respir. Dis.* 134: 688–693.

Barnes, P. J. (1984). The third nervous system in the lung: Physiology and clinical perspectives. *Thorax* 39: 561–567.

Bell, J. A., Bluestein, B. M., Danta, I., and Wanner, A. (1984). Effect of inhaled ipratropium bromide on tracheal mucociliary transport in bronchial asthma. *Mt. Sinai J. Med.* 51: 215–217.

Berger, J., Albert, R. E., Sanborn, K., and Lippmann, M. (1978). Effects of atropine and methacholine on deposition and clearance of inhaled particles in the donkey. *J. Toxicol. Environ. Health* 4: 1–18.

Blari, A. M. J. N., and Woods, A. (1969). The effects of isoproterenol, atropine and disodium cromoglycate on ciliary motility and mucous flow measured in vivo in cats. *Br. J. Pharmacol.* 35: 379p–389p.

Bonini, N. M., Gustin, M. C., and Nelson, D. L. (1986). Regulation of ciliary motility by membrane potential in *Paramecium*: A role for cyclic AMP. *Cell Motil. Cytoskel.* 6: 256–272.

Borson, D. B., Charlin, M., Gold, B. D., and Nadel, J. A. (1982). Non-adrenergic noncholinergic nerves mediate secretion of macromolecules by tracheal glands of ferrets. *Fed. Proc.* 42: 1715.

Borum, P., Mygind, N., and Schultz Larsen, F. (1979). Intranasal ipratropium: A new treatment for perennial rhinitis. *Clin. Otolaryngol.* 4: 407–411.

Bulbring, E., Burn, J. H., and Shelley, H. J. (1953). Acetylcholine and ciliary movement in the gill plates of *Mytilus edulis*. *Proc. R. Soc. Lond.* 141: 445–449.

Burton, J. D. K. (1962). Effect of dry anesthetic gases on the respiratory mucous membrane. *Lancet* 1: 235–238.

Camner, P., Strandberg, K., and Philipson, K. (1974). Increased mucociliary transport by cholinergic stimulation. *Arch. Environ. Health* 29: 220.

Chervinsky, P. (1977). Double-blind study of ipratropium bromide, a new anticholinergic bronchodilator. *J. Allergy Clin. Immunol.* 59: 22–30.

Chopra, K. (1978). Effects of atropine on mucociliary transport velocity in anesthetized dogs. *Am. Rev. Respir. Dis.* 118: 367–371.

Clarke, S. W., Jones, J. C., and Oliver, D. R. (1970). Resistance to two-phase gas–liquid flow in airways. *J. Appl. Physiol.* 29: 464–471.

Cross, C. E., Halliwell, B., and Allen, A. (1984). Antioxidant protection: A function of tracheobronchial and gastrointestinal mucus. *Lancet* 1: 1328–1330.

Davis, S. S., Cox, A., Marriott, C., Readman, A. S., and Barrett-Bee, K. (1985). A new mucotropic agent—in vitro and in vivo evaluation of 2-α-thenoylthiopropionylglycine (Bronchoplus). *Eur. J. Respir. Dis.* 67: 94–102.

Di Benedetto, G., Manara-Shediac, F. S., and Mehta, A. (1991). Effect of cyclic AMP on ciliary activity of human respiratory epithelium. *Eur. Respir. J.* 4: 789–795.

Dunnill, M. S. (1975). The morphology of the airways in bronchial asthma. In *New Directions in Asthma*. Edited by M. Stein. Park Ridge, IL, American College of Chest Physicians, pp. 213–221.

Eckert, R., and Murakami, A. (1972). Calcium dependence of ciliary activity in the oviduct of the salamander *Necturus*. *J. Physiol.* 226: 699–711.

Edwards, G. F., Steel, A. E., Scott, J. K., and Jordan, J. W. (1976). *S*-Carboxymethylcysteine in the fluidification of sputum and treatment of chronic airway obstruction. *Chest* 70: 506–513.

Ericsson, C. H., Juhasz, J., Mossberg, B., Philipson, K., Svartengren, M., and Camner, P. (1987). Influence of ambroxol on tracheobronchial clearance in simple bronchitis. *Eur. J. Respir. Dis.* 70: 163–170.

Foliguet, B., and Pucelle, E. (1986). Apical structure of human respiratory cilia. *Bull. Eur. Physiopathol. Respir.* 22: 43–47.

Foster, W. M., Bergofsky, E. H., Bohning, D. E., Lippmann, M., and Albert, R. E. (1976). Effect of adrenergic agents and their mode of action on mucociliary clearance in man. *J. Appl. Physiol.* 41: 146.

Francis, R. A., Thompson, M. L., Pavia, D., and Douglas, R. B. (1977). Ipratropium bromide: Mucociliary clearance rate and airway resistance in normal subjects. *Br. J. Dis. Chest* 71: 173–178.

Freitag, L., Kim, C. S., Long, W. M., Venegas, J., and Wanner, A. (1989a). Mobilization of mucus by airway oscillations. *Acta Anaesthesiol. Scand.* 33(Suppl. 90): 93–101.

Freitag, L., Long, W. M., Kim, C. S., and Wanner, A. (1989b). Removal of excessive bronchial secretions by asymmetric high-frequency oscillations. *J. Appl. Physiol.* 67: 614–619.

Gibbons, I. R., and Rowe, A. J. (1965). Dynein: A protein with adenosine triphosphatase activity from cilia. *Science* 149: 424–426.

Giordano, A., Holsclaw, D., and Litt, M. (1978). Effects of various drugs on canine tracheal mucociliary transport. *Ann. Otol.* 87: 484–490.

Girard, P. R., and Kennedy, J. R. (1986). Calcium regulation of ciliary activity in rabbit tracheal epithelial explants and outgrowth. *Eur. J. Cell Biol.* 40: 203–209.

Hennessey, T., Machemer, H., and Nelson, D. L. (1985). Injected cyclic AMP increases ciliary beat frequency in conjunction with membrane hyperpolarization. *Eur. J. Cell Biol.* 36: 153–156.

Hidaka, H., and Tanaka, T. (1982). Biopharmacological assessment of calmodulin function: Utility of calmodulin antagonists. In *Calmodulin and Intracellular Ca^{2+} Receptors*.

Edited by S. Kakiuchi, H. Hidaka, and A. R. Means. New York, Plenum Press, pp. 19.

Inness, I. R., and Nickerson, M. (1970). Drugs inhibiting the action of acetylcholine on structure innervated by postganglionic parasympathetic nerves (antimuscarinic or atropinic drugs). In *The Pharmacological Basis of Therapeutics*. Edited by L. S. Goodman and A. Gilman. New York, Macmillan, pp. 524–548.

Iravani, J., and Van As, A. (1972). Mucus transport in the tracheobronchial tree of normal and bronchitic rats. *J. Pathol.* 106: 81–93.

Iravani, J. (1972). Wirkung eines Bronchoschkretolytikums auf die tracheobronchiale Reinigung. *Arzneimittelforschung* 22: 1744–1747.

Keal, E. E. (1971). Biochemistry and rheology of sputum in asthma. *Postgrad. Med. J.* 47: 171.

Kim, C. S., and Eldridge, M. A. (1985). Aerosol deposition in the airway model with excessive mucus secretions. *J. Appl. Physiol.* 59: 1766–1772.

Kim, C. S., Brown, L. K., Lewars, G. G., and Sackner, M. A. (1983). Deposition of aerosol particles and flow resistance in mathematical and experimental airway models. *J. Appl. Physiol.* 55: 154–163.

Kim, C. S., Rodriguez, C. R., Eldridge, M. A., and Sackner, M. A. (1986). Criteria for mucus transport in the airways by two-phase gas–liquid flow mechanism. *J. Appl. Physiol.* 60: 901–907.

Kim, C. S., Iglesias, A. J., and Sackner, M. A. (1987). Mucus clearance by two-phase gas–liquid flow mechanism: Asymmetric periodic flow model. *J. Appl. Physiol.* 62: 959–971.

Kim, C. S., Eldridge, M. A., and Wanner, A. (1988). Airway responsiveness to inhaled and intravenous carbachol in sheep; effect of airway mucus. *J. Appl. Physiol.* 65: 2744–2751.

King, M., and Angus, G. E. (1981). Effect of aerosolized bronchodilators on viscoelastic properties of canine tracheal mucus. *Chest* 80: 852–854.

King, M., Cohen, C., and Viires, N. (1979). Influence of vagal tone on rheology and transportability of canine tracheal mucus. *Am. Rev. Respir. Dis.* 120: 1215–1219.

King, M., Phillips, D. M., Gross, D., Vartian, V., Chang, H. K., and Zidulka, A. (1983). Enhanced tracheal mucus clearance with high frequency chest wall compression. *Am. Rev. Respir. Dis.* 128: 511–515.

King, M., Phillips, D. M., Zidulka, A., and Chang, H. K. (1984). Tracheal mucus clearance in high frequency oscillation. II: Chest wall versus mouth oscillation. *Am. Rev. Respir. Dis.* 130: 703–706.

King, M., Brock, G., and Lundell, C. (1985a). Clearance of mucus by simulated cough. *J. Appl. Physiol.* 58: 1776–1782.

King, M., Kelly, S., and Cosio, M. (1985b). Alteration of airway reactivity by mucus. *Respir. Physiol.* 62: 47–59.

Kobayashi, K., Tamaoki, J., Sakai, N., Kanemura, T., Horii, S., Isono, K., Takeuchi, S., Chiyotani, A., Yamawaki, I., and Takizawa, T. (1991). Guanosine-3′,5′-cyclic monophosphate (cyclic GMP) stimulates ciliary motility in rabbit cultured tracheal epithelium. *J. Jpn. Soc. Bronchol.* 13: 8–12.

Konietzko, N., Muller, N., and Adam, W. E. (1974). Studies of mucociliary clearance following the use of Atrovent by healthy individuals and patients with chronic bronchitis. *Wien Med. Wochenschr.* 124(Suppl. 21): 15–19.

Konietzko, N., Klopfer, M., Adam, W. E., and Matthys, H. (1975). Die mukociliare Klarfunktion der Lunge unter β-adrenerger Stimulation. *Pneumonologie* 152: 203–207.

Krieger, E., and Reitberger, U. (1975). Sputum rheology following treatment with Sch 1000 MDI and orciprenaline MDI. *Postgrad. Med. J.* 51(Suppl. 7): 108.

Landowne, D., and Ritchie, J. M. (1971). On the control of glycogenolysis in mammalian nervous tissue by calcium. *J. Physiol.* 212: 503–517.

Lee, W. I., Verdugo, P., Schurr, J. M., and Blandau, R. J. (1976). Control of oviductal ciliary activity. Effect of extracellular [Ca^{2+}]. *Biophys. J.* 16: 120a.

Leikauf, G. D., Ueki, I. F., Widdicombe, J. H., and Nadel, J. A. (1986). Alteration of chloride secretion across canine tracheal epithelium by lipoxygenase products of arachidonic acid. *Am. J. Physiol.* 250: F47–54.

Leith, D. (1977). Cough. In *Respiratory Defense Mechanisms, Part 2.* Edited by J. D. Brain, D. F. Proctor, and L. M. Reid. New York, Marcel Dekker, pp. 545–592.

Lieberman, J. (1968a). Measurement of sputum viscosity in a cone-plate viscometer. II. An evaluation of mucolytic agents in vitro. *Am. Rev. Respir. Dis.* 97: 662–672.

Lieberman, J. (1968b). Dornase aerosol effect on sputum viscosity in cases of cystic fibrosis. *JAMA* 205: 114–115.

Limber, C. R., Reiser, H. G., Roettig, L. C., and Curtis, G. M. (1952). Enzymatic lysis of respiratory secretions by aerosol trypsin. *JAMA* 149: 816–821.

Lopez-Vidriero, M. T., Costello, J., Clark, T. J. H., Das, I., Keal, E. E., and Reid, L. (1975). Effect of atropine on sputum production. *Thorax* 30: 543–547.

Lopez-Vidriero, M. T., Das, I., Smith, A. P., Picot, R., and Reid, L. (1977). Bronchial secretion from normal human airways after inhalation of prostaglandin $F_{2\alpha}$, acetylcholine, histamine, and cytric acid. *Thorax* 32: 734–739.

Lundgren, J. D., Hirata, F., Marom, Z., Logun, C., Steel, L., Kaliner, M., and Shelhamer, J. (1988). Dexamethasone inhibits respiratory glycoconjugate secretion from feline airways in vitro by the induction of lipocortin (lipomodulin) synthesis. *Am. Rev. Respir. Dis.* 137: 353–357.

Lundgren, J. D., Kaliner, M. A., Logun, C., and Shelhamer, J. H. (1989). Platelet activating factor (PAF) releases lipoxygnase metabolites and glycoconjugates (GC) from human airway tissue in vitro. *FASEB J.* 3: A609.

Marchette, L. C., Marchette, B. E., Abraham, W. M., and Wanner, A. (1985). The effect of systemic hydration on normal and impaired mucociliary function. *Pediatr. Pulmonol.* 1: 107–111.

Marin, M. G., Davis, B., and Nadel, J. A. (1976). Effect of acetylcholine on Cl^- and Na^+ fluxes across dog tracheal epithelium in vitro. *Am. J. Physiol.* 231: 1546–1549.

Marom, Z., Shelhamer, J. H., and Kaliner, M. (1981). Effects of arachidonic acid, monohydroxyeicosatetraeonic acid and prostaglandins on the release of mucous glycoproteins from human airways in vitro. *J. Clin. Invest.* 67: 1695–1702.

Marom, Z., Shelhamer, J. H., Bach, M. K., Morton, D. R., and Kaliner, M. (1982). Slow-reacting substances, leukotrienes C_4 and D_4, increase the release of mucous from human airways in vitro. *Am. Rev. Respir. Dis.* 126: 449–451.

Marom, Z. Shelhamer, J., Alling, D., and Kaliner, M. (1984). The effects of corticosteroids on mucous glycoprotein secretion from human airways in vitro. *Am. Rev. Respir. Dis.* 129: 62–65.

Martin, G. P., Loveday, B. E., and Marriott, C. (1990). The effect of bromhexine hydrochloride on the viscoelastic properties of mucus from the mini-pig. *Eur. Respir. J.* 3: 392–396.

Martin, J., Powell, E., Shore, S., Emrich, J., and Engel, L. A. (1980). The role of respiratory muscles in the hyperinflation of bronchial asthma. *Am. Rev. Respir. Dis.* 121: 441–447.

Matthys, H., Vastag, E., Daikeler, G., and Kohler, D. (1983). The influence of aminophylline and pindolol on the mucociliary clearance in patients with chronic bronchitis. *Br. J. Clin. Pract. [Suppl.]* 23: 10–15.

Millar, A. B., Pavia, D., Agnew, J. E., Lopez-Vidriero, M. T., Lauque, D., and Clarke, S. W. (1985). Effect of oral *N*-acetylcysteine on mucus clearance. *Br. J. Dis. Chest* 79: 262–266.

Mossberg, B., Strandberg, K., Philipson, K., and Camner, P. (1976). Tracheobronchial clearance in bronchial asthma: Response to beta-adrenoreceptor stimulation. *Scand. J. Respir. Dis.* 57: 119.

Murakami, A., Machemer-Rohnisch, S., and Eckert, R. (1974). Stimulation of ciliary activity by low levels of extracellular adenine nucleotides in the amphibian oviduct. *Exp. Cell Res.* 85: 154–158.

Nelson, D. J., and Wright, E. M. (1974). The distribution, activity, and function of the cilia in the frog brain. *J. Physiol.* 243: 63–78.

Pack, R. J., and Richardson, P. S. (1984). The aminergic innervation of the human bronchus: A light and electron microscopic study. *J. Anat.* 138: 493–502.

Pavia, D., and Thompson, M. L. (1971). Inhibition of mucociliary clearance from the human lung by hyoscine. *Lancet* 1: 449–450.

Pavia, D., Thomson, M. L., and Phillipakos, D. (1976). A preliminary study of the effect of a vibrating pad on bronchial clearance. *Am. Rev. Respir. Dis.* 113: 92–96.

Pavia, D., Bateman, J. R. M., Sheahan, N. F., and Clarke, S. W. (1979). Effect of ipratropium bromide on mucociliary clearance and pulmonary function in reversible airways obstruction. *Thorax* 34: 501–507.

Pavia, D., Bateman, J. R. M., Sheahan, N. F., and Clarke, S. W. (1980). Clearance of lung secretions in patients with chronic bronchitis: Effect of terbutaline and ipratropium bromide aerosols. *Eur. J. Respir. Dis.* 61: 245–253.

Peatfield, A. C., and Richardson, P. S. (1983). Evidence for non-cholinergic, non-adrenergic nervous control of mucus secretion into the cat trachea. *J. Physiol.* 342: 335–345.

Petty, T. L., Miercort, R., Ryan, S., Vincent, T. N., Filley, G. F., and Mitchell, R. S. (1965). The function and bronchographic evaluation of postmortem human lungs. *Am. Rev. Respir. Dis.* 92: 450–458.

Phipps, R. J. (1984). Production of airway secretions. *Semin. Respir. Med.* 5: 314–318.

Phipps, R. J., Denas, S., and Wanner, A. (1983a). Leukotriene D_4 stimulates secretion of glycoproteins, ions and water in sheep trachea [Abstract]. *Fed. Proc.* 42: 461.

Phipps, R. J., Denas, S. M., and Wanner, A. (1983b). Antigen stimulates glycoprotein secretion and alters ion fluxes in sheep trachea. *J. Appl. Physiol.* 55: 1593–1602.

Pryor, A., Webber, B. A., Hodson, M. E., and Batten, J. C. (1979). Evaluation of the forced expiration technique as an adjunct to postural drainage in treatment of cystic fibrosis. *Br. Med. J.* 2: 417–418.

Puchelle, E., and Zahm, J. M. (1984). Influence of rheological properties of human bronchial secretions on the ciliary beat frequency. *Biorheology* 21: 265–272.

Puchelle, E., Zahm, J. M. Girard, F., Bertrand, A., Polu, J. M., Aug, F., and Sadoul, P. (1980). Mucociliary transport in vivo and in vitro. Relation to sputum properties in chronic bronchitis. *Eur. J. Respir. Dis.* 61: 254–264.

Puchelle, E. Zahm, J. M., and Duvivier, C. (1983). Spinability of bronchial mucus. Relationship with viscoelasticity and mucous transport properties. *Biorheology* 20: 239–250.

Reas, H. W. (1963). The effect of *N*-acetylcysteine on the viscosity of tracheobronchial secretions in cystic fibrosis of the pancreas. *J. Pediatr.* 62: 31–35.

Ross, S. M., and Corrsin, S. (1974). Results of an analytical model of mucociliary pumping. *J. Appl. Physiol.* 37: 333–340.

Rubin, E. M., Scantlen, G. E., Chapman, G. A., Eldridge, M., Menendez, R., and Wanner, A. (1989). Effect of chest wall oscillation on mucus clearance: Comparison of two vibrators. *Pediatr. Pulmonol.* 6: 122–126.

Ruffin, R. E., Wolff, R. K., Dolovich, M. B., Rossman, C. M., Fitzgerald, J. D., and Newhouse, M. T. (1978). Aerosol Therapy with Sch 1000: Short-term mucociliary clearance in normal and bronchitic subjects and toxicology in normal subjects. *Chest* 73: 501–506.

Rutland, J., Griffin, W. M., and Cole, P. J. (1982). Human ciliary beat frequency in epithelium from intrathoracic and extrathoracic airways. *Am. Rev. Respir. Dis.* 125: 100–105.

Sackner, M. A., Epstein, S., and Wanner, A. (1976). Effect of beta adrenergic agonists aerosolized by Freon propellant on tracheal mucous velocity and cardiac output. *Chest* 69: 593–598.

Sackner, M. A., Chapman, G. A., and Dougherty, R. D. (1977). Effects of nebulized ipratropium bromide and atropine sulfate on tracheal mucous velocity and lung mechanics in anesthetized dogs. *Respiration* 34: 181–185.

Santa Cruz, R., Landa, J., and Hirsch, J. (1974). Tracheal mucous velocity in normal man and patients with obstructive lung disease. *Am. Rev. Respir. Dis.* 109: 458–463.

Satir, P. (1989). The role of axonemal components in ciliary motility. *Comp. Biochem. Physiol.* 94A: 351–357.

Serafini, S. M., and Michaelson, E. D. (1977). Length and distribution of cilia in human and canine airways. *Bull. Eur. Physiopathol. Respir.* 13: 551–559.

Serafini, S. M., Wanner, A., and Michaelson, E. D. (1976). Mucociliary transport in central and intermediate size airways: Effect of aminophyllin. *Bull. Eur. Physiopathol. Respir.* 12: 415–422.

Shim, C., King, M., and Williams, M. H., Jr. (1987). Lack of effect of hydration on sputum production in chronic bronchitis. *Chest* 92: 679–682.

Shimura, S., Sasaki, T., Ikeda, K., Yamauchi, K., Sasaki, H., and Takishima, T. (1990). Direct inhibitory action of glucocorticoid on glycoconjugate secretion from airway submucosal glands. *Am. Rev. Respir. Dis.* 141: 1044–1049.

Sleigh, M. A. (1989). Adaptations of ciliary systems for the propulsion of water and mucus. *Comp. Biochem. Physiol.* 94A: 359–364.

Soliman, S. (1984). Pharmacological control of ciliary activity in the young sea urchin larva. Studies on the role of Ca^{2+} and cyclic nucleotides. *Comp. Biochem. Physiol.* 78C: 183–191.

Stafanger, G., Garne, S., Howitz, P., Morkassel, E., and Koch, C. (1988). The clinical effect and the effect on the ciliary motility of oral *N*-acetylcysteine in patients with cystic fibrosis and primary ciliary dyskinesia. *Eur. Respir. J.* 1: 161–167.

Stommel, E. W., and Stephens, R. E. (1985). Cyclic AMP and calcium in the differential control of *Mytilus* gill cilia. *J. Comp. Physiol.* 157: 451–459.

Sutton, P. P., Pavia, D., Bateman, J. R. M., and Clarke, S. W. (1981). The effect of oral aminophylline on lung mucociliary clearance in man. *Chest* 80: 889–892.

Tamaoki, J., Kobayashi, K., Sakai, N., Chiyotani, A., Kanemura, T., and Takizawa, T. (1989). Effect of bradykinin on airway ciliary motility and its modulation by neutral endopeptidase. *Am. Rev. Respir. Dis.* 140: 430–435.

Thomson, M. L., Pavia, D., Jones, C. J., and McQuiston, T. A. C. (1975). No demonstrable effect of *S*-carboxymethylcysteine on clearance of secretions from the human lung. *Thorax* 30: 669–673.

Van As, A. (1974). The role of selective β-adrenoreceptor stimulants in the control of ciliary activity. *Respiration* 31: 146–151.

Verdugo, P. (1980). Ca^{2+}-dependent hormonal stimulation of ciliary activity. *Nature* 283: 764–765.

Villalon, M., Hinds, T. R., and Verdugo, P. (1989). Stimulus–response coupling in mammalian ciliated cells. Demonstration of two mechanisms of control for cytosolic $[Ca^{2+}]$. *Biophys. J.* 56: 1255–1258.

Vishwanath, S., and Ramphal, R. (1984). Adherence of *Pseudomonas aeruginosa* to human tracheobronchial mucin. *Infect. Immun.* 45: 197–202.

Vorhaus, E. F., and Deyrup, I. J. (1953). The effect of adenosine triphosphate on the cilia of the pharyngeal mucosa of the frog. *Science* 118: 553–554.

Wanner, A. (1977). Clinical aspects of mucociliary transport. *Am. Rev. Respir. Dis.* 116: 73–125.

Wanner, A. (1979). The role of mucociliary dysfunction in bronchial asthma. *Am. J. Med.* 67: 477–485.

Wanner, A., and Rao, A. (1980). Clinical indications for and effects of bland, mucolytic and antibiotic aerosols. *Am. Rev. Respir. Dis.* 122: 79–87.

Weaver, A., and Hard, R. (1985). Newt lung ciliated cell models: Effect of MgATP on beat frequency and waveforms. *Cell Motil.* 5: 377–392.

Wood, R. E., Wanner, A., Hirsch, J., and Di Sant'Agnese, A. (1975). Tracheal mucociliary transport in patients with cystic fibrosis and its stimulation by terbutaline. *Am. Rev. Respir. Dis.* 111: 733–738.

L

707

I

Hypersecretion,
  mucous, 527
  see also Airway hypersecretion
Hypersecretory disease, 192–196

[131I]-albumin, 453
  serum concentration, 535–538
  sputum concentration, 535–538
I/V relationship (*see* Current-voltage
    relationship)
Idiopathic pulmonary fibrosis, 563–666
  airway glandular hyperplasia, 563–566
  airway hypersecretion, 563–566
  prognosis, 563–566
Immunoglobulin A (IgA), 539, 603
  secretory, 232–233, 584
Immunoglobulin E (IgE), 605
Immunoglobulin G (IgG), 605
  sputum, 235
Immunoglobulin M (IgM), 605
Indomethacin, 203, 496
In situ hybridization technique, 228
Integrins, 316–317
Interferon α, 318
Ion channels, 67–68
  anion, 2
  calcium-activated, 2
  cation, 19
  chloride Cl⁻,
    Ca²⁺-activated, 12
    cAMP-activated, 12
  G-protein gated, 68
  nondiscriminating cation, 27–28
  open probability, 5
  potassium K⁺, 5–11, 19
    Ca²⁺-activated, 12
    G-protein gated, 68
    large conductance in acinar cells,
      339–341
  receptor-operated, 29
Ionomycin, 353–354
Isobutylmetylxanthine (IBMX), 27–28
Isoproterenol, 76

K

Keratin, 181
Klebsiella pneumoniae, 609
Kultchitsky cell (*see* Neuroendorine
    cell)

L

Lacrimal acinar cells (*see* Acinar cells)
Lactoferrin, 109, 128, 191
Lamina propria, 160–161
Lectin, 126–128
  histochemistry, 133–134
Leukotrienes, 374, 532
  LTC₄, 413, 443, 632
  LTD₄, 413, 443, 632
Limitation of air flow, 549–561
Lipid, 170
  sputum, 235–237
  tracheobronchial secretions, 236
Lipocortin, 378
Lipocortin-like protein, 234
Lipopolysaccharide (LPS), 495
Low iron diamine (LID), 136
Lymphocyte, 155
  T-lymphocytes, 605
Lysosomes, 57
  cDNAs, 318–320
  genomic clones, 318–320
  lysozyme gene, 318–320
  mRNA, 318–320
Lysozyme, 109, 128, 190–192

M

Macromolecules, 220
Macrophage, 199
Macrophage-derived mucous
      secretagogues (MMS), 532
Major basic protein (*see* Eosinophils)
Mannose, 43
Mast cells,
  chymotrypsin-like enzyme, 606

R

^{86}Rb efflux, 412
Ras gene, 76
Ras-like gene, 56
Receptor,
  adrenergic, 61–62
    α-adrenergic, 3
  subtype, 61–62
    β-adrenergic, 3
  subtype, 61–62
    $β_1$, 61–62
    $β_2$, 61–62
  airway submucosal gland, 344–348
    $α_1$-adrenergic, 345–347
    β-adrenergic, 345–347
    $β_1$-adrenergic, 345–347
    $β_2$-adrenergic, 345–347
    bradykinin, 347
    endothelin, 347
    ET_1-receptor, 347
    H_2-receptor, 347
    histamine, 347
    IP_3-receptors, 347
    M_1-receptor, 345–347, 356–357
    M_3-receptor, 345–347, 350–352,
      356–357
    muscarinic, 345–347
    NK_1-receptor, 347–348
    P_2-receptor, 347
    protein kinase C, 347
    purine, 347
    substance P, 347–348
    tachykinin, 347–348
    vasoactive intestinal peptide (VIP),
      347–348
  desensitization, 63
  muscarinic cholinergic, 1, 61–62
    M_1, 339, 477–479
    M_2, 339, 477–479
    M_3, 339, 477–479
  nicotinic, 61
  peptidergic, 3, 62–63
  purinergic, 113
  substance P, 3, 344–348
  tachykinin, 344–348

[Receptor]
  vasoactive intestinal peptide, 344–348
Recoil,
  elastic, 267
Reid index or gland/wall ratio, 128, 190,
    528–529
Resistance,
  across cell membrane, 4
  electrorite, 4
Rheometer,
  controlled shear rate, 296–297
  double-capillary method, 297
  magnetic, 291, 297–299
  simple capillary, 296
Ribosome, 44
  40S, 42–43
  ribosomal subunit, 42
  ribosome-endoplasmic reticulum
    complex, 44
Rigidity,
  mucin polymer, 107
RNA,
  7S, 44
  messenger, 40–43
  methionyl-t, 42
  polymerase, 40

S

$[^{32}S]$-sulfate, 222
Salivary glands, 2, 12
  see also Glands
Second messenger,
  cyclic adenosine monophosophate
    (cAMP), 28–31, 348–349
  diacylglycerol, 31
  Ins(1,4,5)P_3 IP_3, 21–23, 27
    acinar cells of submucosal glands,
      339–341, 348–355
    monoclonal IP_3-receptor antibody,
      339–34
    receptors, 339–341
  Ins(1,3,4,5)P_4 IP_4, 25, 27
  protein kinase, 352
  protein kinase A (PKA), 518–519